PSYCHOLOGICAL DISORDERS

Clinical Perspectives

2025 RELEASE

SUSAN KRAUSS WHITBOURNE

University of Massachusetts Boston

Mc Graw Hill

PSYCHOLOGICAL DISORDERS: CLINICAL PERSPECTIVES,
2025 RELEASE

Published by McGraw Hill LLC, 1325 Avenue of the Americas, New York, NY 10019.

This book is printed on acid-free paper.

1 2 3 4 5 6 7 8 9 LWI 30 29 28 27 26 25

ISBN 978-1-265-91829-3 (bound)
MHID 1-265-91829-5 (bound)
ISBN 978-1-265-39052-5 (loose-leaf)
MHID 1-265-39052-5 (loose-leaf)

Executive Portfolio Manager: *Ryan Treat*
Senior Product Development Manager: *Dawn Groundwater*
Marketing Manager: *Isfa Syed*
Content Project Managers: *Mary Powers* (core), *Jodi Banowetz* (assessment)
Manufacturing Project Manager: *Laura Fuller*
Content Licensing Specialist: *Sarah Flynn*
Cover Image: *Beautiful landscape/Shutterstock*
Compositor: *MPS Limited*

Library of Congress Cataloging-in-Publication Data

Names: Whitbourne, Susan Krauss, author.
Title: Psychological disorders : clinical perspectives / Susan Krauss Whitbourne, University of Massachusetts, Boston.
Other titles: Abnormal psychology
Description: 2025 release. | New York, NY : McGraw Hill, [2025] | “Now with DSM-5-TR Updates.” | Includes bibliographical references and index.
Identifiers: LCCN 2024031978 (print) | LCCN 2024031979 (ebook) | ISBN 9781265918293 (bound edition ; acid-free paper) | ISBN 9781265390525 (loose-leaf edition) | ISBN 9781265391225 (ebook)
Classification: LCC RC454 .H334 2025 (print) | LCC RC454 (ebook) | DDC 616.08–dc23/eng/20240812
LC record available at https://lccn.loc.gov/2024031978
LC ebook record available at https://lccn.loc.gov/2024031979

mheducation.com/highered

To my wonderful, and growing, family: Stacey, Jenny, Taylor, Erik, Teddy, Scarlett, Logan, and Fallon.

ABOUT THE AUTHOR

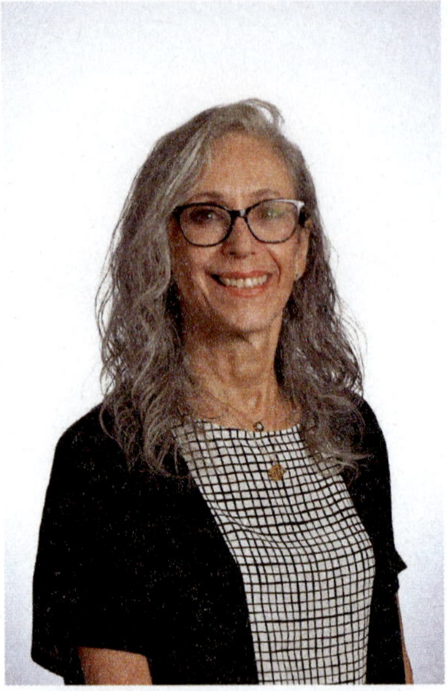

Susan Krauss Whitbourne

Susan Krauss Whitbourne, Ph.D., ABPP (she/her) is professor emerita of Psychological and Brain Sciences at the University of Massachusetts Amherst, and adjunct professor of Gerontology and Faculty Fellow at University of Massachusetts Boston. She has taught large undergraduate classes in addition to teaching and supervising doctoral students in developmental and clinical psychology. Her clinical experience has covered both inpatient and outpatient settings. Professor Whitbourne is a Fellow of the American Psychological Association and a Diplomate of the American Board of Professional Psychology in Geropsychology.

Professor Whitbourne received her PhD from Columbia University in Developmental Psychology. She taught at the State University of New York at Geneseo and the University of Rochester prior to moving to the University of Massachusetts Amherst, where she received the University's Distinguished Teaching Award, the Outstanding Advising Award, and the College of Arts and Sciences Outstanding Teacher Award. In 2001, she received the Psi Chi Eastern Region Faculty Advisor Award, and in 2002, the Florence Denmark Psi Chi National Advisor Award. In 2018, she was recognized as a Psi Chi Distinguished Member. In 2003, she received both the APA Division 20 and Gerontological Society of America Mentoring Awards. As the departmental honors coordinator from 1990 to 2010, Professor Whitbourne was also the Psi Chi faculty advisor from 1990 through 2017, and the director of the Office of National Scholarship Advisement in the Commonwealth Honors College from 1999 through 2017.

The author of 18 books and more than 200 journal articles and book chapters, Professor Whitbourne is regarded as an expert on personality development in middle and late life. She is Co-Principal Investigator of the 50-year-long Rochester Adult Longitudinal Study on psychosocial development from college through later adulthood. She is also a Co-Principal Investigator of the Age-Friendly University study in collaboration with the Gerontology Institute of the University of Massachusetts Boston. Her 2010 book, *The Search for Fulfillment,* was nominated for an APA William James Award. In 2011, she was recognized with a Presidential Citation from APA. In addition to her academic writing, she writes a highly popular blog on *Psychology Today* entitled "Fulfillment at Any Age" and has appeared on numerous media outlets, including *NBC Dateline* and *Today Show, AM Canada,* BBC, and CNN.

She is the President of the Geropsychology Board and a Board of Director of the American Board of Professional Psychology, a past president of the Eastern Psychological Association, and past chair of the Behavioral and Social Sciences Section of the Gerontological Society of America and was a member of the APA Board of Educational Affairs. She served as APA Council Representative to Division 20 (Adult Development and Aging), having also served as Division 20 president. She is a fellow of APA's Divisions 20, 1 (General Psychology), 2 (Teaching of Psychology), 9 (Society for the Psychological Study of Social Issues), 12 (Clinical Psychology), and 35 (Society for the Psychology of Women). In 2019 and 2020, Professor Whitbourne was nominated for president-elect of APA. She was also a member of the Board of Directors of the Massachusetts Psychological Association, and also serves the Nominations and Governance Committee. In 2021, she was a recipient of the Geropsychology Specialty Award of ABPP. She is Chair APA's Committee on Aging.

Professor Whitbourne served as an item writer for the Educational Testing Service, was a member of APA's High School Curriculum National Standards Advisory Panel, wrote the APA High School Curriculum Guidelines for Life-Span Developmental Psychology, and served as an item writer for the Examination for Professional Practice of Psychology.

ABOUT THE CONTRIBUTOR

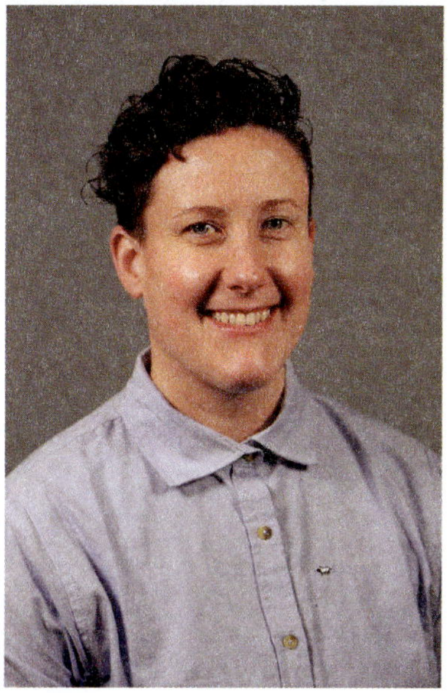

David Tytell

Jennifer L. O'Brien, Ph.D. (she/her) is a clinical psychologist in private practice, based in Cambridge, MA. She previously worked as a staff psychologist at the Massachusetts Institute of Technology's Mental Health and Counseling Service, where she provided psychotherapy to undergraduate and graduate students with a broad range of psychological concerns. She is an adjunct faculty member at the University of Massachusetts, Boston in the Gerontology department of the Manning College of Nursing and Health Sciences. Dr. O'Brien specializes in treating mood and anxiety disorders and has expertise in working with the LGBTQIA+ population.

Dr. O'Brien received her PhD in Clinical Psychology from American University in Washington, D.C. Her dissertation, "Empathic Accuracy and Compassion Fatigue in Therapist Trainees," is published in *Professional Psychology: Research and Practice.* She completed her predoctoral internship at the Durham VA Medical Center in Durham, NC, and her postdoctoral fellowship at the VA Boston Healthcare System, where she worked with military veterans and received extensive training in providing evidence-based treatments for depression, anxiety, PTSD, and substance abuse.

In addition to her clinical expertise, Dr. O'Brien has published chapters in edited volumes on gender and aging and has served as editor of peer-reviewed journals. Dr. O'Brien previously contributed to the last four releases of *Abnormal Psychology: Clinical Perspectives on Psychological Disorders.*

BRIEF CONTENTS

CONTENTS

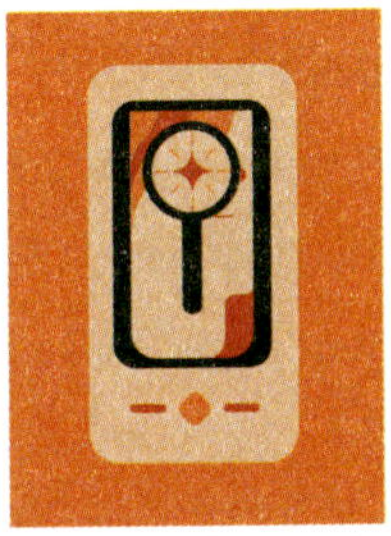

Martin_Mailz/Shutterstock

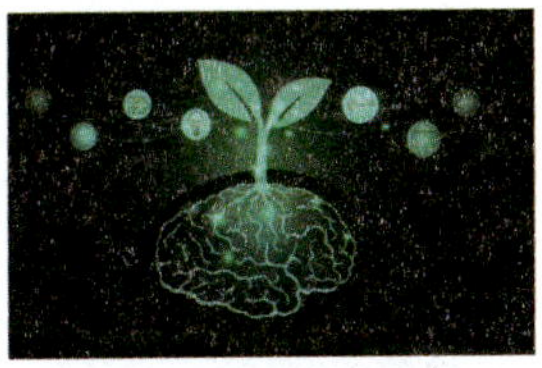

solar22/Shutterstock

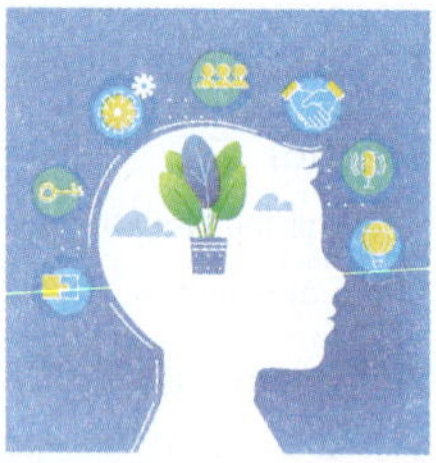

Batshevs/Shutterstock

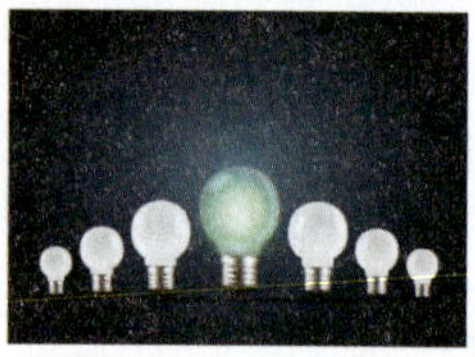

solar22/Shutterstock

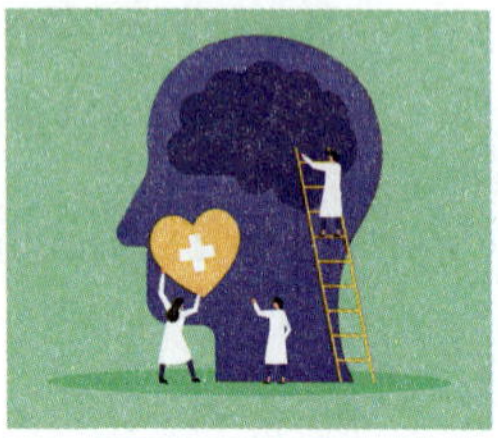

mnaufal design/Shutterstock

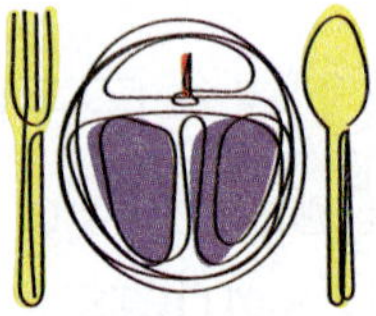

M7Studio/Shutterstock

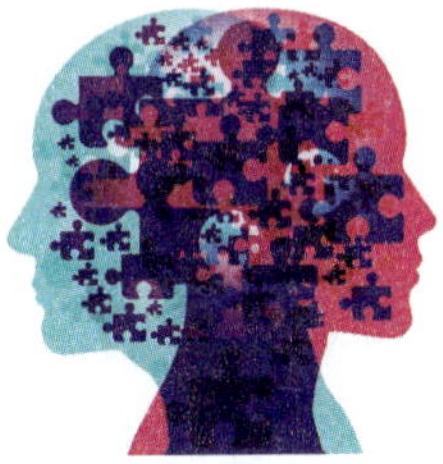
MrSquid/Shutterstock

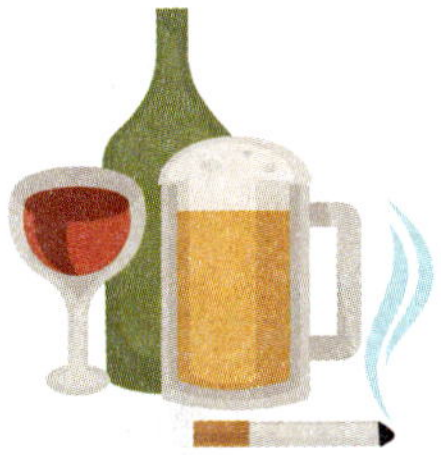
SofiaV/Shutterstock

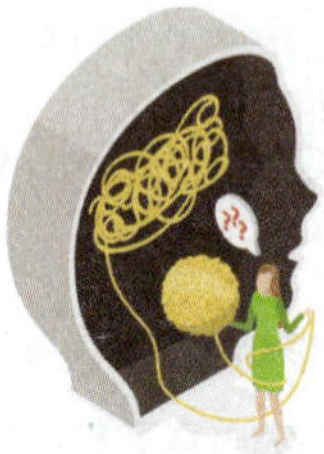

TarikVision/Shutterstock

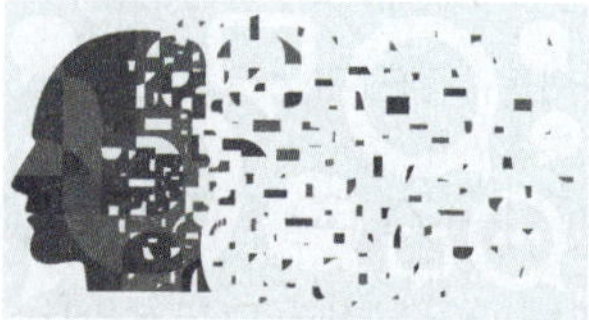

magic pictures/Shutterstock

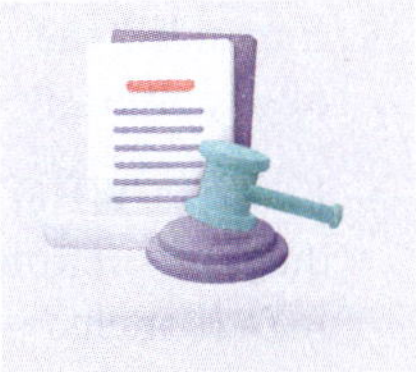

Vector Stock Pro/Shutterstock

GUIDE TO DIVERSITY, EQUITY, AND INCLUSION

Information in this text is informed by research drawn from a wide variety of journals dedicated to investigating the diversity of human psychology. Sources were cited from researchers publishing in such journals as *Current Psychology: A Journal for Diverse Perspectives on Psychological Issues, LGBT Health, Psychology of Sexual Orientation and Gender Diversity, Women and Health, Archives of Women's Mental Health, Hispanic Journal of Behavioral Sciences, Journal of Gender Studies* as well as studies and researchers representing diverse and international samples and issues. Additionally, cultural considerations were added from *DSM-5-TR* where relevant to diagnosis.

In a continuing commitment to capturing the diversity of individuals who experience psychological disorders, the Case Reports and Real Stories feature individuals who reflect a wide range of cultural backgrounds, sexual orientations, and gender expressions.

CHAPTER 1

- Case Report of Rebecca Hasbrouck describes her as a bisexual individual.
- The section on sociocultural contributions to psychological disorders, includes a focus on the roles of culture, discrimination, social injustice, stigma, and racism on mental health with an introduction of themes covered later in the book.
- In the section on causes of psychological disorders, includes coverage of oppression and violence as well as responses to impact of COVID-19 on BIPOC and LGBTQ+ individuals (e.g. Beringer et al., 2023). Includesresearch by Goetter et al. (2020) and Njoroge et al. (2021) on the disproportionate stigma of mental health disorders and how they vary vary by race and ethnicity.
- Discusses oppression of women who practice indigenous methods of healing (Yokushko, 2018) in the section on the history of exorcism and violence committed against women accused of practicing witchcraft from the Middle Ages to 1700s. Includes discussion of beliefs in spiritual possession from research based on Ugandans (Verginer & Juen, 2019).
- Describes World Health Organization's (WHO) Sustainability Development Goals special initiative that includes maximizing human functioning by countering the human rights violations, discrimination, and stigma associated with psychological disorders.
- Discusses problems in careless responding in online surveys with research by Arias et al., (2022).

CHAPTER 2

- Case Report of Pedro Padilla describes him as Mexican American.
- Wayne Brady (depression) is covered in the Real Story.
- Expanded the coverage of cultural formulations and multiculturally competent care.
- Includes WHO's *ICD-11*'s cross-cultural approach in diagnosis, citing work by Reed et al. (2019) noting that *ICD-11* includes cultural considerations in each diagnostic grouping.
- Includes discussion of use of nonbinary terminology in healthcare settings (Drill et al., 2019).
- Describes Veterans Administration Medical Centers as sites for treatment of those with military service.

CHAPTER 3

- Demi Lovato (bipolar, self-harm, and drug abuse) is the subject of the Real Story.
- Uses research by Ford-Paz et al. (2020) to support use by clinicians of evidence-based assessment procedures.
- Refersto research by Oberheim, Swank, and DePue (2017) that notes most current assessment procedures are based on heteronormative language and therefore are not appropriate for individuals of other gender identities.
- The discussion of the WAIS-IV, describes concerns about the language itself, the role of culture, and whether the normative sample is an appropriate one for a given client.
- Cites an example of a study by Dudley et al. (2019) on the Maori of New Zealand raising the issue that administrators and test-takers should ideally be ethnically matched.
- Includes additional research on cross-national validation of the WAIS-IV, and cultural differences toward timing in the WAIS-IV (Melikyan et al., 2021).
- The discussion of multicultural assessment includes the use of research-based instruments that assess cultural identity and degree of acculturation based on study by Leong, Lui, and Kalibatseva (2020).
- Includes research by Oh and Shillingford-Butler (2020) noting that new instruments are being developed to evaluate the extent to which clients believe their clinicians are meeting their needs for culturally informed assessment and treatment.

- Provides information about the MoCA for use with non-English-speaking populations that are becoming increasingly available, citing research by Cesar et al. (2019), Krist et al. (2019), Tang (2020), Quang et al. (2023), and Nasreddine and Patel (2016). Includes use of the MoCA on prison populations (Lima-Pereira et al., 2023).
- Includes research by Diaz-Blancat et al. (2018) supporting the Wisconsin Category Sorting Test as a measure of prefrontal brain functioning and notes that it is being expanded internationally, as shown by research conducted by Miranda et al. (2020), Faustino et al. (2020), and Rammal et al. (2019).
- Discusses the problems of the Boston Naming Test when used for populations for whom English is not the first language as shown by research conducted by Silvestre et al. (2018), Savoie et al. (2019), Na and King (2019) and delCacho-Tena et al., (2023).
- Includes problems in using the Cambridge Neuropsychological Testing Automated Battery (CANTAB) with individuals who are disadvantaged in using computer-based testing, with research by Aran Filipetti et al. (2020). Also includes research on validity of the CANTAB by Campos-Magdaleno et al. (2020).
- Describes problems in research on brain-scanning methods conducted by large international collaboration led by Elliott et al. (2020).
- Includes discussion of the administration of personality assessment measures cross-nationally and to minoritized individuals (e.g. Orjiakor et al., 2023).
- Refers to research by Feinstein et al. (2022) on the importance of standardizing measures across sexual orientation, gender identity and race/ethnicity in members of marginalized or underrepresented communities.
- Discusses the comparison between self-reporting and Rorschach projective tests in refugee populations studied in Norway (Hartmann & Opaas, 2023).
- Includes reference to APA's multicultural guidelines in assessment and discusses the implications of these guidelines for clinicians.
- Provides extensive discussion of neuropsychological testing as adapted for administration to clients from countries other than the U.S. (e.g. Quang et al., 2022).
- Shows how mental status examinations need to be adapted for specific populations within the U.S. based on racial/ethnic status (e.g. Merced et al., 2022).

CHAPTER 4

- Discusses research on endophenotypes conducted by Abhishek et al. (2020).
- Provides research support for the diathesis stress model with work by Nielsen et al. (2020).
- Includes research on environmental factors affecting gene expression by Ciafre et al. (2020) and Palma-Gudiel et al. (2020).
- Discusses the impact on childhood development of maternal sensitivity with research by Dall'Aglio et al. (2020)and Pellicano et al. (2020).
- Includes research by Silva et al. (2021) on the use of neuromodulation in biological treatments.
- Describes research by Mohd Hasim et al. (2023) on attachment style in married couples as an area of research within psychodynamic theories.
- Includes discussion of expanding token economy in helping caregivers in Italy during the COVID-19 lockdown with research by degli Espinosa et al. (2020).
- Cites research by Trombello et al. (2020), discussing the use of homework assignments in telehealth-based behavioral therapy among underserved populations.
- Incorporates the importance of cultural considerations in the administration of Applied Behavior Analysis (Gatzunis et al., 2023).
- The Sociocultural Perspective section of the chapter focuses on social discrimination (Jackson et al., 2019; Hackett et al. 2020), and includes research by Fernandez et al. (2020) on political oppression, poverty, and violence as influences on physical and mental health.
- Discusses the impact of COVID-19 on the mental health of older adults with research by Mushtaq & Khan (2023).
- Describes DBT as a method for high-risk transgender and gender-diverse youth with research by Tilley et al. (2022).
- Describes culturally adapted CBT with research by Silveus et al. (2023).
- Discusses new approaches to group teletherapy by Miu et al. (2020).
- Describes smartphone applications for mindfulness training with research by Gal et al. (2021).

- Discusses the reduction of self-stigma through ACT with research by Kao et al. (2023).
- Includes material on the multicultural approach to treatment with general discussion relating this to need to understand sociocultural context of clients, including the importance of reducing stigmatizing language, and providing treatment to gender-diverse clients.
- Describes post-traumatic stress in the trans community with research by Barr et al. (2022).

CHAPTER 5

- Provides updated prevalence rates of autism spectrum disorder by race/ethnicity and nationality throughout the chapter, including lifetime risks and prevalence.
- Includes research on Tay-Sachs disease in French Canadian populations with research by Sillon et al. (2020).
- Discusses the relationship between maternal alcohol use and damage to frontal areas of the brain with research by Kenton et al. (2020).
- Includes peer training as part of mainstreaming, with research by Nota et al. (2019).
- Summarizes research by Maye et al. (2020) on the role of functional play in treating children with autism spectrum disorder.
- Includes work on virtual reality-based intervention for children with autism spectrum disorder with research by Ip et al. (2018).
- Includes research on biological and psychological interventions for individuals with Rett disorder by Gomathi et al. (2020) and Lim et al. (2020).
- Includes psychosocial interventions for children with specific developmental disorders with work by Musetti et al. (2019).
- Includes research on ADHD in adulthood with work by Wang et al. (2020) and Rosello et al. (2020) and discusses compensatory mechanisms with research by Yap et al. (2021).
- Discusses the need to take sociocultural factors into account in understanding learning disorders (Gyereh & Shukla, 2023).
- Provides a discussion of resilience in individuals with ADHD, citing research by Yap et al., (2021).

CHAPTER 6

- Case Report of David Chen describes him as an individual with non-binary gender identity and queer sexual orientation.
- Includes research by Peralta and Costa (2020) on the validity of first-rank symptoms in schizophrenia.
- Includes research on shared psychotic disorder as observed in children living in socially isolated conditions, with work by Vigo et al. (2019).
- Includes research on the role of the brain in schizophrenia with research by Huang et al. (2020) and Lei et al. (2020).
- Includes discussion of Brief Psychotic Disorder in response to COVID-19 with research by Valdes-Florido et al., (2022).
- Notes that much research on genetics of schizophrenia is conducted on populations of European descent; consequently, investigators are expanding their work to include populations of African and Latinx ancestry (Bigdeli et al., 2020), leading to the identification of more chromosomes involved in schizophrenia than previously reported (Chang et al., 2020).
- Includes research by Banaj et al. (2023) on a worldwide study covering structural abnormalities in schizophrenia.
- Describes research by Suárez Santiago et al. (2023) on the role of GABA in schizophrenia.
- Expands coverage of sociocultural contributors to schizophrenia with research by Lopez et al. (2020) and including research on the vulnerability of migrant populations due to discrimination, exclusion, and language differences (Henssler et al., 2020).
- Includes research on isolation due to COVID-19 as risk factor for schizophrenia, citing research by Sole et al. (2021).
- Discusses the need to adapt Assertive Community Treatment to an individual's culture and mental health resources in the community, based on research conducted in mainland China (Luo et al., 2019).

CHAPTER 7

- Provides updated prevalence data on depressive disorders including variations by gender, race, and ethnicity.
- Describes the Black-White paradox as a relevant concept to understanding race and depression prevalence (Barnes & Barnes, 2017).

- Discusses problems in heritability estimates for research on bipolar disorder, with research by Gordovez and McMahon (2020).
- Shows the potential advantage of pharmacogenetic approaches to bipolar disorder with research by Vecera et al. (2021).
- Includes data on interpersonal and social rhythm therapy in treatment for bipolar disorder, with research by Lam and Cheung (2019).
- Includes sociocultural stresses in relation to prevalence of major depressive disorder, citing research by Monroe et al. (2019).
- Incorporates the minority stress model proposing that individuals in marginalized communities who are affected by societal oppression such as racism and homophobia are exposed to chronic levels of high stress due to this discrimination, citing research by Wilson and Liss (2020).
- Includes prevalence statistics of depressive disorders as varying by race, ethnicity and age with new CDC data.
- Discusses work by Fortuna et al. (2020) showing CBT plus mindfulness as useful interventions for individuals from Latinx communities experiencing ongoing exposure to adversity and stress associated with immigration.
- Includes WHO (2021) data showing suicide rates in low- vs. high-income countries.
- Includes research on Mexican-origin youth by Lawson et al. (2021) showing that a combination of high conscientiousness and low neuroticism predicted an ability to remain positive in the face of stress, which reduced suicide risk compared to that of youths who were lower in both personality traits.
- Includes discussion of oppression trauma based on new research on its role in stress (De Leon et al., 2023).

CHAPTER 8

- Includes research by Delpino et al. (2022) on the global consequences of COVID-19 on anxiety disorders.
- Expands coverage of trauma and effect on separation anxiety disorder from global/diversity perspective, citing evidence that among nearly 39,000 adults studied in 18 countries within the World Health Organization, both childhood adversity and lifetime trauma were shown to increase an individual's likelihood of developing the disorder.
- Includes research by Yeo et al. (2020) on the impact of cognitive style on phobias.
- Discusses role of early life stress and child maltreatment on reactive attachment disorder with model developed by Nakama et al. (2023).
- Discusses virtual reality exposure therapy in treating phobias by Jiang et al. (2020).
- Compares research on cognitive behavioral vs. relaxation-based therapy for anxiety disorder as reported by Montrero-Marin et al. (2018).
- Includes new research on anxiety sensitivity theory of panic disorder conducted by Cho et al. (2021).
- Discusses relaxation training for panic disorder as shown to be effective in research by Sanchez-Meca et al. (2020).
- Cites research by Liu et al. (2020) on role of basal ganglia and frontal lobes in obsessive-compulsive disorder.
- Includes compassion-focused therapy for hoarding disorder as introduced by Chou et al. (2020).
- Includes discussion of cross-cultural aspects of body dysmorphic disorder as reflected in studies conducted in Japan and China by Fang and Hofmann (2010).
- Discusses trauma among women in the military who are victims of sexual assault by Yalch et al. (2018).
- Addresses issues of shaming in Body Dysmorphic Disorder in relation to sexual minority stress based on research by Oshana et al., (2020).
- Includes research on PTSD as related to food insecurity in Latino/Hispanic individuals (Marshall et al., 2023).
- Coverstrauma among medical workers in China treating coronavirus patients during the early months of 2020, citing work by Li et al. (2021).
- Discusses *ICD-11* and the complex post-traumatic stress disorder diagnosis as applied to victims of exposure to such multiple and repeated stressors as torture, slavery, genocide campaigns, prolonged domestic violence, or repeated childhood sexual or physical abuse, including research by Kananian et al. (2020).
- Discusses the role of social support and religious coping in post-traumatic growth, citing research by Yazici et al. (2020).

- Discusses PTSD in rural veterans (Rauch et al., 2023) and veterans who are LGBTQ+ (Shipherd et al., 2021).
- Includes research by Rezay et al. (2020) on PTSD risk created by exposure to natural disasters in early life.
- Covers studies on role of food insecurity as a stressor for PTSD, particularly among individuals from low socioeconomic status and Latino/Hispanic ethnicity (Marshall et al., 2023).
- Includes research showing the effectiveness of holistic treatment for PTSD in underserved areas with research by Rauch et al., (2023).

CHAPTER 9

- Case Report of Rose Marston, a pansexual trans woman gender is described as trans woman and changed sexual orientation from heterosexual to pansexual.
- Referring to Mohajerin et al. (2019), discusses cognitive behavioral therapy in dissociative identity disorder.
- Includes research on illness anxiety disorder in the context of COVID-19 pandemic and need to take health precautions, citing research by Rivera and Carballea (2020) and Nicomedes et al. (2020).
- Discusses research by Yi-Feng Chen et al. (2021) on the "proactive personality," in the context of Chinese health care workers at the height of the pandemic coping with the stress of exposure to patients with the coronavirus.
- Discusses research on minority stress in a study of Hispanic women college students in which a negative university social climate such as racist practices and policies, discrimination based on race, pressures from within one's own race about how to act, and lack of academic confidence were found to be predictors of grade point average and intention to remain in college (Arbona et al., 2018).
- Includes research on compassion fatigue and rumination by Liu et al. (2021).

CHAPTER 10

- Case Report on Maria Nomirez, a Latina individual describes her
- Includes data on ethnic variations in eating disorders by Cheng et al. (2019) and Perez et al. (2021) and discusses comorbidities in eating disorders as discussed by Bahji et al. (2019).
- Includes coverage of eating disorders among LGBTQ+ individuals showing the disproportionately higher prevalence in transgender men and women, reflecting discrimination against these individuals (Nagata et al., 2020; Kamody et al., 2020).
- Describes the nature of eating disorders in older adult women in research by Kilpela et al. (2021).
- Provides global data on prevalence rates of bulimia nervosa (Kessler et al., 2013).
- Examines sociocultural factors in the development of eating disorders in, for example, women college athletes (Thompson et al., 2020) and on-camera journalists (Tran et al., 2020).
- Includes research on the worldwide prevalence of eating disorders (Silén & Keski-Rahkonen, 2022) and variations in eating disorders among ethnic groups (Perez et al., 2021).
- Discusses research findings by Güzel et al. (2023) relating COVID-19 to an increase in worldwide rates of eating disorders.
- Relates early childhood restriction of access to food to emotional and physical neglect and abuse, sexual abuse, and exposure to intimate partner violence, citing research by Coffino et al. (2020).
- Describes the concept of the maltreated ecophenotype as a combined genetic-sociocultural risk factor for eating disorders (Monteleone et al., 2020; Forrest et al., 2020).
- Discusses the stress of living in the COVID-19 lockdown and its impact on sleep disorders as reported by Beck et a. (2021).
- Includes DNA methylation research by Montalvo-Ortiz et al. (2018) on intermittent explosive disorder
- Covers international data on oppositional defiant disorder as discussed by Vasileva et al. (2020) and Osa et al. (2019).
- Cites work by Diaz et al. (2019) on mood and substance disorder risk in children with oppositional defiant disorder.
- Includes epidemiological studies on comorbidity of intermittent explosive disorder by Pereira et al. (2020).
- Discusses the role of trauma in development of conduct disorder as shown by the increasing recognition that

children raised in harsh environments that expose them to trauma, abuse, and neglect are particularly at risk for developing this disorder; pointed to role of undiagnosed physical disease (Kerekes et al., 2020).

CHAPTER 11

- Real Story describes the case of Lamar Odom (sex addiction).
- Covers the United Nations Sustainability Development Goal of achieving gender equality and empowering all women and girls.
- Includes discussion of the prevalence of paraphilic disorders, with citations based on work by Bartova et al. (2020) and Tzeng et al. (2019).
- Describes the more inclusive approach represented by *ICD-11*'s classification of paraphilic disorders, citing Krueger et al. (2017).
- Clarifies work on cisgender men involved in drag performance, citing Knutson and Koch (2019).
- Discusses the side effects of hormonal treatment for paraphilic disorders in men, citing ElSayed and Gupta (2020).
- Notes advantages of CBT for treating paraphilias, citing work by Assumpção et al. (2014).
- Discusses role of chronic health conditions in sexual dysfunctions, citing, Sivaratnam et al. (2021).
- Includes research on personality traits and premature ejaculation by Gao et al. (2021).
- Describes research on sexual dysfunctions in same-sex relationships between men and between women, and between bisexual adults (Barbonetti et al., 2019; Peixoto & Nobre, 2015; Shepler et al., 2018).
- Describes Spanish language translation of the FSFI (Rincón-Hernández et al., 2021).
- Clarifies language in order to describe sexual dysfunctions from a more gender-neutral perspective (i.e., “women” and “men” vs. “males” and “females”), citing APA publication manual (2020).
- Described sexual dysfunctions in trans individuals after gender affirming surgery with research by Kerchof et al (2019) and Zwickl et al. (2023).
- Discussion of the meaning of gender dysphoria as a diagnostic concept.
- Describes diagnostic clarification from *ICD-11*, which uses the term *gender incongruence* rather than *dysphoria.*
- Discusses rates of psychological disorders among individuals with gender dysphoria, citing research by Newcomb et al. (2020).
- Describes the victimization of trans women, particularly those of color, citing work by Ussher et al. (2020).
- Includes transphobia as a form of minority stress, leading transgender individuals to experience feelings of stigma, along with concealment of their transgender identities, citing Lindley and Galupo (2020).
- Coverage of the relationship between transphobia and lack of support for transgender individuals as well as other behaviors contributing to marginalization, citing work by Axt et al. (2021).
- Includes research by Bretherton et al. (2020) and Connolly and Gilchrist (2020) on health inequities faced by transgender individuals that can further contribute to anxiety, depression, and suicidality as well as substance abuse.
- Discusses gender-affirming medical treatment and affirmative psychotherapy with transgender individuals, including work by Morris et al. (2020).
- Includes research on the need for translations of measures of sexual functioning (Rincón-Hernández et al., 2021).
- Discusses cultural influences on sexual disorders including variations by country (Tan, 2023), and attitudes toward sexual sadism and masochism (Lantto & Lundberg, 2022).

CHAPTER 12

- Real Story covers Mary J. Blige (substance use disorder).
- Includes prevalence statistics of substance use disorders with variations by race/ethnicity and gender, citing SAMHSA and NIDA.
- Discusses high rates of substance use disorders among people who are incarcerated, who engage in sex work, or who are unhoused, and how these circumstances place these individuals at risk of extreme health inequities, reflecting their social exclusion, citing research by Aldridge et al. (2018).
- Covers the dual pandemics of COVID-19 and substance abuse, citing work by Dubey et al. (2020).

- Includes the Sustainability Development Goal of building stronger global policies regarding alcohol use.
- Includes research showing the benefits of physical activity as adjunct to CBT in treating alcohol use disorders, citing Cabe et al. (2021).
- Covers the acculturation in terms of "Americanization" citing work by Lui and Zamboanga (2018) in which researchers show that young adult Hispanic and Asian Americans adopt the alcohol use patterns of their age peers.
- Describes the Strong African American Families (SAAF) prevention program, a family-centered program for youth between the ages of 10 and 14 and based in schools, community centers, and churches (Kogan et al., 2019).
- Covers research on e-cigarette use in teens and young adults by Chen et al. (2020).
- Refers to research by Silva et al. (2020) on culturally adapted interventions for substance use disorders.
- Describes research on sociocultural influences in gambling disorder by Badji et al. (2020) and Williams et al. (2023).
- Includes third-wave therapy approaches for people of color as described by Dela Cruz et al. (2023).

CHAPTER 13

- Discusses problems of diagnosing delirium in older adults as reported by Oh et al. (2017).
- Cites research by Manini et al. (2021) on the impact of social isolation due to COVID-19 on psychological symptoms of neurocognitive disorders.
- Discusses the role of antioxidants in reducing neurocognitive disorder risk, citing de Andrade Teles et al. (2018).
- Discusses caregiver interventions using behavioral methods, citing research by Liu et al. (2021).
- Covers research on brain injury associated with football-related head injury, citing Alosco et al. (2020).
- Includes new discussion of the need to tailor assessment procedures for people with Alzheimer's disease based on their language and racial/ethnic status.
- Describes sociocultural contributions to TBI's prevalence and availability of treatment citing information from the CDC.

CHAPTER 14

- Real Story describes the case of Brandon Marshall (borderline personality disorder).
- Includes global prevalence data of personality disorders and distinction between low- and high-income countries as reported by Winsper et al. (2020).
- Describes the problem with use of "histrionic" personality disorder as a outmoded concept, citing Tripathi et al. (2019).

CHAPTER 15

- Chapter information reflects current APA Ethics Code regarding considerations in multicultural treatment.
- Indicates the need for adapting informed consent procedures for non-English speaking individuals as cited by McMillan (2020).
- Includes APA Guidelines for Psychotherapy with Lesbian, Gay, and Bisexual Clients.
- Includes APA Guidelines for Psychological Practice with Older Adults.
- Provides extensive information on the role of psychologists in forensic settings.

PREFACE

With its case-based approach, *Psychological Disorders: Clinical Perspectives* helps students understand the human side of psychological disorders. The 2025 Release ties concepts together with an integrated, personalized learning program, and features updates from the *DSM-5-TR* which was released in 2022.

The decision to change the title from *Abnormal Psychology* to *Psychological Disorders: Clinical Perspectives* reflects a shift towards more clinically accurate and sensitive terminology within the field of psychology. "Abnormal" carries a stigma and can be seen as pejorative, whereas "Psychological Disorders" attempts to highlight the scientific study of mental disorders without attaching judgment or stigma to individuals. This change aligns with modern approaches to mental health education that prioritize inclusivity, destigmatization, and accurate representation of psychological concepts. By changing the title this program aims to create a more respectful and understanding learning environment while maintaining academic rigor in the exploration of mental health disorders.

Importantly, we changed words in the title in this release from "Abnormal Psychology" to "Psychological Disorders," and consistently removed "abnormal" from the language contained in each chapter. This approach reflects the adaptations that the field is making to understand behavior as involving a continuum rather than a categorical distinction between "normal" and "abnormal." "Psychological disorders" now are seen in the field, and by us, as constellations of behavior that receive diagnoses when they are associated with significant impairment and distress.

A Personalized Experience That Leads to Improved Learning and Results

How many students think they know everything about abnormal psychology but struggle on the first exam? Students study more effectively with Connect and SmartBook.

- Connect's assignments help students contextualize what they've learned through application, so they can better understand the material and think critically.
- Connect reports deliver information regarding performance, study behavior, and effort so instructors can quickly identify students who are having issues or focus on material that the class hasn't mastered.
- SmartBook helps students study more efficiently by highlighting what to focus on in the chapter, asking review questions, and directing them to resources until they understand.
- SmartBook creates a personalized study path customized to individual student needs.

SMARTBOOK®

SmartBook is optimized for mobile and tablet and is accessible for students with disabilities. Content-wise, it has been enhanced with improved learning objectives that are measurable and observable to improve student outcomes. SmartBook personalizes learning to individual student needs, continually adapting to pinpoint knowledge gaps and focus learning on topics that need the most attention. Study time is more productive and, as a result, students are better prepared for class and coursework. For instructors, SmartBook tracks student progress and provides insights that can help guide teaching strategies.

Evergreen

Content and technology are ever-changing, and it is important that you can keep your course up to date with the latest content, assessments, and accessibility. That's why we want to deliver the most current and relevant content for your course, hassle-free. Whitbourne, *Psychological Disorders: Clinical Perspectives*, uses an Evergreen delivery model, which is a product delivery model and experience that provides customers with the most relevant and up-to-date content, tools, and accessibility. Engage students and freshen up assignments with up-to-date coverage of select topics and new questions, all without having to switch editions or build a new course.

Powerful Reporting

Whether a class is face-to-face, hybrid, or entirely online, McGraw Hill Connect provides the tools needed to reduce the amount of time and energy instructors spend administering their courses. Easy-to-use course management tools allow instructors to spend less time administering and more time teaching, while reports allow students to monitor their progress and optimize their study time.

- The **At-Risk Student Report** provides instructors with one-click access to a dashboard that identifies students who are at risk of dropping out of the course due to low engagement levels.
- The **Category Analysis Report** details student performance relative to specific learning objectives and goals, including APA learning goals and outcomes and levels of Bloom's taxonomy.
- The **SmartBook Reports** allow instructors and students to easily monitor progress and pinpoint areas of weakness, giving each student a personalized study plan to achieve success.

Informing and Engaging

McGraw Hill Connect offers several ways to actively engage students. McGraw Hill Education Connect is a digital assignment and assessment platform that strengthens the link between faculty, students, and course work. Connect for *Psychological Disorders: Clinical Perspectives* includes assignable and assessable videos, quizzes, exercises, and Interactivities, all associated with learning objectives.

The McGraw Hill Immersive Brain Program provides opportunities for students to learn about the brain and its connection to behavior through interaction. Embedded within the Whitbourne, *Psychological Disorders: Clinical Perspectives* ebook, SmartBook, and ReadAnwhere App are three-dimensional, dynamic figures of the brain. Students have the opportunity to navigate within these dynamic figures to explore key structures and functions to support their understanding of key concepts. Sample figures include: stress & anxiety, sleep, and neural transmission.

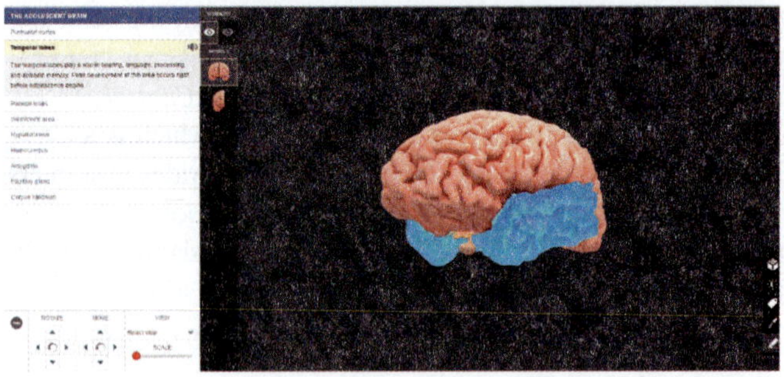

The McGraw Hill Immersive Brain Program is an interactive learning program focused on the brain and its connection to behavior.

Guiding students through the critical reading of current academic and clinical research is facilitated in Connect with our **Critical Thinking Assignment** tool. Critical Thinking Assignment (formerly Power of Process) has been redesigned for an improved user experience and enhanced accessibility (now compliant with WCAG standards). Over 50 new research articles were added as part of our Summer 2024 Evergreen release. Updated functionality supports additional workflows with the following benefits:

- Supports up to two documents for comparing/contrasting
- Side-by-side display of the document and the question for students
- Ability to leave written or audio feedback for students at an assignment-level or question-level
- Ability to create rubrics or use an MH rubric
- Inclusion of a wizard to guide students through the questions

Located in Connect, **NewsFlash** is a multi-media assignment tool that ties current news stories, TedTalks, blogs and podcasts to key psychological principles and learning objectives. Students interact with relevant news stories and are assessed on their ability to connect the content to the research findings and course material. NewsFlash is updated twice a year and uses expert sources to cover a wide range of topics including: DEI guidelines & clinical theory, mental health of Black transgender youth, and many more.

Writing Assignment

Available within McGraw Hill Connect®, the Writing Assignment tool delivers a learning experience to help students improve written communication skills and conceptual understanding. Assign, monitor, grade, and provide feedback on writing more efficiently and effectively.

McGraw Hill GO

McGraw Hill GO is an easy-to-use, quick-to-set-up eBook+ that lives within the Learning Management System (LMS). GO equips instructors and students with essential course materials: trusted, assignable content and auto-graded chapter questions that sync directly into the LMS. GO makes it easier to keep up with student progress and direct attention where it matters.

Thinking Critically About Psychological Disorders

Faces of Abnormal Psychology connects students to real people living with psychological disorders. Through its unique video program, Faces of Abnormal Psychology helps students gain a deeper understanding of psychological disorders and provides an opportunity for critical thinking.

Interactive Case Studies help students understand the complexities of psychological disorders. Co-developed with psychologists and students, these immersive cases bring the intricacies of clinical psychology to life in an accessible, gamelike format. Each case is presented from the point of view of a licensed psychologist, a social worker, or a psychiatrist. Students observe sessions with clients and are asked to identify major differentiating characteristics associated with each of the psychological disorders presented. Interactive Case Studies are assignable and assessable through Connect.

SUPPORTING INSTRUCTORS WITH TECHNOLOGY

With McGraw Hill Education, you can develop and tailor the course you want to teach.

With **Create,** faculty can easily rearrange chapters, combine material from other content sources, and quickly upload content you have written, such as your course syllabus or teaching notes. Find the content you need by searching through thousands of leading McGraw Hill Education textbooks. Arrange your book to fit your teaching style. Create even allows you to personalize your book's appearance by selecting the cover and adding your name, school, and course information. Order a Create book, and you will receive a complimentary print review copy in three to five business days or a complimentary electronic review copy via email in about an hour. Experience how McGraw Hill Education empowers you to teach your students your way. **http://create.mheducation.com**

With **Polling,** every learner has unique needs. Uncover where and when you're needed with the new Polling tool in McGraw Hill Connect®! Polling allows you to discover where students are in real time. Engage students and help them create connections with your course content while gaining valuable insight during lectures. Leverage polling data to deliver personalized instruction when and where it is needed most.

Trusted Service and Support

McGraw Hill Education's Connect offers comprehensive service, support, and training throughout every phase of your implementation. If you're looking for some guidance on how to use Connect, or want to learn tips and tricks from super users, you can find tutorials as you work. Our Digital Faculty Consultants and Student Ambassadors offer insight into how to achieve the results you want with Connect.

Instructor Supplements

Instructor's Manual The Instructor's Manual provides a wide variety of tools and resources for presenting the course, including learning objectives and ideas for lectures and discussions.

Test Bank and Test Builder Organized by chapter, the questions are designed to test factual, conceptual, and applied understanding; all test questions are available within Test Builder.

Available within Connect, Test Builder is a cloud-based tool that enables instructors to format tests that can be printed, administered within a Learning Management System, or exported as a Word document of the test bank. Test Builder offers a modern, streamlined interface for easy content configuration that matches course needs, without requiring a download.

Test Builder allows you to:

- Access all test bank content from a particular title.
- Easily pinpoint the most relevant content through robust filtering options.
- Manipulate the order of questions or scramble questions and/or answers.
- Pin questions to a specific location within a test.
- Determine your preferred treatment of algorithmic questions.
- Choose the layout and spacing.
- Add instructions and configure default settings.

Test Builder provides a secure interface for better protection of content and allows for just-in-time updates to flow directly into assessments.

PowerPoint Presentations The PowerPoint presentations, available in both dynamic, lecture-ready and accessible, WCAG-compliant versions, highlight the key points of the chapter and include supporting visuals. All of the slides can be modified to meet individual needs.

Image Gallery The Image Gallery features the complete set of downloadable figures and tables from the text. These can be easily embedded by instructors into their own PowerPoint slides.

Remote Proctoring and Browser-Locking Capabilities Remote proctoring and browser-locking capabilities, hosted by Proctorio within Connect, provide control of the assessment environment by enabling security options and verifying the identity of the student.

McGraw Hill connect + proctorio

Seamlessly integrated within Connect, these services allow instructors to control students' assessment experience by restricting browser activity, recording students' activity, and verifying students are doing their own work.

Instant and detailed reporting gives instructors an at-a-glance view of potential academic integrity concerns, thereby avoiding personal bias and supporting evidence-based claims.

Clinical Perspectives

The subtitle, *Clinical Perspectives,* reflects the emphasis on the experience of clients and clinicians in their efforts to facilitate each individual's maximum functioning. Each chapter begins with a clinical case study that typifies the disorders in that chapter, then returns to the case study at the end with the outcome of a prescribed treatment on the basis of the best available evidence. Throughout the chapter, the author translates the symptoms of each disorder into terms that capture the core essence of the disorder. The philosophy is that students should be able to appreciate the fundamental nature of each disorder without necessarily having to memorize all of its diagnostic criteria. In that way, students can gain a basic understanding that will serve them well regardless of their ultimate professional goals.

These cases focus on individuals from a variety of ethnicities, nationalities, gender identities, sexual orientations, and ages. In particular, the mini cases in each chapter are intended to reflect the importance of cultural variations that psychologists see in their private offices, clinics, hospitals, and counseling centers.

Above all, the study of psychological disorders is the study of profoundly human experiences. To this end, the author has developed a biographical feature entitled "Real Stories." You will read narratives from the actual experiences of celebrities, sports figures, politicians, authors, musicians, and artists ranging from Lady Gaga to Wayne Brady. Each story is written to provide insight into the particular disorder covered within the chapter. By reading these fascinating biographical pieces, you will come away with a more in-depth personal perspective to use in understanding the nature of the disorder.

The author has developed this text using a scientist-practitioner framework where research is informed by clinical practice. Within each disorder, you will read about research on theories and treatments based on the principles of evidence-based practice. This means that the approaches are tested through extensive research informed by clinical practice. Many researchers in the field of psychological disorders also treat clients in their own private offices, hospitals, or group practices. The results they provide from the lab are informed by the knowledge that their findings can ultimately provide real help to real people.

CHAPTER-BY-CHAPTER CHANGES

This release reflects the most recent revision to the *Diagnostic and Statistical Manual of Mental Disorders* (*DSM*) published the American Psychiatric Association in 2022 and known as *DSM-5-TR*. The *DSM-5-TR* was written following a lengthy process of revising the previous editions, the *DSM-5* and *DSM-IV-TR,* involving hundreds of researchers contributing to task forces intended to investigate each of the major categories of disorders. Changes from these prior editions are highlighted in each chapter with a section entitled "What's in the *DSM-5-TR*."

Throughout the text, the author has incorporated changes based on new terminology, diagnoses, diagnostic information, cultural considerations, and risks associated with suicide and suicidal behavior, as specified in the *DSM-5-TR*. Each section of the text was reviewed specifically to ensure that it is consistent with *DSM-5-TR* and all terminology was revised accordingly as stated both in the introduction to *DSM-5-TR* and each specific set of diagnostic criteria.

The author and contributor have incorporated language suggested by the APA Inclusive Language Guidelines and meets standards based on sensitivity analyses. All references to gender were updated (e.g., woman instead of female), the terms "ethnoracial" and "minoritized" are now used throughout, and other cultural considerations were described where appropriate in keeping with the *DSM-5-TR* diagnostic considerations.

In addition to the *DSM-5-TR* updates, this release includes hundreds of new and updated references, including many international sources, and the mental health impacts of the COVID-19 pandemic have been added throughout. The language has been revised to be more inclusive with respect to gender, gender identity, and race/ethnicity. Many photos have been replaced to update the book and increase diversity, equity, and inclusion.

Specific updates to this release appear below:

CHAPTER 1

- Reworded the introduction with attention to psychological disorders rather than "abnormal" psychology.
- Reorganized presentation of biopsychosocial perspective to provide clearer coverage.
- Introduced the term psychopathology as studied in research.

- Expanded discussion of stigma, including material from new references including stigma toward mental health treatment among older adults.
- Added ageism as a form of discrimination that interacts with other forms of discrimination.
- Pointed out the importance of understanding psychological disorders from a culturally sensitive perspective.
- Revised historical themes, providing greater clarity and connection to present understandings of psychological disorders.
- Added modern-day use of exorcism with example from Poland and other countries.
- Pointed out that beliefs in the spiritual approach still exist today.
- Clarified the biopsychosocial perspective by reorganizing the section in which it is introduced members of marginalized communities with regard to the sociocultural perspective.
- Noted the importance of concern for human rights as modern version of "moral treatment."
- Added meta-analysis as a research method.
- Expanded discussion of importance that research findings be examined from the perspective of scientific validity.
- Added discussion of structural modeling as example of higher-level correlational methods.
- Added discussion of inattentive responders to online surveys and how this affects the findings from those studies.
- Discussed problems of obtaining population statistics based on the source of information and to keep in mind that estimates may not always be accurate depending on how the data were collected.
- Added new references based on case study and focus group methods.

CHAPTER 2

- Expanded discussion of patient vs. client in psychology.
- Added Applied Behavior Analysts to list of master-level clinicians
- Added greater detail to use of inclusive language in case formulations.
- Added Veterans Administration Medical Centers as site for psychological treatment.
- Included new paragraph on community mental health centers (CMHC's) as sites for treament.
- Added college counseling centers as sites for treatment.
- Clarified relationship between counseling and psychotherapy.
- Added new research on measuring remission rates.

CHAPTER 3

- Provided greater clarity regarding the nature of structured clinical interviews.
- Added information regarding newer methods that are becoming available which are normed for expansive gender identities
- Provided clarification regarding clinical interviews, including structured vs. unstructured.
- Added discussion of taking diversity into account in administering and interpreting the WAIS-5.
- Updated WAIS-IV to WAIS-5.
- Described in more detail the history of the MMPI, leading to the current MMPI-3.
- Added description of the Personality Inventory for DSM-5 and discussed its cross-national validity.
- Added the Rorschach Performance Assessment System (R-PAS) as a way to quantify scores.
- Updated the Real Story on Demi Lovato.
- Added paragraph on the American Psychological Association's Multicultural Guidelines (2017).
- Added inhibitory control as a feature of executive functioning.
- Added the SLUMS as a mental status screening instrument.
- Described problems in applying mental status exams to individuals with substance use disorders.
- Showed in detail how the Boston Naming Test is being translated to a number of languages other than English.
- Included discussion of assessments as focusing on both strengths and weaknesses to provide a fuller picture of the client.

CHAPTER 4

- Added description of Default Mode Network.
- Updated description of endophenotypes.
- Added new research on twin studies.
- Added q22.11 deletion syndrome.

- Included concept of intergenerational trauma under section on endophenotypes.
- Improved the discussion of SNP's with new and clearer figure.
- Added third generation antipsychotics, ketamines, and psilocybin to medications.
- Added new concerns about use of ECT based on new studies of long-term risks.
- Included HEXACO 6-factor personality trait model
- Added new references on attachment style and how it is applied in psychotherapy
- Incorporated new reference to the relevance of psychodynamic therapy in current treatment approaches.
- Added Applied Behavior Analysis as a treatment method based on the behavioral perspective
- Provided newer approach to incorporating vicarious reinforcement in treatment using modeling.
- Clarified description of counterconditioning.
- Added culturally-adapted CBT for use with a diverse range of clients.
- Expanded discussion of social discrimination as cause of internalized transphobia in transgender individuals.
- Added new concerns about COVID-19's impact on mental health as well as the effects of climate change.
- Provided expanded approach to describing the acceptance-based approach to theory and treatment and provided fuller description of ACT including the ACT hexaflex with detailed explanation of each point in the hexaflex.
- Added discussion of invalidating early environments that could negatively impact coping skills when individuals reach adulthood.
- Added the Interpersonal Effectiveness module to description of DBT.
- Showed that mindfulness-based cognitive therapy can be successfully used in digital form, which can make it a method accessible to a wide range of clients.
- Expanded discussion of DBT to different populations as well as discussing its long-term effects.

CHAPTER 5

- Included prevalence statistics on intellectual developmental disorder with new global and U.S. estimates.
- Discussed need for greater understanding of the many complex factors that affect the lives of affected individuals and their families.
- Updated statistics on fetal alcohol syndrome disorder including discussion of importance of prevention.
- Included new research on mindfulness training for staff working with individuals with intellectual developmental disorder.
- Added new approach known as "Circle of Security program which incorporates family support as well as treatment of individuals with fetal alcohol syndrome disorder.
- Described Multifaceted Case Management as approach in treatment of individuals with fetal alcohol syndrome disorder.
- Clarified steps in diagnosis of autism spectrum disorder.
- Included new statistics on autism spectrum disorder, including racial/ethnic variations as reported by the CDC.
- Revised the discussion of autistic savant syndrome.
- Described new research on genetics of autism spectrum disorder.
- Included alterations in the DMN as contributor to autism spectrum disorder symptoms.
- Added Applied Behavior Analysis as treatment for autism spectrum disorder.
- Includes new research on augmented virtual reality in treatment of autism specrum disorder.
- Emphasized importance of taking into account personal values of families in treating autistm spectrum disorder.
- Provided greater specificity of the genetics of Rett syndrome.
- Described possible neurological contributions fo high-functioning autism spectrum disorder.
- Added sociocultural factors to risk of the development of a learning disorder.
- Described in more detail the Response to Intervention approach in treatment of learning disorders.
- Updated the role of vocational training for adults with learning disorders including addition of Project Search UK as a successful translation of the U.S-based program.
- Expanded discussion of stuttering and its affect on individuals, but also included new research on resilience.

- Included discussion of effects of social or pragmatic communication disorder on children's academic development.
- Added new prevalence data on ADHD including racial/ethnic variations.
- Presented new data on lifetime prevalance of ADHD.
- Described lifetime outcomes associated with ADHD and associated risks of other psychological disorders.
- Incorporated new genetic research on ADHD.
- Added compensating factors for ADHD as individuals move through adulthood.
- Included new section on treatment of ADHD with nonstimulant medication as well as new research on behavioral and CBT-based treatments.
- Replaced previous section on psychosocial treatment with the ADHD tracking scale as adjunct to behavioral interventions.
- Added further distinction to description of developmental coordination disorder.
- Included new research on video game training for individuals with developmental coordination disorder.

CHAPTER 6

- Provided updated language on categories of delusions.
- Included new global data on COVID-19 and the risk of psychotic disorders.
- Added new research on structural brain changes associated with schizophrenia.
- Added new discussion on neuroplasticity deficits in individuals with schizophrenia and how this could affect their cognitive abilities.
- Expanded discussion of biological treatments for schizophrenia to include third generation anti-psychotics.
- Added new research on Theory of Mind and other social cognitive disturbances in people with schizophrenia.
- Included new meta-analytic data on cognitive behavioral treatments of schizophrenia as well as potential value of third wave forms of therapy.
- Added a revised view of family dynamics as contributors to schizophrenia and the importance of including caregivers in interventions.
- Added the developmental risk factor model in highlighting the contribution of social factors affecting schizophrenia.

CHAPTER 7

- Updated prevalence data with the latest findings from the National Institutes of Health and added the effect of COVID-19 on problems in providing sufficient treatment given prevalence increases in 2023.
- Included new discussion of the risks presented by persistent depressive disorder compared to major depressive disorder.
- Discussed new research on reduced cognitive flexibility of children with disruptive mood dysregulation disorder.
- Included new research on genetics and the history of childhood maltreatment in development of premenstrual dysphoric disorder.
- Added new discussion of whether premenstrual dysphoric disorder should be included as a psychological disorder.
- Incorporated recent research on non-adherence to treatment among individuals with bipolar disorder as presenting a risk factor for negative lifetime health outcomes.
- Discussed new research pointing to the impact of non-adherence to treatment on relapse of individuals with bipolar disorder,
- Included new research on transcranial magnetic stimulation in treatment of depression.
- Expanded discussion of minority stress model after events in the spring of 2020 including the COVID-19 pandemic and oppression-based trauma.
- Added new research showing the benefits of religion in resilience to depressive symptoms following the COVID-19 pandemic.
- Provided updated suicide statistics including variations by race, ethnicity, gender, and age.

CHAPTER 8

- Discusses impact of COVID-19 on the prevalence of anxiety disorders and problems in diagnosis for those clients seen in primary care settings only.
- Adds non-pharmacological interventions for children with selective mutism.
- Provided new research on neurological contributions to specific phobias.
- Adds "fear of falling" as a possible form of specific phobia in older adults.

- Expanded discussion of the use of virtual reality exposure therapy for specific phobias.
- Described One Session Treatment as an effective treatment for children with specific phobias.
- Added short-term psychodynamic therapy for panic disorder and agoraphobia based on new randomized studies.
- Discussed that older adults benefit more from CBT alone than when it is combined with ACT.
- Updated list of compulsions with more recent examples.
- Added new psychological and sociocultural contributors to body dysmorphic disorder.
- Included new research on acceptance-based and compassion-focused therapy in treatment of body dysmorphic disorder.
- Added discussion of the role of discrimination and cultural attitudes toward, members of marginalized communities in body dysmorphic disorder.
- Updated discussion of risk factors for hoarding disorder to include adverse life events associated with childhood and later adulthood.
- Provided new distinctions between forms of hair pulling, adding risk factors in later life.
- Added discussion of comorbidities for hair pulling as well as effects on a number of life domains associated with the disorder.
- Included decoupling as treatment for trichotillomania.
- Added new data on role of personality traits in risk for excoriation disorder.
- Included newer and more expansive model of stress and early life maltreatment as risk factors for reactive attachment disorder.
- Discussed new research on risk factors for PTSD including being LGBTQ+, and exposed to natural disasters, witnessing an overdose, experiencing chronic food insecurity, and working in professions that place people in potentially traumatic situations.
- Added ketamine as a treatment for PTSD.
- Included newer treatments developed by the VA System for PTSD including eye movement desensitization therapy, and specialized forms of CBT.
- Added new information of efficacy of internet-delivered therapy for PTSD.
- Included new research on couples therapy in which one individual is a Veteran.
- Added new data on "dose-response" principle as applied to treatment for PTSD.

CHAPTER 9

- Discussed role of early trauma as effect on developing brain creating risk for dissociative disorders.
- Replaced Herschel Walker with Adam Duritz in the Real Story.
- Added new research on role of COVID-19 as risk factor for somatic symptom disorders.
- Described the role of "COVID anxiety" on illness anxiety.
- Included new discussion of "diabetes distress" in contributing to anxiety and depression in older adults.
- Discussed the impact of *ICD-11* changes in diagnoses of functional neurological disorder on ability of individuals to be able to receive treatment to overcome biases against people with these disorders.
- Added new information on factitious disorder imposed on another as a manifestation of medical abuse.
- Included physical therapy as a possible treatment for individuals with functional neurological disorder.
- Added specificity to life events and hassles as sources of stress.
- Discussed the role of social support as a coping method to manage stress.
- Added the role of personality traits as risk factors for stress, citing a new study on older adults with lymphoma.
- Included new studies on emotional expression as a coping method for managing life stressors.
- Revised the "Type A" behavior pattern section to reflect the retraction of Eysenck's research emerging in a 2019 retraction paper published by Kings College London.
- Substituted the Type A section with research on Five Factor Model traits and their relationship to chronic disease.
- Added management of pain as an application of behavioral medicine.
- Included new studies on wearable technologies in behavioral medicine for chronic diseases.

CHAPTER 10

- Includes updated prevalence data for eating disorders.
- Added discussion of orthorexia with new research distinguishing this pattern from concern with healthy eating.
- Introduces atypical anorexia nervosa which occurs in individuals of higher weight.
- Describes meta-analysis of studies on suicidal self-injury among individuals with anorexia nervosa.
- Changed Real Story from Portia De Rossi to Lily Collins.
- Added discussion of how internalized ageism may lead to increased rates of binge eating in later adulthood.
- Added new research showing benefits of yoga for treatment of eating disorders.
- Included expanded discussion of reclassification in *DSM-5-TR* of disorders covered in this chapter.
- Covered new research showing the role of sociocultural factors in eating disorders as represented by COVID-19.
- Added description of problems in the estimating prevalence of avoidant/restrictive food disorder limiting knowledge of variations accoding to such factors as geographic location and age.
- Described new case study of pica in an adult woman.
- Added new behavioral treatments for pica.
- Reworded descriptions of enuresis and encopresis including outlining subtypes of both.
- Described new method of enhanced toilet training as a treatment for elimination disorders.
- Added new research on the efficacy of devices for treatment of sleep apnea including neurostimulation.
- Included new information on the treatment of oppositional defiant disorder involving collaboration with parents.
- Described a new study showing that early exposure to family violence has different impacts on men and women in the development of intermittent explosive disorder.
- Provided new data on the effectiveness of cognitive behavioral therapy for intermittent explosive disorder including new treatment known as Cognitive, Relaxation, and Coping Skills Training for intermittent explosive disorder,
- Added the "callous/unemotional" set of personality traits as risk factors for disruptive behavior disorders in childhood.
- Included new research on subgroups of individuals who engage in shoplifting along with changes in identity that may accompany being labeled as a shoplifter.
- Described recent research on neuroimaging studies of individuals with kleptomania.
- Added group treatment through cognitive behavioral and mindfulness as showing benefits for people with kleptomania.

CHAPTER 11

- Provided more nuanced introduction to paraphilic disorders and clarified that a "paraphilia" is not necessarily a "psychological disorder."
- Expanded discussion of stigma in paraphilic disorders.
- Added research based on crowdsourcing as a method to estimate the prevalence of sexual interest and offending against children.
- Described a case study of exhibitionism directed against older woman by a caretaker in a long-term care health facility.
- Distinguished "everyday sadism" from the disorders of sexual masochism and sexual sadism.
- Covered new research on the relationship between high sex drive (seven or more orgasms a week for a minimum of six months) and specific paraphilic disorders.
- Described the "off-label" use of SSRI's that may have benefit by working on the dopamine and serotonin systems, thought to contribute to the development of a paraphilia.
- Added new research showing that clinicians may become the focus of treatment if they express pathologizing attitudes toward their clients with paraphilic disorders.
- Described sociocultural influences in paraphilic disorders as shown by research in the U.K. on popular pornography websites.
- Discusses rape supportive culture as an influence on sexual violence against women.
- Included new research on sexual dysfunctions in transgender individuals, including outcomes of studies on changes in sexual dysfunction following gender-affirming care.

- Added pelvic floor therapy as treatment for sexual dysfunctions.
- Added a discussion pointing out that healthcare and mental healthcare professionals should consider addressing sexual concerns expressed by individuals, regardless of their age.
- Clarified distinctions between gender dysphoria and transvestic disorder, including discussion of the term "non-binary."
- Added new data on the effectiveness of gender-affirming medical procedures for individuals with gender dysphoria.
- Included more detail on gender-affirming psychotherapy.

CHAPTER 12

- Expanded discussion of risks associated with substance use disorder.
- Provided updated data from SAMHSA on prevalence of substance use disorders, including variations by race, ethnicity, and age.
- Discussed "generational forgetting" as an influence on the continued use of illicit substances such as LSD as well as changes resulting from new forms of administration.
- Reorganized chapter subheads to make the organization of the chapter easier to follow.
- Discussed life course variations in stress affecting alcohol use.
- Updated research evidence in favor of genetic explanations of alcohol use disorder.
- Updated discussion of alcohol expectancy theory.
- Expanded discussion of alcohol use patterns in individuals who otherwise engage in healthy behaviors.
- Added new research on the effect of long-term marijuana use on cognitive functioning.
- Described the risks associated with comorbidity in Veterans.
- Updated the statistics on deaths and the economic burden associated with prescription drug misuse.
- Described new research on caffeine use in pre-teenage children.
- Updated prevalence statistics on vaping.
- Added third wave therapies as being effective for people of color and individuals from collectivist cultures.
- Included new research on predictors of problem gambling from a large-scale Canadian study.

CHAPTER 13

- Added the need to screen for anesthetic use in assessment of delirium.
- Provided new introduction to the discussion of the prevalence of Alzheimer's disease.
- Used National Institute of Aging summary to differentiate stages of Alzheimer's disease.
- Included a new infographic clarifying the distinction between normal aging and Alzheimer's disease.
- Described specifics of the multi-faceted approach to the diagnosis of Alzheimer's disease.
- Added the "DASH" diet as an approach to reducing the risk of neurocognitive disorders associated with cardiovascular disease and diabetes.
- Included new medications approved by the FDA for the treatment of Alzheimer's disease and discussed the pros and cons of each.
- Added imbic-predominant age-related TDP-43 proteinopathy as another cause of dementia that may resemble Alzheimer's disease.
- Updated statistics on traumatic brain injury.
- Described new research on sociocultural influences on traumatic brain injury.
- Added new research on cognitive impairments associated with COVID-19.

CHAPTER 14

- Added updated research on antisocial personality disorder regarding the AMPD proposal of a "psychochopathic specifier."
- Included a new reference to the "dark tetrad" to update from the "dark triad.
- Discussed the importance of therapeutic alliance when working with individuals with antisocial personality disorder.
- Described the results of research on borderline personality disorder in later adulthood.

- Added a new method of treatment called "Borderline Compass."
- Included new research on longing for connection in avoidant personality disorder.
- Described problems in metacognition that can be experienced by people with avoidant personality disorder.
- Added clarification distinguishing OCPD from OCD.
- Included new research on the long-term health risks of people with OCPD.

CHAPTER 15

- Changed Real Story from *Kahler v. Kansas* to Robert Card.
- Added new discussion of ethics of using artificial intelligence in the provision of psychological treatment.
- Included new material on the ethics of assessment of parents whose children are being seen in mental health settings.
- Updated the Guidelines for Psychological Evaluations in Child Protection Matters.
- Added new material on the APA's recommendations for responding to demands of the legal system in the form of subpoenas.
- Updated the material on duty to warn describing legislation in Pennsylvania, California, and Virginia.
- Described problems faced by parole boards in conducting assessments of prisoners.
- Added recommendation that psychologists involved in forensic examinations do so on the basis of standardized training and performance standards.

Acknowledgments

The following instructors were instrumental in the development of the text, offering their feedback and advice as reviewers:

David Alfano, *Community College of Rhode Island*
Colleen Bartels, *Hudson Valley Community College*
Bryan Cochran, *University of Montana*
Julie A. Deisinger, *Saint Xavier University*
Daniel Dickman, *Ivy Tech Community College*
Angela Fournier, *Bemidji State University*
Perry Fuchs, *University of Texas at Arlington*
Janice Gallagher, *Ivy Tech Community College*
Richard Helms, *Central Piedmont Community College*
Heather Jennings, *Mercer County Community College*
Joan Brandt Jensen, *Central Piedmont Community College*
Christian Johnston, *University of Louisiana*
Cynthia Kalodner, *Towson University*
Patricia Kemerer, *Ivy Tech Community College*
Barbara Kennedy, *Brevard Community College-Palm Bay*
Joseph Lowman, *University of North Carolina-Chapel Hill*
Don Lucas, *Northwest Vista College*
James A. Markusic, *Missouri State University*
Mark McKellop, *Juniata College*
Maura Mitrushina, *California State University-Northridge*
Oswaldo Moreno, *Virginia Commonwealth University*
John Norland, *Blackhawk Technical College*
Karen Clay Rhines, *Northampton Community College*
Ty Schepis, *Texas State University*
William R. Scott, *Liberty University*
Dr. Wayne S. Stein, *Brevard Community College*
Deb Stipp, *Ivy Tech Community College*
Marla Sturm, *Montgomery County Community College*
Terry S. Trepper, *Purdue University-Calumet*
Naomi Wagner, *San Jose State University*
Nevada Winrow, *Baltimore City Community College*

It has been particularly satisfying to work on this release with my daughter, Jennifer L. O'Brien, PhD, who served as my research assistant and author of all the Case Reports and Real Stories in the text. Now in a private group practice in Cambridge, MA she served as a psychologist at the Massachusetts Institute of Technology (MIT) Medical Mental Health and Counseling Services. Jenny received her PhD in 2014 from American University and completed a predoctoral internship at the Durham V.A. Hospital and a postdoctoral internship at the Boston V.A. Hospital. As a clinician, she specializes in working with individuals in the LGBTQIA+ community. Her wide range of experiences with this population as well as veterans and university students from all over the world gives her a unique perspective and set of insights that inform the entire book.

Finally, a great book can't come together without a great publishing team. Ryan Treat, Executive Portfolio Manager, has supported the project with his many invaluable ideas and insights about how best to shape the current release. Dawn Groundwater, our longtime Senior Product Development Manager is someone whose wisdom, honesty, and perspective have proven invaluable. I would also like to thank our Content Project Manager (CPM), Mary Powers, who is incredibly responsive and has guided us through the many complexities involved in supervising all production aspects of the revision. Sarah Flynn, our Content Licensing Specialist, has ably responded to our search for the best possible illustrations and photos that make the pages of the book come alive. Isfa Syed, Marketing Manager, is giving us the feedback we need to ensure that the text meets the needs of both students and instructors. In this latest release, my contributor and I continue to feel very grateful to be part of the McGraw Hill family, whose commitment to student success is truly remarkable.

A Letter from the Author

I am very glad that you are choosing to read my textbook. The topic of psychological disorders has never been more fascinating or relevant. We constantly hear reports of celebrities openly speaking about their mental health issues which lead the media to speculate on their diagnosis, speculation that may or may not be accurate. Given all this misinformation in the mind of the public, I feel that it's important for you to be educated in the science and practice of clinical psychology. At the same time, psychological science grabs almost as many headlines in all forms of news media. It seems that everyone is eager to learn about the latest findings, ranging from the neuroscience of behavior to the effectiveness of the newest treatment methods. Advances in brain-scanning methods and studies of psychotherapy effectiveness are greatly increasing our understanding of how to help treat and prevent psychological disorders.

Particularly fascinating to me was expanding the coverage in this edition to reflect advances in the understanding of sociocultural factors on mental health. Jennifer O'Brien was my resource in ensuring that the treatment of LGBTQ+ issues in this text are up-to-date and relevant. I also found it important to incorporate the influence of COVID-19 on mental health, with its tragic consequences for the lives of everyone in the world during the years 2020–2021. Although the pandemic itself no longer has the same influence on global health, it will continue to have a profound role in affecting people's lives for years to come.

The profession of clinical psychology is also undergoing rapid changes. With changes in health care policy, it is very likely that more professionals, from psychologists to mental health counselors, will be employed in providing behavioral interventions. By taking this first step toward your education now, you will be preparing yourself for a career that is increasingly being recognized as vital to helping individuals of all ages and all walks of life to achieve their greatest fulfillment.

I hope you find this text engaging and thought-provoking. Please feel free to e-mail me at susan.whitbourne@umb.edu with your questions and reactions to the material. As a long-time user of McGraw Hill's Connect in my own teaching, I can also vouch for its effectiveness in helping you achieve mastery of this course. I am also available to answer any questions teachers have, from an instructor's point of view, about how best to incorporate this book's digital media into your own teaching.

Thank you again for choosing to read this book!

Best,
Susan

McGraw Hill connect®

Your complete course platform

Connect enables you to build deeper connections with your students through cohesive digital content and tools, creating engaging learning experiences. We are committed to providing you with the right resources and tools to support all your students along their personal learning journeys.

65%
Less Time Grading

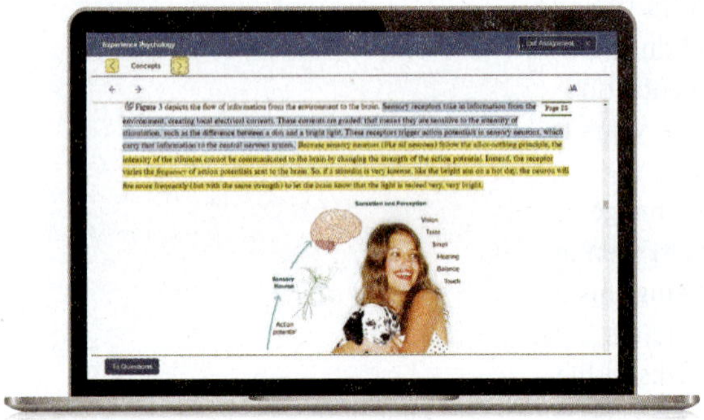

Laptop: Getty Images; Woman/dog: George Doyle/Getty Images

Every learner is unique

In Connect, instructors can assign an adaptive reading experience with SmartBook®. Rooted in advanced learning science principles, SmartBook delivers a personalized experience, focusing students on their learning gaps and ensuring the time they spend studying is time well spent.
mheducation.com/highered/connect/smartbook

Study anytime, anywhere

Encourage your students to download the free ReadAnywhere® app so they can access their online eBook, SmartBook®, or Adaptive Learning Assignments when it's convenient, even when they're offline. Because the app automatically syncs with students' Connect accounts, all their work is available every time they open it.
mheducation.com/readanywhere

"I really liked this app—it made it easy to study when you don't have your textbook in front of you."

Jordan Cunningham, a student at *Eastern Washington University*

Effective tools for efficient studying

Connect is designed to help students be more productive with simple, flexible, intuitive tools that maximize study time and meet students' individual learning needs. Get learning that works for everyone with Connect.

SUPPORT AT every step

Education for all

McGraw Hill works directly with Accessibility Services departments and faculty to meet the learning needs of all students. Please contact your Accessibility Services Office, and ask them to email **accessibility@mheducation.com**, or visit **mheducation.com/about/accessibility** for more information.

Affordable solutions, added value

Make technology work for you with LMS integration for single sign-on access, mobile access to the digital textbook, and reports to quickly show you how each of your students is doing. And with our Inclusive Access program, you can provide all these tools at the lowest available market price to your students. Ask your McGraw Hill representative for more information.

Solutions for your challenges

A product isn't a solution. Real solutions are affordable, reliable, and come with training and ongoing support when you need it and how you want it. Visit **supportateverystep.com** for videos and resources both you and your students can use throughout the term.

Updated and relevant content

Our Evergreen delivery model provides you with the most relevant and up-to-date content, tools, and accessibility. Engage students and freshen up assignments with up-to-date coverage of select topics and new questions, all without having to switch editions or build a new course.

Overview to Understanding Psychological Disorders

CHAPTER 1

OUTLINE

Learning Objectives

1.1 Explain what behavior constitutes a psychological disorder.

1.2 Describe the social impact of psychological disorders.

1.3 Define the characteristics of a psychological disorder.

1.4 Describe the causes of psychological disorders.

1.5 Summarize how explanations of psychological disorders have changed through time.

1.6 Describe research methods pertaining to psychological disorders.

1.7 Summarize the experimental approach to scientific research.

1.8 Describe the correlational design approach to scientific research.

1.9 Describe types of research studies.

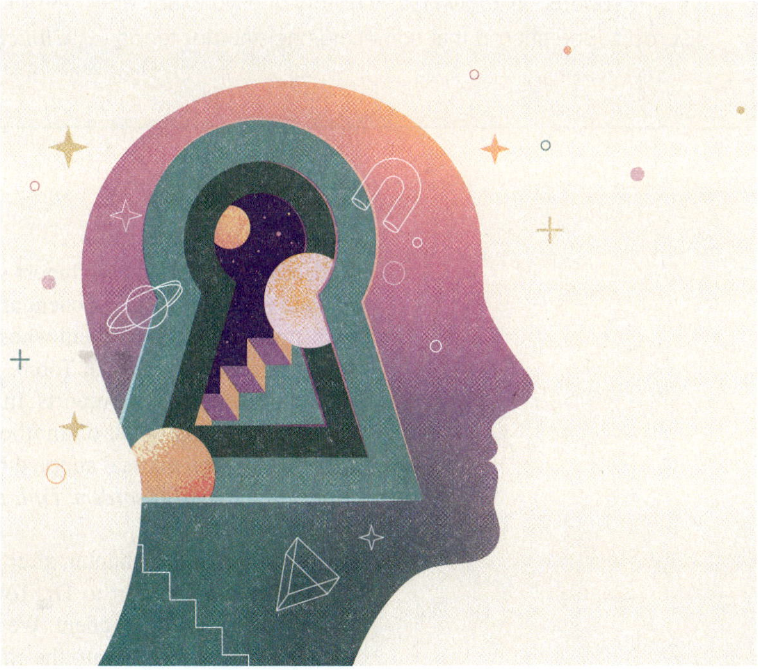

Marish/Shutterstock

Case Report

Rebecca Hasbrouck

Demographic information: 18-year-old White bisexual cisgender woman. Rebecca's pronouns are she/her/hers.

History of present illness: Rebecca self-referred to the university counseling center. She is a first-year college student, living away from home for the first time. Following the first week of classes, Rebecca reports that she is having trouble falling and staying asleep, has difficulty concentrating in her classes, and often feels irritable. She reports she is frustrated by the difficulties of her coursework and worries that her grades are beginning to suffer. She also relays that she is having trouble making friends at school and that she has been feeling lonely because she has no close friends here with whom she can talk openly. Rebecca is very close to her boyfriend of 3 years, though they are attending college in different cities.

Rebecca was tearful throughout our first session, stating that, for the first time in her life, she feels overwhelmed by feelings of hopelessness. She reports that although the first week at school felt like "torture," she is slowly growing accustomed to her new lifestyle, despite her struggles with missing her family and boyfriend, as well as her friends from high school.

Psychiatric history: Rebecca has no prior history of depressive episodes or other mental health concerns, and she reports no known family history of psychological disorders. She shared that sometimes her mother tends to get "really stressed out," though she has never received professional mental health treatment.

Current symptoms: Depressed mood, difficulty falling asleep (insomnia), difficulty concentrating on schoolwork. She described feelings of hopelessness but denied any thoughts of suicide or self-harm.

Risk level: Low risk. Rebecca has no current thought of suicide and no past history of suicidality or suicide attempts.

Case formulation: Although it appeared at first as though Rebecca was experiencing a major depressive episode, she did not meet the diagnostic criteria. While the age of onset for depression tends to be around Rebecca's age, given her lack of a family history of depression and the fact that her symptoms were occurring in response to a major stressor, the clinician determined that Rebecca was suffering from adjustment disorder with depressed mood.

Treatment plan: The counselor will refer Rebecca for weekly psychotherapy. Therapy should focus on improving her mood, and it also should allow her a supportive space to discuss her feelings surrounding the major changes that have been occurring in her life.

Sarah Tobin, PhD
Clinician

Rebecca Hasbrouck's case report summarizes the pertinent features that a clinician would include when first seeing a client after an initial evaluation. Each chapter of this book begins with a case report for a client whose characteristics are related to the chapter's topic. A fictitious clinician, Dr. Sarah Tobin, who supervises a clinical setting that offers a variety of services, writes the case reports. In some instances, she provides the services, and in others, she supervises the work of another psychologist. For each case, she provides a diagnosis using the official manual adopted by the profession, known as the *Diagnostic and Statistical Manual of Mental Disorders, Fifth Edition-Text Revision (DSM-5-TR)* (American Psychiatric Association, 2022).

At the end of this chapter, after you have developed a better understanding of the client's disorder, we will return to Dr. Tobin's description of the treatment results and expected future outcomes for the client. We also include Dr. Tobin's personal reflections on the case to help you gain insight into the clinician's experience in working with individuals with psychological disorders.

The study of psychological disorders is filled with countless fascinating stories of people who suffer from psychological disorders. In this chapter, you will be able to get some sense of the reality that psychological disturbance is certain to touch everyone, to some extent, at some point in life. As you progress through this course, you will almost certainly develop a sense of the challenges people associate with psychological problems. You will find yourself drawn into the many ways that mental health problems affect the lives of individuals, their families, and society. In addition to becoming more personally familiar with the emotional aspects of psychological disorders, you will learn about the scientific and theoretical basis for understanding and treating the people who suffer from them.

1.1 What Is a Psychological Disorder?

Psychological disorders are constellations of behavior that receive diagnoses when they are associated with significant impairment and distress. It is possible that you know someone like Rebecca, who is experiencing more than the average degree of adjustment difficulties in college. Would you consider her to have a psychological disorder, or is she reacting in an ordinary way to her stressful circumstances? Is it necessary to give Rebecca any diagnosis at all? What if she showed up at your door looking as if she were ready to harm herself? Questions such as these therefore are basic to advancing the field's understanding of the nature of psychological disorders.

psychological disorders
Constellations of behavior that receive diagnoses when they are associated with significant impairment and distress.

Researchers in the field of **psychopathology** face these questions as an intrinsic part of their work. The question of what is a psychological disorder and what are simply individual differences in behavior has great practical and theoretical significance. One potential resolution incorporates the concept of "harm," or distress and impairment, as well as "dysfunction," which reflects the internal mechanisms within the individual that produce symptoms along with associated harm (Stein, Palk, & Kendler, 2021).

psychopathology
The scientific study of psychological disorders.

Taking these factors into account, now reflect on either yourself or someone you know whose behavior might form the basis for a diagnosis of a psychological disorder. What might lead you to draw this conclusion? Have there been times in your life when you went through a period of feeling unusually sad or anxious? Are there people you know whose behavior concerns you because they seem so fearful or sad, or because they seem to misuse alcohol or drugs? Even if someone in your immediate circle has never shown signs of such difficulties, there are many examples in social media of famous individuals who have struggled with psychological issues. Indeed, throughout this book, you will read the "Real Stories" of well-known individuals who publicly described their own experiences with psychological disorders.

As you can see from these examples, psychological disorders are part of the human experience, directly or indirectly touching the life of every person. However, they don't have to destroy those lives. As you read about these disorders and the people who live with them, you will find that psychological disorders and the issues associated with them can be treated, and sometimes even prevented.

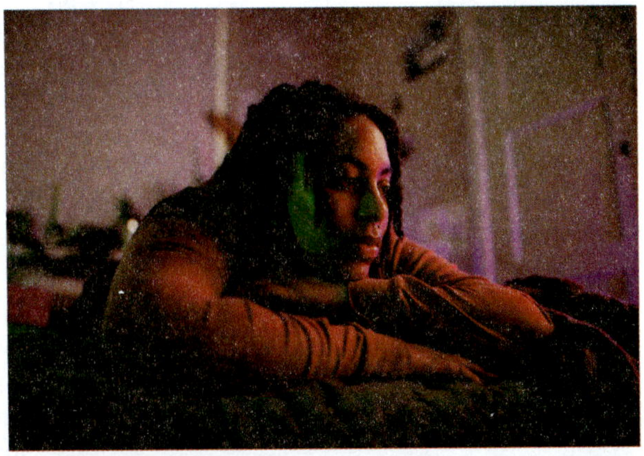

Deciding on whether an individual's behavior reflects symptoms of a psychological disorder is an important focus of the field of psychological disorders.
Maskot/DigitalVision/Getty Images

1.2 The Social Impact of Psychological Disorders

Psychological disorders affect both the individual and the other people in the individual's social world. Put yourself in the following situation. You receive an urgent text from the mother of your best friend, Jeremy. You call her and find out he's been admitted to a behavioral health unit of the local hospital and wants to see you. According to Jeremy's mother, only you can understand what he is going through. The news comes out of the blue and is puzzling and distressing. You had no idea Jeremy had any psychological problems. You ponder what you will say

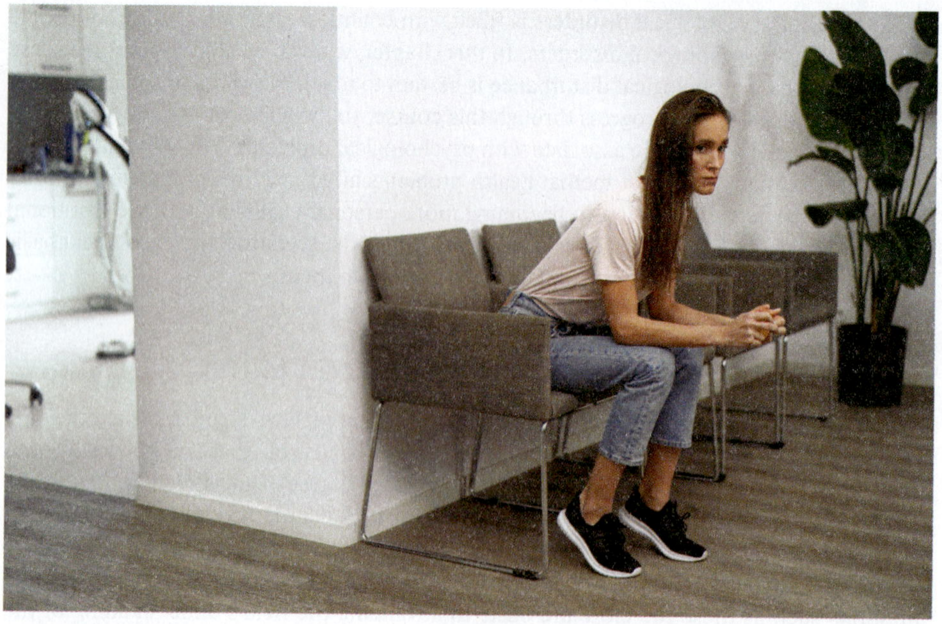

The families of individuals with psychological disorders face significant stress when their relatives must be hospitalized.

Westend61 on Offset/Shutterstock

to him when you see him. Jeremy is your closest friend, but now you wonder how your relationship will change. How much can you ask him about what he's going through? How is it that you never saw it coming? Unsure about what to do when you get there, you wonder what kind of shape he'll be in and whether he'll even be able to communicate with you. What will it be like to see him in this setting? What will he expect of you, and what will this mean for the future of your friendship?

stigma
A negative label that causes certain people to be regarded as different, defective, and set apart from mainstream members of society.

Now imagine the same scenario, but instead you receive news that Jeremy was just admitted to the emergency room of a general hospital with acute appendicitis. You know exactly how to respond when you go to see him. You will ask him how he feels, what exactly is wrong with him, and when he will be well again. Even though you might not like hospitals very much, at least you have a pretty good idea about what hospital patients are like. The appendectomy won't seem like anything special, and you would probably not even consider whether you could be friends with Jeremy again after he is discharged. He'll be as good as new in a few weeks, and your relationship with him will resume unchanged.

Now that you've compared these two scenarios, consider the fact that people with psychological disorders frequently face situations such as Jeremy's in which even the people who care about them aren't sure how to respond to their symptoms. Furthermore, even after their symptoms are under control, individuals like Jeremy continue to experience profound and long-lasting emotional and social effects as they attempt to resume their former lives. Their disorder itself may also bring about anguish and personal suffering. Like Rebecca in our opening example, they must cope with feelings of loneliness and sadness.

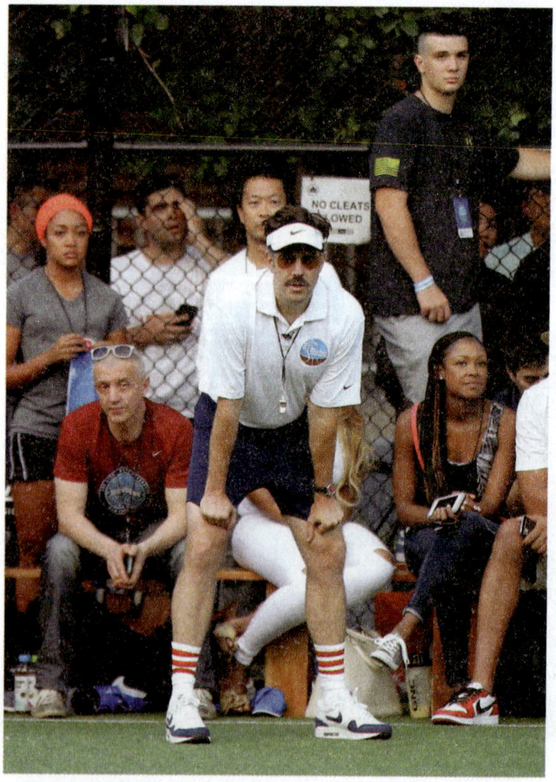

The popular television series, "Ted Lasso," challenged the stigma of psychological disorders.

J. Countess/Getty Images

Psychological disorders are almost inevitably associated with **stigma**, a negative label that causes certain people to be regarded as different, defective, and set apart from mainstream members of society. This stigma exists even in today's society, despite greater awareness of the prevalence of mental health issues. Social attitudes toward people with psychological disorders range from discomfort to outright prejudice. Language, humor, and stereotypes portray psychological disorders in a negative light, and many people fear that those who have these disorders are violent and dangerous.

There seems to be something about a psychological disorder that makes people want to distance themselves from it as much as possible. The result is social discrimination, which serves only to complicate the lives of the afflicted even more. Making matters worse, people experiencing symptoms of a psychological disorder may not avail themselves of the help they could receive from treatment because they too have incorporated stigmatized views of mental illness, as have their caregivers (Ribeiro et al., 2023). Some individuals are able to resist the stigma of psychological disorders due to their ability, for example, to define their identity separate from their disorder and to reject the labels other people apply to them (O'Connor, Yanos, & Firmin, 2018).

In the chapters that follow, you will read about a wide range of disorders affecting mood, anxiety, substance use, sexual functioning, and thought disturbance. Case descriptions will give you a glimpse into the feelings and experiences of real people who have these disorders, and you may find that some of them seem similar to you or to people you know. As you read about the disorders, put yourself in the place of the people who have these conditions. Consider how they feel and how they would like people to treat them, rather than on the diagnoses alone.

1.3 Defining a Psychological Disorder

There is a range of behaviors people can show in adapting to their lives and circumstances. Consider the following list, and try to decide which might reflect a psychological disorder:

- Feeling jinxed when your "lucky" seat in an exam is already occupied when you get to class
- Being unable to sleep, eat, study, or talk to anyone else for days after your romantic partner says, "It's over between us"
- Breaking into a cold sweat at the thought of being trapped in an elevator
- Swearing, throwing pillows, and pounding fists on the wall in the middle of an argument with a roommate
- Refusing to eat solid food for days at a time in order to stay thin
- Engaging in a thorough hand-washing after coming home from a bike ride
- Protesting the rising cost of college by joining a picket line outside the campus administration building
- Being convinced that people are constantly being critical of everything you do
- Drinking a six-pack of beer a day in order to be "sociable" with friends
- Playing video games for hours at a time, avoiding other study and work obligations

If you're like most people, you probably found it surprisingly difficult to decide which of these behaviors might constitute a disorder, because so many of these behaviors are part of everyday life. You can see now why mental health professionals struggle to find an appropriate definition. Yet criteria need to exist so they can provide appropriate treatment in their work with clients.

With this list of behaviors in mind, now consider the five criteria that exist in the field of psychological disorders and their treatment. In reality, no one would diagnose a psychological disorder on the basis of a single behavior, but using these criteria can at least give you some insight into the process that clinicians use when deciding whether a given individual's behaviors would suggest that a diagnosis is appropriate.

The first criterion for a psychological disorder is **clinical significance**, meaning the behavior includes a measurable degree of impairment that a clinician can observe. People who feel jinxed about not having a lucky seat available for an exam would fit this criterion only if they could not concentrate on the exam at all unless they sat in that seat and this happened for every exam they take.

clinical significance
The criterion for a psychological disorder in which the behavior being evaluated includes a measurable degree of impairment that the clinician can observe.

The second criterion is that the behavior must reflect a dysfunction in a psychological, biological, or developmental process. Concretely, this means that even if researchers do not know the cause of that dysfunction, they assume that it can one day be discovered.

The third criterion is that the behavior must be associated with significant distress or disability in important realms of life. This may sound similar to clinical significance, but what distinguishes distress or disability is that it applies to the way the individual feels or behaves, beyond a measurable effect the clinician can observe. The individual either feels negatively affected by the behavior ("distress") or suffers negative consequences in life as a result ("disability"). People may enjoy playing video games to a point, but if they exclude their other obligations, it will negatively affect their lives. They may also feel distressed but unable to stop themselves from engaging in the behavior.

The fourth criterion is that the individual's behavior cannot simply be socially deviant as defined in terms of religion, politics, or other aspects of their identity. The person who refuses to eat meat for ideological reasons would not be considered to have a psychological disorder by this standard. However, if that person restricts all food intake to the point that their health is in jeopardy, then that individual may meet one of the other criteria for a psychological disorder, such as clinical significance and/or the distress-disability dimension.

The fifth and final criterion for a psychological disorder is that it is assumed to reflect a dysfunction within the individual. A psychological disorder cannot be assigned on the basis of differences in political beliefs between citizens and their governments. Campus protesters who want to keep college costs down could not, according to this criterion, be considered psychologically disordered, although they may be putting themselves at other kinds of risk if they never attend a single class or are arrested for trespassing on university property.

As you can see, deciding which behaviors fall into the category of a psychological disorder is a difficult proposition. Furthermore, when it comes to making an actual diagnosis to assign to a client, the mental health professional must also weigh the merits of using a diagnostic label against the disadvantages. The merits are that the individual will receive treatment (and be able to receive insurance reimbursement), but a possible disadvantage is that the individual will be labeled with a psychological disorder that becomes part of their health records. At a later point in life, that diagnosis may make it difficult for the individual to qualify for certain jobs.

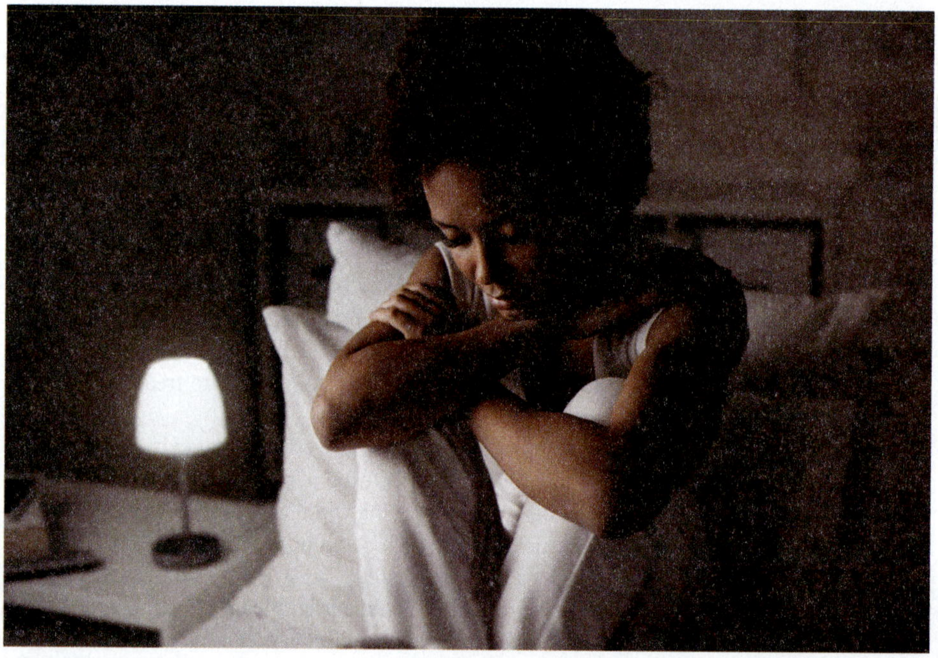

This woman is distressed over her inability to fall asleep, but does this mean she has a psychological disorder?

Andrea De Martin/Alamy Stock Photo

Fortunately, mental health professionals have these criteria to guide them, with extensive manuals that allow them to feel reasonably confident they are assigning diagnoses when appropriate. These five criteria, and the specific diagnoses for the many forms of psychological disorders that can affect people, form the core content of this course.

It is important to acknowledge that the five criteria you just read about exist within a sociocultural lens consistent with current Western views in the field of mental health. These cultural lenses can influence the way a psychological disorder is defined, and, further how professionals provide help to those they treat.

What's in the *DSM-5-TR*

Definition of a Psychological Disorder

Compare what you think constitutes disordered behavior with the five criteria for a psychological disorder described in the text. Which of these criteria were in your own definition? How would you determine whether an individual meets these criteria?

As you will learn in Chapter 2, the diagnostic manual known as the *DSM-5-TR* provides clinicians with considerable guidance when they decide whether an individual's behavior constitutes a psychological disorder and if so, which would provide the correct diagnosis.

1.4 What Causes Psychological Disorders?

Psychological disorders are best conceptualized from multiple vantage points, reflecting a combination of biological, psychological, and sociocultural factors as these evolve during the individual's growth and development over time.

Within the **biopsychosocial perspective**, we see sociocultural factors interacting with biological and psychological contributions, in that environmental influences such as exposure to toxic substances or stressful living conditions can also lead individuals to experience psychological disorders. Environmental deprivation caused by poverty, malnutrition, or social injustice can also place individuals at risk for psychological disorders by contributing to adverse physiological outcomes.

biopsychosocial perspective
A model in which the interaction of biological, psychological, and sociocultural factors is seen as influencing the development of the individual over time.

Biological Contributions

We start with the biological part of the equation. The factors within the body that can contribute to disordered behavior include genetic aberrations that, alone or in combination with the environment, influence the individual's psychological functioning. Biological contributions can also include physical changes that occur as part of normal aging, illnesses an individual develops, and injuries or harm caused to the body.

The most relevant genetic influences for our purposes are inherited factors that alter the functioning of the nervous system. However, psychological disorders can also be produced by environmental influences alone if these affect the brain or related organs of the body. For example, brain injury resulting from a head trauma can result in altered thoughts, memory loss, and changes in mood. Additionally, changes in other organ systems in the body can affect an individual's psychological functioning as in, for example, pain due to a chronic medical condition.

Psychological Contributions

The idea that psychological disorders have psychological contributions is probably not one that you believe requires a great deal of explanation. Within the biopsychosocial perspective, however, psychological causes are not viewed in isolation. They are seen as part of a larger constellation of factors influenced by physiological alterations interacting with exposure to a certain environment.

Psychological contributions can include the effects of a person's individual experiences. For example, an individual who was bullied as a child may develop extreme anxiety while

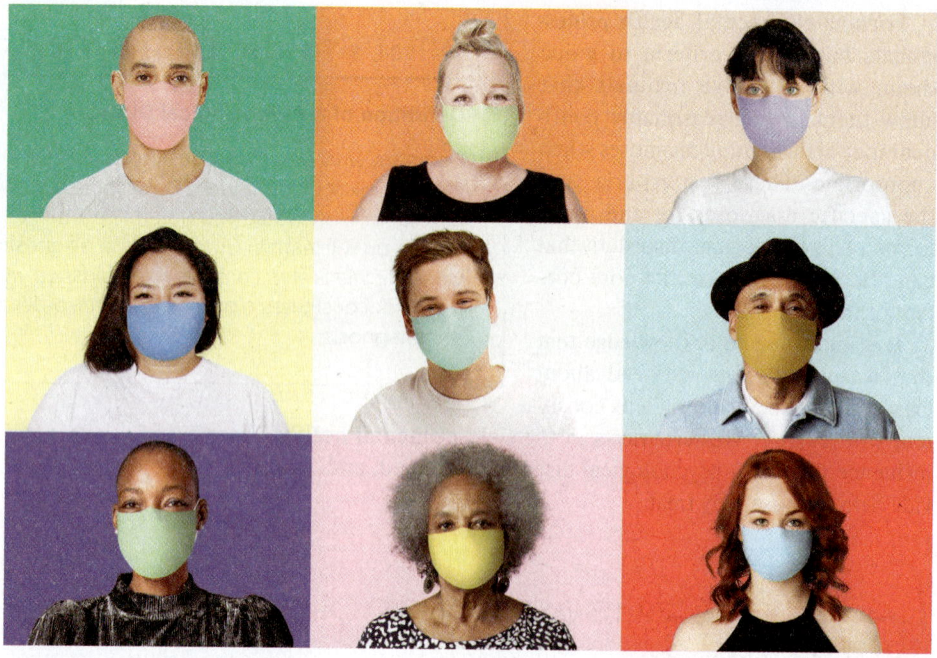

The social distancing and masking required during the COVID-19 pandemic was a sociocultural influence on the population's mental health.
Rawpixel.com/Shutterstock

being around other people. They may also express emotional instability as the result of feeling that their parents or caretakers could not be relied on to watch over them.

Although there are no purely psychological causes in the biopsychosocial perspective, we can think of those that reflect learning, life experiences, or exposure to key situations in life as reflecting predominantly psychological influences. These can also include difficulty coping with stress, illogical fears, susceptibility to uncontrollable emotions, and a host of other dysfunctional thoughts, feelings, and behaviors that lead individuals to meet the criteria for psychological disorder.

Sociocultural Contributions

sociocultural perspective
The theoretical perspective that emphasizes the ways that individuals are influenced by people, social institutions, and social forces in the world around them.

The **sociocultural perspective** looks at the various circles of influence on the individual, ranging from close friends and family, to instances of discrimination (e.g., racism), to the institutions and policies of a country or the world as a whole. These influences interact in important ways with biological processes and with the psychological contributions that occur through exposure to particular experiences.

One important and unique sociocultural contribution to psychological disorders is discrimination, whether based on such factors as social class, income, race and ethnicity, nationality, sexual orientation, age, disability, or gender. Discrimination, as well as oppression that those in marginalized groups face, not only limits people's ability to experience psychological well-being, but can also have direct effects on physical health and development. For example, people of color in the United States—especially Black and African American people—experience higher instances of oppression and violence due to systemic racism that has a very real impact in terms of increasing daily stress and anxiety for these individuals. During the COVID-19 pandemic, statistics showed the disproportionate effect of the coronavirus on Black and Indigenous People of Color (BIPOC) and LGBTQ+ groups in terms of virus rates, economic impact, and mortality (Beringer, de Vries, Gill, & Gutman, 2023). Due to systemic inequality associated with COVID-19, LGBTQ+ individuals particularly LGBTQ+ people of color had higher rates of a range of mental health issues, including suicidality and substance use, than their non-LGBTQ+ counterparts (Njoroge, Forkpa, & Bath, 2021).

As you learned earlier, people diagnosed with a psychological disorder are likely to be stigmatized as a result of their symptoms and diagnostic label. The stress of carrying the stigma of mental illness increases the emotional burden for these individuals and their support systems. Because it may prevent them from seeking badly needed help, it also perpetuates a cycle in which people in need of support become increasingly at risk and hence develop more serious symptoms.

The stigma of psychological disorders seems to vary by ethnicity and race. For example, among individuals with two forms of disorders involving anxiety, shame and stigma can become barriers to receiving treatment (Goetter et al., 2020). Variations in the willingness to acknowledge mental health issues also occur across age and gender lines. Older individuals, by gaining more exposure to psychotherapy through various forms of media, continue to be more likely to hold stigmatized views about mental health treatment (Hannaford, Shaw, & Walker, 2019).

The existence of multiple forms of discrimination (such as racism, ageism, transphobia, and higher rates of violence and police brutality against BIPOC individuals) also means that individuals must cope not only with their symptoms and the stigma of their symptoms, but also with the negative attitudes toward their socially defined group. This often means that individuals in need of mental health treatment do not seek care. In some cases, as with transgender people (and particularly trans people of color), this reluctance can stem from a perception that they will encounter transphobic attitudes and discriminatory behaviors in the treatment setting. Clinicians working with individuals from discriminated-against groups are increasingly learning the importance of considering these factors in both diagnosis and treatment. You will learn later in the book about the specific guidelines mental health experts are developing to help ensure that clinicians receive adequate training in translating theory and understanding of stigma and discrimination into practice.

The Biopsychosocial Perspective

Table 1 summarizes the three categories of causes of psychological disorders you just learned about. These reflect the varying contributions in the biopsychosocial perspective of biological, psychological, and sociocultural influences. As you have seen, disturbances in any of these areas of human functioning can contribute to the development of a psychological disorder. This breakdown is helpful, but keep in mind that there are many possible interactions among these influences.

Although all three sets of factors interact in their impact on individuals, the degree of influence of each of these variables differs among disorders. For some disorders, such as schizophrenia, biology seems to play a particularly dominant role. For other disorders, such those involving extreme changes in mood, psychological factors may predominate. Disorders involving reactions to stressful events may reflect sociocultural influences such as exposure to racial injustice or living in a war-torn country.

TABLE 1 **Causes of Psychological Disorders**

Biological	Genetic inheritance Physiological changes Exposure to toxic substances
Psychological	Past learning experiences Maladaptive thought patterns Difficulties coping with stress
Sociocultural	Social policies Discrimination Stigma

The biopsychosocial perspective also incorporates a developmental component. This means we must understand how these three sets of influences change over the course of an individual's life. Some circumstances endanger the individual more at certain times than at others. Young children may be especially vulnerable to such factors as inadequate nutrition, harsh parental criticism, and neglect. Protective factors, on the other hand, such as loving caregivers, adequate health care, and early life successes can reduce an individual's likelihood of developing a disorder. These early risk-protective factors become part of the individual's susceptibility to developing a disorder, and they remain influential throughout life.

Later in life, risk factors change in their specific form and potential severity. Individuals who experience physical health problems due to a lifetime of poor dietary habits may be more likely to develop psychological symptoms related to altered cardiovascular functioning. On the other hand, if the older individual has developed an extensive social support network, this can somewhat offset the risk presented by their poor physical health.

At all ages, the biological, psychological, and sociocultural factors continue to interact and affect the individual's mental health and well-being as well as the expression of a particular psychological disorder (Whitbourne & Meeks, 2011). We can use the biopsychosocial framework to develop an understanding of the causes of psychological disorders and, just as importantly, the basis for treatment.

spiritual explanations
Explanations that regard psychological disorders as the product of possession by evil or demonic spirits.

humanitarian explanations
Explanations that regard psychological disorders as the result of cruelty, stress, or poor living conditions.

scientific explanations
Explanations that regard psychological disorders as the result of causes that we can objectively measure, such as biological alterations, faulty learning processes, or emotional stressors.

1.5 Prominent Themes in Psychological Disorders Throughout History

The greatest thinkers of the world, from ancient times to the present, have attempted to explain the varieties of human behavior that now are regarded as evidence for a psychological disorder. Throughout history, three prominent themes recur: the spiritual, the humanitarian, and the scientific.

Spiritual explanations regard disturbances in behavior as the product of possession by evil or demonic spirits. **Humanitarian explanations** view psychological disorders as the result of cruelty, stress, or poor living conditions. **Scientific explanations** look for causes that researchers can objectively measure, such as biological alterations, faulty learning processes, cultural and environmental influences, and emotional stressors.

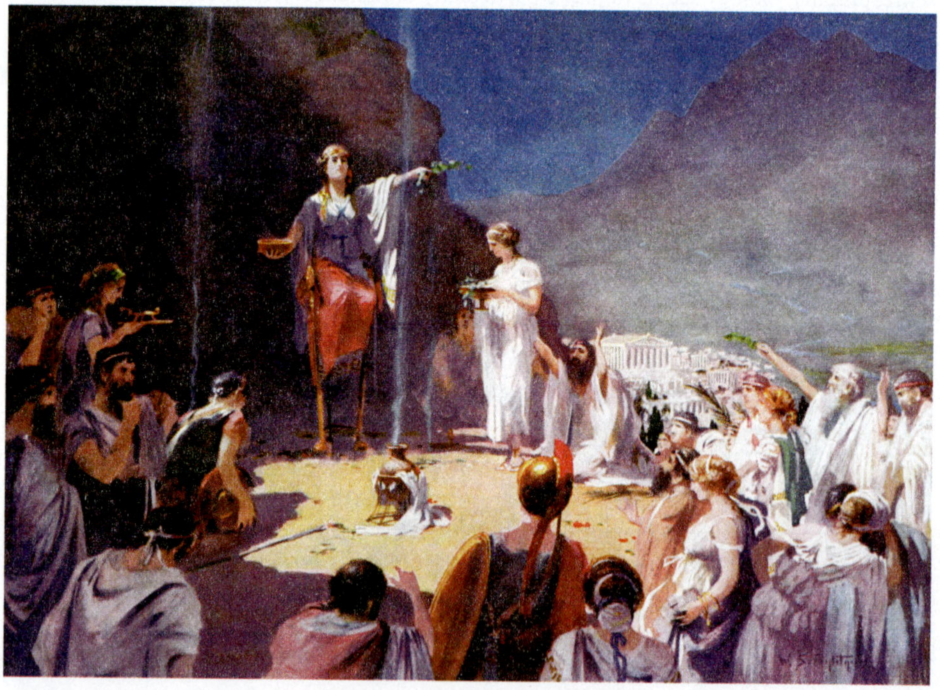

The ancient Greeks sought advice from oracles, wise advisors who made pronouncements from the gods.
World History Archive/Alamy Stock Photo

As you will see, each approach has had its period of major influence, but in some ways the issues are the same today as in ancient times, in that the actual causes of psychological disorders remain unknown. The scientific approach will undoubtedly provide the key to discovering what causes psychological disorders, but it will nevertheless be important for mental health professionals to follow the principles of the humanitarian approach. Spiritual explanations may never completely disappear from the horizon, particularly within certain cultures. Consequently, an understanding of all three themes remains important for mental health practitioners to consider in order to provide the best prospects for treatment.

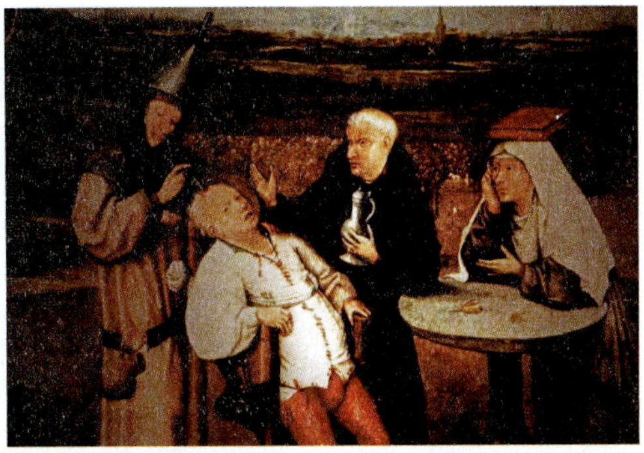

Hieronymus Bosch's *Removal of the Stone of Folly*, painted in the 1490s, depicted a medieval "doctor" cutting out the presumed source of madness from the skull, the prevailing belief at the time.

Arterra Picture Library/Alamy Stock Photo

Spiritual Approach

As the oldest approach to psychological disorders the spiritual approach dates back to prehistoric times. Archeologists have discovered evidence from about 8000 B.C.E. suggesting that the people in these ancient times believed that psychological disorders were caused by spiritual possession that needed to be eliminated from the brain. The existence of these beliefs led prehistoric peoples to cut holes into the skull, a procedure known as **trephining**.

Trephining continued to be practiced throughout history and even into modern times, but its use during ancient times seems to be specifically associated with beliefs that the individual experiencing psychological symptoms was possessed by evil spirits.

The ritual of **exorcism** is another practice that stems from a belief in spiritual possession as the cause of psychological disorders. In an exorcism, a shaman, priest, or person entrusted with the task carries out rituals that attempt to drive out demons by putting the individual under extreme physical and mental duress. Exorcism continues to exist into the present day. For example, Vietnamese people with psychological symptoms are reported to seek exorcism and spirit-calling as forms of healing at Buddhist temples (Nguyen, 2014). There are also reports from modern day Poland of exorcism used to "treat" individuals who appear to possess multiple identities (Pietkiewicz, Kłosińska, Tomalski, & van der Hart, 2021).

trephining
The process of cutting a hole in the skull to allow so-called, "evil spirits" to escape.

exorcism
A ritual believed to cure psychological disturbance by ritually driving away evil spirits.

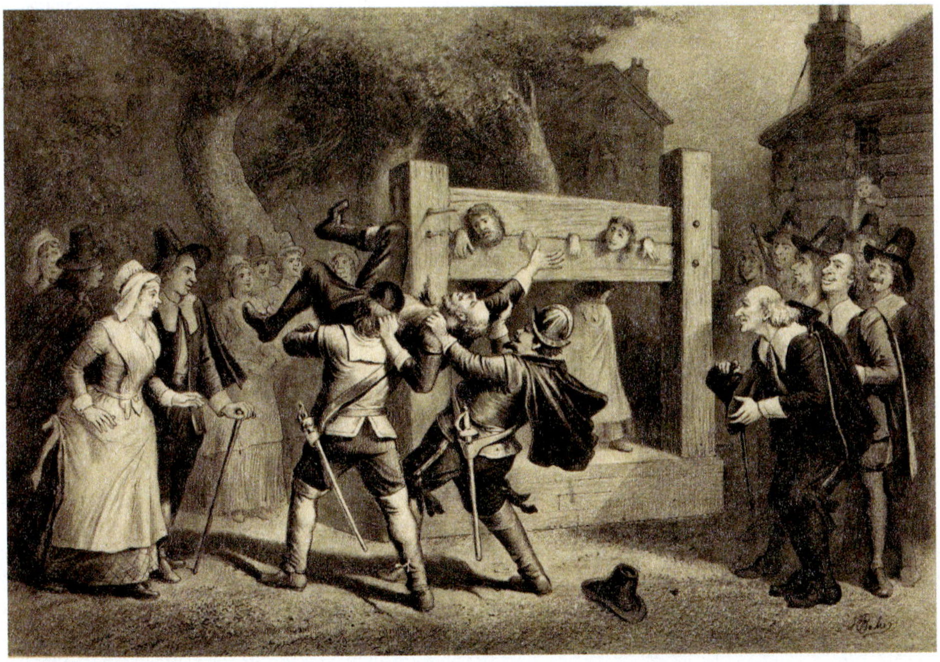

Witch-burning was a common practice in sixteenth-century Germany, as shown in this rendering.

GL Archive/Alamy Stock Photo

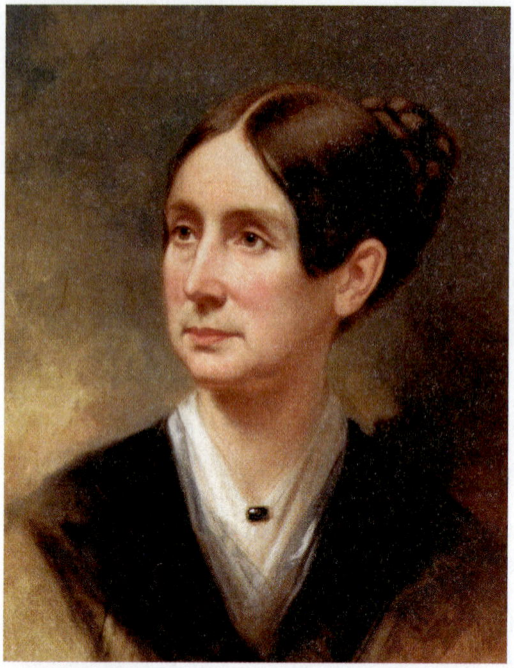

Dorothea Dix was a Massachusetts reformer who sought to improve the treatment of people with psychological disorders in the mid-1800s.

IanDagnall Computing/Alamy Stock Photo

Beliefs in spiritual possession reached a peak during the Middle Ages in European countries. People used a variety of magical rituals to "cure" people with psychological disorders, when it took the form of casting these individuals as sinners, witches, or personifications of the devil. The view that people with psychological disorders are possessed by evil spirits is apparent in the 1486 book *Malleus Maleficarum*, in which two German Dominican monks used it to justify their harsh punishment of women deemed as "witches." Depicting them as heretics and devils whom the Church had to destroy in the interests of preserving Christianity, the book's authors recommended "treatments" such as deportation, torture, and burning at the stake.

From the 1500s to the late 1600s, individuals punished for witchcraft, primarily women, were often those who practiced indigenous methods of healing or whose behavior did not conform to social norms. In the United States, these punishments culminated in the infamous Salem witchcraft trials (1692–1693). The practice ended when townspeople began to doubt the authenticity of the charges. However, remnants of the oppression of women who practice indigenous methods of healing remain today in both Western and non-Western cultures (Yakushko, 2018).

The spiritual approach is no longer the prevalent explanation for psychological disorders in Western culture. Yet, because there remain certain pockets of believers, it is important to keep in mind the possibility that beliefs in possession may exist within some cultures and philosophies (Verginer & Juen, 2019).

Humanitarian Approach

The humanitarian approach to psychological disorders developed in part as a reaction against the spiritual approach and its associated punishment of people with psychological disorders. The roots of the humanitarian approach can be traced to the Middle Ages, with the establishment of shelters to house these individuals, who often were ostracized by their families. The shelters were typically located within poorhouses and monasteries.

Although shelters could not offer treatment, they initially provided some protection from a harsh outside world. However, they increasingly became overcrowded and conditions within grew intolerable. Rather than providing protection, shelters then became places of neglect, abuse, and maltreatment. A widespread belief that people with psychological disorders lacked ordinary sensory capabilities led to such practices as not providing them with heat, clean living conditions, or appropriate food.

During the sixteenth and seventeenth centuries, views about medicine were generally uninformed. Thus, like treatments for physical illness, the treatment of people with psychological disorders included bleeding, forced vomiting, and purging. However, with the newer sciences that had already begun to develop in the Renaissance, therapeutic healing based on compassionate support began to emerge (Dreher, 2013).

By the end of the eighteenth century, the humanitarian approach gained further strength as a few courageous people working in hospitals in France, Scotland, and England began to recognize the inhumanity of the conditions in the poorhouses and monasteries housing those with psychological disorders. The idea of **moral treatment** began to take hold based on the belief that people had a right to humane care and that they would benefit the most in their recovery from a quiet and restful environment. Asylums became the institutions following this model, offering shelter and support, and patients were put in restraints only if absolutely necessary. Even in those cases, the patient's comfort came first.

moral treatment
The belief that people could develop self-control over their behaviors if they had a quiet and restful environment.

Yet again, however, conditions in the institutions originally formed to protect patients began to worsen in the early 1800s due to overcrowding and the increasing use of physical punishment as a means of control. In 1841, Boston schoolteacher Dorothea Dix (1802–1887) took up the cause of reform. Horrified by the overcrowding and appalling conditions in the asylums, Dix appealed to the Massachusetts legislature for more state-funded public hospitals to provide humane treatment for people with psychological disorders. From Massachusetts, she then spread her message throughout North America and Europe.

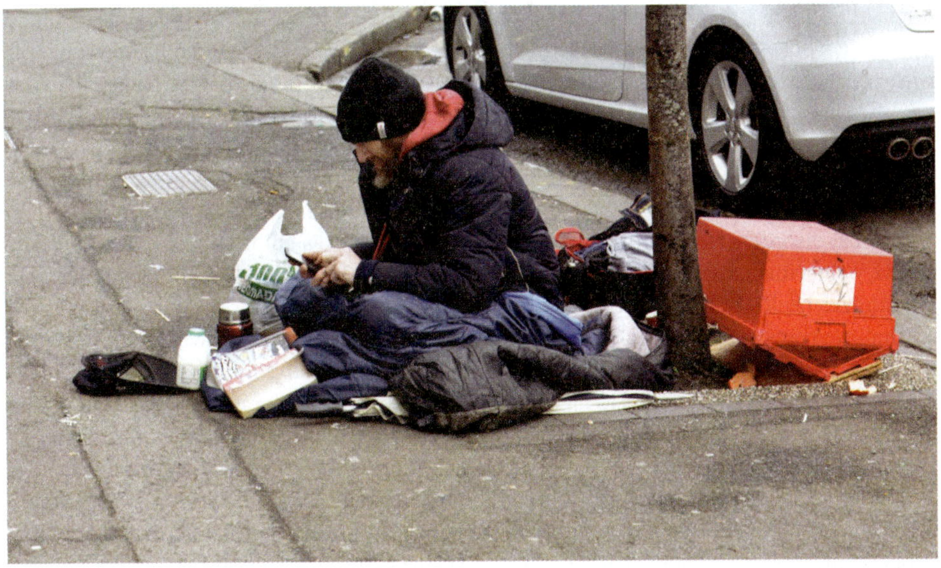

Although deinstitutionalization was designed to enhance the quality of life for people who had been held for years in public psychiatric hospitals, many individuals left institutions only to find a life of poverty and neglect on the outside.

Charles Stirling/Alamy Stock Photo

Over the next 100 years, governments built scores of state hospitals throughout the United States following the humanitarian model originally advocated by Dix. Her work was carried forward into the twentieth century by advocates of the **mental hygiene** movement, the goal of which was to improve the care and treatment of people living in mental hospitals. The mental hygiene movement placed an emphasis on preventing the development of psychological disorders through early intervention (Toms, 2010).

mental hygiene
The focus within psychiatry on helping individuals maintain mental health and prevent the development of psychological disorders.

Once again, however, it was only a matter of time before the hospitals became overcrowded and understaffed. It simply was not possible to cure people by providing them with the well-intentioned but ultimately ineffective interventions proposed by moral treatment. Public outrage over the worsening situation in mental hospitals eventually led to a more widespread realization that mental health services required dramatic changes.

In 1963, the U.S. government took emphatic action with the passage of groundbreaking legislation. The Community Mental Health Act of that year initiated a series of changes that would affect mental health services for decades to come. This legislation paved the way for the **deinstitutionalization movement**, the release of hundreds of thousands of patients from mental hospitals starting in the 1960s. The legislation mandated that people living in mental hospitals be moved into less restrictive programs in the community, such as vocational rehabilitation facilities, day hospitals, and psychiatric clinics. These facilities included **halfway houses**, community treatment facilities designed for deinstitutionalized clients leaving a hospital who are not yet ready for independent living.

deinstitutionalization movement
The release of hundreds of thousands of patients from mental hospitals starting in the 1960s.

halfway house
A community treatment facility designed for deinstitutionalized clients leaving a hospital who are not yet ready for independent living.

Also making deinstitutionalization possible was the development, in the 1950s, of pharmacological treatments that could successfully control the symptoms of many psychological disorders. Now patients could receive treatments that would allow them to live on their own outside psychiatric hospitals for extended periods of time. By the mid-1970s, state mental hospitals that once overflowed with patients were practically deserted. Hundreds of thousands of institutionally confined people were free to begin living with greater dignity and autonomy.

The deinstitutionalization movement did not completely fulfill the dreams of its originators, however. Rather than eliminating inhumane treatment, it created another set of woes. Many of the promises and programs hailed as alternatives to institutionalization ultimately failed to materialize because of inadequate planning and insufficient funds. Many patients were shuttled back and forth between hospitals, halfway houses, and shabby boarding homes, never gaining a sense of stability or respect. A great number spend long periods of time as homeless and marginalized members of society. Although the intention behind releasing patients from psychiatric hospitals was to restore basic human rights to those with psychological disorders, the result may not have been as liberating as many had hoped.

Advocates of the humanitarian movement today suggest new forms of compassionate treatment for people with psychological disorders. This latest approach encourages what are now called mental health consumers to take an active role in choosing their treatment. Various advocacy groups have worked tirelessly to change the way the public views people with psychological disorders and the way society deals with them in all settings. Primary among these groups is the U.S. National Alliance for the Mentally Ill (NAMI) with its grassroots-based local and regional chapters.

positive psychology
Perspective that emphasizes the potential for growth and change throughout life.

The humanitarian approach is also reflected in the **positive psychology** movement, which emphasizes the potential for growth and change throughout life. The movement views psychological disorders as difficulties that inhibit the individual's ability to achieve highly subjective well-being and feelings of fulfillment. In addition, the positive psychology movement emphasizes health over illness and prevention over intervention.

Improvements in mental health care from a human rights perspective have become a central feature of the World Health Organization's (WHO) Special Initiative for Mental Health (2019–2023), intended to ensure access to high-quality and affordable care for mental health conditions at a global level by the year 2023 (WHO, 2019b). Consistent with WHO's Sustainability Development Goals (SDGs), this special initiative is intended to maximize human functioning by countering the human rights violations, discrimination, and stigma associated with psychological disorders. The wide-ranging program is intended to directly benefit more than two billion people living around the world, particularly those living in the 40 countries that the WHO refers to as fragile, conflict-affected, or vulnerable settings.

It is clear that the humanitarian approach remains a central feature of mental health care in the twenty-first century. Although having shifted its focus from the earlier centuries, which was based on such concepts as moral treatment, concern for human rights remains a central issue in the provision of humane and equitable treatment.

Scientific Approach

Looking next at the scientific approach, we now return to ancient times when it was the early Greek philosophers who first took an analytic approach to understanding psychological disorders. Hippocrates (ca. 460–377 B.C.E.), considered the founder of modern medicine, believed that mental health depended on a balance of four so-called bodily "humors" based on the elements of air, water, fire, and earth. These physical qualities determined all behavior originating from the body. Although his theory itself would eventually be proven wrong, Hippocrates was far ahead of his time in putting forth the notion that mental health reflected factors within the body rather than possession by evil spirits.

Several hundred years later, the Roman physician Claudius Galen (130–200 C.E.) carried this view of bodily humors forward, also expanding medical knowledge by conducting anatomical studies of the human body. This approach helped to advance the position that diseases had their source in irregular bodily functioning.

The scientific approach to psychological disorders receded for hundreds of years in favor of explanations rooted in the spiritual perspective. It next emerged in the writings of Dr. Benjamin Rush (1745–1813), the founder of U.S. psychiatry and a signer of the Declaration of Independence. In 1783, Rush joined the medical staff of Pennsylvania Hospital. Appalled by the poor treatment of "psychologically disturbed" patients there, Rush advocated for improvements such as placing patients in their own wards, giving them occupational therapy, and prohibiting hospital visits by curiosity seekers looking for entertainment.

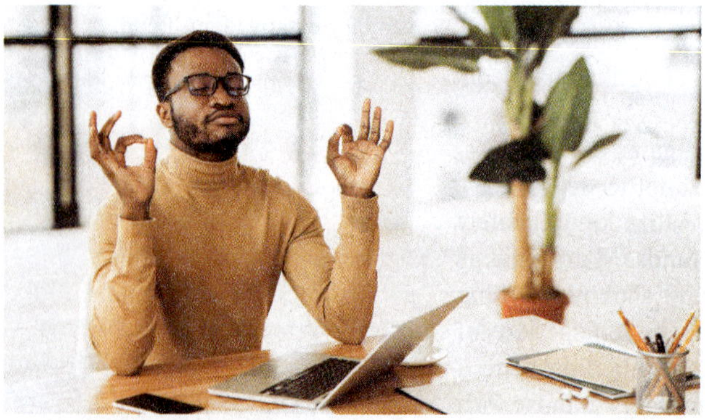

Positive psychology emphasizes personal growth through meditation and other alternate routes to self-discovery.

Prostock-Studio/iStock/Getty Images

Reflecting the prevailing methods of the times, though, Rush also supported the use of bloodletting and purging in the treatment of psychological disorders, as well as the so-called tranquilizer chair, intended to reduce blood flow to the brain by binding the patient's head and limbs. Rush also recommended submerging patients in cold shower baths and frightening them with death threats. He thought that by inducing fear, he could counteract their sometimes violent behavior. However, even while advancing these seemingly unscientific methods, Rush also advocated for the use of medicinal herbs in treating psychological disorders (Forcen, 2017). These can be seen as precursors to modern pharmacological, scientifically based interventions.

The next major advance in the scientific approach occurred in 1844, when a group of 13 mental hospital administrators formed the Association of Medical Superintendents of American Institutions for the Insane. This organization eventually changed its name to the American Psychiatric Association and is now a leading internationally recognized scientific and professional society.

In 1845, the scientific approach received another impetus with the publication of *The Pathology and Therapy of Mental Disorders* by the German psychiatrist Wilhelm Griesinger. He proposed that "neuropathologies" were the cause of psychological disorders, and in so doing, recognized the role of the nervous system in disordered behavior. Further advances occurred when the German psychiatrist Emil Kraepelin (1856-1926) promoted a classification system for psychological disorders that paralleled those applied to medical diseases, focusing on documenting the patterns of symptoms associated with specific disorders. Ultimately, this work provided the scientific basis for current diagnostic systems.

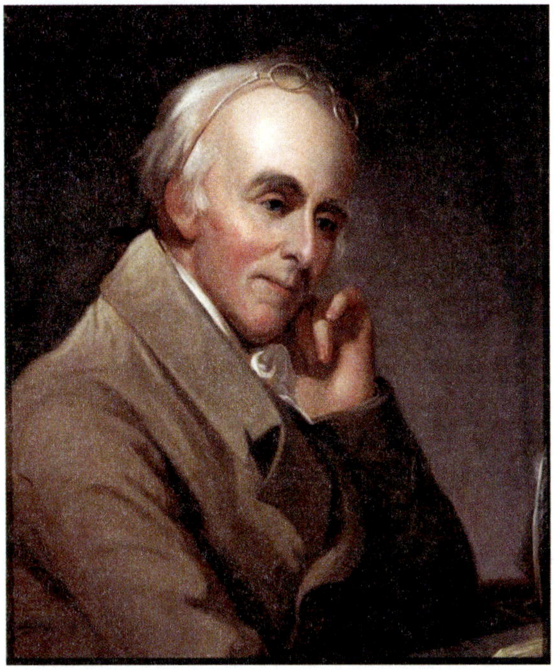

Dr. Benjamin Rush, founder of American psychiatry, was an ardent reformer who promoted the scientific study of psychological disorders.

GL Archive/Alamy Stock Photo

While these advances in medical science and psychiatry were taking place, the origins of a psychological approach to disordered behavior began to emerge in the early 1800s, when European physicians experimented with hypnosis for the treatment of people showing symptoms of psychological disorders. Eventually, these efforts led to the groundbreaking work of Viennese neurologist Sigmund Freud (1856-1939), who in the early 1900s developed psychodynamic theory, based originally in neurology but ultimately becoming focused on the concepts of the unconscious mind, inhibited sexual impulses, and early development.

Throughout the twentieth century, psychologists continued to develop models based on observations of the behavior of laboratory animals. The work of Russian physiologist Ivan Pavlov (1849-1936), known for his discovery of classical conditioning, became the basis for the behaviorist movement begun in the United States by John B. Watson (1878-1958). B. F. Skinner (1904-1990) formulated a systematic approach to operant conditioning, specifying the types and nature of reinforcement and its use as a way to modify behavior. In the twentieth century, these models continued to evolve into theories that would have more direct relevance to psychological disorders, including those of Albert Bandura (1925-2021), Aaron Beck (1921-2021), and Albert Ellis (1913-2007).

These newer models, along with integrative models that take a biopsychosocial approach, are leading to promising empirical (evidence-based) ways to understand the causes of psychological disorder. Although not all may prove useful, they will help ensure that our application of the scientific perspective results in treatments that are both humane and based in solid research.

1.6 Research Methods in Psychological Disorders

As you've just learned, the scientific approach led to significant advances in the understanding and treatment of psychological disorders. The essence of the **scientific method** is objectivity: the process of testing ideas about the nature of psychological phenomena without bias before accepting these ideas as adequate explanations.

scientific method
The process of testing ideas about the nature of psychological phenomena without bias before accepting these ideas as adequate explanations.

The scientific method relies on a progression of steps, from posing questions of interest to sharing the results with the scientific community. Throughout their application of the scientific method, researchers maintain the objectivity that is the hallmark of the scientific approach. This means they do not let their personal biases interfere with the collection of data or the interpretation of findings. They remain open to alternate explanations that could account for their findings. Toward this end, researchers are now making their data available in open-access repositories that allow other scientists to examine their procedures, analyses, and conclusions.

Although the scientific method is based on objectivity, this does not mean scientists have no personal interest in what they are studying. In fact, many researchers pursue knowledge in areas that relate to their own lives, particularly in the field of psychological disorders. They may have relatives diagnosed with certain disorders, or they may have developed this interest through their clinical work. Regardless of what motivated them to study a particular topic, researchers studying psychological disorders must maintain their distance and be able to look at their findings without bias.

In posing questions of interest, psychological researchers may wonder whether a particular kind of experience led to an individual's symptoms, or they may speculate about the role of particular biological factors. Clinical psychologists are also interested in finding out whether a certain treatment will effectively manage the symptoms of a disorder. In either case, the ideal approach is to progress through the scientific method's steps, in which the researcher proposes a hypothesis, conducts a study, collects the data, and performs empirical analyses of the data. When these phases have been completed, researchers communicate results by publishing them in scientific journals, ideally after obtaining peer review to ensure the study's validity.

meta-analysis
A statistical approach that evaluates significance of findings across multiple studies and samples.

Increasingly common in the field of clinical psychology is the use of the research method known as **meta-analysis**, a statistical approach that evaluates significance of findings across multiple studies and samples. In choosing studies to include in their analyses, researchers using this approach set so-called "inclusion criteria" to ensure that the findings from these previous studies were obtained using well-established methods and representative samples, with data that are either previously published or available from the original researchers. Findings based on meta-analyses, such as demonstrations of the value of a particular intervention, can provide strong support, given that they incorporate more than one research group's results.

1.7 Experimental Design

independent variable
The variable whose level is adjusted or controlled by the experimenter.

dependent variable
The variable whose value is the outcome of the experimenter's manipulation of the independent variable.

In the experimental approach to scientific research, an investigator sets up a test of a hypothesis to determine whether one variable or factor influences a second variable. The experimental method is the only approach that can test cause and effect because it allows investigators to change variable A to see how this affects variable B. For example, the investigator may wish to determine whether a particular form of therapy reduces anxiety levels in people seeking treatment. The investigator then provides some people with therapy and other people with no therapy. In this case, therapy is the **independent variable**, which is the variable whose level is adjusted or controlled by the experimenter. The "experimental" group receives the treatment, and the "control" group receives no treatment. The level of anxiety people report serves as the **dependent variable**, which is the variable whose value is the outcome of the experimenter's manipulation of the independent variable. The investigator may hope that the anxiety levels of the participants decrease more in the experimental than the control group if they are both compared before and after treatment, but must wait for the findings to be analyzed before drawing any firm conclusions. Depending on the nature of the particular study, there may be more than one experimental group. For example, an investigator may want to compare two different treatments against each other, evaluating both in comparison to a third control group. In that case, the independent variable takes on three values: treatment one, treatment two, and no treatment.

randomized controlled trial (RCT)
Experimental method in which participants are randomly assigned to intervention groups.

evidence-based treatment
Treatment in which clients receive interventions based on the findings of controlled clinical studies.

The gold standard for research in clinical psychology is the **randomized controlled trial (RCT)**, an experimental method in which participants are randomly assigned to intervention groups. The key to this method is the use of randomization, which minimizes the chances that bias can enter into the decision about which participants receive which treatment. Because this is such a powerful design, RCT is the foundation for **evidence-based treatment**, in which clients receive interventions based on the findings of controlled clinical studies.

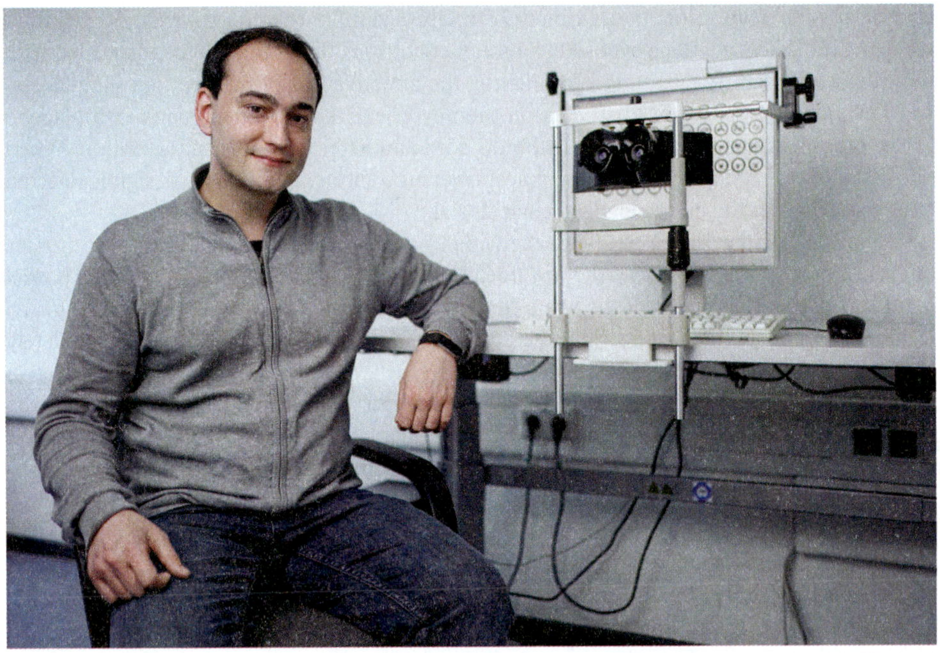

This researcher is demonstrating the equipment being used for a study on reducing spider phobia.
picture alliance/Getty Images

Ideally, in an RCT, before conducting the study the investigators define a single primary outcome (i.e., a specific dependent variable). They may also define secondary outcomes, but at the outset they need to be clear about their primary focus, such as levels of anxiety in the previous example. Otherwise, they may make the mistake of picking and choosing the results they report in a way that distorts the findings. Imagine if a researcher found no effect of a clinical treatment for anxiety on anxiety levels of the participants but instead found that it alleviated depression. This may be of interest, but because it was not predicted based on the study's underlying theory, it has no sound rationale and could have been due to chance factors.

To ensure that RCT-based studies conform to acceptable standards, researchers are increasingly being required to enter their work in a public trial registry before they begin. If they do not, their research will not be eligible for publication in any of the most prestigious research journals, which report only findings that are reviewed by other experts in the field. When researchers describe their randomization methods, however, the majority fail to report the exact procedures they used in assigning participants to treatment as compared to control groups (Cañedo-Ayala et al., 2020). Consumers are therefore well-advised to check how well a given study adheres to these guidelines before seeking a new intervention based on its results.

Consumers should also be wary of findings published in open-access journals that do not implement rigorous peer review. Researchers pay an often sizable fee to publish their findings in these journals, making them more open to skeptical reading than is true for articles that appear in journals sponsored by scientific associations or well-established editorial boards. Some of these journals are now called "predatory," because they literally prey on researchers, offering to publish their work but requiring high submission fees (Omer et al., 2019). Even worse, articles published in these journals may end up in large-scale studies intended to synthesize findings across multiple investigations, which then can present misleading findings (Barker et al., 2023).

You should also be critical of findings you read about in the news or in daily online digests, because these too may also fall short of peer-reviewed scrutiny. These may contain misleading information about the efficacy of new treatments, particularly if they are written in a way to capture public attention.

Keep in mind, too, that well-controlled research in clinical psychology includes a **placebo condition** in which participants receive a treatment similar to the experimental treatment but

placebo condition
Condition in an experiment in which participants receive a treatment similar to the experimental treatment, but lacking the key feature of the treatment of interest.

lacking the key feature of the treatment of interest. Unlike the control group, the group receiving the placebo will be exposed to a set of conditions that mimic those associated with the treatment itself. If the study is evaluating the effectiveness of medication, the placebo will have inert ingredients. In studies on therapy effectiveness, participants in a placebo group may meet with experimenters who do not administer the actual intervention. When participants are randomly assigned to placebo versus treatment group, the design is referred to as a **placebo-controlled randomized clinical trial**.

placebo-controlled randomized clinical trial
Experimental method in which participants are randomly assigned to a placebo versus treatment group.

As you might imagine, it can be challenging to design the placebo in a way that mimics but is not the same as the actual therapy. Ideally, researchers would want the placebo participants to receive treatments of the same frequency and duration as the experimental group participants who are receiving psychotherapy. Even in studies with medication, a completely inert placebo may not be sufficient to establish true experimental control. In an "active placebo" condition, researchers build the experimental medication's side effects into the placebo. If they know that a medication produces dry mouth, difficulty swallowing, or upset stomach, then the placebo must also mimic these side effects, or participants will know they are receiving placebos.

Expectations about the experiment's outcome can affect both the investigator and the participant. These so-called "demand characteristics" can compromise the conclusions about the intervention's true effectiveness. Obviously, the investigator should be as unbiased as possible, but there still may be subtle ways that they communicate cues that affect the participant's response. The participant may also have a personal agenda in trying to prove or disprove the study's supposed true intent. The best way to eliminate demand characteristics is to use a **double-blind** method, an experimental procedure in which neither the person giving the treatment nor the person receiving the treatment knows whether the participant is in the experimental or control group. To accomplish this, the investigator hires a research assistant or investigator who is not familiar with the study's purpose to run participants through the conditions.

double-blind
An experimental procedure in which neither the person giving the treatment nor the person receiving the treatment knows whether the participant is in the experimental or control group.

The problem with the experimental method in the study of psychological disorders is that many variables of greatest interest to psychologists are factors the investigator cannot control; hence, they are not truly "independent." For example, depression can never be an independent variable because the investigator cannot manipulate it. A researcher interested in the effects of aging cannot make one group older than the other by randomly assigning people to the groups.

Studies that investigate differences among groups not created by random assignment are known as "quasi-experimental." In such studies, researchers can compare older and younger groups, for instance, but cannot say that aging caused any differences the investigator observes between them.

1.8 Correlational Design

correlational design
Study in which researchers test the relationships between variables that they cannot experimentally manipulate.

Studies based on a **correlational design** test relationships between variables that researchers cannot experimentally manipulate. In a positive correlation, as the scores on one variable increase, so do the scores on the other. In a negative correlation, as scores on one variable increase, scores on the other decrease. For example, because one aspect of depression is that it causes a disturbance in normal sleep patterns, you would expect scores on a measure of depression to be positively correlated with scores on a measure of sleep disturbance. If the measure of sleep used in this study were the number of hours asleep, we could predict that the relationship would be negative. It is also possible that there is no correlation between two variables. In other words, two variables show no systematic relationship with each other. For example, depression is unrelated to the individual's height, and there would be no reason to expect the two variables to exhibit any correlation at all.

The statistic used in correlational studies is a number, expressed in decimals, between +1 and −1. Positive numbers (e.g., +0.43) represent positive correlations, meaning that, as scores on one variable increase, scores on the second variable increase as well. Negative numbers (e.g., −0.43) represent inverse relationships, so that as one variable increases, the

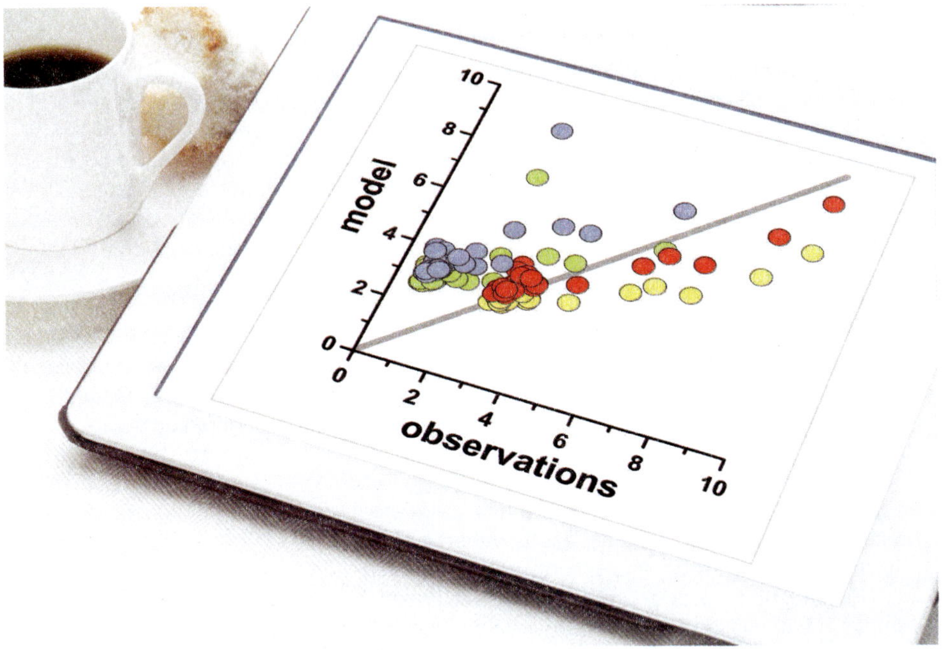

A correlation indicates the relationship between two variables, as shown in this scatterplot.
marekuliasz/Shutterstock

other decreases to a similar extent. The number itself must be presented along with an indication of its statistical significance, meaning that based on the number of participants in the research (among other factors), the relationship has a low probability of occurring due to chance.

Regardless of the size or significance of a correlation, the key feature of studies using this method is that they cannot establish cause and effect. Just knowing that there is a correlation between two variables does not tell you whether one variable causes the other. The correlation simply tells you that the two variables are associated with each other in a particular way. Sleep disturbance might cause a higher score on a measure of depression, just as a high degree of depression might cause more disturbed sleep patterns. Or, a third variable that you have not measured could account for the correlation between the two variables that you have studied. Both depression and sleep disturbance could be due to an underlying process that alters the body's hormones, such as an undetected medical condition, which causes both physiological and psychological disturbances.

You Be the Judge

Being Sane in Insane Places

In the early 1970s, psychologist David Rosenhan embarked upon a groundbreaking study that was to shatter people's assumptions about the difference between "sane" and "insane." Motivated by what Rosenhan regarded as a psychiatric diagnostic system that led to the hospitalization of people inappropriately diagnosed as having schizophrenia, he and his co-workers decided to conduct their own experiment to put the system to the test. See whether you think their experiment proved the point.

Eight people with no psychiatric history of symptoms of any kind, employed in a variety of professional occupations, checked themselves into psychiatric hospitals complaining about hearing voices that said, "Empty," "Hollow," and "Thud." These were symptoms that psychiatric literature never reported. In every other way, the "pseudopatients" provided factual information about themselves except their names and places of employment. Each was admitted to their respective hospital; once admitted, they showed no further signs of experiencing these symptoms. However, the hospital staff never questioned their need to be hospitalized; quite the contrary, their behavior on the hospital wards, now completely "normal," was taken as further evidence of their need for continued hospitalization. Despite the efforts of the pseudopatients to convince the staff that there was nothing wrong with them, it took from 7 to 52 days for all to be discharged. Upon their release, they received the diagnosis of "schizophrenia in remission" (meaning that for the moment they no longer would have a diagnosis of schizophrenia).

There was profound reaction to the Rosenhan study in the psychiatric community. If it was so easy to institutionalize people who had no actual disorder, wasn't there something wrong with the diagnostic system? How about the tendency to label people as "schizophrenic" when there was nothing wrong with them, and to hang on to the label even when they no longer showed any symptoms? The pseudopatients also reported that they felt dehumanized by the staff and failed to receive any active treatment. Once on the outside, they could report to the world at large about the failure of psychiatric hospitals to provide appropriate treatment. True patients would not have received so much sympathetic press, and therefore this study's findings could have a much broader impact on attitudes toward institutionalization.

Now, you be the judge. Do you think it was unethical for Rosenhan to devise such a study? The mental health professionals at the hospitals had no idea they were the actual subjects of a study. They had responded to what seemed to them to be serious psychological symptoms exhibited by individuals voluntarily seeking admission. At the point of discharge, the fact that the doctors labeled the pseudopatients as in remission implied that they were symptom-free, but there was no reason for the staff to doubt the truth of their symptoms. On the other hand, had the staff known they were in a study, they might have reacted very differently, and as a result, the study would not have had an impact.

How about the quality of this study from a scientific point of view? There was no control condition, so it was not truly an experiment. Moreover, the study did not take objective measures of the staffs' behavior, nor were there direct outcome measures that the researchers could statistically analyze. It's important to take these criticisms into account when interpreting the study's findings (Bartels & Peters, 2017).

Q: *You be the judge:* With all its flaws, was Rosenhan's study worthwhile? Did the ends justify the means?

Investigators who use correlational methods in their research must always be on guard for the potential existence of unmeasured variables influencing the observed results. However, increasingly sophisticated statistical modeling procedures are making it possible to go beyond simply linking two variables to see whether they are correlated. For example, one research team used the procedure known as "structural modeling," an advanced correlational technique, to take into account the multiple roles of adverse experiences in childhood with sleep disturbances as influence on the development of psychopathology (Liu et al., 2023). Such studies can move the field well beyond the linking of two variables into an understanding of underlying mechanisms.

1.9 Types of Research Studies

Now that we've reviewed the basic analytical procedures, let's take a look at how investigators gather the data they use for analysis. Depending on the question under investigation, the resources available to the investigator, and the types of participants the investigator wants to study, the data gathering method may take one or more of several forms. Table 2 summarizes these methods.

TABLE 2 **Research Methods: Psychological Disorders**

Type of Method	Purpose	Example
Survey	Obtain population data	Researchers working for a government agency attempt to determine disease prevalence through questionnaires administered over the telephone.
Laboratory study	Collect data under controlled conditions	An experiment is conducted to compare reaction times to neutral and fear-provoking stimuli.
Case study	An individual or a small group of individuals is studied intensively	A therapist describes the cases of members of a family who share the same unusual disorder.
Single-case experimental design	The same person serves as subject in experimental and control conditions	Researchers report on the frequency of participants' behavior while they are being given attention (experimental treatment) vs. being ignored (control condition) for aggressive outbursts in a psychiatric ward.
Behavioral genetics	Attempt to identify genetic patterns in inheritance of particular behaviors	Genetic researchers compare the DNA of people with and without symptoms of particular psychological disorders.

Survey

Investigators use a **survey** to gather information from a sample of people representative of a particular population. Typically, an investigator uses a survey to gather data that will be analyzed through correlational statistics. In a survey, investigators design sets of questions to tap into these variables, using questions to be answered with rating scales ("agree" to "disagree"), open-ended answers, or multiple choice. For example, a researcher may conduct a survey to determine whether age is correlated with subjective well-being, controlling for the influence of health. In this case, the researcher may hypothesize that subjective well-being is higher in older adults, but only after taking into account the role of health. The survey questions provide responses that can be translated into variables and subjected to statistical analysis.

survey
A research tool used to gather information from a sample of people considered representative of a particular population, in which participants are asked to answer questions about the topic of concern.

If you've ever taken an online survey, either as part of a research project or as a consumer of a particular product, you know that the process can become quite tedious. This so-called "response burden" means that researchers must balance the value of gaining extensive information in a survey against the possibility that participants either leave missing responses, quit, or even fabricate answers just to get to the end (Arias, Ponce, & Martínez-Molina, 2022). In reading reports based on surveys, then, it's important to consider whether the researchers instituted controls for inattentive or false responding (Sun et al., 2023).

Researchers also use surveys to gather statistics about the frequency of psychological symptoms. For example, the Substance Abuse and Mental Health Services Administration of the U.S. government (SAMHSA) conducts yearly surveys to establish the frequency of use of illegal substances within the population. By asking approximately the same questions on each occasion, such agencies, and users of the data set, can track changes in health and health-related behaviors over time. Some of the most important survey data come from large-scale epidemiological studies. This is how it becomes possible to know how many people are likely to develop a disorder and who is at risk.

The **incidence** of a disorder is the frequency of *new* cases within a given time period. Respondents providing incidence data state whether they now have a disorder they have never had before and are experiencing for the first time. Incidence information can cover any time interval; epidemiologists tend to report it in terms of 1 month, 6 months, and 1 year. Investigators use incidence data when they are interested in determining how quickly

incidence
The frequency of new cases within a given time period.

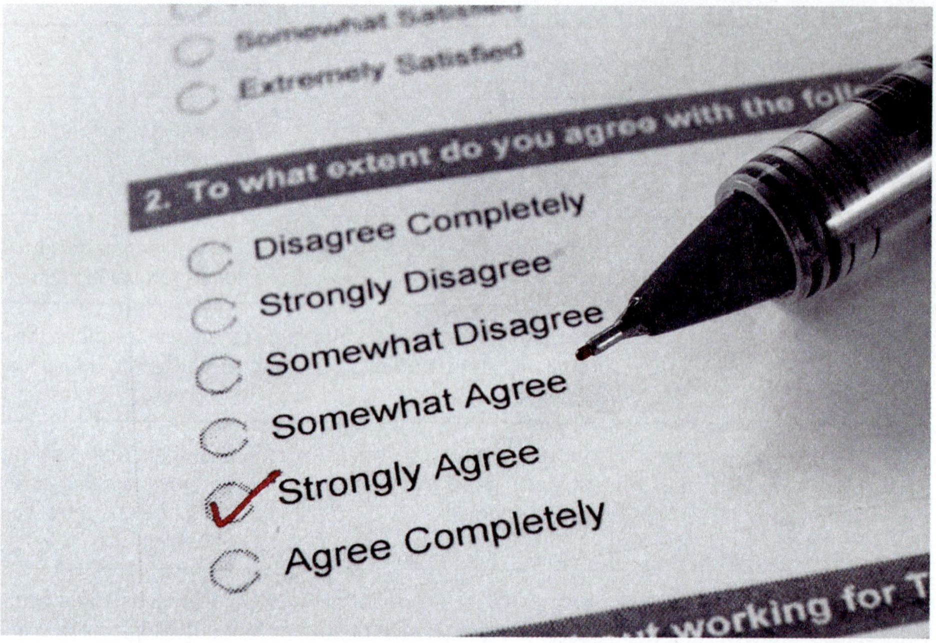

In a study using the survey technique, researchers ask participants to complete rating scales or provide brief information on questionnaires.
zimmytws/Shutterstock

a disorder is spreading. For example, during the COVID-19 pandemic, which by definition was caused by a "novel" virus, the only relevant data researchers could collect starting in 2020 came from tracking new cases.

prevalence
The number of people who have ever had a disorder at a given time or over a specified period.

The **prevalence** of a disorder refers to the number of people who have *ever* had the disorder over a specified period of time. To collect prevalence data, investigators ask respondents to state whether, during this period of time, they experienced the symptoms of the disorder. The time period of reference can be the day of the survey, in which case we call it "point prevalence." There is also "1-month prevalence," which refers to the 30 days preceding the study, and "lifetime prevalence," which refers to the entire life of the respondent. For example, researchers may ask respondents whether they smoked cigarettes at any time during the past month (1-month prevalence) or whether they ever used cigarettes in their lifetime (lifetime prevalence). Typically, lifetime prevalence is higher than 1-month or point prevalence because the question captures all past experiences of a disorder or a symptom.

comorbidity
Co-occurrence of two (or more) disorders within the same individual.

Epidemiological research can also discover the frequency of co-existing disorders, a situation referred to as **comorbidity**, which literally means these diagnoses co-occur within the same individual. Diagnoses of comorbidity are remarkably common. The National Comorbidity Survey (NCS), conducted in the United States between 1990 and 1992, and its Replication (NCS-R), conducted between 2001 and 2002, documented the extent to which psychiatric diagnoses co-occur in the general population. Data from the NCS-R continue to be reported, because this survey represents one of the largest and most comprehensive epidemiological studies conducted in psychiatry to date (National Institute of Mental Health, 2020). It is important to point out that, due to such issues as recall bias among survey participants, who may not accurately recall or report their symptoms, these prevalence estimates are, indeed, estimates rather than absolute numbers (Kessler et al., 2012). Additionally, multiple prevalence reporting sources can differ in their precise estimates. The estimates you read about in this text are reported based on the latest sources available.

Laboratory Studies

Research carried out in psychological laboratories allows for the gathering of data under controlled conditions. For example, investigators may show participants stimuli on computer screens and ask them to respond based on what the stimuli call for, such as the presence of a certain word or letter, or an arrow facing left or right that would have to be identified as such. The collected data might include speed of reaction or memory for different types of stimuli. Laboratory studies may also compare brain scan recordings taken while participants were responding under differing conditions or instructions (such as to press a button when they see an "A" but not a "C"). Another type of laboratory study may observe people in small-group settings while investigators study their interactions to a given instruction or prompt, such as to discuss a controversial issue or resolve a disagreement.

Although laboratories are ideal for conducting such experiments, they may also be appropriate settings for self-report data in which participants respond to questionnaires, especially if the researcher is seeking to collect those responses in a fixed period of time or under conditions offering a minimum of distractions. The laboratory may also be a desirable setting for investigators to ask respondents to complete self-report instruments via computer, allowing the investigator to collect data in a systematic and uniform fashion across respondents. Increasingly, though, online experiments are used to simulate laboratories, because of their convenience and ability to expand their samples beyond those who can physically enter the laboratory.

Case Study

Many early classic studies of psychological disorders used the **case study** method, in which the researcher or clinician intensively interviews, observes, and tests an individual or small group of individuals. For example, Freud based much of his theory on reports of his own patients, trying to trace the relationship between their recalled experiences, the development of their symptoms, and ultimately their progress in therapy.

case study
An intensive study of a single person described in detail.

Currently, investigators conduct case studies because they afford researchers the opportunity to report on rare cases or to chronicle the way a disorder evolved over time in a closely studied individual. As an example, a therapist in one study reported on the treatment she provided to a 3-year-old child who had recently suffered the loss of his mother, recounting vignettes to document the course of therapy (Dunbar, 2023).

The in-depth nature of the case study is also a potential disadvantage, in that it does not rely on the types of experimental control or sample size that would make it a useful addition to the literature. Investigators using case studies must therefore be extremely precise in their methods and, as much as possible, take an objective and unbiased approach. They are likely to seek publication in a journal that specializes in the case study approach rather than one that relies on large sample or experimental data.

Researchers may also use methods in which they expand on single cases, using focus groups or interviews to collect descriptive information about a particular topic. In this type of **qualitative research**, researchers use rigorous methods to code the data and summarize information in a way that reflects an objectively applied set of standards. Recent improvements in statistical software for analyzing qualitative data now make it possible to develop reliable coding schemes that other researchers can replicate. As an example, one set of researchers collected data through focus groups which they analyzed through this software to understand what led grandparents to provide healthy food choices to their grandchildren (Jongenelis, Morley, Worrall, & Talati, 2021).

qualitative research
A method of analyzing data in which researchers use rigorous methods to code the data and summarize information in a way that reflects an objectively applied set of standards.

One consideration in qualitative research is the need to protect the rights of participants. For example, researchers interested in a particular group to which individuals belong, such as families from economically disadvantaged backgrounds, may inadvertently elicit negative experiences by virtue of the nature of the questions they ask (Summers, 2020).

Single-Case Experimental Design

In a **single-case experimental design (SCED)**, the same person serves as the subject in both the experimental and the control conditions. Particularly useful for studies of treatment effectiveness, a single-case design typically alternates between the baseline condition ("A") and the intervention ("B"). Another term for SCEDs is *ABAB designs*, reflecting the alternation between conditions A and B. Figure 1 shows an example of an SCED studying self-injurious behavior.

single case experimental design (SCED)
Design in which the same person serves as the subject in both the experimental and control conditions.

REAL STORIES

Sir Elton John (1947–Present)

In 2020, Sir Elton John, regarded as one of the most successful singer-songwriters in pop music history, celebrated 30 years of sobriety. He has talked openly in interviews and memoirs about the arc of his drug and alcohol addictions and his road to recovery, which have spanned his astonishing musical career.

John, born Reginald Dwight in a suburb outside London, England, has been making music and performing for more than 50 years. In a 2019 memoir (John, 2019a), he recalls discovering his talent for piano as a child in his parents' home. As he grew up, he expanded his musical horizons to blues and rock and roll, and as a teenager he built his performing skills playing in local pubs. In 1967, when he was 20, John began working with a local record company and was introduced to a lyricist Bernie Taupin, who was 17 at the time. John and Taupin started collaborating on songs, with John writing music and Taupin the lyrics. Their combined talents launched John's career and started a decades-long musical partnership (John, 2019a).

While his musical career climbed to dizzying heights, during the 1980s John started to feel that his addictions to drugs and alcohol were bringing him to the point of despair and hopelessness. He also struggled with an eating disorder and sex addiction, and at one point he attempted to take his own life by drowning in his swimming pool.

Speaking about this time in a 2019 *Variety* interview (2019b), John recalls: ". . . I wasn't thinking too much about being an artist. I had reached the lowest ebb in my life–the absolute bottom. I hated myself so much. I was consumed with shame."

In a 2012 memoir *Love Is the Cure*, John, who is gay, reflected that the lowest point of his drug and alcohol addiction coincided with the AIDS epidemic in the 1980s: "I was a drug addict and self-absorbed. . . . You know, I was having people die right, left, and center around me, friends. And yet I didn't stop the life that I had, which is the terrible thing about addiction. It's that–you know, it's that bad of a disease."

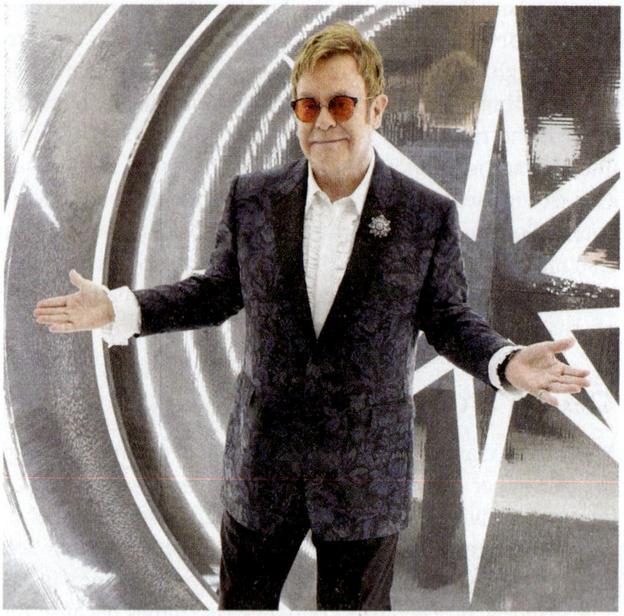

Sir Elton John in 2017 at the 25th Annual Elton John AIDS Foundation's Academy Awards Viewing Party.

Dimitrios Kambouris/Staff/Getty Images

Eventually, in 1989, John came to a realization when his partner at the time confronted him about his issues. In his words, he "surrendered" to the process of recovery, and threw himself into it fully (John, 2013). John has spoken about how his participation in Alcoholics Anonymous and Narcotics Anonymous (AA and NA) helped him to start over in a sense. He learned to give up his need for control, and found for the first time he was able to slow down and reprioritize his life (John, 2019b).

After starting his recovery, John struggled at first to get back into music. He took a year off from working, and once he returned, he felt shaky about his ability to perform and write, having grown used to working under the influence of drugs and alcohol for nearly two decades. However, he knew that his sobriety had to come first and to this day he considers it his top priority.

Despite his initial struggles when re-entering the pop music world, John's career indeed continued to climb to new levels of stardom following his recovery from addiction. He started to write for movies and musical theater and continued to release chart-topping music. Among his many accomplishments, John's career highlights include more than 50 albums, 38 of which went multiplatinum and one diamond, 50 top-40 hits, and a total of 300 million records sold. John holds the current record for the best-selling single of all time, "Candle in the Wind," which has sold more than 33 million copies. His performances number somewhere around 4,000, and in 2018 he embarked on a 3-year worldwide farewell tour.

In addition to his music career, John has a long history of humanitarian work, most notably with his Elton John AIDS Foundation, which has helped to raise over $450 million for research and programs for AIDS treatment. He and his husband David Furnish, who were married in 2014, have two young sons together. John's life story was depicted in the acclaimed 2019 film *Rocketman*, which focused on the star's long battle with and recovery from addiction. Following a highly successful "farewell" tour around the world which marked the end of his performing days, John has continued to make hit music, recently releasing chart-topping songs with current pop stars including Britney Spears and Dua Lipa. His continued success shows that he remains relevant and iconic, many decades into his career.

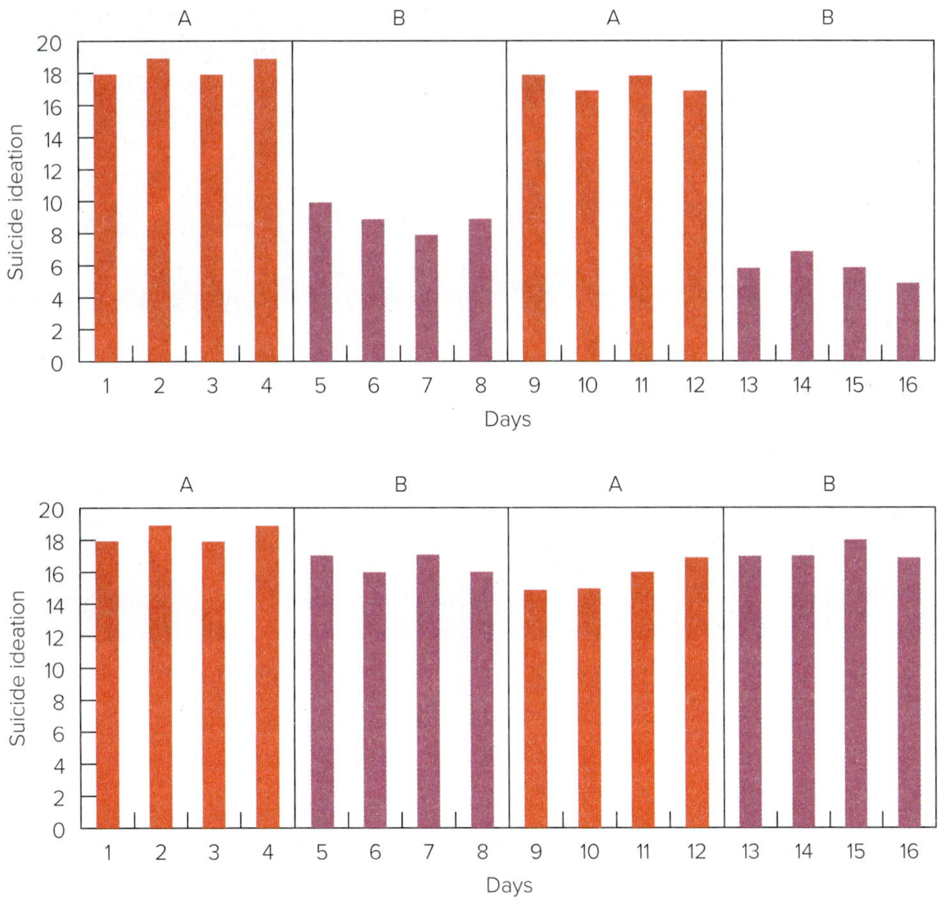

FIGURE 1 ABAB Design

In an ABAB design, researchers observe behaviors in the "A" phase, institute treatment in the "B" phase, and then repeat the process. In this hypothetical study, suicide ideation seems to improve with treatment in the top set of graphs but shows no effect of treatment in the bottom set of graphs.

SOURCE: Rizvi, S. L., & Nock, M. K. (2008). Single-case experimental designs for the evaluation of treatments for self-injurious and suicidal behaviors. *Suicide and Life-Threatening Behavior, 38*, 498–510.

In cases where withholding the treatment in the "B" phase would present an ethical problem because the researcher would be eliminating an effective treatment, the variation known as multiple baseline method is substituted. Here the researcher alternates between treatment and withdrawal of treatment across different subjects, for different behaviors, or in different settings. For example, in treating a client with suicidal ideation, an investigator may first target suicidal thoughts, and second, target suicidal behaviors. The power of the design lies in showing that the behaviors change only when the researcher introduces specific treatments directed at altering those specific behaviors. However, researchers must be certain to make clear when over the course of the study the treatments are introduced, or the results will be difficult to interpret (Coon & Rapp, 2018). Furthermore, because multiple factors can affect treatment outcomes, researchers are also advised to take into account such influences as intervening life events, personality, and potential familial influences (Maric & Kok, 2023).

Research in Behavioral Genetics

The goal of research in **behavioral genetics** is to identify the role of hereditary factors in psychological disorders by examining genetic variations and connecting them to performance on psychological tests or diagnosis of specific disorders. This area of research is becoming increasingly important in the field as investigators attempt to understand the biological component of biopsychosocial contributions to psychopathology.

The data produced by studies in behavioral genetics are based in part on the **heritability index**, a decimal that can range from 0 to 1. To calculate the heritability index, researchers compare rates in individuals varying in degree of genetic closeness, an approach known as **genetic epidemiology**. Another way to express heritability is as a percentage of the variability in the trait in a population that is due to genetic factors.

behavioral genetics
Research area focused on identifying the role of hereditary factors in psychological disorders.

heritability index
A decimal ranging from 0 to 1 that shows the extent to which test scores or other measurements are accounted for by genes. Heritability can also be expressed as the percent of variation in a trait accounted for by genetic factors.

genetic epidemiology
Study of the role of genetic factors in disease by studying rates in individuals varying in degree of genetic closeness.

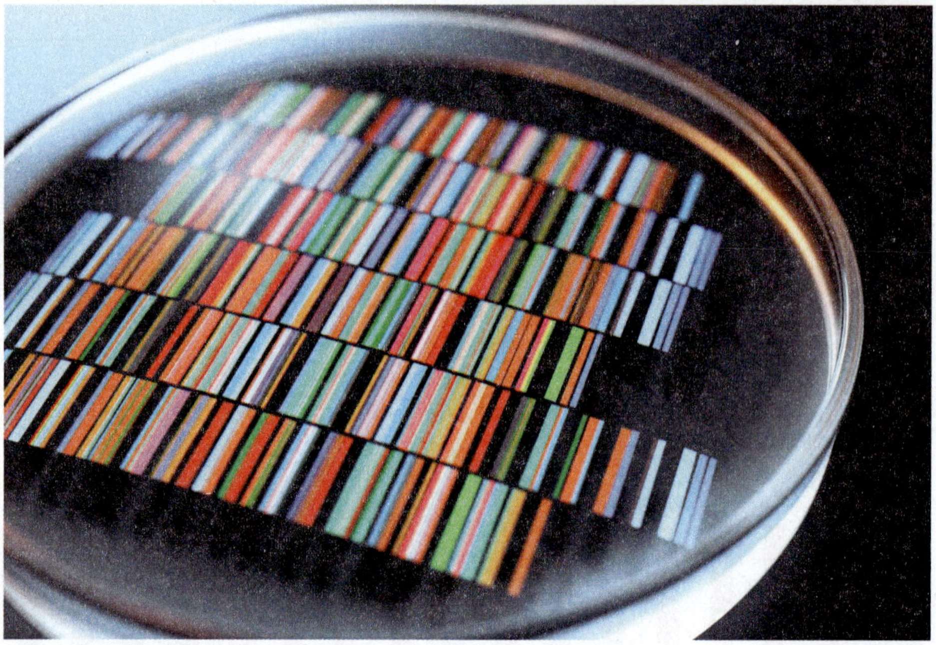

Gene mapping is revolutionizing the way scientists understand and treat psychological disorders.
Connect world/Shutterstock

gene mapping
The approach used by biological researchers in which they examine genetic variations and connect them to performance on psychological tests or diagnosis of specific disorders.

molecular genetics
The study of how genes translate hereditary information.

After examining evidence of a disorder's heritability, researchers can then use **gene mapping** to identify particular sequences of genes along each chromosome that may be associated with that disorder. This process becomes the basis for **molecular genetics**, in which researchers use molecular genetics to understand the link between a disorder's heritability and the possible genes that are affected in that disorder. Particular areas of focus in this field relevant to psychological disorders include studies that connect genes with the operation of given functions of the brain in people with specific psychological disorders (e.g., Langevin et al., 2019).

Return to the Case: Rebecca Hasbrouck

An intern met with Rebecca at the counseling center once a week for 12 consecutive weeks. During the first few sessions Rebecca was often tearful, especially when talking about her boyfriend and how lonely she was feeling. In therapy, she and the intern worked on identifying her emotions and finding coping skills for dealing with stress. Eventually, Rebecca's feelings of sadness lifted as she became accustomed to her life on campus and was able to make a few close friends. Because she was feeling better, her sleep also improved, which helped her to concentrate in class more easily, allowing her to perform better and thus feel more confident in herself as a student.

Dr. Tobin's Reflections: It was clear to me in our initial session that Rebecca was a young woman who was having a particularly difficult time dealing with ordinary adjustment issues in adapting to college. She was overwhelmed by the many new experiences confronting her as well, and she seemed particularly unable to cope with being on her own and being separated from her support network including her family and boyfriend. Her high academic standards added to her stress, and because she didn't have social support, she was unable to talk about the difficulties she was having, which surely perpetuated her problems. I am glad she sought help early, before her difficulties became exacerbated, and that she responded so well to treatment.

SUMMARY

- Questions about impairment and distress are basic to understanding the nature of psychological disorders.
- Social attitudes toward people with psychological disorders range from discomfort to prejudice. Language, humor, and stereotypes all portray psychological disorders in a stigmatized fashion. Stereotypes then result in social discrimination, which only serves to complicate the lives of the affected even more.
- There are five diagnostic criteria for what is considered a psychological disorder: (1) clinical significance, (2) dysfunction in psychological, biological, or developmental processes, (3) significant distress or disability, (4) behavior that cannot be defined as deviant in terms of politics, and (5) behavior that reflects dysfunction in the individual.
- Causes of psychological disorders incorporate biological, psychological, and sociocultural factors. The term *biopsychosocial* refers to the interaction among these factors and their role in the development of an individual's symptoms.
- The three prominent themes in explanations of psychological disorders that recur throughout history are spiritual, humanitarian, and scientific explanations. Spiritual explanations regard disturbances in as the product of possession by evil or demonic spirits. Humanitarian explanations view psychological disorders as the result of cruelty, stress, or poor living conditions. Scientific explanations look for causes in objectively measured phenomena, such as biological alterations, faulty learning processes, emotional stressors, or other qualities that can be empirically observed.
- Researchers use various methods to study the causes and treatment of psychological disorders. The two basic research designs include experimental design, which involves random assignment to conditions, and correlational design, which tests relationships between variables that researchers cannot experimentally manipulate.
- Researchers collect data through methods that include surveys, laboratory studies, and case studies. Surveys enable researchers to estimate the incidence and prevalence of psychological disorders. In a laboratory, participants are exposed to conditions based on the nature of the experimental manipulation. Case studies enable the researcher to intensively study a few individuals. A case study can also be a single-case experimental design, in which the researcher studies one person at a time in both the experimental and control conditions, in alternating phases.
- Investigations in the field of behavioral genetics attempt to determine the extent to which people inherit psychological disorders. Family inheritance studies enable researchers to draw inferences about the relative contributions of biology and family environment to the development of psychological disorders. Genetic mapping is making it possible to identify specific genes involved in the transmission of psychological disorders.

KEY TERMS

Behavioral genetics
Biopsychosocial perspective
Case study
Clinical significance
Comorbidity
Correlational design
Deinstitutionalization movement
Dependent variable
Double-blind
Evidence-based treatment
Exorcism
Gene mapping
Genetic epidemiology
Halfway house
Heritability index
Humanitarian explanations
Incidence
Independent variable
Mental hygiene
Molecular genetics
Meta-analysis
Moral treatment
Placebo condition
Placebo-controlled randomized clinical trial
Positive psychology
Prevalence
Psychological disorders
Psychopathology
Qualitative research
Randomized controlled trial (RCT)
Scientific explanations
Scientific method
Single-case experimental design (SCED)
Sociocultural perspective
Spiritual explanations
Stigma
Survey
Trephining

CHAPTER 2

Diagnosis and Treatment

OUTLINE

Learning Objectives

2.1 Describe the experiences of the client and the clinician.
2.2 Summarize the process for diagnosing psychological disorders.
2.3 Explain the steps of the diagnostic process.
2.4 Describe treatment planning and goals.
2.5 Explain the course of treatment.
2.6 Explain the outcome of treatment.

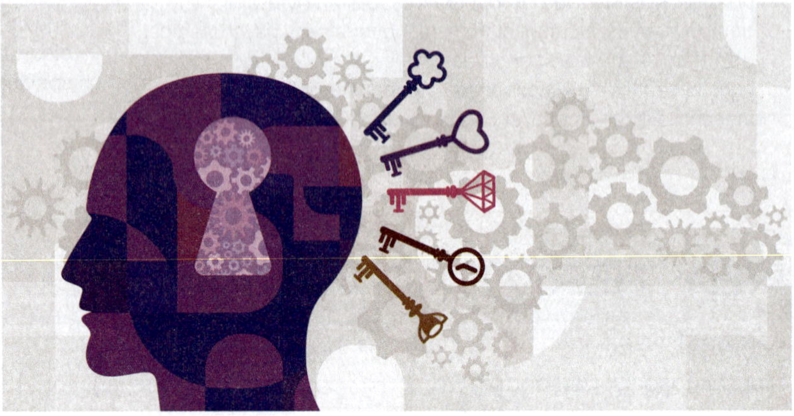

magic pictures/Shutterstock

Case Report

Pedro Padilla

Demographic information: 28-year-old Mexican American heterosexual cisgender man. Pedro's pronouns are he/him/his.

History of present illness: Pedro's girlfriend, Natalia, referred Pedro to an outpatient mental health clinic in the community. He is in his second year as a defense attorney at a small law firm. Natalia reported that about 6 months ago, Pedro's parents began divorce proceedings, at which point she noticed some changes in his behavior. Although his job had always been challenging, Pedro was a hard worker who devoted himself to his studies throughout his academic career and had been just as motivated at his current job. Since the divorce, however, Natalia reported that Pedro had been sleeping only a few hours a night and was having trouble keeping up with his caseload at work. It had gotten so bad that the firm considered firing him.

When he was seen at the outpatient clinic, Pedro reported that the past 6 months had been very difficult for him. Although he stated he had always been a "worrier," he couldn't get his parents' divorce off his mind, and it was interfering with his ability to focus and perform well at his job. He described most of his worries as fears that his parents' divorce would destroy their lives as well as his. He said that he worried that somehow their divorce was his fault, and that once the thought entered his mind, it would play on repeatedly like a broken record. He also explained that Natalia had threatened to break up with him if he didn't "get it together," an ultimatum about which he was also spending a great deal of time worrying. Finally, he stated that he constantly worried that he had ruined her life and that this thought was also very repetitive.

Pedro was noticeably anxious and irritable throughout the session, especially when talking about his parents or about Natalia. Early in the session, he expressed that he had been feeling very tense all day and that his stomach was "in knots." Throughout the session, his legs and hands were fidgety, and he stood up and sat down in his chair several times. He stated that since starting his new job, he had become very short-tempered with people and often felt "wired" and tense, and as a result he had a difficult time concentrating on his work and sleeping soundly. He explained that he couldn't remember the last time he felt calm or didn't worry about anything for an entire day.

He also stated that he could barely think about anything other than his parents' divorce and his relationship problems with Natalia, even if he tried to get his mind off these worries. He reported that prior to learning of his parents' divorce, he was mainly "obsessive" about his work, which he noted was similar to the way he behaved as an undergraduate and in law school. He said he was usually afraid he would make an error and would spend more time worrying about failing than actually doing his work. As a result, he said, he often had little time for friends or romantic relationships because he would feel guilty if he were engaging in pleasurable activities rather than focusing on his work. A serious relationship of 4 years ended after his ex-girlfriend grew tired of what she called his "obsession" with working and his neglect of their relationship. Currently, faced with losing his job and another important relationship, Pedro stated that he realizes for the first time that his anxiety might be interfering with his life.

Psychiatric history: Pedro reported that he is not sure whether there is any family history of anxiety. He stated that his family "never" discusses mental health or emotions in depth, and further that he never felt comfortable talking with others (except Natalia) about his anxiety. He said that ever since he could remember, he had "always" felt anxious and often worried about things more than other people. He remembered a particular instance in high school when he barely slept for 2 weeks because he was preparing an argument for his school's debate team. Pedro stated he has never had any psychotherapy or taken any psychiatric medication, and that in general there is a strong stigma in his family against mental health treatment, which he attributed in part to cultural norms (his parents are immigrants from Mexico). He reported that although his worrying often makes him feel "down," he has never felt severely depressed and has no history of suicidal ideation.

Symptoms: Over a period of approximately 6 months, Pedro had increased difficulty sleeping through the night, restlessness, difficulty concentrating, and irritability. He said he found it difficult to control the worry and spent most of his time worrying about either his parents' divorce, work, or his relationship with Natalia.

Risk level: Low. Pedro has no current suicidal ideation or thoughts of self-harm, and no past history of suicidality or suicide attempts.

Case Report *continued*

Case formulation: Pedro meets all the required *DSM-5-TR* criteria for generalized anxiety disorder (GAD). He had been displaying excessive worry for more days than not for at least the past 6 months, was unable to control his worry, and presented four of the six main symptoms associated with GAD. Pedro's worry was not related to fears of having a panic attack (as in panic disorder), or about being in social or public situations (as in social anxiety disorder). His anxiety was causing him significant problems at work and in his relationship with Natalia. Finally, his anxiety was not the result of substance use.

Treatment plan: Pedro's treatment plan will rely on a combination of two approaches. First, he will be referred to a psychiatrist for antianxiety medication to ease the physical symptoms of his anxiety. Cognitive behavioral psychotherapy will also be recommended, because this has been shown to be the most effective current therapeutic modality for treating GAD.

Sarah Tobin, PhD
Clinician

Pedro's life was thrown into havoc by the worsening of his anxiety symptoms, putting him at risk of losing his job and his relationship. Dr. Tobin's treatment plan suggests a set of steps to address Pedro's immediate symptoms and ultimately to bring him longer-term relief. In this chapter, you will learn about how clinicians proceed through the steps of diagnosis and treatment planning. In order to help you understand these steps, we will introduce you to the fundamental concepts that guide these key processes.

2.1 Psychological Disorder: Experiences of Client and Clinician

Professionals working in the field of mental health come from a wide range of backgrounds. Their work is directed toward both examining the causes of psychological disorders and understanding the complex issues in the therapeutic process. In this chapter, we focus on treatment, beginning by introducing you to the relevant players, "client" and "clinician."

The Client

client
A person seeking psychological treatment.

patient
In health care settings, a person who receives treatment.

People working in the area of psychological disorders refer to individuals seeking psychological intervention alternately as **client** and **patient**. There are advantages and disadvantages to each term, both from the perspective of the individual receiving treatment and the mental health care professional, as well as the cultural context in which treatment occurs (Costa et al., 2019). Reflecting the idea that the individual in treatment is an active participant in the process, our approach is to use the term *client.*

Within health care settings, however, psychologists may find it preferable to use the term *patient.* In a 2018 resolution, the American Psychological Association put forth the policy that psychologists working with other professionals in these settings refer to those they treat as "patients" rather than "clients" (American Psychological Association, 2018). At the same time, the resolution notes that services provided in health care settings should be "person-centered, . . . which recognizes access to clear and concise health information, equitable access to health care, and supports the involvement of all individuals in their own health care decision making" (p. 2).

Whatever terminology you use to refer to people in treatment, it is important to be sensitive to the language you use to refer to those with a given disorder. We highly recommend that you refer to people as "clients" or "patients" who *have* a certain disorder, and not refer to them by the name of their disorder. In other words, if you call someone a "schizophrenic" you equate the person with the disorder. People are more than the sum of their disorders, nor are all individuals with a given disorder exactly the same. By using your language carefully, you communicate greater respect for the total person.

The Clinician

The person who provides the treatment in a mental health setting is the **clinician**. This is a broad category that includes several types of providers who reflect a variety of training experiences and orientation. **Psychologists** are licensed health care professionals offering psychological services. **Psychiatrists** are physicians (MDs) who receive specialized advanced training in diagnosing and treating people with psychological disorders. **Clinical psychologists** are mental health professionals with training in the behavioral sciences who provide direct service to clients. As of 2023, psychologists have prescribing privileges in Colorado, Iowa, Idaho, Illinois, New Mexico, and Louisiana, as well as in the Public Health Service, the Indian Health Service, the U.S. military, and Guam. Psychologists with prescribing privileges are required to obtain specialized training that goes beyond the clinical coursework they complete as part of their education to be psychologists. This training may vary by state, but in all cases, it is rigorous.

There are three types of doctorates in psychology. The Doctor of Philosophy (PhD) is typically awarded for individuals who complete graduate training in a research-based program. In order to be able to practice, people who get their PhDs in clinical or counseling psychology must also complete an internship and at least 1 year of supervised postdoctoral training. The Doctor of Psychology (PsyD) is the degree that professional schools of psychology award and typically involves less training in research. Individuals with a PsyD also must complete an internship in order to practice. Counseling psychologists, with either a doctorate in education (EdD) or a PhD, also serve as clinicians. In order to qualify for a license to practice, all doctoral-level clinicians must pass an examination, a process that varies by state. Beyond their degree, individuals with doctorates in psychology can receive Specialist status in their field of expertise by receiving board certification from the American Board of Professional Psychology (ABPP).

Professionals with Master's degrees also provide psychological services. These include social workers (licensed independent clinical social workers or LICSWs), Master's-level counselors (LMHCs, LPCs, or MSWs), marriage and family therapists (licensed marital and family therapists or LMFTs), Applied Behavior Analysts, nurse clinicians (LPNs, LPRNs, or PMHNPs), and school psychologists. The mental health field also includes a large group of individuals who do not have graduate-level training but serve a critical role in the functioning and administration of the mental health system. Included in this group are occupational therapists, recreational therapists, and counselors who work in institutions, agencies, schools, and homes. Clinicians within each specialty must train according to the standards of their discipline and maintain credentials, such as licenses, required by their state, province, or country in order to provide mental health services.

clinician
The person providing treatment.

psychologist
Licensed health care professional offering psychological services.

psychiatrist
Person with a degree in medicine (MD) who receives specialized advanced training in diagnosing and treating people with psychological disorders.

clinical psychologist
A mental health professional with training in the behavioral sciences who provides direct service to clients.

2.2 The Diagnostic Process

In order to treat people with psychological disorders, clinicians must first be able to diagnose the disorder for which they will seek care. The diagnostic process requires that clinicians use a systematic and evidence-based approach to understanding and ultimately classifying the disorders they see in their clients. Therefore, clinicians rely on diagnostic manuals, which make it possible to provide consistent diagnoses across people based on the presence or absence of a set of specific symptoms.

Systematic methods of diagnoses are also important for researchers to follow when reporting their findings. These may be the same manuals as those used by clinicians. In other cases, however, researchers may base their findings on research-based criteria specific to the disorder under investigation. For example, in studies on anxiety disorders, researchers might use checklists of symptoms based on interviews or questionnaires rather than adopt a formal diagnostic process. In these cases, the researchers must be clear in reporting that their findings apply not to diagnosed cases but to individuals showing symptoms of the disorder.

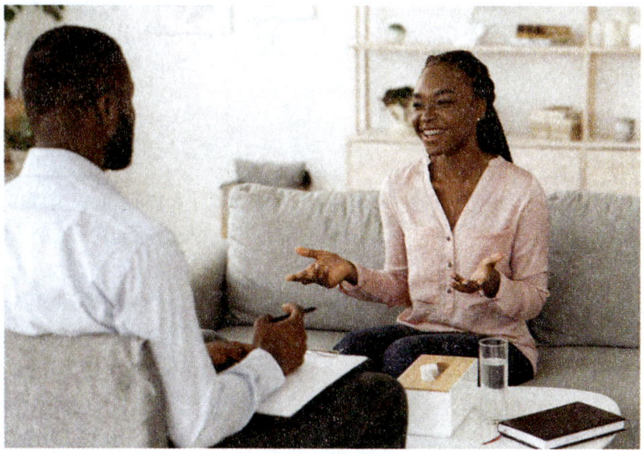

A trusting, positive relationship between clinician and client is crucial to a good therapeutic outcome.

Prostock-studio/Alamy Stock Photo

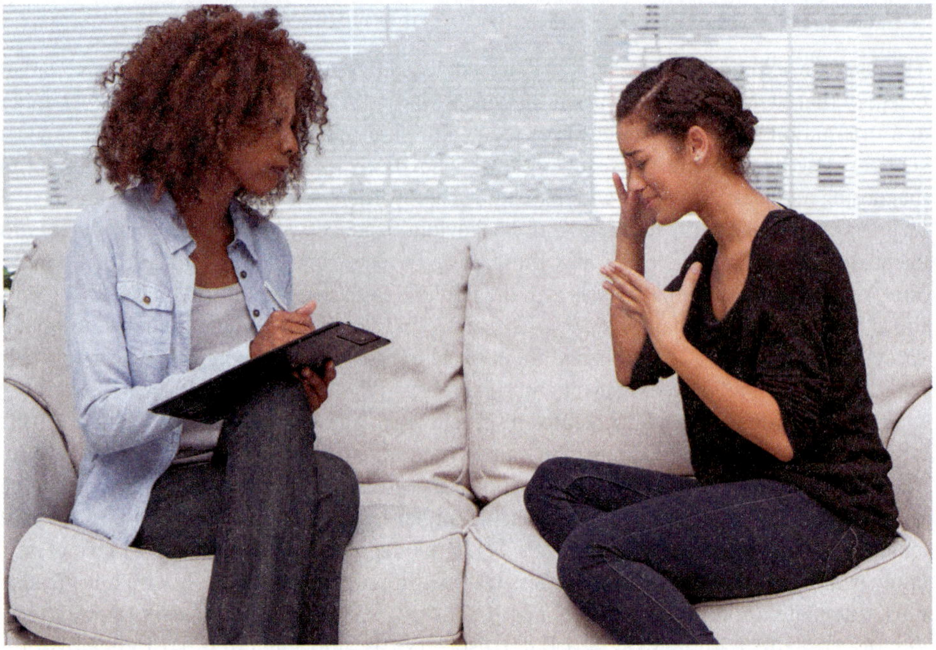

The diagnostic process requires that clinicians conduct an assessment in a sensitive and thorough manner.
wavebreakmediamicro/123RF

reliability
When used with regard to diagnosis, the degree to which clinicians provide diagnoses consistently across individuals who have a particular set of symptoms.

validity
The extent to which a test, diagnosis, or rating accurately and distinctly characterizes a person's psychological status.

Whether based on a formal diagnostic process or on a research-based measure, the instrument itself must meet two sets of criteria. The first is **reliability**, meaning that the instrument yields consistent results across different individuals, or when administered to the same person more than once. Clinicians rating similar clients need to be consistent, and different clinicians also need to be able to arrive at diagnoses that agree with each other. Similarly, in research, people scoring high on one set of items should also score high on related items, or on those same items administered 1 or 2 weeks later.

The second criterion for a diagnostic instrument is **validity**, which is the extent to which a test, diagnosis, or rating accurately and distinctly characterizes a person's psychological status. People receiving high scores on a research-based measure of anxiety should, if the measure is valid, also receive high scores on other measures of anxiety or related indexes, such as restlessness or inability to sleep. A diagnostic manual, to be valid, should be based on prior testing that has demonstrated its ability to differentiate between people who have a particular diagnosis and those who do not.

In addition to guiding treatment, diagnostic manuals have practical importance. Insurance plans require that the clinician report the individual's diagnosis in standard terms when billing for appointments. Without such a classification, the individual will not be able to receive mental health benefits, often referred to as "behavioral health coverage."

Diagnostic and Statistical Manual (DSM-5-TR)

Diagnostic and Statistical Manual of Mental Disorders, Fifth Edition-Text Revision (DSM-5-TR)
A book published by the American Psychiatric Association that contains standard terms and definitions of psychological disorders.

The primary diagnostic manual used in the United States is the ***Diagnostic and Statistical Manual of Mental Disorders (DSM)*** published by the American Psychiatric Association. The most recent version is the *DSM-5-TR*, or fifth edition text revision (American Psychiatric Association, 2022).

Reflecting the increasing reliance of mental health professionals on online tools and mobile applications, the *DSM-5-TR* is available for use on Apple and Android devices. These online versions have the advantage of being easier to navigate than the paper version, which is 1,050 pages long. Rather than having to search through the print version, clinicians can now scroll through screens that guide them more readily through the diagnostic process.

Divided into 22 chapters, the *DSM-5-TR* covers the entire realm of psychological conditions that meet the criteria of being considered "disorders." It also contains additional chapters that provide suggestions for further review as well as general usage guides. Furthermore, because psychological disorders and biological diseases often relate to each other, a number of diagnoses in *DSM-5-TR* have embedded within them a medical diagnosis such as a neurological disease that produces cognitive symptoms. You can read examples of disorders in each category in Table 1.

TABLE 1 **Disorders in *DSM-5-TR***

Category	Description	Examples of Diagnoses
Neurodevelopmental disorders	Disorders that usually develop during the earlier years of life, primarily involving atypical development and maturation	Autism spectrum disorder Specific learning disorder Attention-deficit hyperactivity disorder
Schizophrenia spectrum and other psychotic disorders	Disorders involving symptoms of distortion in perception of reality and impairment in thinking, behavior, affect, and motivation	Schizophrenia Brief psychotic disorder
Bipolar and related disorders	Disorders involving elevated mood	Bipolar disorder Cyclothymic disorder
Depressive disorders	Disorders involving sad mood	Major depressive disorder Persistent depressive disorder
Anxiety disorders	Disorders involving the experience of intense anxiety, worry, fear, or apprehension	Panic disorder Agoraphobia Specific phobia Social anxiety disorder
Obsessive-compulsive and related disorders	Disorders involving obsessions and compulsions	Obsessive-compulsive disorder Body dysmorphic disorder Hoarding disorder
Trauma and stressor-related disorders	Responses to traumatic events	Post-traumatic stress disorder Acute stress disorder Adjustment disorder
Dissociative disorders	Disorders in which the normal integration of consciousness, memory, sense of self, or perception is disrupted	Dissociative identity disorder Dissociative amnesia
Somatic symptom and related disorders	Disorders involving recurring complaints of physical symptoms that may or may not be associated with a medical condition	Illness anxiety disorder Functional neurological symptom disorder
Feeding and eating disorders	Disorders characterized by severe disturbances in eating behavior	Anorexia nervosa Bulimia nervosa Binge eating disorder
Elimination disorders	Disorders involving bladder and bowel disturbances	Enuresis (bladder) Encopresis (bowel)
Sleep-wake disorders	Disorders involving disturbed sleep patterns	Insomnia disorder Narcolepsy

Sexual dysfunctions	Disorders involving disturbance in the expression or experience of sexuality	Erectile disorder Female orgasmic disorder Premature ejaculation
Gender dysphoria	Mismatch between experienced/expressed gender and sex assigned at birth	Gender dysphoria
Disruptive, impulse-control, and conduct disorders	Disorders characterized by repeated expression of impulsive or disruptive behaviors	Kleptomania Intermittent explosive disorder Conduct disorder
Substance-related and addictive disorders	Disorders related to the use of substances	Substance use disorders Substance-induced disorders
Neurocognitive disorders	Disorders involving impairments in thought processes caused by substances or medical conditions	Mild neurocognitive disorder Major neurocognitive disorder
Personality disorders	Disorders in an individual's personality	Borderline personality disorder Antisocial personality disorder Narcissistic personality disorder
Paraphilic disorders	Disorder in which a paraphilia causes distress and impairment	Pedophilic disorder Fetishistic disorder Exhibitionistic disorder
Other mental disorders	Conditions or problems for which a person may seek professional help	Other specified mental disorder due to another medical condition
Medication-induced movement disorders and other adverse effects of medication	Disturbances that can be traced to use of medication	Tardive dyskinesia Medication-induced postural tremor
Other conditions that may be a focus of clinical attention	Conditions or problems for which a person may seek medical help	Problems related to abuse or neglect Suicidal behavior

SOURCE: From the *Diagnostic and Statistical Manual of Mental Disorders, Fifth Edition-TR.* 2022 American Psychiatric Association.

DSM-5-TR contains a "Section III" that includes assessment measures and issues not covered within the diagnostic chapters. These chapters include an alternative approach to diagnosing personality disorders, conditions for further study, and a discussion of culture and psychiatric diagnoses.

axis
A class of information in previous *DSMs* regarding one dimension of an individual's functioning.

multiaxial system
A multidimensional classification and diagnostic system in previous *DSMs* summarizing relevant information about an individual's physical and psychological functioning.

International Classification of Diseases (ICD)
The diagnostic system of the World Health Organization (WHO).

The *DSM-5* (which preceded the *DSM-5-TR* by 9 years) was a major revision of the *DSM-IV-TR,* which organized diagnoses using five separate "axes." Each **axis** represented a category of information regarding one dimension of an individual's functioning. This **multiaxial system** was intended to summarize all relevant information about an individual's physical and psychological functioning.

Mental health professionals outside the United States base their diagnoses on the World Health Organization's (WHO) diagnostic system, the ***International Classification of Diseases (ICD).*** WHO developed the *ICD* as a tool for comparing disease rates among its 194 member states, providing assurance that countries employ the same terminology when reporting epidemiological data. Thus, the *ICD* includes all health conditions, not just psychological disorders.

The *ICD-11* took effect as the official reporting tool for member states in early 2022 (WHO, 2019a). Like the *DSM-5-TR,* this international system reflects the work of a large panel of experts. With approximately 55,000 separate codes to classify all diseases, disorders, injuries, and causes of death, the *ICD-11* has the advantage of allowing for a high level of specificity in the assignment of diagnoses. It is also intended to be used cross-culturally, and its translations in 43 languages facilitates use by health care workers around the world. Reflecting its international focus, the *ICD-11* also includes cultural considerations into each diagnostic grouping (Reed et al., 2019). An accompanying *Clinical Descriptions and Diagnostic Guidelines* publication (CDDG) assists clinicians in the initial stages of the diagnostic process.

What's in the *DSM-5-TR*

Changes from the *DSM-IV-TR* in the *DSM-5* Structure

All editions of the *DSM* have generated considerable controversy, and the fifth edition was no exception. The need for a diagnostic manual meeting criteria of reliability and validity forms the heart of controversy regarding the *DSM-5-TR*. In its revised form, it remains the collective wisdom of clinicians and researchers who believed they were providing criteria that would result in the consistent application of diagnoses (reliability) to classify disorders that individuals actually experience (validity).

The most significant changes in the *DSM-5-TR* that distinguish it from its predecessors concern the decision by its scientific panels to eliminate the multiaxial system. Axis I of the *DSM-IV-TR* contained major "syndromes," or illness clusters. Axis II contained diagnoses of personality disorders and what was then called mental retardation. Axis III was used to note the client's medical conditions. Axis IV rated the client's psychosocial stresses, and Axis V rated the client's overall level of functioning.

The *DSM-5-TR* authors had considered using a dimensional model in which disorders are viewed along a continuum rather than being divided into separate diagnostic categories. However, in the end, they chose not to do so. The current organization begins with neurodevelopmental disorders and then proceeds through "internalizing" disorders (characterized by anxiety, depressive, and somatic symptoms) to "externalizing" disorders (characterized by impulsive, disruptive conduct and substance-use symptoms). The hope is that eventually there will be new research allowing future diagnostic manuals to be based on underlying causes rather than symptoms alone.

Additional Diagnostic Information

As part of the diagnostic process, clinicians may wish to add information about the medical status of their clients. If illnesses that are primarily medical are not specified in *DSM-5-TR*, clinicians may use the standard *ICD-11* diagnoses for the conditions. By specifying these illnesses, clinicians transmit information that has important therapeutic implications. For example, many medications aimed at treating certain medical conditions have side effects that can alter a client's cognitive status, mood, or levels of alertness. In addition, knowing about a client's medical condition can provide the clinician with insights about the individual's

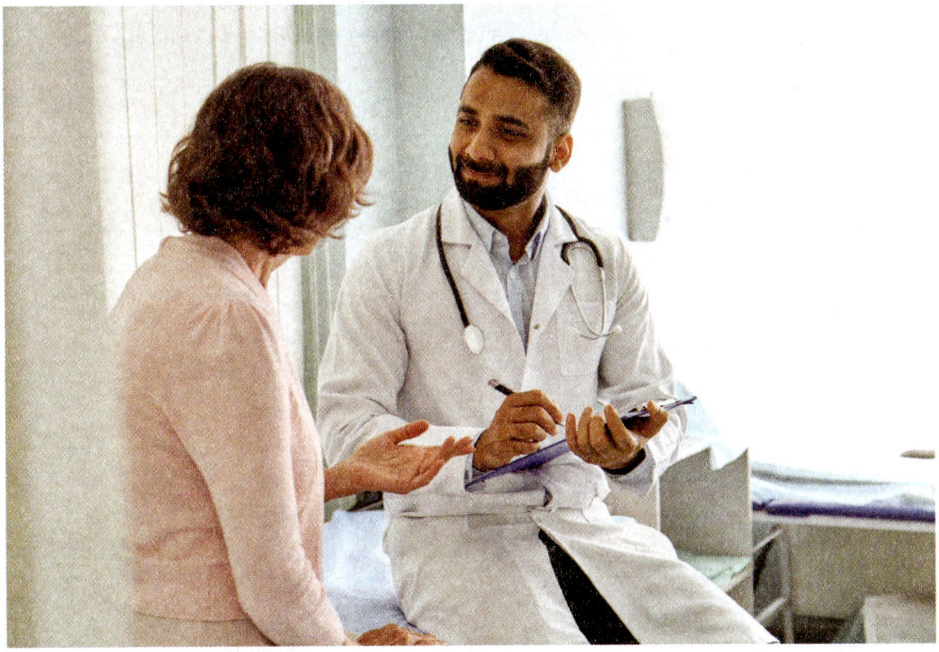

Mental health professionals include relevant medical diagnoses when making diagnoses of psychological disorders.

Ground Picture/Shutterstock

psychological symptoms. It would be useful to know that a middle-aged individual appearing in treatment for a depressive disorder for the first time had a heart attack 6 months ago. The heart attack may have constituted a risk factor for the development of depression, particularly in a person with no previous psychiatric history.

In providing a total diagnostic picture of the client's psychological disorder, clinicians may also decide it is important to specify factors that influence the individual's health status or reason for contacting health services. Formerly referred to as "Z" codes in the *ICD-10*, such circumstances now receive "Q" codes in the *ICD-11*. Several of these are summarized in Table 2.

Clinicians also may want to include their overall judgment of a client's psychological, social, and occupational functioning. An instrument known as the WHO Disability Assessment Schedule (WHODAS) is included as a section of the *DSM-5-TR* so clinicians can provide such a rating. An example of a question from the WHODAS the clinician might ask is, "In the past 30 days, how much difficulty have you had in concentrating on doing something for 10 minutes?" The client indicates whether the difficulty is None, Mild, Moderate, or Severe. Other questions ask about the client's difficulty taking care of household duties, engaging in community activities, and performing activities such as washing and getting dressed.

Cultural Concepts of Distress

cultural concepts of distress
Ways that individuals in specific cultural groups experience, understand, and communicate their suffering, behavioral problems, or troubling thoughts and emotions.

Within particular cultures are idiosyncratic patterns of symptoms, many of which have no direct counterpart to a specific diagnosis. *DSM-5-TR* incorporates **cultural concepts of distress**, the ways that individuals in specific cultural groups experience, understand, and communicate their suffering, behavioral problems, or troubling thoughts and emotions. The three main categories of the cultural concepts of distress are cultural syndromes, idioms of distress, and explanations. You can read about each of these key concepts in Table 3.

As you can see, the cultural concepts of distress take into account a broad range of factors that need to be considered in order for the clinician to get a full understanding of each client. These factors include race, religion, immigration status, and relationships with family and community as potential sources of not only symptoms but also support.

TABLE 2 **Examples from Q Codes in *ICD-11***

Problem Area	Examples
Problems associated with interpersonal interactions	Difficulties with friends Relationship distress with partner Inadequate social skills
Problems associated with absence, loss, or death of partner	Absence of family member Disappearance or death of family member
Problems associated with harmful or traumatic events	Victim of crime or terrorism Exposure to disaster, war, or other hostilities Personal history of physical abuse
Problems associated with employment or unemployment	Chronic workplace stress ("burnout")
Problems related to family support group	Inadequate family support Disruption of family by separation or divorce Dependent relative needing care at home
Problems associated with upbringing	Inadequate parental supervision or control Removal from home in childhood Events resulting in loss of self-esteem in childhood

TABLE 3 **Cultural Concepts of Distress in *DSM-5-TR***

Component of Cultural Concept of Distress	Problem	Examples
Cultural syndromes	Clusters of symptoms and attributions that tend to occur among individuals in specific groups who share the same culture	*Ataque de nervios,* a syndrome in Latinx cultural contexts, reflected in such symptoms as intense emotional upset, aggressive behaviors, and fainting episodes.
Cultural idioms of distress	Ways of expressing distress in a particular culture or group	*Kungfungisisa,* meaning "thinking too much" among the Shona of Zimbabwe, referring to depression, anxiety, and physical symptoms.
Cultural explanations or perceived causes	How people in the culture label or attribute causes to symptoms, illness, or distress	*Dhat syndrome,* the belief in South Asia that semen loss causes diverse symptoms in young men such as fatigue, anxiety, weight loss, and depressive mood.

SOURCE: From the *Diagnostic and Statistical Manual of Mental Disorders, Fifth Edition-TR.* 2022 American Psychiatric Association.

2.3 Steps in the Diagnostic Process

As you have just learned, clinicians assign a diagnosis to their clients using a standard set of criteria. The diagnostic process consists of systematic procedures to ensure that this diagnosis is one that best seems to fit the client's symptoms.

Diagnostic Procedures

The key to the diagnostic process is that the clinician gains as clear a description as possible of a client's symptoms, both those the client reports and those the clinician observes. Dr. Tobin, when hearing Pedro describe himself as "anxious," starts with the premise that he *may* have an anxiety disorder. However, she recognizes that clients do not always label their internal states accurately. Therefore, the clinician also must attend carefully to the client's behavior, emotional expression, and apparent state of mind.

At the outset of the diagnostic process, clinicians listen to clients describe the experience of their symptoms in their own words. This initial stage leads into the more systematic approach to diagnosis, which allows clinicians to arrive at a provisional understanding of the client's symptoms.

As you will learn in the chapter "Assessment," a variety of diagnostic tools give the clinician a framework for determining the extent to which a client's symptoms coincide with the diagnostic criteria of a given disorder. The clinician must determine the exact nature of a client's symptoms, the length of time the client has experienced these symptoms, and any other behaviors, thoughts, or feelings that may represent important symptoms that the client may not report. In the process, the clinician also obtains information about the client's personal and family history as well as cultural background and identity. By asking questions in this manner, the clinician begins to formulate the **principal diagnosis**–namely, the disorder or disorders most closely aligned with the primary reason the individual is seeking professional help.

Similarly, the clinician needs to rule out systematically the possibility of alternate diagnoses, a process referred to as **differential diagnosis.** The clinician conducts a differential diagnosis by comparing the client's symptoms to those associated with disorders sharing similar symptoms until other possibilities can be eliminated. This is important primarily so that the

principal diagnosis
The disorder most closely aligned with the primary reason the individual is seeking professional help.

differential diagnosis
The process of systematically ruling out alternative diagnoses.

clinician can be sure to embark on the appropriate treatment. The clinician must also rule out medical diagnoses that could produce symptoms similar to those of a psychological disorder.

In Pedro's case, the predominant symptom is anxiety, which would suggest that he should receive the diagnosis of an anxiety disorder. Dr. Tobin must then determine which anxiety disorder most closely fits Pedro's symptoms. At the same time, she needs to consider whether Pedro has a medical disorder that could produce similar symptoms. It is also possible that Pedro's symptoms represent adjustment difficulties related to the divorce of his parents or the stress he encounters at work. He may have a comorbid psychological disorder related to substance use. Dr. Tobin's initial diagnosis must be tested against these possibilities, as well as take into consideration relevant cultural factors that may be important in understanding his symptoms. If she is unable to provide this level of competency and sensitivity, she is ethically bound to refer Pedro to another clinician who has the appropriate experience and can provide him with competent care.

The diagnostic process can take anywhere from a few hours to weeks depending on the complexity of the client's presenting symptoms. The client and clinician need not wait until the diagnostic process is complete to begin doing therapeutic work, particularly if the client is in crisis. The course of therapy would then be adjusted as the diagnosis is more firmly established.

Case Formulation

case formulation
A clinician's analysis of the client's development and the factors that might have influenced his or her current psychological status.

Once clinicians make a formal diagnosis, they are still left with a formidable challenge–to piece together a picture of how the disorder evolved. The **case formulation** provides an analysis of the factors that might have influenced the client's current psychological status. With this descriptive information, the clinician can more confidently design a treatment plan that is attentive to the client's symptoms, unique past experiences, and future potential for growth.

The cornerstone of a thorough case formulation is an understanding of the client from a biopsychosocial perspective that goes beyond the symptoms and takes into account such factors as the client's prior development, family history, and cultural or socially relevant information about the client.

In her work with Pedro, Dr. Tobin starts to flesh out the details of her case formulation as she gets to know him better in the initial therapy phases. Her case formulation will expand to include Pedro's family history, focusing on the divorce of his parents, as well as the possible causes of his perfectionism and concern over his academic performance. She will try to understand why he feels so overwhelmed at work and gain a perspective on why his relationship with Natalia has been so problematic. Finally, she will need to investigate the possible role of his mother's panic attacks and how they relate to Pedro's experience of anxiety symptoms. To aid in differential diagnosis, Dr. Tobin will also evaluate Pedro's pattern of substance use as well as any possible medical conditions that she did not detect during the initial assessment phase. As we will see below, Dr. Tobin will also want to include information based on her cultural formulation of Pedro's case.

Cultural Formulation

cultural formulation
A tool that includes the clinician's assessment of the client's degree of identification with the culture of origin, the culture's beliefs about psychological disorders, the ways in which the culture interprets particular events, and the cultural supports available to the client.

Making a diagnosis requires taking multiple factors from the client's life into account that include the relevant sociocultural context. A **cultural formulation** includes the clinician's assessment of the client's degree of identification with their culture of origin, the culture's beliefs about psychological disorders, the ways in which people in the culture interpret particular events, and the cultural supports available to the client.

You might expect cultural norms and beliefs to have a stronger impact on clients who strongly identify with their culture of origin. The client's familiarity with and preference for using a certain language is one obvious indicator of cultural identification. A culture's approach to understanding the causes of behavior may influence clients who strongly identify with their culture. Exposure to these belief systems may, in turn, influence the expression of a client's symptoms.

Even if a client's symptoms do not specifically represent a culture-bound syndrome, clinicians must consider the individual's cultural background as a framework for interpreting these symptoms. For example, members of a given culture attach significant meanings to particular events. In certain Asian cultures, an insult may provoke the condition known as *amok*, in which an individual broods over the insult, becomes outraged, and then forgets the episode entirely. Without taking this background into account, the clinician may very well draw the wrong conclusions, assuming that the symptoms reflect a disturbance within the individual when they in fact reflect the playing out of a culturally influenced scenario.

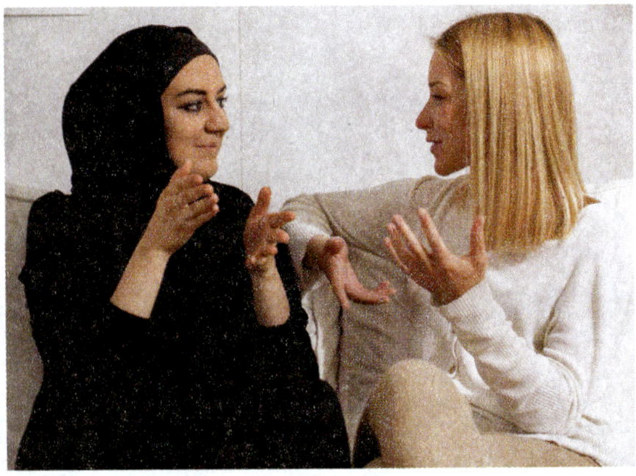

Ground Picture/Shutterstock

According to the principle of **multiculturally competent care**, clinicians should be able to demonstrate awareness of and skill in addressing culturally relevant factors when working with individuals from cultural backgrounds that differ from their own.

multiculturally competent care
A clinician's ability to demonstrate awareness of and skill in addressing culturally relevant factors when working with individuals from cultural backgrounds that differ from their own.

In Pedro's case, cultural factors influenced his views on mental health and seem to have acted as a barrier to his seeking treatment sooner. Pedro mentions that his parents, who are Mexican immigrants, attach stigma to mental health problems and particularly to talking openly about such struggles and seeking help for them. Pedro seems to have internalized these feelings, despite being raised in a different cultural context in the United States. It seems it was his girlfriend's concerns that pushed him to finally seek help, without which it is unclear how much longer he might have put off treatment. The clinician in this case should pay attention to Pedro's feelings about having anxiety and how they might affect the outcome of treatment.

As in Pedro's case, clinicians should look within the client's cultural background not only for diagnostic purposes but also as a way of identifying cultural supports that may be available to them. Clients from cultures that incorporate extended family networks and religious connections can draw on emotional resources to help them cope with stressful life events.

Along with sensitivity to a client's cultural background, clinicians need to ensure that their use of language reflects this sensitivity. For example, terminology reflecting binary gender distinctions within health care settings can create obstacles to health care among LGBTQ+ communities (Drill et al., 2019). The American Psychological Association's Inclusive Language Guidelines (2021) clearly spell out the terms both to avoid and to use in communicating respectfully to individuals of diverse backgrounds. As stated in its foreword, these guidelines include, but are not limited to, sexism, ableism, ageism, heterosexism, classism, and religious bigotry.

Cultural formulations are critical in understanding psychological disorders from a biopsychosocial perspective. The fact that psychological disorders, and beliefs about them, vary from one culture to another supports the claim of the sociocultural perspective that cultural factors play a role in influencing the expression of psychological disorders. It is imperative that clinicians are culturally competent in their work with multicultural clients in order to address this influence and to ensure that clients have optimal outcomes.

2.4 Planning the Treatment

Clinicians typically follow up the diagnostic phase by developing a **treatment plan**, the outline for how therapy should take place. In the treatment plan, the clinician describes the treatment goals, treatment site, modality of treatment, and theoretical approach. The decisions the clinician makes while putting the treatment plan together reflect what they know at the time about the client's needs and the available resources; however, clinicians often revise the treatment plan once they see how the proposed intervention methods are actually working.

treatment plan
The outline for how therapy should take place.

Goals of Treatment

The first step in treatment planning is the establishment of treatment goals, ranging from those that have immediate consequence to those of a more long-term nature. Ideally, treatment goals reflect what the clinician knows about both the disorder and the recommended therapy, and the particular needs and concerns of the individual client.

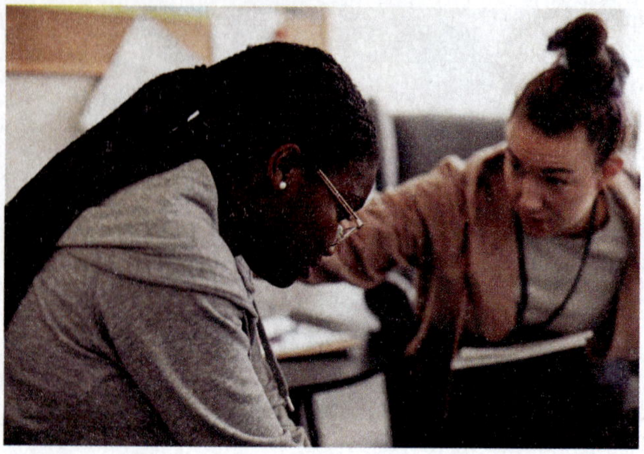

Clinicians working with clients who are in crisis seek to manage their immediate symptoms.
Maskot Images/Shutterstock

The immediate goal of treating clients in crisis is to ensure that their symptoms are managed, particularly if they are at risk of harm to themselves or others. Pedro, for example, needs psychiatric treatment in order to bring his anxiety symptoms under control. The clinician may need to hospitalize a client who is severely depressed and suicidal. However, the treatment plan may include this immediate goal only until the clinician gains a broader understanding of the client's situation.

Short-term goals are aimed at alleviating the client's symptoms by addressing problematic behavior, thinking, or emotions. The plan at this point includes establishing a working relationship between the clinician and the client, as well as setting up specific objectives for therapeutic change. Another short-term goal might be to stabilize a client taking medications, a process that could take several weeks or longer if the first round of treatment is unsuccessful. In Pedro's case, Dr. Tobin will need to ensure that the medications he is receiving are in fact helping to alleviate his anxiety. She will also need to work with the psychiatrist on the case to monitor any adverse side effects. Her short-term goals with Pedro will also include beginning to examine the nature of his anxiety and how he can start to manage his symptoms using psychological interventions.

Long-term goals include more fundamental and deeply rooted alterations in the client's psychological health. These are the ultimate aims of therapeutic change. Ideally, the long-term goals for any client are to achieve recovery, or at least to learn to cope with the symptoms of the disorder. Depending on the nature of the client's disorder, available supports, and life stressors, these long-term goals can take some time to accomplish. Dr. Tobin's long-term goals with Pedro are to take him off the medication. At the same time, she would plan to help him gain an understanding of the causes of his symptoms and, in the process, reduce their severity if not eliminate them altogether.

In many cases, clinicians carry out treatment goals in a sequential manner. The clinician first deals with the crisis, then handles problems in the near future, and finally addresses issues that require extensive work in the months ahead. Many clients, however, experience a cyclical unfolding of stages. New sets of immediate crises or short-term goals may arise in the course of treatment; or there may be a redefinition of long-term goals as the course of treatment progresses. It is perhaps more helpful to think of the three stages not as consecutive stages, but as steps with different levels of treatment focus that can change in priority over time. This is particularly true when considering disorders that can take on a chronic quality, requiring perhaps several years to show lasting improvement (Beutel et al., 2022).

Treatment Sites

Clinicians must take into account a number of issues when recommending which treatment site will best serve the client. Treatment sites vary in the degree to which they provide a controlled environment and in the nature of the services that clients can receive. Clients who are in crisis or are at risk of harming themselves or others need to be in controlled environments. However, there are many other considerations including cost and insurance coverage, the need for additional medical care, availability of community support, and the projected length of treatment. Depending on the symptoms and the availability of these supports, clinicians recommend in-patient settings, outpatient settings, schools, or the workplace.

Psychiatric Hospitals

In a psychiatric hospital, a client receives medical interventions and intensive forms of psychotherapy. These settings are most appropriate for clients at risk of harming themselves or others and who seem incapable of self-care. In some cases, clinicians may involuntarily hospitalize clients through a court order until they can bring the symptoms under control (you will read about this in more detail in the chapter "Ethical and Legal Issues").

In the United States, veterans can receive inpatient care at Department of Veterans Affairs Medical Centers, primarily but not limited to treating conditions related to their military service.

Specialized Inpatient Treatment Centers Clients may need intensive supervision but not actual hospital care. For these individuals, specialized inpatient treatment centers provide both supportive services and round-the-clock monitoring. Included in this category are recovery treatment centers for adults seeking to overcome substance addiction. Clinicians may also recommend this treatment site to children who need constant monitoring due to severe behavioral disturbances.

Outpatient Treatment By far the most common treatment site is an outpatient clinic or a therapist's private practice office. **Community mental health centers (CMHCs)** are outpatient clinics that provide psychological services on a sliding fee scale for individuals who live within a certain geographic area. Professionals in private practice offer individual, couples, family, or group sessions. Types of private practice include group practices (in which multiple clinicians see clients), individual practices, or remotely in virtual practices. Some prepaid health insurance plans cover the cost of such visits, either to a private practitioner or to a clinician working in a health maintenance organization (HMO). Clinicians in private practice may also opt to offer services at an out-of-pocket cost and not accept insurance. Medicare is available to support the costs of outpatient mental health services for individuals in the United States who are 65 and older. Veterans may be seen for these services in outpatient clinics within U.S. Veterans Affairs clinics. Other agencies supported partially or completely by public funds may also offer outpatient treatment. With regard to Pedro, it is an outpatient treatment that Dr. Tobin will choose because his symptoms are not sufficiently severe to justify hospitalization.

community mental health center (CMHC)
Outpatient clinic that provides psychological services on a sliding fee scale for individuals who live within a certain geographic area.

Clients receiving outpatient services will, by necessity, receive more limited care than what they would encounter in a hospital, in terms of both the time involved and the nature of the contact between client and clinician. Consequently, clinicians may advise that their clients receive additional services, including psychiatric medication, vocational counseling, in-home services, group therapy, or the support of a self-help organization, such as Alcoholics Anonymous.

Clients with serious psychological disorders who are able to live in the community may require the additional support of facilities intended to serve the needs of this specific population. These facilities may be connected with a hospital, a public agency, or a private corporation.

Halfway houses are designed for clients who have been discharged from psychiatric facilities but who are not yet ready for independent living. A halfway house provides a living context with other deinstitutionalized people, and it is staffed by professionals who work with clients in developing the skills they need to become employed and to set up independent living situations. **Day treatment programs** are designed for formerly hospitalized clients, as well as for clients who do not need hospitalization but do need a structured program during the day, similar to what a hospital provides.

halfway house
A community treatment facility designed for deinstitutionalized clients leaving a hospital who are not yet ready for independent living.

day treatment program
A structured program in a community treatment facility that provides activities similar to those provided in a psychiatric hospital.

Telemental Health Services The newest treatment site in psychological treatment is a platform offered through virtual client-clinician contact. **Telemental health** or **telepsychology** is the provision of psychological services using videoconferencing or telephone. Telemental health can also be conducted via smartphone applications that allow clients to track their mood states or communicate with their clinician over e-mail. Li ke online learning, telemental health can be provided either in real time or in an asynchronous manner over digital platforms (American Psychological Association, 2014).

Although already used increasingly prior to the COVID-19 pandemic, telemental health saw exponential growth beginning in 2020, due to restrictions on face-to-face sessions in a majority of settings. The advantages of telemental health's portability and ease of access will undoubtedly lead to its becoming a permanent fixture as a treatment site option. For example, individuals living in isolated rural areas will gain new access to mental health services,

telemental health
Also referred to as telepsychology, the provision of psychological services using the platform of videoconferencing or telephone.

telepsychology
Also referred to as telemental health, the provision of psychological services using the platform of videoconferencing or telephone.

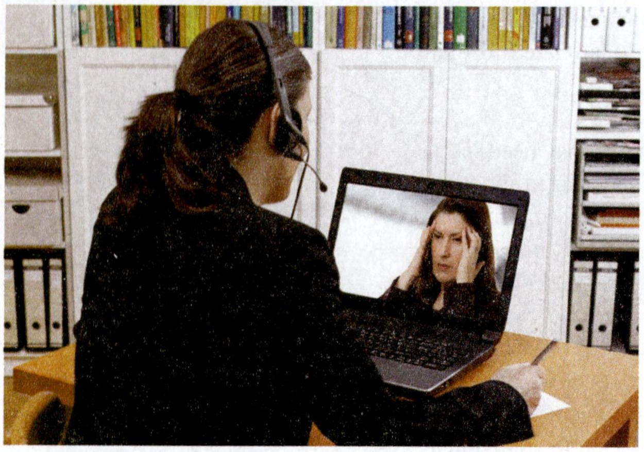

Telemental health services are the newest treatment sites for people with psychological disorders.
Agenturfotografin/Shutterstock

as will those with physical disabilities. Even individuals who have no physical barriers to attending in-person sessions may become less likely to miss a virtual session, given its ease of access (Silver, Coger, Barr, & Drill, 2020). And as third-party payers move to reimburse mental health services provided in a virtual format, the use of telemental health will only continue to gain strength.

Other Treatment Sites Clients may also receive treatment in the places where they work or go to school, which helps to reduce barriers to accessing necessary treatment and other resources. School psychologists are trained to work with children and teenagers who require further assessment or behavioral interventions. In the workplace, employee assistance programs (EAPs) provide employees with a confidential setting in which they can seek individual help in the form of counseling, assistance with substance abuse, and family treatment. College counseling centers are housed on the campus of a college or university, and can provide a range of treatment options for students, such as outpatient therapy, psychiatric medication management, and assistance with referrals for long-term treatment off-campus.

Modality of Treatment

modality
Form in which the clinician offers psychotherapy.

counseling
Short-term, problem-focused treatment.

psychotherapy
Treatment modality that focuses on development of a working relationship between clinician and client

The **modality**, or form in which the clinician offers psychotherapy, is another crucial component of the treatment plan. Clinicians recommend one or more modalities depending on the nature of the client's symptoms and whether or not other people in the client's life should be involved.

You may see treatment modalities referred to as "counseling" or "psychotherapy"–which is often shortened to therapy, and this depends on the general goal or the treatment. **Counseling** is typically short term in nature and problem focused, whereas **psychotherapy** typically entails longer-term treatment and there is a greater emphasis on development of a working relationship between clinician and client.

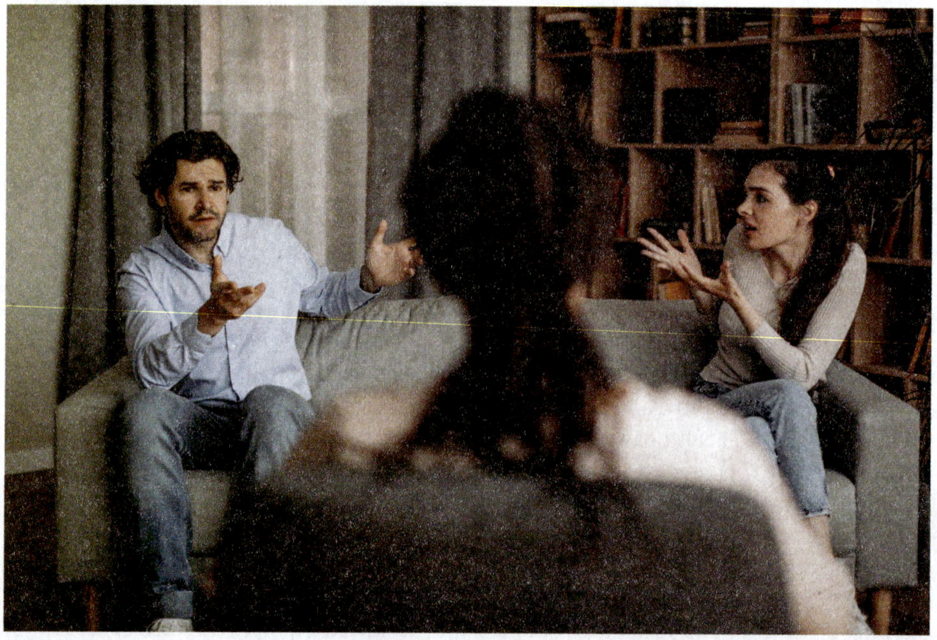

In couples therapy, clinicians involve both partners in seeking to understand their relational issues.
Prostock-studio/Shutterstock

Clients receive treatment on a one-to-one basis in **individual psychotherapy**. In **couples therapy** (sometimes referred to as "relational therapy") both or all partners in a relationship meet with a clinician, and in **family therapy**, several or all family members are involved in treatment. Although in family therapy, one person may be identified as the "patient," the therapist views the whole family system as the target of the treatment.

Group therapy is a psychological treatment in which the therapist facilitates discussion in a structured fashion among several clients who talk together about their problems. In this way, clients have the opportunity to share their difficulties with others, receive feedback, develop trust, and improve their interpersonal skills.

A clinician may recommend any or all of these modalities in any setting. Specific to psychiatric hospitals is **milieu therapy**, which is based on the premise that the milieu, or environment, is a major component of the treatment. Ideally, the milieu is organized in a way that allows clients to receive consistent therapeutic and constructive reactions from all who live and work there. In addition to traditional psychotherapy, clients participate in other therapeutic endeavors through group or peer counseling, occupational therapy, and recreational therapy.

individual psychotherapy
Psychological treatment in which the therapist works on a one-to-one basis with the client.

couples therapy
Treatment provided for both partners in a relationship.

family therapy
Psychological treatment in which the therapist works with several or all members of the family.

group therapy
Psychological treatment in which the therapist facilitates discussion among several clients who talk together about their problems.

milieu therapy
A treatment approach, used in an inpatient psychiatric facility, in which all facets of the milieu, or environment, are components of the treatment.

Determining the Best Approach to Treatment

Whatever treatment modality a clinician recommends, it must be based on the choice of the most appropriate theoretical perspective or combination of perspectives. Many clinicians are trained according to a particular set of assumptions about the origins of psychological disorders and the best methods of treating these disorders. Often, this theoretical orientation forms the basis for the clinician's treatment decisions. However, just as frequently, clinicians adapt their theoretical orientation to fit the client's needs.

After decades of debate regarding which treatments are most effective, and for whom, psychologists adopted the principles of **evidence-based practice in psychology**—clinical decision making that integrates the best available research evidence and clinical expertise in the context of the cultural background, preferences, and characteristics of clients (American Psychological Association Presidential Task Force on Evidence-Based Practice, 2006). Evidence-based practice now forms the basis for training in graduate programs and postdoctoral continuing education (e.g., Barrett, Gonsalvez, & Shires, 2019). However, there remains a lag in research examining evidence-based practice in student-trainee supervision (Barrett, Gonsalvez, & Shires, 2020).

evidence-based practice in psychology
Clinical decision making that integrates the best available research evidence and clinical expertise in the context of the cultural background, preferences, and characteristics of clients.

As you read in this book about various disorders and the most effective treatments, keep in mind that clinicians need to abide by the findings of empirically based research. However, evidence-based practice also implies that clinicians should base their treatments on state-of-the-art research findings that they adapt to the particular features of the client, taking into account the client's background, needs, and prior experiences.

You Be the Judge

Psychologists as Prescribers

In 2002, New Mexico became the first state to approve prescription privileges for psychologists. Louisiana followed shortly thereafter (2004), as did Illinois (2014), Iowa (2016), Idaho (2017), and most recently (after over 12 years of debate) Colorado (2023). These landmark pieces of legislation are paving the way for other states to take similar action.

There are several arguments against the granting of prescription privileges to psychologists. Unlike psychiatrists, psychologists do not receive medical training and therefore do not have the undergraduate premedical training or the years of medical school, internship, and residency that physicians receive. Philosophically, research-oriented psychologists argue that the granting of prescription privileges will refocus the profession away from science and instead emphasize the role of psychologists as practitioners. Psychologists should not be in the business, they argue, of handing out medication. A second argument against prescription privileges concerns the role of medication in psychological treatment. From this perspective, psychologists should be focused on psychotherapy. The long-term benefits of psychotherapy, these critics argue, are equal to if not greater than the long-term benefits of medication for the majority of disorders including major depression, anxiety disorders, and other nonpsychotic disorders. In the exceptional cases of serious mental illness, such as schizophrenia and bipolar disorder, psychologists can work as a team with psychiatrists to maintain their clients on long-term medication regimens.

The arguments in favor of prescription privileges are also compelling. If psychologists have the power to prescribe medications, they can do a better job than psychiatrists do in integrating medication into psychotherapy. From the client's point of view, there is greater continuity of care, in that the individual does not need to see more than one mental health practitioner. Psychologists in favor of prescription privileges also point to the fact that with prescription privileges, psychologists can also intervene to reduce or discontinue a patient's medications. A second argument in favor of prescription privileges is that there are other nondoctoral-level health professionals with this legal power including psychiatric nurse practitioners and psychiatric nurse specialists, among others, although the exact nature of their privileges varies across states. In any case, specialized training is required for a clinical psychologist to meet the legal requirements for prescribing psychotherapeutic medications.

Practitioners who belong to the American Psychological Association continue to lobby in favor of more widespread acceptance of prescription privileges across the United States. As the Oregon case demonstrates, however, this legislation is likely to face a rocky road in other states.

Q: *You be the judge:* Does having prescription privileges reduce the scientific status of psychology as a profession? Would you prefer that the psychologist you might see for treatment can also incorporate medications into your treatment?

2.5 The Course of Treatment

Progress in psychological treatment is a function of the joint efforts of the clinician and client working together toward an improvement in the client's state of mental health and well-being. Each individual has a part to play in determining the outcome of the case, as does the unique interaction of their personalities, abilities, expectations, and backgrounds.

The Clinician's Role in Treatment

Above and beyond whatever treatment techniques a clinician uses, the quality of the relationship between the client and the clinician is a crucial determinant of therapy's outcome. A good clinician does more than mechanically administering treatment to a client. The best clinicians infuse a deep personal interest, concern, and respect for the client into the therapeutic relationship.

Dr. Tobin will work with Pedro in the initial weeks of therapy to establish this solid basis for their further work together. As treatment proceeds, she will continue to evaluate the effectiveness of her intervention and make adjustments accordingly.

The Client's Role in Treatment

In optimal situations, psychotherapy is a joint enterprise in which the client plays an active role. It is largely up to the client to describe and identify the nature of their disorder, to articulate their personal reactions as treatment progresses, and to initiate and follow through on changes as they emerge over time.

Throughout treatment, the client's attitudes toward therapy and the therapist are an important part of the contribution the client makes to the therapeutic relationship. There is a special quality to the help the client is requesting; it requires revealing potentially painful, embarrassing, and personal material that the client is not accustomed to sharing with a professional. For some clients, then, part of the work in treatment is learning to be more comfortable discussing their symptoms with a therapist or other mental health professional.

Social attitudes toward psychological disorders based on their cultural backgrounds can also affect how readily clients engage in treatment. The client may come from a culture in which it is taboo to admit to being sad or anxious. The client's family may communicate the idea that people should not need to rely on therapists to get better. They may think there's something wrong with them because they are in need of help. Although attitudes toward therapy are becoming more accepting in current Western culture, there is still a degree of potential shame or embarrassment that clients must confront. To someone who is already troubled by severe problems in living, the added anxiety caused by worrying about what it means to seek psychotherapy can be further inhibiting.

With so many potential forces driving the individual away from seeking therapy, the initial step is sometimes the hardest to take. Thus, the therapeutic relationship requires the client to be willing to work with the clinician in a partnership and to be prepared to endure the pain and

REAL STORIES

Wayne Brady (1972–Present)

As an accomplished comedian, actor, singer, and game show host, Wayne Brady has been known to the world as a funny and quick-witted entertainer who brings his playful personality to a diverse range of projects. In 2014 he revealed that he had been suffering in silence with clinical depression for many years. He went public with this revelation on an episode of the television show *Entertainment Tonight* (Bueno, 2014), when he shared that on the night of his 42nd birthday he had what he believes was a "complete breakdown." News of the interview rippled through the entertainment world and spurred a journey of treatment and healing for Brady, as he bravely shared with the world what lay beneath his public persona.

Brady was born in Columbus, Georgia, to parents who immigrated from the West Indies. He was raised largely by his grandmother in Orlando, Florida and started performing in community theater when he was 16. In 1996 Brady made his television debut at the age of 24, in the comedy competition *Kwik Witz*. He then started appearing in the original British version of the long-running sketch comedy show *Whose Line Is It Anyway*, and later in the U.S. version. From there he went on to host his own talk show, *The Wayne Brady Show*, and he has been the host of the popular TV game show *Let's Make a Deal* since 2009. Brady is also musically gifted; he starred on Broadway in the musical *Kinky Boots* and released a full studio album in 2008. Brady has received 16 Emmy nominations, 5 Emmy wins, and a Grammy nomination.

In the *Entertainment Tonight* interview, Brady recalls his 2013 breakdown: "I was there by myself, in my bedroom, and I had a complete breakdown . . . go ahead and imagine for yourself a brother in his underwear, in his room; you got snot . . . and that birthday was the beginning of, 'OK, I've got to make a change!'" Brady acknowledged that due to his public persona and success as a comedian, there was a sense that he could not be seen as someone who struggles with depression, noting, "People think Wayne Brady's always happy. . . . No I'm not always happy because I'm human!" (Bueno, 2014).

Brady has also revealed that the suicide of comedian and actor Robin Williams was another inspiration to seek help (CBS News, 2014). Remarking on the similarities between himself and Williams, he noted that the public can have a difficult time understanding that comedians may inhabit a private world in which they are suffering, and that they are indeed capable of experiencing great sadness, despite an ability to make others laugh.

In a 2017 interview with Dr. Freda Lewis-Hall, Brady (2017) reflected on his decision to share his diagnosis of depression with the world. "The reason that I wanted to speak, is that I happened to struggle with depression. A lot of people have. . . . [I]t shouldn't be a secret." While talking about the stigma of depression, Brady also spoke to the ways that building coping tools for himself, combined with being open and frank about his depression with himself and publicly, have proved to be healing. Through speaking publicly he hopes to inspire others, particularly other men of color, to be open and acknowledge when they are suffering.

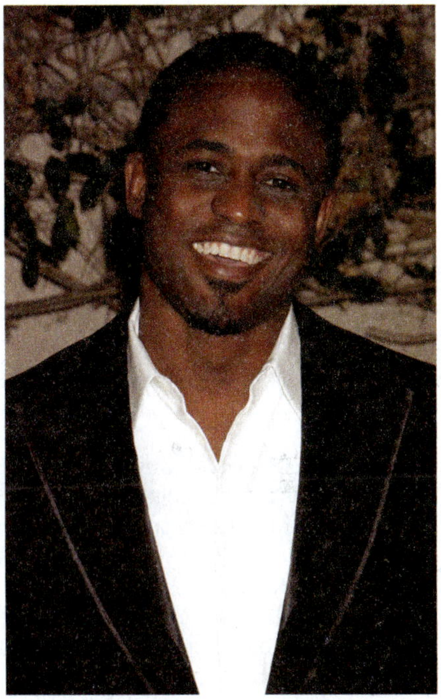

Wayne Brady arriving at Celebrity Fight Night in Phoenix, AZ in 2004.

Helga Esteb/Shutterstock

Since going public with his struggles, Brady has gone on to become a spokesperson for mental health awareness and continues to share his own insights about his journey. In a 2017 social media post (Child Mind Institute, 2017), he expressed his desire to help others confront their issues with hope: "To anyone who is struggling with depression and who feels like they're in that dark box, what I would say to you is just know that you can get help. There's light."

embarrassment involved in making personal revelations. Moreover, it also requires a willingness to break old patterns and to try new ways of viewing the self and relating to others.

2.6 The Outcome of Treatment

remission
Situation in which the individual's symptoms no longer interfere with his or her behavior and are below those required for a *DSM* diagnosis.

In the best of all possible worlds, the treatment works. The client remains in treatment until the treatment has run its course; then, they show improvement and maintains this improved level of functioning. **Remission** is said to occur when the individual's symptoms no longer interfere with their behavior and are below those required for a *DSM* diagnosis. Although this is obviously the most desirable outcome, the road to remission is often not so smooth, and either the client does not attain the treatment plan goals or unanticipated problems arise. Remission rates also depend on the specific disorder and treatment methods used for that disorder. For example, one large-scale review of prior studies showed variations in remission rates according to mode of treatment, criteria for remission, and diagnosis (Jonsson et al., 2023).

Change is very difficult, and many clients have become so accustomed to living with their symptoms that the effort necessary to solve the problem seems overwhelming. Clinicians find it particularly frustrating when they encounter these negative attitudes or when clients do not seem willing to follow through on their expressed desire to change. At times, clinicians also face frustration over practical constraints. They may recommend a treatment that they are confident can succeed but that would exceed available insurance reimbursement or would otherwise not be feasible, given the client's current living situation. In other cases, people in the client's life refuse to support the client throughout the treatment, even though they play central roles.

Over time, those in the mental health field learn that they are limited in how effective they can be in changing the lives of people who go to them for help. However, as you will discover in this book, therapy is effective, and the majority of treatments do result in significant improvement in the lives of clients and their families.

Return to the Case: Pedro Padilla

Pedro, a young lawyer, was prescribed antianxiety medication through the psychiatrist at the mental health clinic. Within 4 weeks, he reported that he was able to sleep through the night and was feeling less restless. His psychotherapy focused on relaxation techniques such as deep breathing as well as cognitive techniques such as labeling and challenging his worrying, and coming up with various ways to cope with stress rather than worrying excessively. Therapy was also helpful for Pedro to discuss and sort through his feelings about his parents' divorce, and to understand how his anxiety affected his romantic relationships.

Dr. Tobin's reflections: Typical of many individuals with GAD, Pedro has always felt like a constant "worrier," but this anxiety was recently aggravated by a stressful event: his parents' divorce. Additionally, his lack of sleep was likely contributing to his difficulty with the concentration necessary for keeping up with the standards of work required in his career. Since he had been doing well at work up until this point, Pedro may not have felt that his anxiety was a problem. His anxiety may have also gone unnoticed due to the intense pressure and sacrifice that all individuals face who work in Pedro's career area. Further, he may have internalized cultural beliefs from his family about discussing and seeking help for mental health concerns.

It was clear, however, that Pedro worried about many issues to a greater degree than others did in his situation. At the time he presented for treatment, his inability to control his worry over his parents and his girlfriend was causing major problems in his work and social life. Not only that, but his past anxiety had caused problems that he did not recognize at the time. For many people who suffer from GAD, the longer it goes untreated, the worse it may get.

Fortunately for Pedro, his girlfriend recognized that he was struggling and he was able to obtain help for his overwhelming anxiety. I am pleased with the progress of therapy so far. It will be important to talk with Pedro during treatment about his beliefs around having anxiety, as well as his experience of seeking out mental health treatment, which understandably might feel very challenging and uncomfortable at first. However I have hope that, given his many strengths, Pedro will be able to manage his symptoms through the psychological methods over which he is gaining mastery. Pedro has the potential to be a successful lawyer, and given his strong relationship with Natalia, I am hopeful that he will be able to turn his life around with only a slight chance of re-experiencing these symptoms.

SUMMARY

- People working in the field of mental health use both *client* and *patient* to refer to those who use psychological services. Our preference is to use the term *client*, reflecting the view that clinical interventions are a collaborative endeavor.
- The person providing the treatment is the clinician. There are many types of clinicians who approach clinical work in a variety of ways based on training and orientation. These include psychiatrists, clinical psychologists, social workers, counselors, therapists, and nurses. The field also includes those who do not have graduate-level training. These include occupational therapists, recreational therapists, and counselors who work in institutions, agencies, schools, and homes.
- Clinicians and researchers use the *Diagnostic and Statistical Manual of Mental Disorders, Fifth Edition-Text Revision* (*DSM-5-TR*) to diagnose psychological disorders. In recent editions, authors of the *DSM* have strived to meet the criterion of reliability so that a clinician can consistently apply a diagnosis to anyone showing a particular set of symptoms. At the same time, researchers have worked to ensure the validity of the classification system so that the various diagnoses represent real and distinct clinical phenomena.
- The *DSM-5-TR* presents diagnoses organized into 22 chapters. The classification system is descriptive rather than explanatory, and it is categorical rather than dimensional. Additional chapters provide usage guides and suggestions for alternative diagnostic approaches requiring further testing.
- The diagnostic process uses all relevant information to arrive at a label that characterizes a client's disorder. Key to diagnosis is gaining as clear a description as possible of a client's symptoms, both those the client reports and those the clinician observes. Differential diagnosis, the ruling out of alternate diagnoses, is a crucial step in the diagnostic process.
- To gain full appreciation of the client's disorder, the clinician develops a case formulation: analysis of the client's development and the factors that might have influenced his or her current psychological status.
- A cultural formulation accounts for the client's cultural background in making diagnoses.
- Culture-bound syndromes are behavior patterns that are unique to particular cultures.
- Clinicians typically follow up the diagnostic phase by setting up a treatment plan, the outline for how therapy should take place. The first step in a treatment plan is for the clinician to establish treatment goals, ranging from immediate to long term.
- Treatment sites vary in the degree to which they provide a controlled environment and in the nature of the services that clients receive. These include psychiatric hospitals, inpatient treatment centers, and outpatient treatment ranging from a private therapist's office or telemental health site to a community-based mental health center. Other treatment sites include halfway houses, Veterans Affairs Medical Centers, day treatment programs, schools, and workplaces.
- Modality, or the form in which one offers psychotherapy, is also a crucial component of the treatment plan. It can be individual, family, group, or milieu therapy. Whatever treatment or modality a clinician recommends, it must be based on the choice of the most appropriate theoretical perspective or combination of perspectives.
- In optimal situations, psychotherapy is a joint enterprise in which clients play an active role. In the best of all possible worlds, the client remains in treatment until the treatment runs its course, and the client shows improvement and maintains the improved level of functioning. Although not always successful, the majority of treatments do result in significant improvement.

KEY TERMS

Axis
Case formulation
Client
Clinical psychologist
Clinician
Community mental health center (CMHC)
Counseling
Couples therapy
Cultural concepts of distress
Cultural formulation
Day treatment program
Diagnostic and Statistical Manual of Mental Disorders, Fifth Edition-Text Revision (DSM-5-TR)
Differential diagnosis
Evidence-based practice in psychology
Family therapy
Group therapy
Halfway house
Individual psychotherapy
International Classification of Diseases (ICD)
Milieu therapy
Modality
Multiaxial system
Multiculturally competent care
Patient
Principal diagnosis
Psychiatrist
Psychologist
Psychotherapy
Reliability
Remission
Telemental health
Telepsychology
Treatment plan
Validity

CHAPTER 3

Assessment

OUTLINE

Learning Objectives

3.1 Define key concepts of assessment.

3.2 Describe clinical interviews.

3.3 Identify mental status examination.

3.4 Explain intelligence testing.

3.5 Describe personality testing.

3.6 Recognize behavioral assessment.

3.7 Identify multicultural assessment.

3.8 Explain neuropsychological assessment.

3.9 Describe neuroimaging.

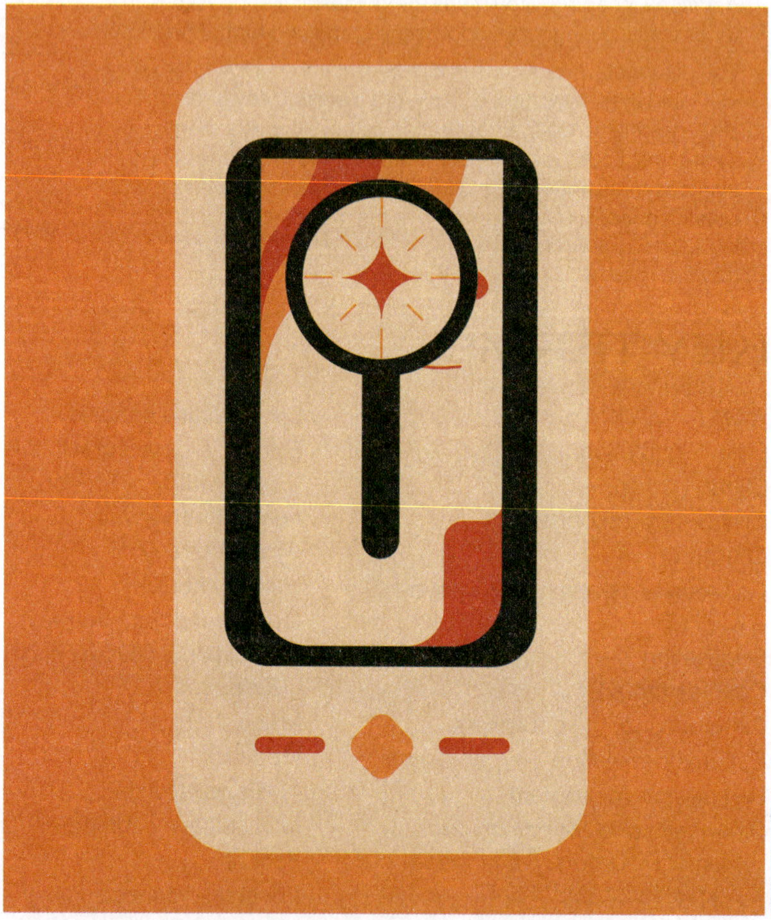

Martin_Mailz/Shutterstock

Case Report

Ben Robsham

Demographic information: 22-year-old Black gay cisgender man. Ben's pronouns are he/him/his.

History of present illness: Ben's supervisor referred him for an assessment at his employer's employee assistance program following an incident in which Ben hit his head while operating a subway train. When driving aboveground, Ben reported that the brakes jammed as he was coming to an intersection where pedestrians were crossing. Using the emergency brake, Ben was able to stop the train, but the abrupt halt caused him to hit his head on the glass window and temporarily lose consciousness. He is unable to recall what happened directly after he hit his head. Ben took a 2-week leave of absence after the incident and avoided going to work for an additional 2 weeks. When his supervisor called him, Ben stated, "I can't leave my house. They'll come and get me."

Psychiatric history: Ben has no history of psychiatric treatment. He stated that he has never experienced depression or anxiety, and that he typically feels "just fine," which has made the recent changes in his psychological state all the more disturbing to him. Ben reported that he has never used drugs and only occasionally drinks when he is in a social environment. Additionally, Ben reported that his maternal grandfather and uncle had both been diagnosed with schizophrenia. Finally, Ben reported having no remarkable past or current medical history.

Risk level: Low risk. Ben denies any current suicidal ideation, and has no past history of suicide attempts.

Case formulation: Because Ben's symptoms emerged following the incident, Ben will be referred for neuropsychological testing to rule out possible traumatic brain injury.

Diagnosis: Rule out mild neurocognitive disorder due to traumatic brain injury with behavioral disturbance.

Treatment plan: After an initial intake interview at the employee assistance program, Ben was referred for further psychological evaluation and psychiatric consultation to Dr. Antwan Washington, a neuropsychologist. The tests administered by Dr. Washington are in Table 1.

Sarah Tobin, PhD
Referring Clinician

TABLE 1 **Tests Administered to Ben**

Clinical Interview
Wechsler Adult Intelligence Scale, Fifth Edition (WAIS-5)
Trail-Making Test, Parts A and B
Clock Drawing Test
Paced Auditory Serial Addition Test (PASAT)
Boston Naming Test, Second Edition (BNT)
Wechsler Memory Scale (WMS)
Minnesota Multiphasic Personality Inventory-2 (MMPI-2)

3.1 Characteristics of Psychological Assessments

psychological assessment
A broad range of measurement techniques, all of which involve having people provide scorable information about their psychological functioning.

standardization
A psychometric criterion that clearly specifies a test's instructions for administration and scoring.

evidence-based assessment
Assessment that requires the identification of strategies that maximize diagnostic accuracy, informs treatment planning, and makes efficient use of clinician and patient time and resources.

A **psychological assessment** is a broad range of measurement techniques, all of which involve having people provide scorable information about their psychological functioning. You will see as we discuss Ben's case that a comprehensive assessment proved valuable in helping to understand the nature of his symptoms and potential directions for treatment.

Although the basic principles are the same across assessment methods, there are several types of assessments that vary according to the purpose toward which clinicians will use them. A diagnostic assessment provides a diagnosis, or at least a tentative diagnosis, of an individual's psychological disorder. Forensic assessments are used in the context of criminal cases where legal determinations are made on the basis of the psychologist's findings. In employment settings, an assessment provides information that an employer can use to evaluate whether a job applicant is suited for a position. Other assessments are conducted to evaluate whether an individual has suffered brain damage due to an accident or disease. Whatever the exact purpose of the assessment, the psychologist who conducts it is required to be objective, thorough, and knowledgeable about the most appropriate tools.

In Ben's case, the clinician must evaluate the potential contribution of the injury itself as well as the appearance of symptoms unrelated to the train incident. Dr. Tobin provided an initial evaluation, and as a result of this assessment, she decided to refer Ben to a specialist in the area of traumatic brain injury.

As you learned in Chapter 2, the tests that clinicians use in the assessment process must be held to high standards of consistency and accuracy. Just to remind you, to be reliable, the test should produce the same results regardless of when it is given, and the individual should answer items within the same subscale of a test in reasonably similar fashion. The validity of a test reflects the extent to which a test measures what it is designed to measure. An intelligence test should measure intelligence, not personality. Before using a given test, clinicians should be aware of its reliability and validity, information that is readily available in the published literature about the measurement.

A test will be reliable and valid only to the extent that it is administered and scored similarly from person to person. In other words, it should meet the criterion of **standardization**, meaning that the test has clear instructions for administration and scoring. Each person conducting the assessment should do so in accordance with instructions. Similarly, test scores should be calculated in the same manner for everyone according to the same predefined criteria. Furthermore, clinicians must have a consistent way of interpreting scores based on a clear statistical set of formulas.

In addition to ensuring a test's reliability and validity, clinicians should take into account its applicability to the diversity of people who will be taking the test. Test publishers design their measures for use by individuals from a range of ability levels, first languages, cultural backgrounds, and age. Clinicians need to ensure that they are using the most appropriate instrument for a given client. For example, it would not be appropriate to use a test standardized for young adults to conduct an assessment on an older adult unless the test's equivalence across age groups has been firmly established (Kiosses & Marino, 2019).

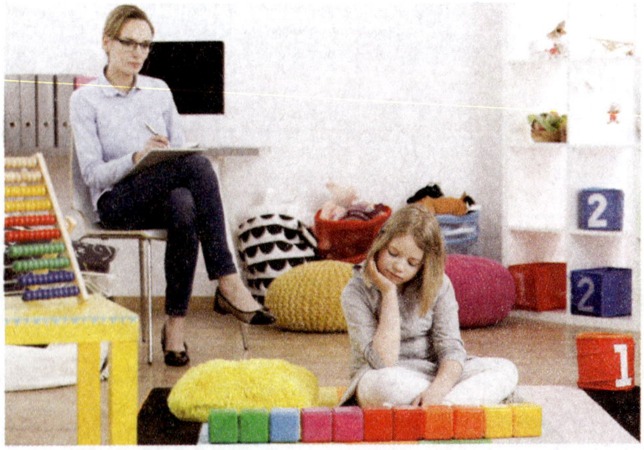

A psychologist assesses a child with a form of autistic disorder.
Photographee.eu/Shutterstock

As is true for evidence-based practice, clinicians need to ensure that their assessments follow certain guidelines, known as **evidence-based assessment**. To conform with these principles, an assessment instrument should maximize the accuracy of the diagnosis, be usable in treatment planning for the client, and make efficient use of the time and resources available both to the clinician and to the client (Ford-Paz et al., 2020). By following these guidelines, clinicians ensure that they will evaluate their clients using the most current and appropriate materials available.

Consider the case of a seasoned clinician who remains attached to the assessment methods they learned about in graduate school

20 or 30 years ago because they are comfortable using them and feel confident about their validity. Although the method might still be appropriate for the purposes of their work, they should continue to evaluate them critically, particularly given the availability of newer procedures that could better serve the purpose. To be consistent with cultural factors in assessment, clinicians should also consider the possibility that newer assessment methods have become available that take these factors into account. For example, most current assessment procedures are based on heteronormative language (in which heterosexuality and gender identities along the gender binary are the default) and therefore are not appropriate for individuals with expansive gender identities (Oberheim, Swank, & DePue, 2017). As newer instruments become available that are normed for these expansive gender identities (e.g., Feinstein et al., 2022), clinicians should begin to incorporate them into their assessments.

3.2 Clinical Interview

Clinicians typically begin their assessment with the **clinical interview**, a series of questions that they administer in face-to-face or virtual interaction with the client. The answers to these questions provide important background information, allow clients to describe their symptoms in their own words, and enable clinicians to make observations of their clients to help guide decisions about the next steps, which may include further testing.

clinical interview
A series of questions that clinicians administer in face-to-face interaction with the client.

Unstructured Interview

The least formal version of the clinical interview is the **unstructured interview**, which consists of a series of open-ended questions regarding the client's symptoms, health status, family background, life history, and reasons for seeking help. In addition to noting the answers to these questions, the clinician also observes the client's level of comfort, apparent mood, extraneous comments, and any other behaviors that might inform the clinician in understanding the client's psychological state. For example, people with major depressive disorder may show a range of behaviors indicating sadness such as frowning, avoiding eye contact, and a tendency to stay as far away as possible from the clinician (Fiquer et al., 2018).

unstructured interview
A series of open-ended questions aimed at determining the client's reasons for being in treatment, symptoms, health status, family background, and life history.

The clinician may also use cues from the client's appearance that give further indication of the client's symptoms. A person with an unusually disheveled appearance may be experiencing cognitive symptoms that interfere with their ability to care for personal hygiene. Other cues given by a person's clothing and overall appearance may also suggest their attitudes, values, and interests.

The typical unstructured clinical interview covers the areas outlined in Table 2. Because the clinical interview allows for more freedom of administration than a test with preset questions and response categories, the clinician can vary the order of questions and the exact wording they use during the interview. Furthermore, its length can be adjusted based on what the clinician finds out, although the typical length is 30 to 45 minutes. The main feature of the unstructured interview is that it does not have a preset order, although each clinician may have certain preferences about which questions to ask and how to word them.

In Ben's case, the clinical interview provided Dr. Tobin with key information about his history including his education, vocational background, and relationship history. She determined that, prior to the incident, he enjoyed engaging with others, so his current isolation is a change from his previous pattern of social functioning. He appeared slightly disheveled in his clothing and general grooming status. It is difficult to know exactly what this might mean without knowing Ben's typical appearance prior to the incident, so Dr. Tobin may make note of these features but reserve judgment on their meaning.

Dr. Washington obtained more detailed information from Ben in his initial interview with him. Ben stated that he has difficulty concentrating, and that his main symptom is the

TABLE 2 Areas Covered in a Clinical Interview

Topic	Purpose
Age, gender, race, sexual orientation, and pronouns	Obtain basic demographic information and material to center important aspects of the individual's identity.
Reason for referral	Hear client's reason for seeking treatment, in their own words.
Education and work history	Obtain socioeconomic status and gain understanding of client's occupational and educational context.
Current social situation	Find out whether client is currently in a relationship and how much social support is potentially available.
Cultural considerations	Obtain information about gender identity, religious and spiritual identity, racial identity, and other sociocultural factors such as nationality, languages spoken, and immigration status (if applicable) to help with cultural formulation.
Physical and mental health history	Determine whether client has any medical illnesses and whether there has been a recent change in health.
	Find out about history of present problem including past diagnoses and treatments and whether treatment was helpful or not.
Drug/alcohol use and current medication	Ascertain whether client is using psychoactive substances (including alcohol and caffeine). Obtain list of prescriptions to avoid potential interactions with any psychotropic medications.
Family history	Find out whether client's family has medical and psychological disorders, particularly any relevant to client's current symptoms.
Behavioral observations	Note behaviors, including nonverbal behaviors, that indicate whether client is experiencing anxiety or altered mood. Also note whether client seems to be experiencing difficulties in attention or compliance. Attempt to determine client's mental status. Compare client's appearance with stated age. Determine whether client is oriented to time, place, and person. Observe any unusual motor behaviors.

occurrence of "very strange thoughts" that have been quite troubling to him. Specifically, he stated that he feels too afraid to leave his apartment because he believes that the police will apprehend and arrest him as punishment for "what [he] did." Although there were no fatalities, Ben worries that others blame him for killing passengers and if he returned to work the passengers would turn on him, thus resulting in his apprehension. He states that he spends several hours a day worrying about the consequences of the incident and sometimes hears accusatory voices blaming him for hurting people and telling him that he is a "monster." He reported that he has heard these voices only a few times in the past 4 weeks.

Though Ben reports that he feels distressed about his recent psychological problems, he stated that he had no thoughts of hurting or killing himself. He also stated that he has been unable to get a full night's sleep since the incident. In response to Dr. Washington's further questioning, Ben reports that he has difficulty falling asleep, and when he does sleep, he is awakened by frequent nightmares about the incident. He feels that those he believes he killed are "haunting" him.

Ben stated that although he was worried about what he had been experiencing recently, he had been too embarrassed to tell anyone, worrying that he was "going crazy." Since he had not spent time with friends or family and had not been to work, the people in his life were unaware of the extent of his recent psychological difficulties. Ben took a leave of absence for the first 2 weeks following the incident and has since been calling in sick daily. He seemed somewhat relieved to be seen clinically, hoping this process might help reveal the nature of his troubling symptoms.

As you can see from Ben's case, the clinical interview can become a key step in the diagnostic process because of the information it provides regarding the client's current symptoms, history, and availability of social support. In addition, this interview had the added benefit of providing Dr. Washington with the chance to establish the rapport with Ben that would be necessary as the assessment progressed.

Structured Interview

Unlike the clinical interview, the **structured interview** uses a series of assessment questions that follow a predetermined wording and order. A structured interview can either provide a diagnosis on which to further base treatment or classify the client's symptoms into a *DSM* disorder. Structured interviews have the advantage of being standardized, making them less subject to variation from clinician to clinician.

structured interview
A standardized series of assessment questions that follow a predetermined wording and order.

The **Structured Clinical Interview for *DSM-5* Disorders-Clinical Version (SCID-5-CV)** (First, Williams, Karg, & Spitzer, 2016) provides clinicians with a step-by-step pathway through the diagnostic process. The SCID-5-Research Version is a companion instrument used for research purposes, such as in epidemiological studies on particular disorders or as a way to ensure that participants in a given study meet the diagnostic criteria for the condition being investigated. There is also a version of the SCID-5 designed specifically to assess personality disorders. Although written based on the *DSM*-5, the SCID-5-CV is the instrument's current form.

Structured Clinical Interview for *DSM-5* Disorders (SCID-5)
A structured clinical interview developed to assess *DSM-5* symptoms.

The SCID-5-CV is structured to guide the clinician along each step of *DSM-5* diagnostic process. The clinician begins by reading the interview questions provided for each corresponding *DSM-5* criterion, noting whether each symptom is present or absent. As the interview proceeds, the clinician adapts the questions based on prior responses from the client. For example, if a client states that they have symptoms of anxiety, the interviewer would follow up with questions about these symptoms but otherwise would skip down or move on to the next area of the interview. The SCID-5-CV takes 45 to 90 minutes to administer, depending on the complexity of the client's symptoms.

There is empirical support for use of the SCID-5-CV. A large-scale international study found that the instrument has high levels of reliability in terms of agreement across multiple raters. The instrument also provides diagnoses that correspond to those arrived at through longer-term, more intense clinical methods (Osório et al., 2019).

One key practical advantage is that anyone with proper training can administer the SCID-5-CV. This means that the instrument can be administered as part of an initial screening by, for example, licensed mental health professionals. Similarly, its companion instrument used for research can also be administered by an interviewer without an advanced psychology degree.

3.3 Mental Status Examination

A clinician uses a **mental status examination** to assess objectively a client's behavior and functioning in a number of spheres, with particular attention to the symptoms associated with psychological disturbance. In conducting a mental status examination, the clinician systematically assesses a number of features of the client, including appearance, attitudes, behavior, mood and affect, speech, thought processes, content of thought, perception, cognition, insight, and judgment. You can read more about instruments used in mental status examinations later in this chapter.

mental status examination
A method of objectively assessing a client's behavior and functioning in a number of spheres, with particular attention to the symptoms associated with psychological disturbance.

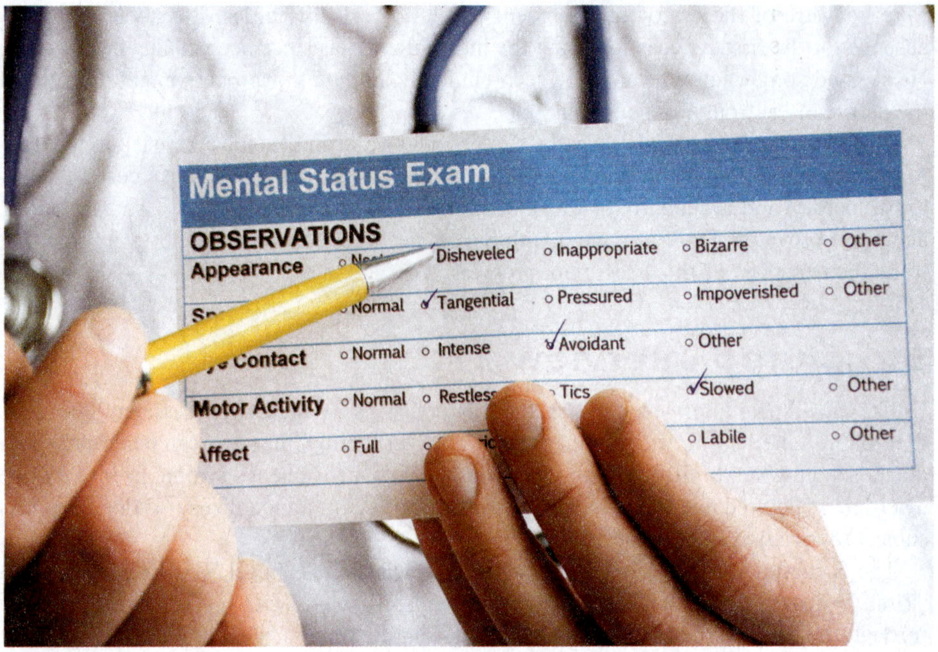

In a mental status examination, clinicians objectively document a client's behavior and functioning.

Shidlovski/Shutterstock

In Ben's case, Dr. Washington utilized a mental status exam, and through this tool, he noted that Ben was not experiencing an altered mental state at the time of the interview. He arrived on time and was alert, had no difficulty with his memory, and was fully aware of his surroundings. His speech was normal in tone, rhythm, volume, and rate; in other words, he spoke to Dr. Washington without any apparent limitation on his ability to carry out a conversation.

Ben also showed no deficits in his ability to understand Dr. Washington, and he was able to follow the instructions for each of the tests that he went on to complete. His affect was appropriate, meaning that his apparent emotional state matched that expected in the situation, though he made a few self-deprecating jokes when he became frustrated during the administration of a test he found difficult. In general, though, he cooperated with the examiner and appeared motivated and interested in the tests themselves. Dr. Washington then proceeded directly to the next, more comprehensive, phase of testing.

3.4 Intelligence Testing

Clinicians use intelligence tests to serve a variety of functions, including diagnosis of learning disabilities, determination of giftedness or intellectual developmental disorder, and prediction of future academic achievement. These tests have a long history in psychology, dating back to 1905, when the French psychologist Alfred Binet (1857–1911) devised a test for use in school children. Current tests continue to draw from the original scales even while updating the basis for scoring and many of the subtests (Gibbons & Warne, 2019).

Intelligence tests can also aid clinicians in the diagnosis of neurological and psychiatric disorders as a component of a more comprehensive assessment procedure. Those working in human resource departments within business and industry can administer intelligence tests in order to evaluate the potential for employees to perform in specific conditions. Of course, intelligence tests continue to be administered in educational settings, particularly when decisions must be made about grade or classroom placement.

The most commonly used intelligence tests in clinical settings are administered on a one-to-one basis, providing a comprehensive view of the client's knowledge of words and facts, and abilities to perform a range of perceptual, memory, reasoning, and timed tasks. There are also paper-and-pencil, or computer-administered, intelligence tests that can provide scores to be used in research, group, or employment settings.

Stanford-Binet Intelligence Test

First developed in the early 1900s by Alfred Binet (1857–1911) to measure the intelligence of children, the Stanford-Binet is now in its fifth edition, known as the **Stanford-Binet 5 (SB5)**. The SB5 produces what is known as a **deviation intelligence (IQ)** score. The test administrator records the scores from each test and then converts them to standardized scores that reflect where the individual stands in relationship to others of similar age and gender. The average deviation IQ score is set at 100 with a standard deviation of 15. If a child receives an SB5 IQ score of 115, this means the child stands at or above the IQ of 84 percent of the population.

In addition to yielding an overall IQ score, the SB5 yields scores on measures of scales labeled Fluid Reasoning, Knowledge, Quantitative Reasoning, Visuospatial Reasoning, and Working Memory (Table 3). As you can see from these descriptions, the scales provide a more in-depth understanding of the child's cognitive strengths and weaknesses than can be conveyed in an overall IQ score.

Stanford-Binet 5 (SB5)
Individually administered test of intelligence, most commonly used in assessing children.

deviation intelligence (IQ)
An index of intelligence derived from comparing the individual's score on an intelligence test with the mean score for that individual's reference group.

Wechsler Intelligence Scales

The first comprehensive individual test specifically designed to measure adult intelligence was the **Wechsler Adult Intelligence Scale (WAIS)**. Originally developed in 1939 by Bellevue Hospital (New York City) psychologist David Wechsler (1896–1981), the WAIS is now in its fifth edition (WAIS-5) (Wechsler, 2024).

Wechsler Adult Intelligence Scale (WAIS)
The first comprehensive individual test that researchers specifically designed to measure adult intelligence.

TABLE 3 Types of Abilities Assessed by the Stanford-Binet 5 (SB5)

Scale	Definition	Example
Fluid Reasoning	Ability to solve novel problems	Sort picture chips into groups of three
Knowledge	Accumulated fund of general information	Show how to perform a given action
Quantitative Reasoning	Ability to solve problems with numbers or numerical concepts	Count a set of items
Visual-Spatial Reasoning	Ability to analyze spatial relationships and geometric concepts	Assemble puzzle-like forms
Working Memory	Ability to store, transform, and retrieve information in short-term memory	Recall a sequence of taps

SOURCE: Roid, G. H., & Barram, R. A. (2004). *Essentials of Stanford-Binet Intelligence Scales (SB5) assessment.* Hoboken, NJ: Wiley.

The WAIS has its counterparts in parallel tests for children that use the same format as the adult scales. These include the Wechsler Intelligence Scale for Children–Fifth Edition (WISC-V) (Wechsler, 2014) and the Wechsler Preschool and Primary Scale of Intelligence–Fourth Edition (WPPSI-IV) (Wechsler, 2012).

Wechsler originally sought to develop a tool that he could use in clinical settings for understanding an adult's intellectual functioning. He believed that it was important to include not only tests of vocabulary and knowledge but also those that would tap into an individual's intelligence through pictures and actions. Originally he labeled these two categories of tests as "Verbal" and "Performance." For many years, clinicians reported the WAIS scores in terms of these two categories of subtests; however, over time it became increasingly evident that these two categorical scores did not adequately capture the full complexity of intellectual functioning. The WAIS-5 includes new test items, several new tests, and a completely different scoring system compared to its predecessors. Administered on a tablet, the WAIS-5 also provides precise timing of responses, allowing measures of speed to accurately be factored into scale scores.

The WAIS-5, like its predecessors and the SB5, can produce an overall IQ score based on an age-normed mean of 100 and standard deviation of 15. The full scale score is not as useful for clinical purposes as are the primary index scores, The five index scale scores allow clinicians to examine in depth the client's cognitive functioning along these key dimensions.

Figure 1 illustrates the structure of the WAIS-5 along with its index scores. At the top is the Full Scale IQ (FSIQ), which reflects general cognitive functioning and, as mentioned earlier, provides the least amount of specificity. In general, the Verbal Comprehension scales measure knowledge gained through educational experiences, corresponding to crystallized intelligence. Visual spatial scales include problem-solving with computer-presented blocks or puzzles. Fluid reasoning scales tap into an individual's ability to solve problems, particularly those that are nonverbal and mathematical. Working Memory scales include Running Digits, in which individuals must recall the last string of a set of numbers. Digits forward and backward involve recalling either in order, or backwards, a short series of numbers. Processing Speed tests use nonverbal symbols that the test taker must learn to associate with digits (Coding) or to find among a more complex array (Symbol Search).

Because the WAIS-5 is given on an individual basis, clinicians have ample opportunities to observe the test-taker's behavior during the test, possibly gaining valuable diagnostic information to complement the test scores. In fact, the instructions for WAIS scoring

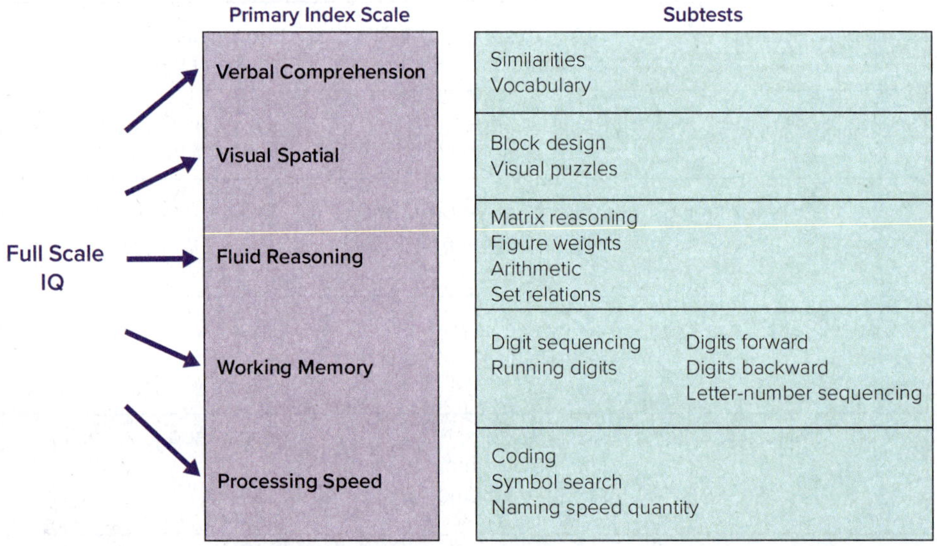

FIGURE 1 Structure of the WAIS-5

*Supplemental subtest

procedures have included for the examiner to include behavioral observations such as the individual's native language fluency; physical appearance; problems with vision, hearing, or motor behavior; difficulties with attention and concentration; motivation for testing; and any unusual behaviors that the test-taker shows.

Researchers and clinicians alike who use the WAIS-5 recognize the importance of ensuring its applicability to test-takers from a variety of diverse backgrounds. There have long existed controversies about the meaning of differences in intelligence test scores among racial and ethnic groups on the various versions of the WAIS. Test-taking biases can result in invalid placement and decisions about diagnoses, especially if the test norms were developed on samples that differ culturally from those of the individual test-taker (Shuttleworth-Edwards, 2016).

In addition, clinicians should take into account whether, based on language, the normative sample is an appropriate one for a given client. For example, a study comparing rural adults living in Russia and the United States showed that the Russian test-takers placed less value on their timed performance than did the Americans (Melikyan, Puente, & Agranovich, 2021). If nothing else, as suggested by a study of Māori of New Zealand (Dudley, Barker-Collo, Wilson, & Garrett, 2019), administrators and test-takers should ideally be ethnically matched. Such an approach can help to maximize rapport and reduce anxiety on the part of the test-taker, leading to a more accurate estimate of abilities.

Table 4 shows Ben's performance on the WAIS-IV which was the predecessor to the WAIS-5, many of whose tests remain in place with the most recent version. Ben's FSIQ was 115, indicating that he has an above-average level of performance (higher than 84 percent of the population). If you look across the entire pattern of his scores, however, you'll notice that Ben demonstrated high variability among the index scores that make up the FSIQ. This type of variability suggests a wide range to Ben's cognitive abilities. The clinician found it noteworthy that Ben's Processing Speed cluster score was low (higher than only 40 percent of the population), suggesting that Ben struggles with the perception of visual patterns and stimuli, particularly when speed is a factor. The appearance of this low test score where he should have performed well given his job suggests possible injury to the areas of his brain involved in processing of spatial information.

While administering the WAIS-IV, Dr. Washington carefully recorded Ben's behaviors, further fleshing out the picture provided by the test scores themselves. Ben stated several times throughout the testing session that "they give you fake confidence early on," referring to his frustration as the test became more difficult. Despite his frustration, Ben remained determined to complete the test. For example, he took nearly 6 minutes to complete the

TABLE 4 **Ben's WAIS-IV Scores**

Full Scale:	115		
Verbal Comprehension Index	132		
Perceptual Reasoning Index	107		
Working Memory Index	111		
Processing Speed Index	97		
Individual Subtests:			
Vocabulary:	15	Picture Completion:	12
Similarities:	17	Coding:	7
Arithmetic:	13	Block Design:	10
Digit Span:	11	Matrix Reasoning:	14
Information:	14	Symbol Search:	12
Comprehension:	18	Figure Weights:	13
Letter-Number Seq.:	10	Visual Puzzles:	10
		Cancellation:	12

final Block Design item (far longer than average) and finally stated, "It doesn't make sense—there aren't enough blocks." On the Matrix Reasoning subtest, Ben took nearly 1 minute for each response toward the end of the task. While completing the Figure Weights subtest, Ben commented on what the shapes in the stimulus book looked like and made several jokes throughout the subtest administration. On the Letter-Number Sequencing task, before giving his response to each item, Ben described how each correlated with the name of a different type of army ship or plane. As the tests became more difficult toward the end of the testing session, Ben appeared visibly restless and began to tap his fingers and tap on his legs. On tasks requiring verbal responses, Ben provided long elaborations, and when the test required a short answer, he would sometimes respond in a sing-song voice.

3.5 Personality Testing

Tests of personality provide insight into a person's thoughts, behaviors, and emotions. There are a variety of personality tests that clinicians adapt for such purposes as diagnosis, case formulation, or research. The choice of a personality test to use may reflect not only its potential applications, but the particular theoretical orientation guiding the clinician's work. Clinicians may also choose which personality tests to use based on a client's presenting problem, as in the case of assisting in the diagnosis of a personality disorder.

Outside the clinical realm, personality tests provide valuable information that researchers use to test predictions related to their own particular area of investigation. For example, researchers might examine whether scores on a personality test measuring self-esteem are related to scores on another measure of optimism.

Self-Report Tests

self-report clinical inventory
A psychological test with standardized questions having fixed response categories that the test-taker completes independently, self-reporting the extent to which the responses are accurate characterizations.

Perhaps the most common form of personality test for use in diagnosis, a **self-report clinical inventory** contains standardized questions with fixed response categories that the test-taker completes independently either in paper-and-pencil or, increasingly, in online format. In a self-report inventory, test-takers rate the extent to which the items apply to them on a fixed scale of, for example, 7 = strongly agree to 1 = strongly disagree.

A major advantage of self-report inventories is that they are relatively easy to administer and score. Consequently, large numbers of people can take them in an efficient manner. Using predetermined criteria to interpret the scores, computers can even produce brief explanatory reports. Clinicians can incorporate some or all of these reports in their case formulations based on the additional material they collect through other assessment methods.

Self-report tests also have the advantage of providing clinicians with a wealth of information about the validity and reliability of the better-known self-report inventories when interpreting the scores of their own clients. At the same time, the clinician can determine whether the test meets the criteria of cultural fairness that has been validated in samples of similar age, ethnicity, and cultural background as that of the client (Melikyan, Agranovich, & Puente, 2019).

Minnesota Multiphasic Personality Inventory-3 (MMPI-3)
Self-report personality inventory containing 335 true/false items, all in the form of statements that describe the individual's thoughts, behaviors, feelings, and attitudes.

MMPI-3 The most widely used self-report clinical instrument is the **Minnesota Multiphasic Personality Inventory-3 (MMPI-3)**, the most recent version of the test originally published in 1943. Developed as a tool intended to provide clinical diagnoses, the original MMPI contained 10 scales corresponding to specific diagnoses, such as depression, schizophrenia, and hypomania. The MMPI also was designed to detect inconsistent or fabricated responding through additional "validity" scales.

The current version of the test is the 2020 revision known as the MMPI-3 (Ben-Porath & Tellegen, 2020). After undergoing a set of prior improvements, including versions known as the MMPI-2 and the MMPI-2-RF, the MMPI-3 represents the first major revamping of the instrument since 1989. There are 335 true/false items on the MMPI-3, all in the form of statements that describe the individual's thoughts, behaviors, feelings, and attitudes. These items represent a combination of items on the original MMPI and items added during subsequent revisions. The new items not only replaced outdated language used in the original instrument but also addressed limitations in the clinical scale scores, which had become apparent in the decades after its publication and subsequent widespread use. Primarily, these scores did not correspond to the original clinical categories, meaning that the test's administrators could not interpret them as evidence of specific diagnoses. In other words, a high "Schizophrenia" scale score did not imply that the individual had a diagnosis of schizophrenia.

Additionally, the MMPI-3 scales themselves changed from an original set of 10 designed to correspond to psychiatric diagnoses to an expanded set of 52, building on those from later revisions, and adding new scales designed to tap into particular so-called "specific problems" such as eating concerns, cognitive complaints, and overall malaise or sense of physical debilitation. Table 5 contains the current eight clinical scales. There are also three so-called "higher-order" scales that address the underlying dimensions represented by the clinical scales. These higher-order scales include Emotion/Internalizing Dysfunction (problems with mood and affect), Thought Dysfunction (disordered thinking), and Behavior/Externalizing Dysfunction (under-controlled behavior) (Ben-Porath & Tellegen, 2020).

Another key change in the MMPI-3 was the use of a broader normative sample than the ones used in prior revisions. The 1,620 U.S. adults in the current MMPI-3 normative sample were chosen on the basis of the U.S. Census projections of 2020 for race and ethnicity, education, and age. Spanish-language norms for use in the United States are now also available. Increasingly, researchers are testing the MMPI-3's applicability across diverse samples, and finding support for its utility as a diagnostic instrument (e.g., Anestis et al., 2023). As a result of the inclusion of these new normative samples, the MMPI-3's score for a given client should therefore be more interpretable than was true in the past, when clinicians had to rely on the less representative samples.

Other Self-Report Inventories The SCL-90-R (Derogatis, 1994) measures the test-taker's current experiencing of 90 physical and psychological symptoms. There are nine overall symptom scales, such as Depression, Anxiety, and Hostility. Additionally, the SCL-90-R produces an overall global severity index and the number and intensity of the individual's symptoms. Unlike measures that have no defined target period, the SCL-90-R focuses on the client's current status. Because it is sensitive to the client's state, the SCL-90-R can be administered on multiple occasions, making it well suited for use by clinicians who wish to track the progress of their clients throughout the course of treatment.

TABLE 5 Restructured Clinical Scales on the MMPI®-3

Scale	Scale Name	Type of Content
RCd	Demoralization (DEM)	General unhappiness and dissatisfaction
RC1	Somatic Complaints (SOM)	Diffuse physical health complaints
RC2	Low Positive Emotions (LPE)	Lack of positive emotional responsiveness
RC4	Antisocial Behavior (ASB)	Rule breaking and irresponsible behavior
RC6	Ideas of Persecution (PER)	Belief that others pose a threat to the self
RC7	Dysfunctional Negative Emotions (DNE)	Maladaptive anxiety, anger, and irritability
RC8	Aberrant Experiences (ABX)	Unusual thoughts or perceptions
RC9	Hypomanic Activation (HPM)	Over-activation, aggression, impulsivity, and grandiosity

Restructured Clinical Scales listing. Excerpted from the *Minnesota Multiphasic Personality Inventory®-3 (MMPI®-3) Manual for Administration, Scoring, and Interpretation* by Yossef S. Ben-Porath and Auke Tellegen.

Its brief format and sensitivity to the test-taker's current state makes the SCL-90-R a useful research tool. For example, Chinese researchers used this instrument in a study of COVID-19's impact on levels of anxiety in cancer survivors. These individuals showed a pronounced increase in scores compared to their own family members and Chinese norms (Han et al., 2020).

A second widely used self-report instrument plays a prominent role in research on personality, and also has utility in the study of personality disorders. The NEO Personality Inventory (Revised) (NEO-PI-R) (Costa & McCrae, 1992) is a 240-item questionnaire that measures five personality dimensions, or sets of traits. The scales are designed so the test-taker can complete them as well as individuals who know the test-taker, such as spouses, partners, or relatives (Form R). Various forms of the NEO-PI-R are available online, some in briefer versions. There is also a free online version, known as the IPIP-NEO which provides similar trait scores that can be used in clinical as well as research-based sample (e.g., Hobbs et al., 2023).

Uses of the NEO-PI-R beyond research on personality and personality disorders can include clinical applications. For example, in a study on therapy effectiveness, Delgadillo and colleagues (Delgadillo et al., 2020) reported that personality traits of therapists were predictive of the outcomes of treatment for clients with depression and anxiety disorders.

Clinicians and researchers can also use specific self-report inventories designed to investigate a given disorder or area of interest for which a general test may not be as relevant. The Personality Inventory for the DSM-5 (PID-5) considered an "emerging measure" in the DSM-5-TR provides scores on domains within the personality disorders. As shown in a recent study comparing White U.S. college students with Black Nigerian college students, the PID continues to receive support across diverse populations (Orjiakor, Sellbom, Keeley, & Bagby, 2023). It also is shown to have utility cross-nationally, as shown in a study of Iranian adults (Ghamkhar Fard et al., 2021) and in older adults (Stone, Segal, & Krus, 2021).

Returning to Ben, you can see his MMPI-2-R scores in Figure 2. He has slightly elevated scores on the Ideas of Persecution scale and endorsed several critical items relating directly to psychosis such as "I have no enemies who really wish to harm me" (False), "I have strange and peculiar thoughts" (True), and "At times my thoughts have raced ahead faster than I could speak them" (True). According to his responses, he may have unusual thought content and may often feel suspicious that others are saying bad things about him. As a result, he may feel disconnected from reality. He may believe that his feelings and thoughts are controlled by others. His unusual thought content was evidenced at times throughout the WAIS-IV administration in his atypical reactions to certain test items. His scores on the MMPI-2-R, however, indicate that he does not tend to be impulsive or take physical risks and generally follows rules and laws. These may be protective factors for Ben, in that he may be able to maintain some control of his thoughts, which may differentiate him from those with diagnosable psychotic disorders.

Based on his scores on the MMPI-2-R (which was the current version at the time of testing), it appears that Ben has a traditional sense of masculinity and may have stereotypically masculine preferences in work, hobbies, and other activities. In the clinical interview, he reported having had no previous significant romantic relationships, which may be a result of his tendency to be guarded and hostile in his relationships with others. Ben's scores on the MMPI-2-R also suggest that he does endorse aberrant experiences, but his score on persecution is within the normative range. He also received scores above the norm on somatic complaints.

Looking at Ben's scores, Dr. Washington concluded that his limited coping resources may be a more situational than long-standing problem. Further, Ben's clinical profile suggests that he may be excessively sensitive and overly responsive to the opinions of others. He may overemphasize rationality and be moralistic and rigid in his attitudes and opinions. As a result, he may be argumentative and have a tendency to blame others and act suspicious, hostile, and guarded in relationships. This may account for his report of having few close friends at school and his preference for being alone in his dorm room.

Clinicians typically interpret MMPI scores in the context of other test scores. They also may use the content scales to flesh out the profiles provided by the basic 10 clinical scales. The Restructured MMPI-2 and MMPI-3 provide a different perspective on a client's current psychological state, because the content scales provide a more descriptive summary of the client's symptoms. Dr. Washington noted that Ben's score was high on the Demoralization scale, suggesting that Ben felt discouraged and hopeless about his current life situation.

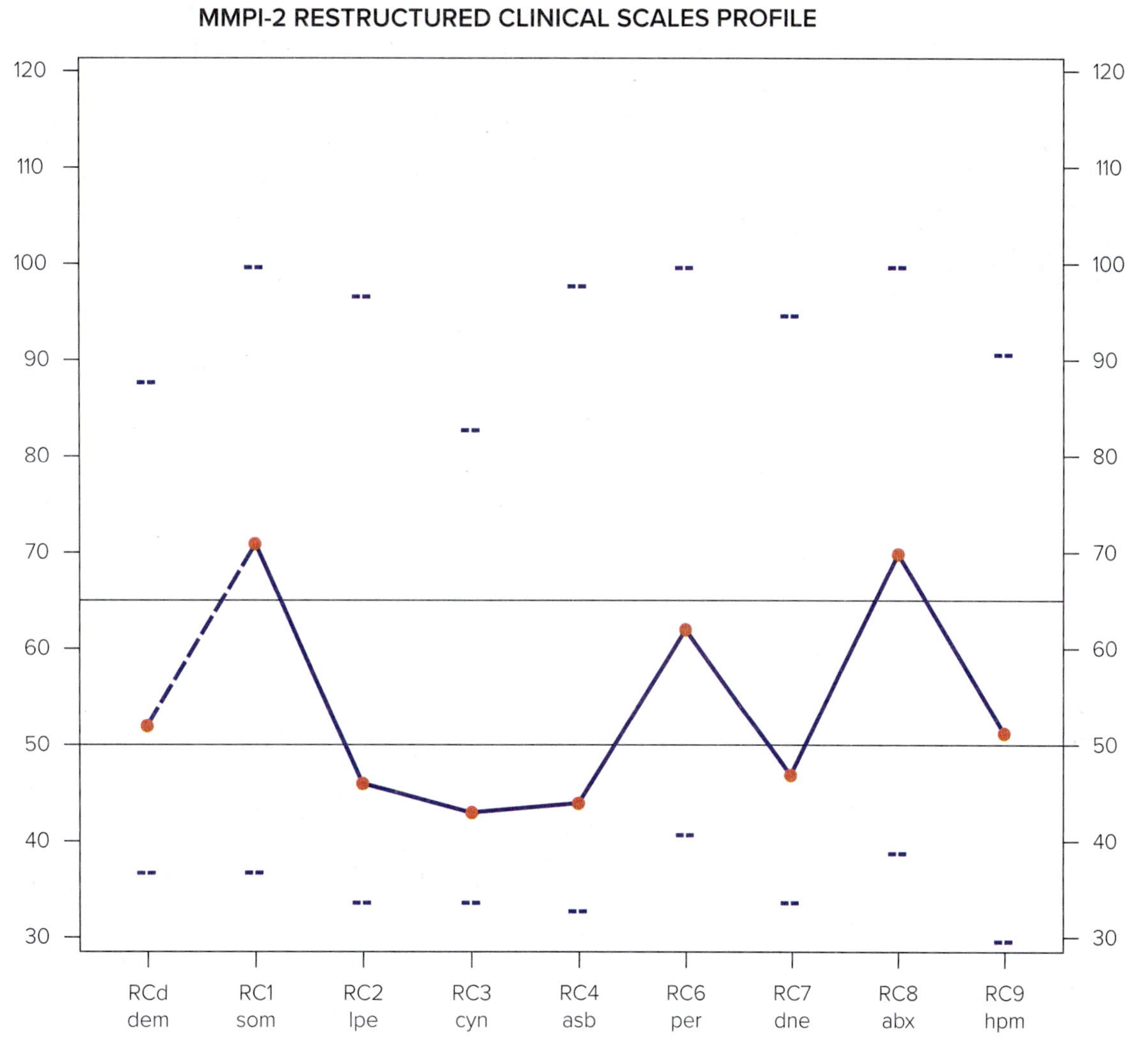

	RCd dem	RC1 som	RC2 lpe	RC3 cyn	RC4 asb	RC6 per	RC7 dne	RC8 abx	RC9 hpm
Raw score:	4	10	3	3	3	2	4	7	14
T score (plotted):	52	71	46	43	44	62	47	70	51
Non-gendered T score:	51	68	47	44	46	63	46	69	53
Response %:	100	100	100	100	100	100	100	100	100

Note: The highest and lowest uniform T scores possible on each scale are indicated by a "--".

Legend

dem = Demoralization	cyn = Cynicism	dne = Dysfunctional negative emotions
som = Somatic complaints	asb = Antisocial behavior	abx = Aberrant experiences
lpe = Low positive emotions	per = Ideas of persecution	hpm = Hypomanic activation

FIGURE 2 Ben's MMPI-2-R Profile

Projective Testing

A **projective test** is a technique in which the test-taker is presented with an ambiguous item or task and is asked to respond by providing their own meaning or perception. The underlying idea behind projective tests is that they could overcome the potential bias that exists when clients report on their own inner experiences. For example, clients may not wish to say outright that they are experiencing unusual symptoms or have qualities that could be construed in a negative light. On projective tests, clients may be less guarded about their responses because they do not know how the assessor will interpret their answers.

projective test
A technique in which the test-taker is presented with an ambiguous item or task and is asked to respond by providing his or her own meaning or perception.

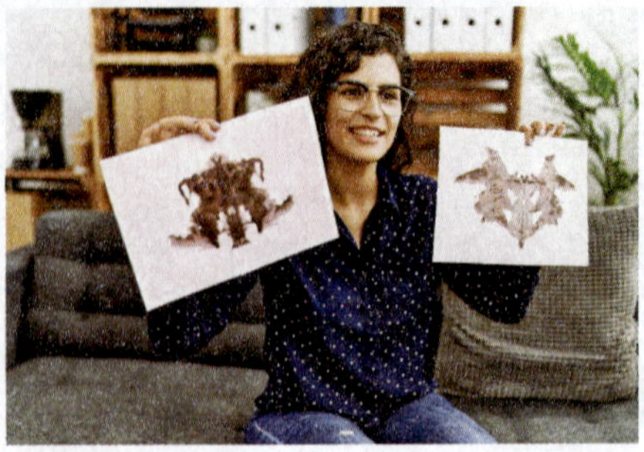

Two of the cards on the Rorschach Inkblot test.
Krakenimages.com/Shutterstock

Rorschach Inkblot Test
Projective assessment method in which individuals describe their perceptions of each of a set of symmetrical inkblots.

Thematic Apperception Test (TAT)
A projective test in which individuals invent a story to explain what is happening in a set of ambiguous pictures.

Rorschach Inkblot Test

The most famous projective technique is the **Rorschach Inkblot Test**, named after Swiss psychiatrist Hermann Rorschach, who developed the method in 1911. To administer the test, the examiner shows the test-taker a set of 10 cards one by one (5 are black and white; 5 have color). The test-taker's job is to describe what the inkblot looks like. Although the method sounds simple enough, over the last century researchers and clinicians have continued to refine the scoring methods; now there is an elaborate interpretative system in place known as the Rorschach Performance Assessment System (R-PAS) based on the idea that test itself measures behaviors in response to a specific set of stimuli (Meyer & Eblin, 2012). Researchers continue to provide data on the convergence between R-PAS scores and self-report, as shown in one study of traumatized refugees living in Norway. After undergoing psychotherapy, their scores on the two sets of measures converged, suggesting they had developed greater self-insight into their traumatic experiences (Hartmann & Opaas, 2023).

Like other clinical measures, the Rorschach has value for researchers interested in aspects of personality not necessarily tapped by self-report scales. For example, Gritti et al. (2020) found that scales derived from the Rorschach were more sensitive than self-report scales in a study of the reactions of people high in narcissism in response to threats to their self-esteem.

Thematic Apperception Test (TAT)

The **Thematic Apperception Test (TAT)** presents test-takers with a very different task than the Rorschach. Test-takers look at black-and-white drawings that portray people in a variety of ambiguous situations such as standing in a dark hallway or sitting in a bedroom. The test-taker is asked simply to tell a story about what is happening in each scene, focusing on such details as what the characters in the picture are thinking and feeling. The TAT's original purpose was to evaluate motivational needs, such as the need for achievement or the need for power. Its use has expanded to clinical settings and, like the Rorschach, better scoring systems are available to reduce the role of subjectivity in interpreting the stories that clients tell about the pictures (Jenkins, 2017).

Like the Rorschach, the TAT can provide a useful approach in studies that have clinical applications. For example, Joo and Park (2019) found that, as predicted, individuals with depressive symptoms provided TAT-based narratives higher in negative emotional tone. Those high in depression produced narratives indicating a lack of agency, or the ability to effect changes in their environment.

Projective tests are most useful when combined with self-report inventories rather than as the sole basis for diagnosing or evaluating a client. In Ben's case, Dr. Washington decided not to conduct projective testing until the neuropsychological assessment was completed. Clinicians typically do not administer these instruments as part of a standard battery, particularly if the client's symptoms might be related to a trauma or injury.

REAL STORIES

Demi Lovato (1992–Present)

From a young age, Demi Lovato—who uses they/them and she/her pronouns—has had two very distinct but intertwined personas: a beloved entertainer and a person in a deep struggle with mental health and addiction. In the 2017 documentary *Simply Complicated*, Lovato details her early challenges, beginning with her parents' divorce resulting from her father's struggles with addiction and abusive behavior. Lovato recalls starting to feel depressed around the age of 5, the same time they started modeling, singing, and participating in beauty pageants with the support of their mother.

While privately battling depression and dealing with bullying in school, Lovato landed their first acting role on the popular children's show *Barney and Friends*. They soon began playing guitar and writing songs and recalls that music felt like "an outlet to pour my emotions out and create something beautiful." The pressure to continue getting roles mounted as she continued to focus on developing their talents through acting classes and working on their music. Lovato got a part in a Disney Channel television series, which led to two more roles in *Sonny with a Chance*, and the *Camp Rock* and *Camp Rock 2* movie franchise with the Jonas Brothers. At 15, they had their first major career break, which eventually blossomed into a successful solo pop music career.

Lovato recalls in *Simply Complicated* that at this point "I definitely felt the pressure increase, when the fame started to creep into my life." She has described herself as a perfectionist who wanted to live up to

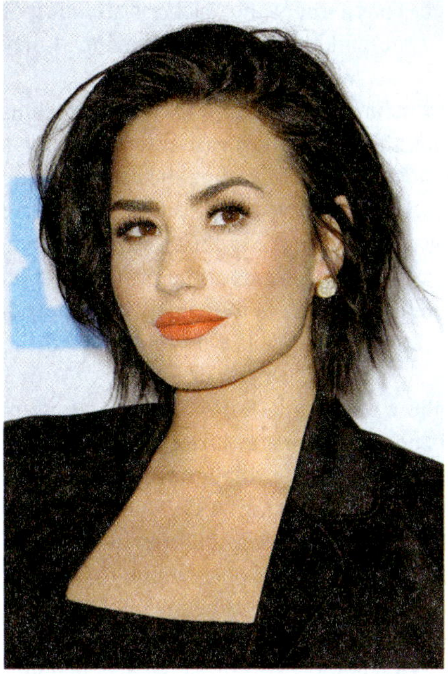

Demi Lovato attending the WE Day California in April, 2016.

Tinseltown/Shutterstock

others' expectations, despite the pressure this put on them and the compromises they were forced to make as a teenager. In the documentary, Lovato's management team describes the changes they started to notice in them, as the feelings of pressure turned into anxiety, which cascaded into concerns about their mood and overall well-being.

Then Lovato developed addictive behaviors, starting with alcohol use, which they say began when they were trying to fit in with other teenagers. She recalls trying cocaine for the first time with friends while they were 17 and working for the Disney Channel. To her, the drug felt simultaneously thrilling and frightening, as if she could easily lose control.

A particularly difficult point came when Lovato was on a promotional tour with the Jonas Brothers for *Camp Rock 2*. When her management team learned she had been abusing Adderall, alcohol, and marijuana they confronted her, and she lashed out by punching one of her backup dancers whom she suspected of having revealed her secret. This marked the onset of their greater struggles with mood and addiction.

Following this turning point, Lovato first sought treatment for their addiction and then was admitted to a psychiatric hospital, where she was diagnosed with bipolar disorder. She was 18 at the time. Lovato recalls that this diagnosis provided some sense of clarity, noting in a 2012 documentary *Stay Strong* (Russo, 2012): "I didn't realize I was sick. . . . I thought that writing seven songs in one night was normal. I thought that staying up until 5:30 in the morning is normal. Last night, I stayed up until five in the morning. I just couldn't sleep. My mind was racing and it's an ongoing thing and I still learn how to cope with it."

Despite embarking on treatment, Lovato continued to struggle with addiction and in particular with cocaine and alcohol use, about which she maintained tremendous secrecy. While she was publicly stating she were sober, her addiction raged on and she continued daily heavy substance use. She remembers faking drug tests, lying, and manipulating others so that she could continue her substance use undetected. She recalls this as a time that was particularly "chaotic–physically, and emotionally."

Eventually her management team confronted Lovato and helped her acknowledge the serious risks to her well-being and career. She began to take her recovery seriously and moved into a sober house, initiating her first long period of recovery.

Lovato started speaking more honestly in interviews, and in their *New York Times* best-selling book *Staying Strong: 365 Days a Year* (Lovato, 2013), they include journal entries over an entire year, acknowledging the importance of openness about their experiences. In *Simply Complicated,* they recall that "I've learned that secrets make you sick."

During this period, Lovato continued to act, starred as a judge on the popular television show *The X Factor*, released new music, and toured the world. In 2018, after 6 years of sobriety, they revealed publicly that they had relapsed, and in July of that year they were hospitalized for an opioid overdose from a combination of oxycodone and fentanyl. They later attributed the relapse to their ongoing struggles with bulimia. In their words, "I'm six years sober and I'm miserable. I'm even more miserable than I was when I was drinking. Why am I sober?"

In their first public performance after their 2018 relapse, Lovato performed at the 2020 Grammy Awards, singing a previously unreleased song they had written just prior to their overdose (GMA Team, 2020). They received a standing ovation and critical praise from the press and their fans for continuing to fight their struggles openly while sharing their gifts with the world. In 2021, Lovato released an online docu-series in which they and their friends and family openly recount their history of substance abuse, chronicling their darkest years of addiction, as well as their road to recovery. In addition to their mental health advocacy, Lovato, who identifies as non-binary, has been a fierce advocate for LGBTQ+ rights.

Lovato continues to record music and perform around the world. Her most recent album of original material was released in 2022, and became a number one hit on the Billboard US Top Rock and Top Alternative Albums lists. In 2023, she released an album of her past hits re-imagined as rock anthems, to critical acclaim.

In a 2023 interview with radio host Howard Stern, Lovato summed up what her battle with addiction has taught her. "Now, I understand the pitfalls of how deep and dark it can get, and how desperate I can get, and I never want to feel that again" (Howardstern.com, 2023).

3.6 Behavioral Assessment

A **behavioral assessment** is a form of measurement based on objective recording of the individual's behavior. Unlike psychological tests, behavioral assessments record actions rather than responses to rating scales or questions.

In a behavioral assessment, the **target behavior** is a behavior of interest or concern, and is what the client and clinician wish to change. Behavioral assessments include descriptions of the antecedents, or events that precede the behaviors, and consequences, which are the outcomes of those behaviors. For example, a child in a classroom may be unusually disruptive immediately following recess, but not immediately following lunch. The antecedent is

behavioral assessment
A form of measurement based on objective recording of the individual's behavior.

target behavior
A behavior of interest or concern in an assessment.

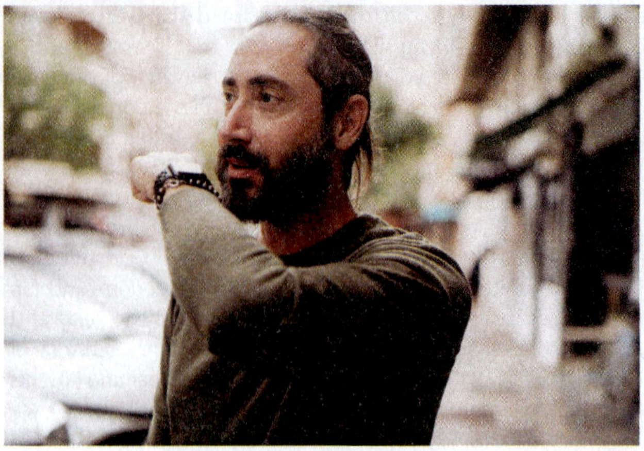

Wearable technology can facilitate the process of behavioral recording.

Westend61 on Offset/Shutterstock

recess, and the consequences are perhaps the teacher's attention or reactions of classmates to the child's disruptive behavior at play but not during a meal.

When clinicians record behavior in its natural context, such as the classroom or the home, this is called ***in vivo* observation**. This approach has the obvious advantage of providing the most realistic measurement of the target behavior. However, it is a time-intensive approach that may not always be practical. In these cases, the clinician could enlist the help of others to conduct the observation on forms designed by the clinician. Returning to the above example, a teacher or teacher's aide could conduct the observation on the child's behaviors.

Analog observations allow for simulation of the situations in which the target behaviors occur. These may take place in a setting or context such as a clinician's office or a laboratory specifically designed for observing the target behavior. A clinician assessing the disruptive child would need to arrange a situation as comparable as possible to the natural setting of the classroom for the analog observation to be valid.

Clients may also report on their own behavior rather than having someone observe them. A **behavioral self-report** is a method of behavioral assessment in which the individual provides information about the frequency of particular behaviors. This self-report also includes the antecedents and consequences of the behavior.

Self-monitoring is a form of behavioral self-report in which the client keeps a record of the frequency of specified behaviors, such as the number of cigarettes smoked or calories consumed, or the number of times in a day that a particular unwanted thought comes to the client's mind.

Clinicians may also obtain information from their clients using **behavioral interviewing** in which they ask questions about the target behavior's frequency, antecedents, and consequences. All these methods would be more appropriate when it is the adult seeking treatment rather than the child, as long as the adult is capable of monitoring his or her own behavior.

Taking advantage of wearable technology, clinicians may also incorporate reports from fitness monitors tracking activity and exercise, sleep patterns, and heart rate. Such data can be useful in diagnosing stress-related, sleep, and eating disorders and can also provide valuable information about treatment progress (e.g., van Kraaij et al., 2020).

in vivo observation
Process of recording behavior in its natural context, such as the classroom or the home.

analog observations
Assessments that take place in a setting or context such as a clinician's office or a laboratory specifically designed for observing the target behavior.

behavioral self-report
A method of behavioral assessment in which the individual provides information about the frequency of particular behaviors.

self-monitoring
A self-report technique in which the client keeps a record of the frequency of specified behaviors.

behavioral interviewing
Assessment process in which clinicians ask questions about the target behavior's frequency, antecedents, and consequences.

multicultural assessment
Assessment process in which clinicians take into account the person's cultural, ethnic, and racial background.

Cultural Formulation Interview (CFI)
A set of questions that assess the impact of culture on key aspects of the client's clinical presentation and care.

3.7 Multicultural Assessment

When psychologists conduct a **multicultural assessment** they take into account the person's cultural, ethnic, and racial background.

The **Cultural Formulation Interview (CFI)** is a set of questions that assess the impact of culture on key aspects of the client's clinical presentation and care. The CFI assesses the client's cultural identity, the individual's cultural conceptualizations of distress, the way the client's culture defines vulnerability and resilience, and any cultural differences between the client and clinician. Questions on the CFI include, "For you, what are the most important aspects of your background or identity?" and "Why do you think this is happening to you?" Background or identity, in turn, refers to "the communities you belong to, the languages you speak, where you or your family are from, your race or ethnic background, your gender or sexual orientation, or your faith or religion" (American Psychiatric Association, 2022).

In addition to the CFI, clinicians may also take advantage of research-based instruments that assess cultural identity and degree of acculturation (Leong, Lui, & Kalibatseva, 2020). It is important for clinicians to ensure that the assessment instruments provide multicultural normative data to assist in the interpretation of scores (Achenbach, 2020).

In the American Psychological Association's Multicultural Guidelines (2017), Guideline #9 specifies that psychologists conduct culturally appropriate assessments that apply not only to diagnosis but to the evaluation that psychologists conduct of their efficacy in this domain.

These guidelines apply to psychologists involved in research as well as service provision, meaning that they also have implications for scientific advances in understanding and treating psychological disorders (Clauss-Ehlers, Hunter, Morse, & Tummala-Narra, 2024). In these areas, cultural sensitivity and cultural humility are essential for psychologists to best fit the needs of clients from diverse backgrounds, and to avoid missing important information that can help in their assessments. Without a sensitive multicultural approach, psychologists may risk biasing or skewing results or findings, which can lead to misdiagnosis and lack of trust within different client populations. Toward this end, psychologists must work hard to recognize their own cultural lenses and biases that might impact their assessments, particularly when a client's background is different than their own.

To ensure that their assessments meet current multicultural assessment criteria, clinicians can seek continuing education (Edwards, Burkard, Adams, & Newcomb, 2017). Additionally, new instruments are being developed to evaluate the extent to which clients believe their clinicians are meeting their needs for culturally informed assessment and treatment (Oh & Shillingford-Butler, 2020).

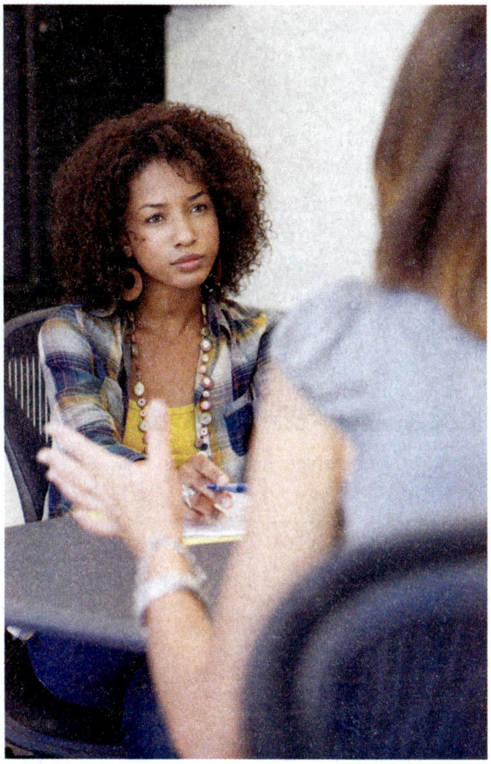

It is important for psychologists to take multicultural considerations into account throughout each part of the assessment process.

Eric Audras/Onoky/Getty Images

3.8 Neuropsychological Assessment

Neuropsychological assessment is a performance-based method used to make it possible for psychologists to understand the cognitive consequences of brain damage, brain disease, and severe mental illness. The assessment consists of a set of tests that the clinician draws from to measure a variety of cognitive functions, focusing on such areas as attention, memory, processing speed, verbal reasoning and comprehension, visual reasoning, verbal memory, and visual memory.

A number of tests evaluate what clinicians call **executive functioning**, the ability to formulate goals, make plans, carry out those plans, and then complete the plans in an effective way. These abilities rely on the adequate functioning of the prefrontal areas of the brain's frontal lobes (Suchy, 2023). Executive functioning also includes the ability to exert **inhibitory control,** in which the individual maintains focus rather than attending to irrelevant information. Measures of inhibitory control can prove useful in understanding a variety of neurocognitive disorders, including those resulting from severe traumatic brain injury (Filipčíková & McDonald, 2023).

You might be surprised to learn that there is no one set procedure for conducting a neuropsychological assessment. Instead, clinicians tailor the tests they administer to a given client based on the diagnostic question and what they believe will be the most effective method to assess the client's strengths and weaknesses. To interpret the test scores, the clinician compares a client's responses on a particular test with normative data from individuals of that age, cultural, or linguistic background who are known to have certain types of injuries or disorders.

Due to the impact of COVID-19 on face-to-face visits between clinicians and clients, the field of teleneuropsychology is gaining increasing importance. Many tests, particularly those involving computer-based administration, appear to show promise as alternatives to in-person assessments (Marra, Hamlet, Bauer, & Bowers, 2020). Additionally, using telehealth methods, clinicians can obtain vital neuropsychological assessment information from caregivers (Farros, Legaspi, & Wallace, 2023).

neuropsychological assessment
A performance-based method assessing cognitive functioning used to examine the cognitive consequences of brain damage, brain disease, and severe mental illness.

executive functioning
The ability to formulate goals, make plans, carry out those plans, and then complete the plans in an effective way.

inhibitory control
The ability to maintain focus rather than attend to irrelevant information.

Brief Screening Tests

A clinician may conduct a brief neuropsychological assessment to screen for neurocognitive disorders. These tools are intended not to lead to a diagnosis but instead to guide the neuropsychologist to next steps in a more thorough assessment.

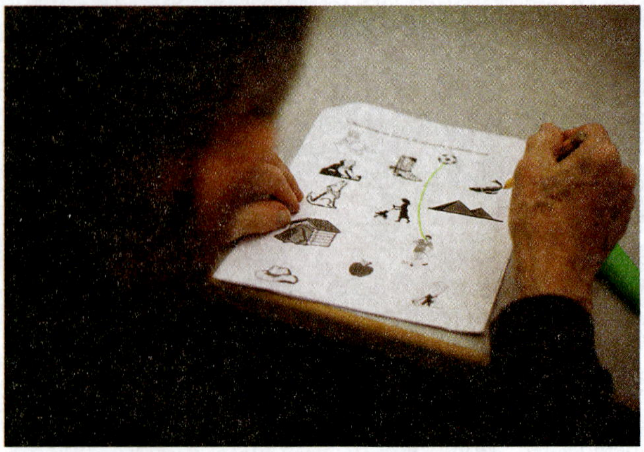

A neuropsychological assessment evaluating the memory, logic, and concentration of an individual with Parkinson's disease.

AMELIE-BENOIST/IMAGE POINT FR/BSIP/Alamy Stock Photo

Mini-Mental State Examination (MMSE)

The **Mini-Mental State Examination (MMSE)** (Folstein, Folstein, & McHugh, 1975) is a structured tool that clinicians use as a brief screening device to assess clients with suspected neurocognitive disorders. Its original purpose was to serve as a quickly administered test that a clinician could administer to individuals who might not be able to complete a full neuropsychological exam. Questions on the MMSE ask the test-taker to follow instructions, remember a set of three unrelated items, copy a picture, and name the current date and location.

Although widely used for initial neurocognitive screening, the MMSE cannot identify the cause of a neurocognitive disorder. Moreover, it is not designed to be administered to individuals who cannot read or write the language of the exam, and it is biased toward people with greater than an eighth-grade education. These limitations mean that the MMSE may not always be appropriate, whether used alone or in combination with other cognitive tests (Merced et al., 2022). Clinicians using the MMSE must weigh the advantages of its brevity against its ability to provide more than a snapshot of an individual's mental state as well as its applicability to a given client.

Mini-Mental State Examination (MMSE)
A structured tool that clinicians use as a brief screening device to assess neurocognitive disorders.

Montreal Cognitive Assessment (MoCA)
Brief cognitive screening device used as part of a neuropsychological assessment.

Montreal Cognitive Assessment (MoCA)

A second brief cognitive screening device, the **Montreal Cognitive Assessment (MoCA)** (Nasreddine et al., 2005) is designed for use by a wide range of clinicians, ranging from nurses to psychologists in the detection of potential cognitive impairment. The MoCA contains a set of short tasks, ranging from exhibiting short recall of the names of objects to drawing the face of an analog clock.

Compared to the MMSE, the MoCA appears to have fewer limitations in terms of its applicability to individuals of varying educational levels (Sala et al., 2020). Versions of the MoCA for use with non-English speaking populations are becoming increasingly available, including in Portuguese (Cesar et al., 2019), Turkish (Krist et al., 2019), Chinese (Tang, 2020), Vietnamese (Quang et al., 2023), and French (Nasreddine & Patel, 2016). It has also been shown to have validity in prison populations (Lima Pereira, Freitas, Simões, & Gerardo, 2023).

Veterans Affairs Saint Louis University Mental Status Exam (SLUMS)

The Veterans Affairs Saint Louis University Mental Status exam (SLUMS; Tariq et al., 2006) is another brief screening tool intended to be sensitive to mild memory loss in older adults that includes enhanced tasks corresponding to attention, numeric calculation, immediate and delayed recall, animal naming, digit span, clock drawing, figure recognition and size differentiation, and immediate recall of facts from a paragraph. Its advantage compared to other mental status examinations is that it can detect cognitive impairment in individuals with less than a high school education (Aiello et al., 2022), and is also particularly useful in testing younger clients who have experienced a traumatic brain injury (Wu et al., 2023).

Executive Functioning

Moving now into tests that tap specific areas of neurological impairment, those that assess executive functioning rely on abilities that require decision making, abstraction, and planning. These key functions are essential in everyday life, and deficits revealed by neurocognitive tests can assist both in diagnosing and in helping to plan treatment for individuals who score below the range of normal functioning.

Trail Making Test (TMT)
A simple test of executive functioning involving the ability to trace a path among a set of related stimuli.

Clock Drawing Test
Simple neuropsychological test in which a test-taker draws a picture of an analog clock.

Trail Making Test (TMT)

The **Trail Making Test (TMT)** is a widely used simple test of executive functioning assessing the ability to trace a path among a set of related stimuli. Although originally designed as a paper-and-pencil measure, it can now be administered on a tablet or with use of a digital pen.

Figure 3 shows a sample item from Trail Making Test Part A. In this example, the task is to draw a line connecting the numbers in order. Although this may seem simple enough, individuals with damage to the frontal lobes of the brain may find it challenging. The abilities tapped by the Trail Making Test include paying attention, scanning visual stimuli, and sequencing numbers.

Clock Drawing Test There are a large number of instruments that measure visuospatial ability. One very simple test used in screening for neurocognitive impairment is the **Clock Drawing Test** (Sunderland et al., 1989). The examiner gives the individual being tested a sheet of paper with a large predrawn circle on it. The client's task is to draw the numbers around the circle to look like the face of an analog clock. Finally, the examiner asks the client to draw the hands of the clock to read "10 after 11." The clinician then rates the client's drawing according to the number of errors. The most impaired clients are unable to reproduce a clock face at all, or they make mistakes in writing the numbers or placing them around the clock. Like the TMT, the Clock Drawing Test can also be administered using digital tools including a digital pen (Binaco et al., 2020).

Researchers are developing assessment instruments that combine elements of these brief screening scales, potentially allowing for greater precision in the screening process (Gonzalez Aguilar & Alba Ferrara, 2020). However, it remains important for clinicians to be aware of their limitations, including the possibility that the screening tests are not appropriate for detecting the potential diagnosis under consideration. For example, their validity for clients with substance use disorders appears to be limited (Ko et al., 2022).

What's in the *DSM-5-TR*

Section III Assessment Measures

DSM-5-TR's Section III contains a set of assessment measures that clinicians can use to enhance their decision-making process. These tools include a "cross-cutting" interview that reviews symptoms across all psychological disorders such as emotional distress, anger, and repetitive thoughts that either the client or someone close to the client can complete. This review of symptoms would allow clinicians to draw attention to symptoms that may not fit precisely into the categorically based diagnoses. Such questions could be incorporated into a mental status examination. One set of questions contains a brief survey of 13 domains for adults and 12 for children. The follow-up questions go into more depth in domains that seem to warrant further attention.

The *DSM-5-TR* authors recognize that dimensional approaches are increasingly being supported by the literature due to the fact that categorical distinctions among disorders may, at times, seem arbitrary. In addition, there are disorders that combine features of two disorders. Many clients also have more than one disorder or diagnoses that do not fit easily into one category. Eventually, a dimensional approach could be combined with the *DSM*'s categorically based diagnoses. This approach would allow clinicians to indicate the severity of a client's disorder, making it possible to evaluate a client's progress during treatment.

In addition to these tools, Section III includes the WHODAS (as presented in the chapter "Diagnosis and Treatment" and a section providing clinicians with tools to perform a cultural formulation. This is a comprehensive semi-structured interview that focuses on the client's experience and social context. The *DSM-5* authors emphasize that the interview should be conducted in a way that allows the client to report his or her subjective experiences. This is intended to reduce the chances that the clinician's stereotypes or pre-existing biases will affect the diagnostic process.

The *DSM-5* authors hope that by providing these tools and techniques, they will not only improve the diagnostic process but also contribute to the research literature on the nature and causes of psychological disorders.

Wisconsin Card Sorting Test (WCST)
Test used in neuropsychological assessment involving the ability to form higher-order abstract concepts.

Wisconsin Card Sorting Test (WCST) The **Wisconsin Card Sorting Test (WCST)** taps the client's ability to form higher-order abstract concepts. Its basic premise is that individuals with deficits in executive functioning will be unable to form these concepts but also show difficulty when having to switch from one set of concepts to another.

A typical trial in the WCST appears in Figure 4. The clinician reveals one card at a time, and the client's job is to indicate which of the cards in the top row matches this card. The test was originally developed using physical cards, but now clinicians typically administer the test in its computerized format. There are 64 cards in the series. In the example shown here, the two red plus signs could match either Card 1 (color), Card 2 (number), or Card 4 (shape). The test-taker chooses one card from the four options, and then receives feedback about whether the choice was correct or not (e.g., the client chose the red circle, guessing color). On the next trial, this feedback would inform the client's choice of card, and if the client was capable of forming concepts, would choose whatever card was red on the next trial. After several trials, the concept shifts (e.g., to

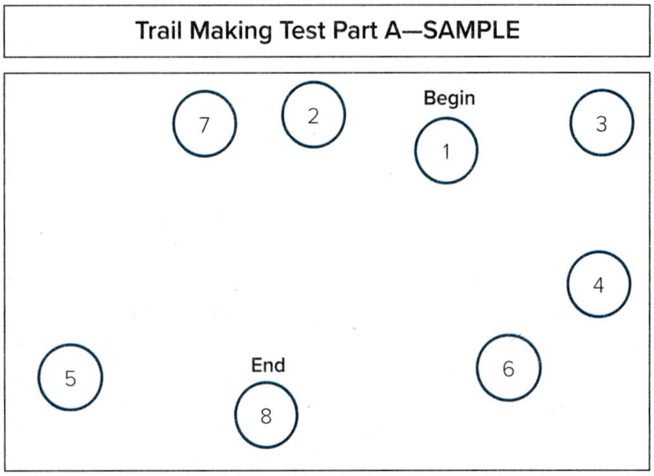

FIGURE 3 Trail Making Test

SOURCE: Adapted from Reitan, R. M. (1958). Validity of the Trail Making Test as an indicator of organic brain damage. *Perceptual and Motor Skills, 8*, 271–276.

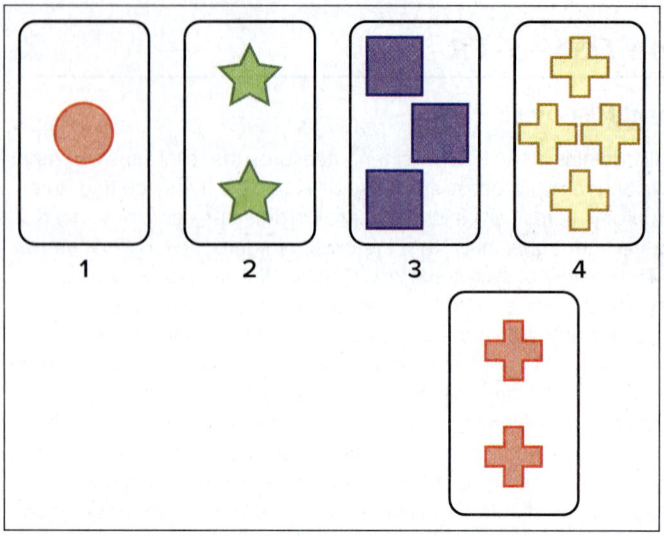

FIGURE 4 Sample Item from the Wisconsin Card Sorting Test

shape) and now the client must switch to choosing cards that match on shape regardless of color.

Brain imaging data support the ability of the WCST to tap into the functioning of the prefrontal areas of the brain (Díaz-Blancat, García-Prieto, Maestú, & Barceló, 2018). Researchers are expanding its use internationally through the publication of normative data from countries such as Argentina (Miranda et al., 2020), Portugal (Faustino, Oliveira, & Lopes, 2022), and Lebanon (Rammal et al., 2019).

Paced Auditory Serial Addition Test (PASAT) The **Paced Auditory Serial Addition Test (PASAT)** assesses the components of executive functioning involved in auditory information processing speed, flexibility, and calculation ability. The client hears a recording of numbers between 1 and 9 every 3 seconds. The task is to add the number just heard with the number that preceded it. If the recording was "1-3-5-2-6-7," the correct response would be "4-8-7-8-13." In addition to assessing traumatic brain injury, the PASAT also serves to test the functioning of individuals with multiple sclerosis, because it appears to tap areas of the brain affected by this disease (Covey et al., 2023).

Paced Auditory Serial Addition Test (PASAT)
Neuropsychological test used to assess processing speed, flexibility, and calculation ability.

Boston Naming Test (BNT)
Neuropsychological test intended to assess word retrieval abilities.

Other Neuropsychological Tests Neuropsychologists use the **Boston Naming Test (BNT)** to assess the word retrieval abilities of children with learning disabilities and adults who have suffered brain damage. Each of the 60 items on the BNT contains a picture of an object, and the test-taker must retrieve its name. The BNT moves from simple items such as *bed*, *tree*, and *pencil* to difficult items at the end such as *palette* and *abacus*. Incorrect answers include the individual's failure to name the item, but also to give a related name (e.g., "mouth organ" for "harmonica") or to name only a part of the item.

Originally written in English for native English speakers, the BNT is now available in a number of translations appropriate for various populations, including Dominican (Silvestre, Iglesias, & Silvestre, 2018), Spanish Latin-American (delCacho-Tena et al., 2023), Italian (Vestito et al., 2023), and Brazilian (Studart-Neto et al., 2022). Yet, clinicians should interpret BNT scores of bilingual adults with caution (Savoie et al., 2019). Furthermore, even when assessing native English-speaking populations, clinicians should be familiar with potential threats to validity in applying the BNT to minoritized individuals (Na & King, 2019).

Glascow Coma Scale (GCS)
Neuropsychological test intended to assess immediate aftermath of brain trauma.

Used to assess the immediate aftermath of brain trauma, the **Glasgow Coma Scale (GCS)** measures impairment of conscious level in response to defined stimuli. The GCS tests the individual's ability to open the eyes, to be oriented to his or her surroundings, and to obey commands. In use for more than 40 years, the GCS remains the most widely accepted measure for detecting coma as a sign of traumatic brain injury (Teasdale et al., 2014). It is particularly useful for clinicians to give the GCS over a period of time following suspected trauma, to track progressive changes over time in the individual's level of consciousness. Because it is available in 32 languages, the GCS has the advantage of being highly useful in multicultural settings.

Other neuropsychological tests investigate a variety of memory functions. The Wechsler Memory Scale, Fourth Edition (WMS-IV; Wechsler, 2009) includes tests of working (short-term) and long-term memory for visual and verbal stimuli. Examiners can choose from among the WMS-IV subscales according to the areas they believe are most critical to evaluate in particular clients. For example, there is an Older Adult Battery appropriate for individuals 65 to 90 years of age that includes only the scales assessing Logical Memory (recall of a story), Verbal Paired Associates (ability to remember the second word in pairs of words), and Visual Reproduction (ability to draw a visual stimulus).

adaptive testing
Testing in which the client's responses to earlier questions determine the subsequent questions presented to them.

Computerized test batteries, which contain a range of tests adaptable to the possible brain damage in the client, provide the opportunity for **adaptive testing**, in which the client's

You Be the Judge

Psychologists in the Legal System

Psychologists working within the legal system are frequently called on to serve as expert witnesses, and their testimony often relies on psychological assessments. Unlike the therapeutic setting, the forensic setting does not necessarily involve a positive relationship between the client and clinician. In fact, the psychologist may face a malpractice suit from the clients if they disagree with an assessment that led to a conviction or unfavorable decision, as in custody cases.

Knapp and VandeCreek (2001) present an interesting case history of a psychologist involved in a custody case who wrote in his report that the father had "authoritarian tendencies and could benefit from participating in parenting classes" (pp. 244–245). However, the psychologist had not actually interviewed the father; he based this statement on what the children told him. As a result, the psychologist was reprimanded by his state licensing board.

Psychologists are also mandated by the APA Ethical Principles of Psychologists and Code of Conduct (also called the Ethics Code) to practice within their field of competence. If they have not received training in forensic psychology, they are required to seek consultation from an expert colleague. A second case example presented by Knapp and VandeCreek involved the testimony by a psychologist proficient in assessment, but not forensic assessment, who testified that on the basis of elevated scores on the MMPI-2 scales 6 and 9, the defendant was indeed "insane." However, legal insanity is not the same as being diagnosed with a psychological disorder, and therefore the psychologist's testimony was discredited in court.

Informed consent is another key ethical principle that applies not only to research but also to assessment and treatment. When a defendant with a psychological disorder is interviewed for a forensic assessment, the psychologist must take all possible precautions to let the defendant know about the limits of confidentiality in this context. In another example presented by Knapp and VandeCreek, a defendant was genuinely startled to hear the psychologist report on the interview, because the defendant had not understood the nature of the informed consent.

As a final example, Knapp and VandeCreek cite the case of a psychologist treating the children of a separated couple. The children stated that they preferred to live with their mother. The mother later requested that the psychologist write a letter to her attorney. In turn, the attorney asked the psychologist to "share your opinions as to where the children should live" (p. 250). This request, because it involves a child custody case would violate APA's Guidelines for Psychological Evaluations in Child Protection Matters (2013); see also Chapter 15.

Q: *You be the judge:* As you can see, the APA Ethics Code clearly states the proper course of action in each case. The question for you to judge is not which course of action is proper, because this is clearly stated in the APA Ethics Code. Instead, consider the complexities psychologists face when interacting in the legal system. These examples are only a handful from the many possible scenarios that can ensue, placing psychologists in situations that require them to be entirely familiar with the principles that guide the profession.

responses to earlier questions determine the subsequent questions presented to them. For example, the **Cambridge Neuropsychological Testing Automated Battery (CANTAB)** consists of 22 specific tests that assess visual memory, working memory, executive function and planning, attention, verbal memory, and decision making and response control. The CANTAB has been shown useful for predicting changes in cognitive status over time as its subtests can be selected based on the specific function under study (Campos-Magdaleno et al., 2020).

Cambridge Neuropsychological Testing Automated Battery (CANTAB)
Computerized neuropsychological test battery offering 22 specific tests.

Before deciding whether to move to a computerized test, the clinician must weigh the advantages of ease of administration and scoring against the potential disadvantages that may exist for clients who are disadvantaged in their ability to use computers, including children (Arán Filippetti, Krumm, & Raimondi, 2020).

Looking now at Ben's tests, Dr. Washington chose to administer tasks that would be sensitive to the type of injury that Ben might have sustained given his low WAIS-IV coding score, which suggested that Ben may have experienced brain damage that led to changes in his ability to focus his visual attention and perform quickly on a psychomotor speed task. Because Dr. Washington did not see Ben at the scene of the accident or in the ER, he could not administer the GCS.

Ben's completion time on Trail Making Test Part A was in the marginally impaired range. On the Clock Drawing Test, Ben received a score of 5 of a possible 10, erroneously crowding the numbers at one end of the clock. He received a score within the normal range on the PASAT, suggesting that the injury did not affect his auditory attentional functioning. On the WCST, Ben showed evidence of perseverative errors, meaning that he was unable to switch mental sets in categorizing the cards according to different criteria. Ben's performance on the WMS-IV was within normal range, a finding consistent with his relatively high scores on the Verbal scales of the Wechsler, indicating that he had not experienced either short- or long-term memory loss.

neuroimaging
Assessment method that provides a picture of the brain's structures or level of activity and therefore is a useful tool for "looking" at the brain.

electroencephalogram (EEG)
A measure of changes in the electrical activity of the brain.

computed axial tomography (CAT or CT) scan
A series of X-rays taken from various angles around the brain that are integrated by computer to produce a composite picture.

3.9 Neuroimaging

Neuroimaging provides a picture of the brain's structures or level of activity and therefore is a useful tool for "looking" at the brain. Psychologists use several types of neuroimaging methods, both in clinical work and research, that vary in the types of results they provide.

The **electroencephalogram (EEG)** measures electrical activity in the brain. EEG activity reflects the extent to which an individual is alert, resting, sleeping, or dreaming. The EEG pattern also shows particular patterns of brain waves when an individual engages in particular mental tasks. Clinicians use EEGs to evaluate clients for conditions such as epilepsy, sleep disorders, and brain tumors.

Computed axial tomography (CAT or CT) scan uses a series of X-rays taken from various angles around the brain that are integrated by computer to produce a composite picture. CT scans of the brain provide a static image of the fluid-filled areas called the ventricles. The method is useful when clinicians are looking for structural damage to the brain because enlarged ventricles would signify loss of vital brain tissue.

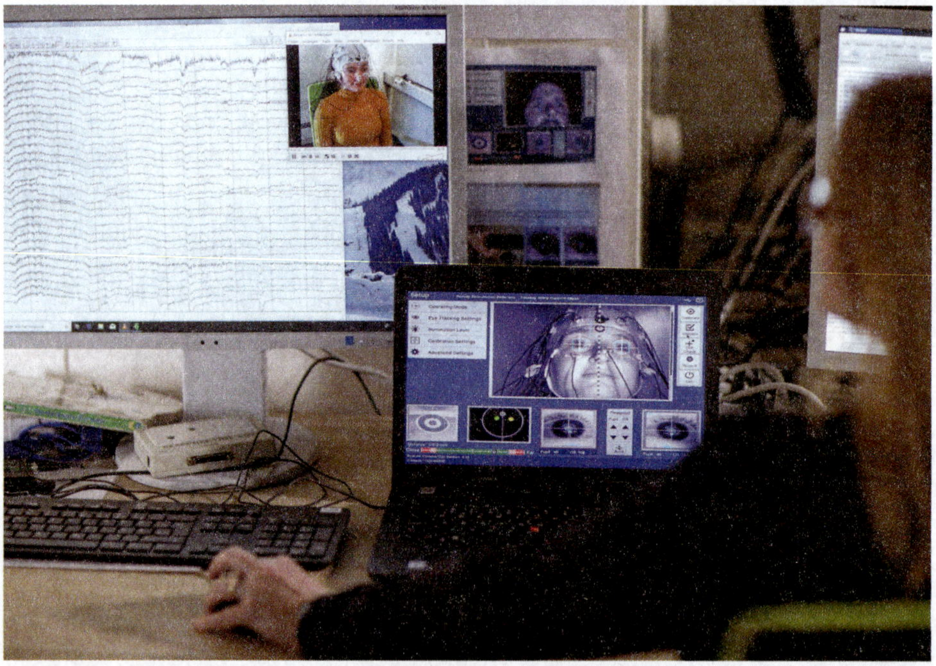

A CAT scan of a patient's brain helps neuropsychologists to find brain structure aberrations that may be causing cognitive dysfunction.
picture alliance/Getty Images

Magnetic resonance imaging (MRI) uses radio waves rather than X-rays to construct a static picture of the living brain based on the water content of various tissues. To conduct an MRI of the brain, the individual is placed inside a capsule that contains a powerful electromagnet. Magnetic force causes the nuclei in hydrogen atoms to transmit electromagnetic energy (hence the term *magnetic resonance*). A computer produces a high-resolution picture of the scanned area based on activity recorded from thousands of angles. The picture from the MRI differentiates areas in the brain of white matter (nerve fibers) from gray matter (nerve cells) and is useful for diagnosing diseases that affect the nerve fibers that make up the white matter. However, because the MRI uses magnetism to detect brain activity, people who have metallic joints, pacemakers, or other permanent metallic implants cannot use this testing method.

A **positron emission tomography (PET) scan** is a measure of brain activity in which a small amount of a radioactive compound is injected into an individual's bloodstream, following which a computer measures the various levels of radiation in different parts of the brain and yields a multicolored image.

In the variant known as **single photon emission computed tomography (SPECT) scan**, a longer and more detailed imaging analysis can be performed. In both methods, the compounds travel through the blood into the brain and emit positively charged electrons called positrons, which act very much like X-rays in a CT scan. The images, which represent the accumulation of the labeled compound, can show blood flow, oxygen or glucose metabolism, and concentrations of brain chemicals. Vibrant colors at the red end of the spectrum represent higher levels of activity, and colors at the blue-green-violet end of the spectrum represent lower levels of brain activity. **Proton magnetic resonance spectroscopy (MRS)** is another scanning method that measures metabolic activity of neurons.

Functional magnetic resonance imaging (fMRI) provides a picture of how areas of the brain react to stimuli in real time, making it possible to precisely monitor the individual's response during, for example, a cognitive task. Researchers are increasingly using fMRIs to understand the brain areas active in the processing of information. One major advantage of the fMRI is that it does not require injection of radioactive materials, like the PET or SPECT scan. However, it cannot be administered to clients with any type of metal implants, including pacemakers or artificial joints. Conversely, children may need some type of behavioral intervention to reduce their head motion while the MRI is being conducted (Greene et al., 2018).

Researchers also use **diffusion tensor imaging (DTI)**, a method to investigate aberrations in the white matter of the brain. DTI scans show the activity of water molecules as they diffuse along the length of axons, making it possible to investigate aberrations in neural pathways.

magnetic resonance imaging (MRI)
The use of radio waves rather than X-rays to construct a static picture of the living brain based on the water content of various tissues.

positron emission tomography (PET) scan
A measure of brain activity in which a small amount of radioactive compounds is injected into an individual's bloodstream, following which a computer measures the varying levels of radiation in different parts of the brain and yields a multicolored image.

single photon emission computed tomography (SPECT) scan
A variant of the PET scan that allows a longer and more detailed imaging analysis to be performed.

proton magnetic resonance spectroscopy (MRS)
A scanning method that measures metabolic activity of neurons and therefore may indicate areas of brain damage.

functional magnetic resonance imaging (fMRI)
Provides a picture of how areas of the brain react to stimuli in real time.

diffusion tensor imaging (DTI)
A method to investigate aberrations in the white matter of the brain.

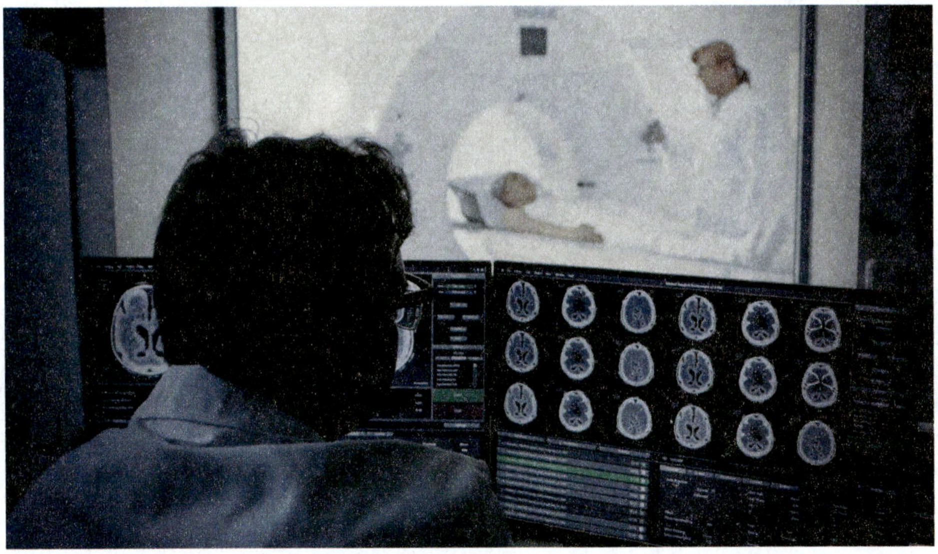

Using an fMRI, clinicians can monitor brain activity to understand the brain areas active when patients process information.

Gorodenkoff/Shutterstock

Keep in mind that brain scans can produce evidence of specific areas of damage, but they do not necessarily correspond to a specific loss of behavioral functioning. Moreover, the measures themselves may fail to achieve one criteria of standardization, namely reliability. A large international collaboration investigating the findings of 90 experiments using brain scanning methods showed low levels of consistency over time as well as across different measures (Elliott et al., 2020).

Upon evaluating Ben through neuropsychological testing, Dr. Washington ordered a CT scan because Ben showed some signs of frontal lobe damage (personality changes, some perseveration on the WCST, and marginal errors on the TMT). However, it was necessary to rule out parietal lobe damage, which can also contribute to this performance pattern and to visual attentional deficits. The CT scan revealed that Ben had experienced a traumatic brain injury as a result of the incident, perhaps in the form of a brain hemorrhage.

3.10 Putting It All Together

As you have just seen in Ben's case, clinicians face a formidable task when attempting to develop a diagnosis from the evidence they obtain through the assessment process. They must evaluate each client on an individual basis and determine which combination of tests will help them most closely identify the nature and cause of that client's behavioral symptoms. In addition, clinicians performing assessments attempt to understand a client's strengths, so they can make recommendations to build on the client's existing abilities and help address treatment to maximize the client's functioning in everyday life.

Return to the Case: Ben Robsham

Given the potential cause of Ben's symptoms, Dr. Washington recommended that Ben receive rehabilitation to strengthen his existing skills so that he can return to his previous employment. Ben will also receive supportive therapy and possibly vocational counseling if he continues to demonstrate deficits in visual and spatial processing speed, skills he clearly needs for his present job.

Dr. Tobin's Reflections: It is somewhat reassuring to know that Ben's injury, though currently interfering with his ability to go to work, will most likely resolve on its own. A neuropsychological assessment was clearly called for in this case; unfortunately, with increases in traumatic brain injuries in recent years, this type of assessment will be even more necessary. Ben's injury occurred at work, but many other young people are experiencing such injuries in areas of activity as diverse as playing hockey or football and fighting in war. With the development of more sophisticated neuroimaging and computerized testing, we will be better prepared to assess individuals like Ben in the future, as well as those clients we see whose disorders are primarily psychological in nature.

SUMMARY

- A psychological assessment is a procedure in which a clinician provides a formal evaluation of an individual's cognitive, personality, and psychosocial functioning. Clinicians conduct assessments under a variety of conditions. In many cases, clinicians use the assessment process to provide a diagnosis, or at least a tentative diagnosis, of an individual's psychological disorder.
- To be useful, clinicians must hold assessments to standards that ensure that they provide the most reproducible and accurate results. The reliability of a test indicates the consistency of the scores it produces. The test's validity reflects the extent to which a test measures what it is designed to measure.
- Clinicians should use the best assessment methods possible. Evidence-based assessment includes (1) relying on research findings and scientifically viable theories, (2) using psychometrically strong measures, and (3) empirically evaluating the assessment process.
- The clinical interview is a series of questions that clinicians administer in face-to-face interaction with the client. The

answers the client provides to these questions provide important background information on clients, allow them to describe their symptoms, and enable clinicians to make observations of their clients that can guide decisions about the next steps, which may include further testing. The format can be structured or unstructured.

- A clinician uses a mental status examination to assess a client's current state of mind. The clinician assesses a number of features of the client including appearance, attitudes, behavior, mood and affect, speech, thought processes, content of thought, perception, cognition, insight, and judgment. The outcome of the mental status examination is a comprehensive description of how the client looks, thinks, feels, and behaves.
- Intelligence tests such as the Stanford-Binet Intelligence Test, but particularly the Wechsler scales, provide valuable information about an individual's cognitive functioning.
- Clinicians use tests of personality to understand a person's thoughts, behaviors, and emotions. There are two main forms of personality tests: self-report and projective. Tests include the Minnesota Multiphasic Personality Inventory (MMPI), the SCL-90-R, the NEO Personality Inventory, and other specific self-report inventories designed to investigate specific disorders or research questions for which a general test may not be relevant.
- In projective tests, the examiner asks questions about an ambiguous stimulus. The most common are the Rorschach and the TAT.
- Behavioral assessments record actions rather than responses to rating scales or questions. The target behavior is what the client and clinician wish to change. Behavioral assessments include descriptions of the events that precede or follow the behaviors. *In vivo* observation takes place when clinicians record behavior in its natural context, such as the classroom or the home. Analog observations take place in a setting or context such as a clinician's office or a laboratory specifically designed for observing the target behavior. In a behavioral self-report the client records the target behavior, including the antecedents and consequences of the behavior. Self-monitoring is a form of behavioral self-report in which the client keeps a record of the frequency of specified behaviors.
- When psychologists conduct a multicultural assessment, they must take into account the person's cultural, ethnic, and racial background.
- Neuropsychological assessment is the process of gathering information about a client's brain functioning on the basis of performance on psychological tests. Clinicians use neuropsychological assessment measures to attempt to determine the functional correlates of brain damage by comparing a client's performance on a particular test with normative data from individuals who are known to have certain types of injuries or disorders. Brief screening methods often provide the first step in conducting a neuropsychological assessment. There are a number of formal assessment tests that neuropsychologists can use depending on the nature of the potential diagnosis. These include tests to assess verbal recall and auditory attention. Neuroimaging methods may also be part of the assessment process, including EEG, CT scan, MRI, fMRI, PET scan, and DTI.

KEY TERMS

Adaptive testing
Analog observations
Behavioral assessment
Behavioral interviewing
Behavioral self-report
Boston Naming Test (BNT)
Cambridge Neuropsychological Testing Automated Battery (CANTAB)
Clinical interview
Clock Drawing Test
Computed axial tomography (CAT or CT) scan
Cultural Formulation Interview
Deviation intelligence (IQ)
Diffusion tensor imaging (DTI)
Electroencephalogram (EEG)
Evidence-based assessment
Executive functioning
Functional magnetic resonance imaging (fMRI)
Glasgow Coma Scale (GCS)
In vivo observation
Inhibitory control
Magnetic resonance imaging (MRI)
Mental status examination
Mini-Mental State Examination (MMSE)
Minnesota Multiphasic Personality Inventory-3 (MMPI-3)
Montreal Cognitive Assessment (MoCA)
Multicultural assessment
Neuroimaging
Neuropsychological assessment
Paced Auditory Serial Addition Test (PASAT)
Positron emission tomography (PET) scan
Projective test
Proton magnetic resonance spectroscopy (MRS)
Psychological assessment
Rorschach Inkblot Test
Self-monitoring
Self-report clinical inventory
Single photon emission computed tomography (SPECT) scan
Standardization
Stanford-Binet 5 (SB5)
Structured Clinical Interview for *DSM-5* Disorders (SCID-5)
Structured interview
Target behavior
Thematic Apperception Test (TAT)
Trail Making Test (TMT)
Unstructured interview
Wechsler Adult Intelligence Scale (WAIS)
Wisconsin Card Sorting Test (WCST)

CHAPTER 4

Theoretical Perspectives

OUTLINE

Learning Objectives

4.1 Summarize theoretical perspectives on psychological disorders.

4.2 Assess theories of the biological perspective and identify treatments.

4.3 Describe trait theory.

4.4 Compare and contrast Freud's theory to post-Freudian psychodynamic views and identify treatments.

4.5 Assess theories of the behavioral perspective and identify treatments.

4.6 Assess theories of the cognitive and cognitive behavioral perspectives and identify treatments.

4.7 Assess theories of the humanistic perspective and identify treatments.

4.8 Assess theories of the sociocultural perspective and identify treatments.

4.9 Explain the acceptance-based perspective.

4.10 Explain the biopsychosocial perspective.

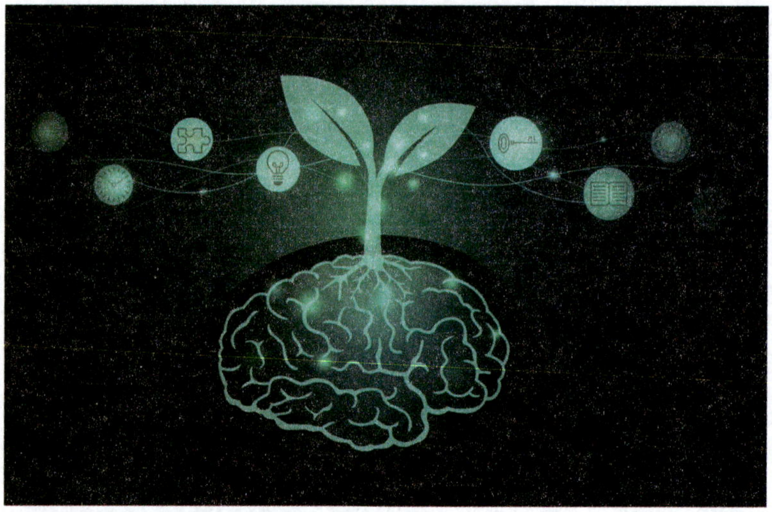

solar22/Shutterstock

Case Report

Meera Krishnan

Demographic information: 26-year-old South Asian heterosexual cisgender woman. Meera's pronouns are she/her/hers.

Presenting problem: Meera self-referred to my outpatient private practice upon the urging of a friend. For the past 3 weeks she reports feeling, in her words, "profoundly sad for no reason at all," lethargic, and preoccupied with feelings that she would be better off dead, though she states she has no specific plan or intent to commit suicide. She stated she oversleeps on most days, has decreased appetite on most days, resulting in weight loss of about 2–3 pounds, and tries to avoid any social contact. She further describes feeling that she has greatly let down her family and friends. As a result of these symptoms, Meera believes her work performance has suffered and notes that she has used all her sick days; she is on warning from her employer that her contract will be reviewed if she misses any more days of work.

Psychiatric history: This is Meera's third depressive episode since her junior year of high school. Each episode has lasted approximately 2 months or slightly longer. She has not previously sought treatment.

Psychosocial history: A college graduate, Meera works as a biologist in a hospital research laboratory. She is the younger of two daughters and reports having a long-standing belief that her parents favor her older sister. She feels that her parents, who immigrated to the United States from India before Meera and her sister were born, disapprove of her current lifestyle in comparison to that of her sister, who married the son of family friends. Although Meera and her sister were once very close, they no longer maintain regular contact, and she rarely visits her parents, although they live in a neighboring town. Meera reports that she rarely drinks alcohol and has never used recreational drugs. She has no medical conditions and reports that, in general, her health is very good. Prior to the onset of her current depressive episode, Meera reports that she exercised regularly by participating in a long-distance running club and enjoyed cooking with her friends and listening to music.

Symptoms: For nearly every day of the last 3 weeks, Meera has been experiencing overwhelming feelings of sadness most of the day, not accounted for by bereavement, substance use, or a medical condition. Her symptoms include feelings of worthlessness, tearfulness, loss of interest, sleep disturbance (oversleeping), and loss of appetite.

Risk level: Low risk. Meera has experienced recurrent thoughts about death and passive suicidal ideation, but she denies intent or planning. She has no past history of suicide attempts.

Case formulation: Because Meera has experienced two previous depressive episodes, each of which have been at least 2 months apart, and the symptoms of her current episode are interfering with her ability to carry out her normal daily functioning, she meets *DSM-5-TR* criteria for major depressive disorder (MDD), recurrent.

Treatment plan: The principles of evidence-based practice suggest that the best treatment for Meera's depression is cognitive behavioral therapy (CBT). Following the intake appointment, she will receive a complete psychological assessment. Given the severity of her symptoms, I will recommend a referral to a psychiatrist for consultation and medical evaluation to determine whether psychiatric medication could be beneficial.

Sarah Tobin, PhD

4.1 Theoretical Perspectives on Psychological Disorders

To guide their work, researchers and clinicians use a set of underlying **theoretical perspectives**, orientations to understanding the causes of human behavior and the treatment of psychological disorders. In this chapter, you will learn about the major theoretical perspectives that inform contemporary psychological research and practice.

theoretical perspective
An orientation to understanding the causes of human behavior and the treatment of psychological disorders.

To facilitate your understanding of these perspectives, you can learn from Meera's case as an example to show how clinicians working within each perspective would address her treatment. Although Meera's plan calls for treatment within the cognitive behavioral perspective, her case has many facets that each of the major theories address and therefore warrants discussion.

4.2 Biological Perspective

biological perspective
A theoretical perspective in which it is assumed that deviations in the body's functioning are responsible for the symptoms of psychological disorders.

Psychologists working within the **biological perspective** believe that deviations in the body's functioning are responsible for the symptoms of psychological disorders. In particular, they seek to trace the causes of psychological symptoms primarily due to disturbances in the nervous system or other bodily systems that have an impact on the nervous system.

Theories

Biological approaches to psychological disorders focus on the roles of the nervous system, the body's physiological functioning, and genetics. The ways in which these interact through life become important pieces of the biopsychosocial perspective.

neurotransmitter
A chemical substance released from a neuron into the synapse, where it can become absorbed by the receiving neuron.

Default Mode Network
Connections of areas within the cortex involved in the processing of internally-generated stimuli.

Role of the Nervous System The transmission of information throughout the nervous system takes place at synapses, or points of communication between neurons.

Neurotransmitters are chemical substances released from a neuron into the synapse, where they can become absorbed by the receiving neuron. Neuroscientists assume that neurons that transmit and respond to the same neurotransmitters operate as pathways responsible for specific functions.

Table 1 shows the proposed role of several major neurotransmitters in psychological disorders. The "serotonin pathway," for example, consists of neurons involved in regulating mood, among other functions. As you can see from the table, however, several neurotransmitters may be relevant to the same function. Conversely, some functions are served by more than one neurotransmitter. In other words, there is not a one-to-one mapping of functions and neurotransmitters, which greatly adds to the challenge of understanding the role neurotransmitters play in psychological disorders. Researchers hope that it may be possible for these links to be understood, and for practitioners to treat irregularities in neurotransmitters that could alleviate psychological symptoms.

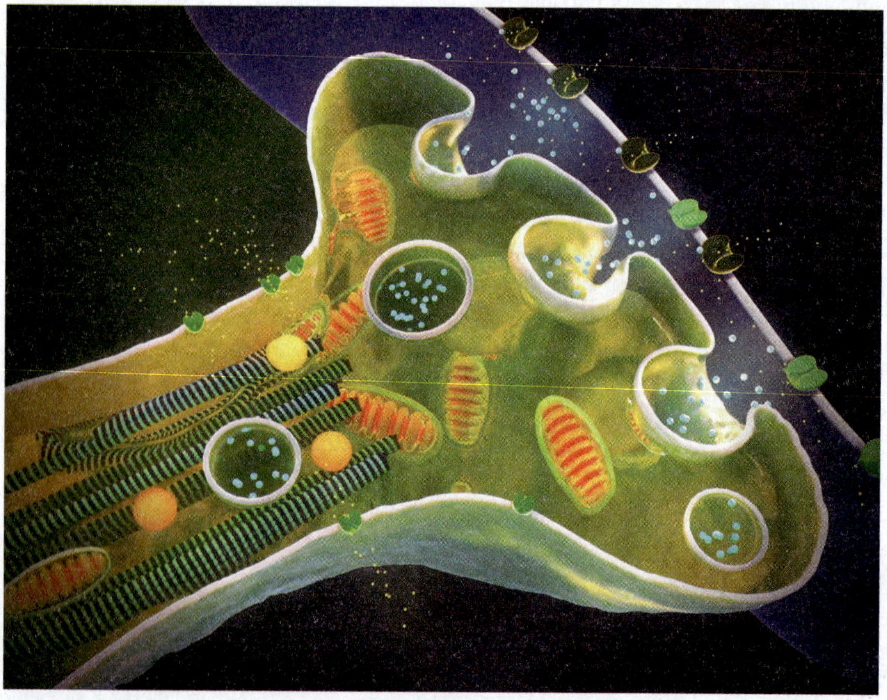

Neurotransmitters released at the synapse are the basic units of communication between neurons.
NANOCLUSTERING/SCIENCE PHOTO LIBRARY/Getty Images

Alterations in brain structures that occur through injury or are present at birth may also play a role in psychological disorders. The role of structural alterations in the brain is getting greater attention with the availability of the increasingly sophisticated brain scanning methods discussed in the chapter "Assessment."

One important set of brain structures with relevance to psychological disorders is the area of activation in the brain known as the **Default Mode Network (DMN)**, which is involved in thinking about the "self" in relation to other people. It also processes internally generated thoughts and images (such as daydreaming).

TABLE 1 **Selected Neurotransmitters Involved in Psychological Disorders**

Neurotransmitter	Related Disorders
Norepinephrine	Depressive disorders Anxiety disorders (panic disorder)
Serotonin	Depressive disorders Anxiety disorders Schizophrenia Anorexia nervosa Substance use disorders
Gamma-aminobutyric acid (GABA)	Anxiety disorders Substance use disorders
Dopamine	Neurocognitive disorder due to Parkinson's disease Schizophrenia Eating disorders Substance use disorders
Acetylcholine	Neurocognitive disorder due to Alzheimer's disease
Opioid peptides	Substance use disorders

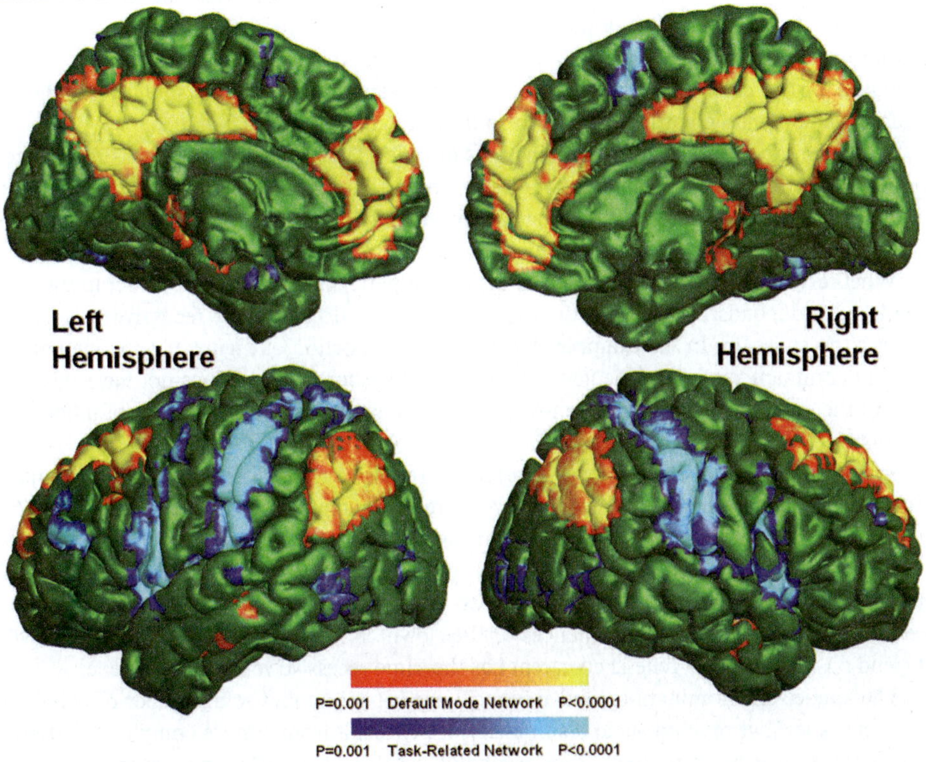

The default mode network (top) is activated by internally-produced stimuli and deactivated (bottom) while the brain processes external stimuli.

Shim, G., Oh, J.S., Jung, W.H. et al. Altered resting-state connectivity in subjects at ultra-high risk for psychosis: an fMRI study. Behav Brain Funct 6, 58 (2010). https://doi.org/10.1186/1744-9081-6-58

The Default Mode Network, as shown in this set of brain scan images, is active when an individual is not engaged in a task (top images) and inactive when the individual is working on a task requiring cognitive resources (Source: Shim G, Oh JS, Jung WH, et al. (2010). Altered resting-state connectivity in subjects at ultra-high risk for psychosis: an fMRI study. *Behavioral and Brain Functions: BBF, 6,* 58. doi:10.1186/1744-9081-6-58. https://www.ncbi.nlm.nih.gov/pmc/articles/PMC2959003/).

Role of Genetics

genes
The instructions for forming proteins contained within each of the body's cells.

genotype
The genetic makeup of an organism.

phenotype
The expression of the genetic program in the individual's physical and psychological attributes.

endophenotype
The expression of a heritable trait that is not outwardly visible.

Basics of Genetics **Genes** are the instructions for forming proteins contained within each of the body's cells. These instructions, in turn, determine how the cell performs. In the case of neurons, genes control the manufacturing of neurotransmitters, as well as the way the neurotransmitters behave in the synapse. Genes also determine, in part, how the brain's structures develop throughout life. Any factor that can alter the genetic code can also alter the way these structures perform.

Your **genotype** is your genetic makeup, which contains the form of each gene you inherit. It is made up of particular sequences of chemical compounds represented by the letters A, G, T, and C (adenine, guanine, thymine, and cytosine).

Your **phenotype** is the expression of your genetic program in your physical and psychological attributes. Some phenotypes are relatively close to their genotype, meaning that they are unaffected by the environment. Eye color is a good example of this situation because your eye color does not reflect environmental influences.

In contrast to the phenotype, an **endophenotype** is the expression of a heritable trait that is not outwardly visible but can be detected in a laboratory task. For example, certain deficits in executive functioning involving the ability to exert inhibitory control appear, across populations of differing ancestry, to be related to a genetic risk for schizophrenia (Arnatkeviciute et al., 2023).

Inherited disorders result when the genes from each parent combine in such a way that the ordinary functioning of a cell is compromised. Certain genetic alterations can themselves produce the neurotransmitter and structural brain variations that can be tied to psychological disorders. For example, the deletion of only a few genetic components on chromosome 22, known as 22q11.2 deletion syndrome, occurring in one out of 2,000 to 6,000 live births, can result in a variety of physical disabilities, immune system dysfunctions, neurodevelopmental disorders, and schizophrenia (Parker et al., 2023).

The inheritance of particular combinations of genes, faulty copying when cells reproduce, or mutations that a person acquires over the course of life may all contribute to genetic alterations that have an effect on psychological functioning. These genetic alterations may also interact with damage caused by exposure to environmental agents such as toxins or injury.

Whether you get a genetically caused disease in patterns determined by alterations in a single gene depends on whether the disease reflects a dominant or recessive pattern of genetic transmission. In the example shown in the top portion of Figure 1, only one parent has the dominant version of the gene. As long as the second parent does not have this version of the gene, each child of these two parents will have a one in two chance of inheriting the disease.

In contrast, if the disease follows a pattern of recessive transmission, both parents must carry the same version of the gene in order to produce a child with the genetic disorder. As you can see in Figure 1, neither parent has the disease but both are carriers of the disease-producing, recessive version of the gene. This means that each child has a one in four chance of developing the genetic disorder. However, two of the children carry the disease-associated version of the gene, so that the chances of their own children developing the disorder will depend on whether their genetic co-parent has the same recessive version of the gene.

polygenic
A model of inheritance in which more than one gene participates in the process of determining a given characteristic.

The single-gene dominant-recessive inheritance model applies to a number of acquired characteristics, but psychological disorders typically result from a more complex set of processes. Thus, it is far more likely that psychological disorders reflect a **polygenic** model, a model of inheritance in which more than one gene participates in the process of determining a given characteristic. There are other characteristics that reflect maternal linkages only, meaning they transmit only through the mother. These disorders occur with defects in the

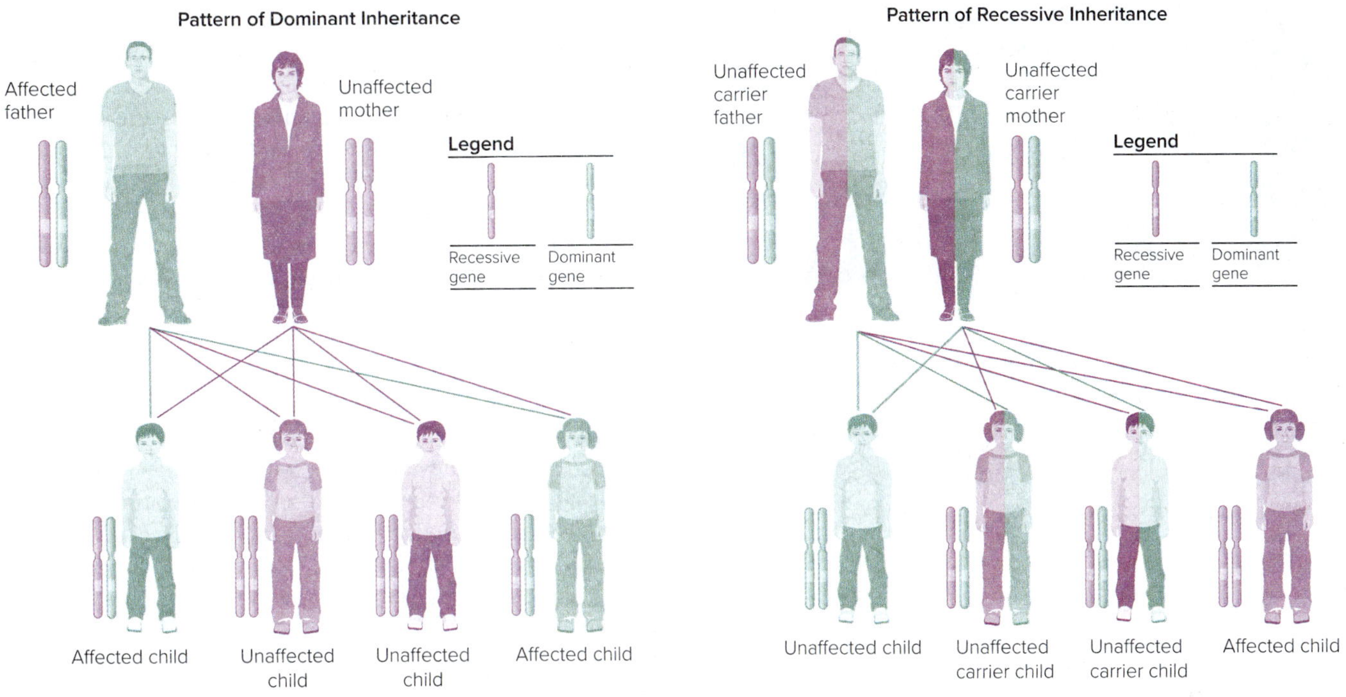

FIGURE 1 Pattern of Dominant-Recessive Trait Inheritance

When a genetic disease is dominant, a child who receives one copy of the disease-producing gene will get the disease (top); when a genetic disease is recessive, only a child who receives two copies of the affected gene will get the disease (bottom).

SOURCE: NHGRI, www.genome.gov

mitochondrial DNA, which is the DNA that controls protein formation in the cell's mitochondria (energy-producing structures).

When researchers study patterns of genetic transmission, they attempt to identify the specific version of each gene that helps make up the individual's genome. This version is known as the **allele**. By following the transmission of the allele along with its associated characteristics, such as presence of a given disease, researchers can then understand its contribution to the disorder.

allele
One of two or more different variations of a gene.

Genetics is becoming big business as DNA analyses made available through online companies make it possible for people to gain a view into their likelihood of developing a particular genetically based disease. People who send in their DNA samples may learn they have an elevated risk of developing blindness or even whether they are likely to consume less caffeine than the average person. Some of the findings these tests produce are rather trivial (such as whether you have dimples), but other results could help inform people's future health decisions. However, an understanding of the genes involved in specific psychological disorders could pave the way for treatments that use "genome editing," in which the genes that cause the disease are repaired or replaced.

Gene-Environment Interactions The environment to which people are exposed heavily influences brain development throughout life, potentially even altering an individual's genome. Consequently, even though researchers working within the genetic perspective focus on inheritance, they realize that they must also take these environmental factors into account.

A very basic way in which genes and the environment interact pertains to the role of parents as they raise their children. The characteristics of the parents influence the environment they provide for their children, which becomes the environment that influences the child's development of interests and abilities. As they get older, children in turn select environments that match those interests and abilities, a process referred to as **niche-picking**.

niche-picking
The selection by children of environments that match their interests and abilities.

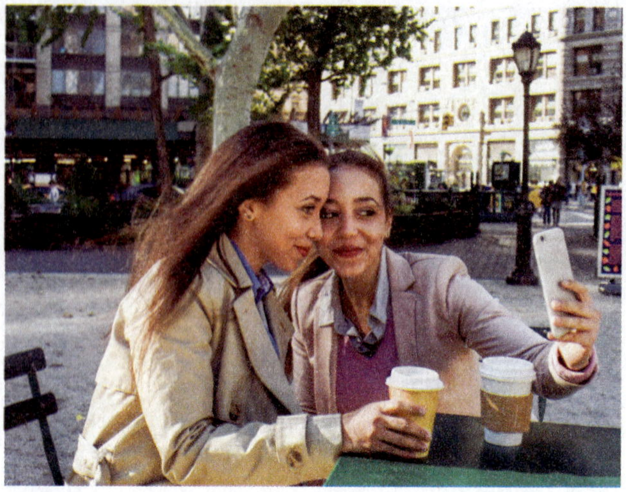

Studies of twins can provide important data regarding genetic influences on psychological disorders

Leland Bobbe/Cultura Creative RF/Alamy Stock Photo

As an example, consider a study conducted on music training in children. The decision to continue music lessons among children 7 to 9 years of age reflected a combination of the personality of the child and the personality of the parents. It was the parents who initially exposed their children to music training, but the child's personality influenced whether that training continued (Corrigall & Schellenberg, 2015).

Gene-environment interactions can also differ according to the individual's developmental status. Researchers studying anxiety and depression in a large sample of twins found that parents had a larger influence on the emergence of these symptoms in the preadolescent compared to adolescent years (Nikstat, Beam, & Riemann, 2023).

Estimates of genetic contributions to psychological disorders may also be made more complex in family inheritance studies by the existence of **assortative mating** in which an individual with a psychological disorder enters into a long-term relationship with another individual who also has that disorder. The offspring of these parents may have a higher risk of the disorder by virtue of their inheritance of genes from both their mother and father (Post et al., 2020).

assortative mating
Entry by a person with a psychological disorder into a long-term relationship with a partner who has the same psychological disorder.

diathesis-stress model
The proposal that people are born with a predisposition (or "diathesis") that places them at risk for developing a psychological disorder if exposed to certain extremely stressful life experiences.

epigenesis
The process of inheriting alterations in gene regulation and expression.

DNA methylation
The process that can turn off a gene when a chemical group, methyl, attaches itself to the gene.

Genetic predispositions may also interact with environmental influences when both alter the effect or expression of the other. For example, people with high genetic risk are more likely to show depressive symptoms when placed under high-stress conditions than are those with low genetic risk. Thus, the same stress has different effects on people with different genetic predispositions. Conversely, the genetic risk of people exposed to higher stress levels becomes higher than that of people who live in low-stress environments. In other words, a person may have a latent genetic predisposition or vulnerability that manifests itself only when that individual comes under environmental stress (Coleman et al., 2020).

According to the **diathesis-stress model**, people are born with a diathesis or genetic predisposition to developing a disease. If they are exposed to harsh or stressful early environments, they become increasingly likely to develop the disorder when they are older. In a protective environment, in contrast, the diathesis will not manifest itself and they will not develop the disorder (e.g., Nielsen, Mennies, & Olino, 2020).

Environmental factors can influence the expression of an individual's genotype through alterations in gene regulation and expression (Ciafrè et al., 2020), a process referred to as **epigenesis**. One of the most significant forms of epigenesis involves the process of **DNA methylation** in which a gene is turned off when a chemical group, methyl, attaches itself to the gene (Figure 2). Such genetic changes may affect the development of psychological disorders, as was shown in a study of anxiety and depression in a large sample of Dutch adults (Hettema et al., 2023).

MINI CASE

Biological Approaches to Treating Meera

A prescribing clinician (such as a psychiatrist or psychiatric nurse practitioner) who works within a biological perspective would treat Meera's depression with antidepressant medications, beginning, most likely, with selective serotonin reuptake inhibitors (SSRIs). Because these medications do not take effect for several weeks, the clinician would monitor Meera closely during this period to ensure she remains stable, meeting with her at least weekly to monitor her progress, learn of any side effects she is experiencing, and make adjustments as necessary, particularly after 4 to 6 weeks. Meera is not a suitable candidate for more radical interventions because, although she has suicidal thoughts, she does not have intent or plans and does not appear to be at significant risk. The clinician may also recommend that Meera attempt to resume her prior exercise routines to help augment the therapeutic effects of her medications.

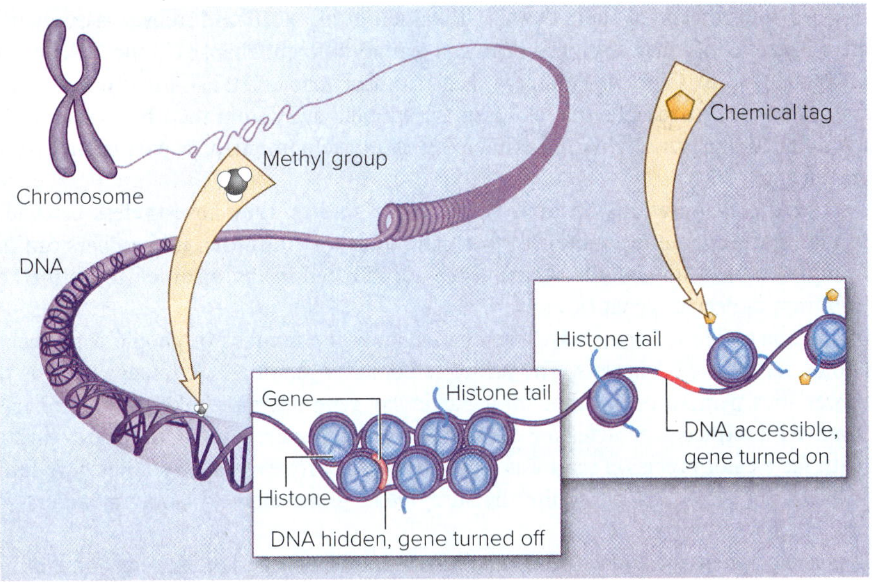

FIGURE 2 Epigenesis

The epigenome can mark DNA in two ways, both of which play a role in turning genes off or on. The first occurs when certain chemical tags, called methyl groups, attach to the backbone of a DNA molecule. The second occurs when a variety of chemical tags attach to the tails of histones, which are spool-like proteins that package DNA neatly into chromosomes. This action affects how tightly DNA is wound around the histones.

SOURCE: National Institute on Aging. (2010). *2009 progress report on Alzheimer's disease*. U.S. Department of Health and Human Services.

Through the epigenetic processes of DNA methylation, features of maternal care, such as the mother's sensitivity toward her infant, can have a lasting impact (Dall' Aglio et al., 2020). In the months after birth, qualities of the father can also alter the process of methylation (Pellicano et al., 2020). The effects of DNA methylation can also be passed down to subsequent generations, which has been demonstrated in studies of offspring of survivors of the Holocaust (Bierer et al., 2020) as well as other conflicts and wars (Hoffman et al., 2023). This phenomenon is often referred to as intergenerational trauma.

Research Methods in Genetics To understand the contributions of genetics to psychological disorders, researchers use three methods: family inheritance studies, DNA linkage studies, and genomics combined with brain scan technology. The methods often complement each other as researchers attempt to tease apart the relationships that underlie the inheritance of complex traits.

Behavioral geneticists typically begin their investigations by using **family inheritance studies**, in which they compare the disorder rates across relatives who have varying degrees of genetic relatedness. This part of the process requires that researchers obtain complete family histories from people whom they can identify as having symptoms of the disorder. The investigators then calculate the **concordance rate**, or agreement ratio, between people diagnosed as having the disorder and their relatives. For example, a researcher may observe that 6 of a sample of 10 twin pairs have the same diagnosed psychological disorder. This would mean that, among this sample, there is a concordance rate of 0.60 (6 of 10).

family inheritance study
Research method in genetics that compares disorder rates across relatives with varying degrees of genetic relatedness.

concordance rate
Agreement ratios between people diagnosed as having a particular disorder and their relatives.

The highest degree of genetic relatedness exists between identical or monozygotic (MZ) twins, who share 100 percent of their genotype, and dizygotic (DZ) or fraternal twins, who share, on average, 50 percent of their genomes, but both types of twins share the same familial environment as long as they were reared together. Therefore, although MZ-DZ twin comparisons are useful, they do not allow researchers to rule out the impact of the environment.

In order to separate the potential impact of the environment in studies comparing MZ and DZ twins, researchers turned long ago to adoption studies in which different families raised MZ twins without having any contact, and therefore the twins experienced different environments. **Cross-fostering studies**, conversely, compares MZ twins reared apart in which one of the adoptive parents had a disorder for which neither child was genetically predisposed. If the children have the same disorder as their biological parents, this suggests that genetic factors play a stronger role than the environment.

cross-fostering study
A type of adoption study in which researchers examine the frequency of the disorder in children whose biological parents had no disorder, but whose adoptive parents do.

There are two important limitations in twin and adoption studies. The first is that MZ twins do not share the same amniotic sac during prenatal development, and they may not even share 100 percent of their DNA (Ollikainen et al., 2010). Moreover, as previously noted, epigenetic influences prior to birth can lead to different changes in the DNA of each twin (Palma-Gudiel, Córdova-Palomera, Navarro, & Fañanás, 2020). Finally, in adoption studies, there may be reasons that children are adopted away from their biological parents that play an unmeasured role in influencing the development of a particular disorder (Marceau et al., 2016).

Despite these limitations of family inheritance studies, they nevertheless provide an important first step in understanding the genetic basis for a disorder. Researchers can then go on to attempt to understand which genes are affected in the disorder, using methods derived from molecular genetics.

genome-wide linkage study
Genetic method in which researchers study the families of people with specific psychological traits or disorders.

In a **genome-wide linkage study**, researchers study the families of people with specific psychological traits or disorders. The principle behind a genome-wide linkage study is that characteristics near to each other on a particular gene are more likely to be inherited together. With refined genetic testing methods available, researchers can now carry this task out with far greater precision than was true in the past. However, such studies have limitations primarily because they require the study of large numbers of family members with differing degrees of relatedness.

genome-wide association studies (GWAS)
Genetic method in which researchers scan the entire genome of individuals who are not related to find the associated genetic variations with a particular disease.

single nucleotide polymorphism (SNP)
A small genetic variation that can occur in a person's DNA sequence.

In **genome-wide association studies (GWAS)**, researchers scan the entire genome of individuals who are not related to find the associated genetic variations with a particular disease. They are looking for a **single nucleotide polymorphism (SNP)** (pronounced "snip"), which is a small genetic variation that can occur in a person's DNA sequence. A SNP variation occurs when a single nucleotide, such as an A, replaces one of the other three. For example, a SNP is the alteration of the DNA segment CTAAGTA to CTAGGTA in which a "G" replaces the second "A" in the first snippet.

As you can see from Figure 3, the genetic sequence of the father contains A, C, T, and C within the SNP, the mother's is G, A, A, and T. Their child's SNP consists of A, A, A, and C. One of these small variations may represent a predisposition to acquiring a particular disease.

With high-tech genetic testing methods now more readily available, researchers have more powerful tools to find SNPs that occur with particular traits (or diseases) across large numbers of people. Although many SNPs do not have measurable effects, researchers believe that other SNPs may predispose people to disease and even influence their response to drug regimens. For example, an international study of SNPs in specific proteins found links to a cluster of characteristics associated with the development of antisocial personality disorder (Tielbeck et al., 2022).

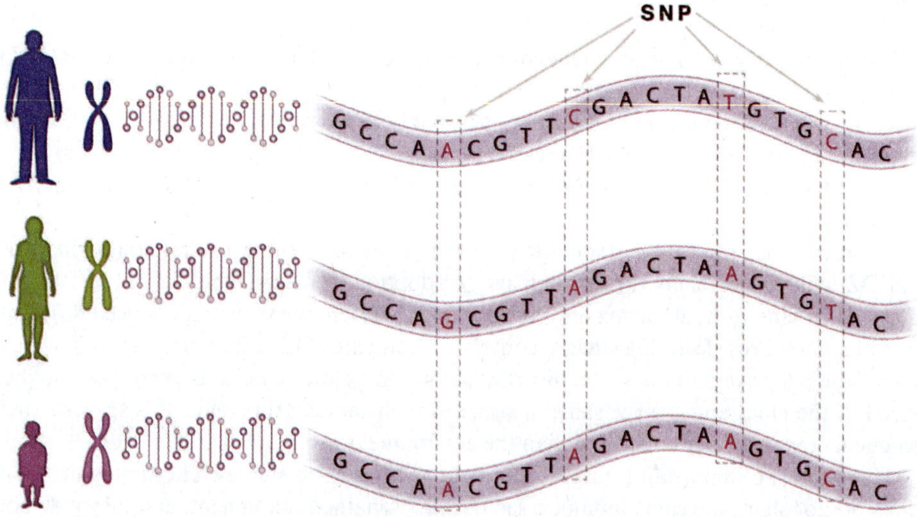

FIGURE 3 Example of the inheritance pattern for a SNP.

A single nucleotide polymorphism (SNP) plays a role in a variety of diseases.

Science History Images/Alamy Stock Photo

Treatment

Treatment of psychological disorders based on the biological perspective primarily consists of the administration of **psychotropic medications**, intended to reduce the individual's symptoms by altering the levels of neurotransmitters hypothesized to be responsible for the disorder. Psychotropic medications first came into use in 1950, when a French chemist, Paul Charpentier, synthesized chlorpromazine (Thorazine). This medication gained widespread acceptance in the 1960s and led the way toward the development of a wider range of psychotropic agents.

psychotropic medications Medications intended to reduce the symptoms of a psychological disorder by altering the levels of neurotransmitters hypothesized to be involved in the disorder.

Currently, the major categories of psychotropic agents are antipsychotics, antidepressants, mood stabilizers, anticonvulsants, antianxiety medications, and stimulants (Table 2). Antipsychotic medications include agents that block dopamine receptors,

TABLE 2 **Major Psychotropic Medications**

Category	Category
Antipsychotics	"Typical," "First generation": -Chlorpromazine -Haloperidol -Perphenazine -Fluphenazine "Atypical," "Second generation": -Risperidone -Olanzapine -Quetiapine -Ziprasidone -Aripiprazole -Paliperidone -Lurasidone "Third generation": -Cariprazine
Antidepressants	Selective serotonin reuptake inhibitors (SSRIs) Serotonin and norepinephrine reuptake inhibitors (SNRIs) Buproprion Tricyclics Tetracyclics Monoamine oxidase inhibitors (MAOIs) Ketamines
Antianxiety medications	Benzodiazepines Buspirone
Stimulants	Methylphenidate Amphetamine Dextroamphetamine Lisdexamfetamine dimesylate
Mood stabilizers	Lithium Carbamazepine Lamotrigine Oxcarbazepine

SOURCE: The National Institute of Mental Health (NIMH). Mental health medications. http://www.nimh.nih.gov/health/publications/mental-health-medications/complete-index.shtml

and they may carry with them side effects that affect an individual's movement, although newer forms of these medications are intended to mitigate somewhat against these side effects.

Some medication categories that researchers developed to treat one disorder, such as SSRIs, also serve to treat other ones, such as anxiety disorders. That clinicians can use the same medications to treat different disorders suggests that alterations involving similar neurotransmitter actions may mediate these disorders.

Ketamines are a class of medications that target the glutamate system. Although ketamines are used as anesthetics, in sub-anesthetic doses they have antidepressant effects (Bahji, Vazquez, & Zarate, 2021). They must be administered intravenously over a 45- to 60-minute period, potentially as often as two to three times a week. Used in the treatment of major depressive disorder when other forms of therapy are ineffective, ketamines also appear to have potential in the treatment of bipolar disorder (Fancy et al., 2023).

The hallucinogenic drug psilocybin is the latest to be tested as a treatment for individuals with major depressive disorder who do not respond to other medications. Psilocybin works by activating serotonin receptors in the parts of the brain involved in processing internally generated stimuli, including the individual's sense of self. For treatment with psilocybin to be effective, the clinician must also provide support through psychotherapy, which may include exploring with the client their readiness for psychadelic interventions (Modlin et al., 2023).

All medications can have serious side effects, unfortunately, leading clients experiencing adverse drug reactions to discontinue their use and seek treatment with a different medication, perhaps from a different category. The Federal Drug Administration (2023) maintains a constantly updated watch list of side effects associated with prescription medications. Individuals and their families can check their medications on this website or sign up for monthly updates.

Treatment based on the biological perspective may also include **psychosurgery**, in which a neurosurgeon operates on brain regions thought to be responsible for the individual's disorder. The first modern use of psychosurgery was a **prefrontal lobotomy**, developed by Portuguese neurosurgeon Egas Moniz in 1935. This method severs the prefrontal lobes from the rest of the brain, a radical procedure that seemed to calm the behavior of a patient experiencing psychotic symptoms but that also created significant personality changes. The technique became widely practiced throughout the next two decades, and although Moniz received a Nobel Prize in 1949 for his work, the method is now discredited on scientific and humanitarian grounds (Dittrich, 2016).

psychosurgery
A form of brain surgery, the purpose of which is to reduce psychological disturbance.

prefrontal lobotomy
A form of biological treatment in which a neurosurgeon severs the patient's prefrontal lobes from the rest of the brain.

Modern psychosurgery relies on targeted interventions designed to reduce symptoms in patients who have proven otherwise unresponsive to less radical treatment (Figure 4). Each type of psychosurgery targets a specific region of the brain that researchers believe is implicated in the symptoms. With higher levels of precision that reflect advances in surgical techniques, including brain visualizations, neurosurgeons can produce a targeted lesion in a specific brain region to provide symptom relief.

For individuals with severe obsessive-compulsive or major depressive disorder, such lesions target the cortex, striatum, and thalamus. **Deep brain stimulation (DBS)**, also called **neuromodulation**, is another form of psychosurgery for individuals with obsessive-compulsive disorder, in which a neurosurgeon implants a microelectrode that delivers a constant low electrical stimulation to a small region of the brain, powered by an implanted battery (Silva et al., 2021).

deep brain stimulation (DBS)
Also called neuromodulation, a treatment in which a neurosurgeon implants a microelectrode that delivers a constant flow electrical stimulation to a small region of the brain, powered by an implanted battery.

neuromodulation
A treatment in which a neurosurgeon implants a microelectrode that delivers a constant low electrical stimulation to a small region of the brain, powered by an implanted battery.

Electroconvulsive therapy (ECT) relies on the application of electric shock to the head for the purpose of inducing therapeutically beneficial seizures. Ugo Cerletti, an Italian neurologist seeking a treatment for epilepsy, developed this method in 1937, and it became used for psychiatric disorders because of its seemingly therapeutic side effects. ECT became increasingly popular in the 1940s and 1950s, but, as the movie *One Flew over the Cuckoo's Nest* famously depicts, staff in psychiatric hospitals also misused it as a way to restrain violent patients.

electroconvulsive therapy (ECT)
The application of electric shock to the head for the purpose of inducing therapeutically beneficial seizures.

Psychiatric Neurosurgery

A handful of medical centers have been conducting several experimental brain surgeries as a last resort for severe obsessive-compulsive disorders that are beyond the range of standard treatment.

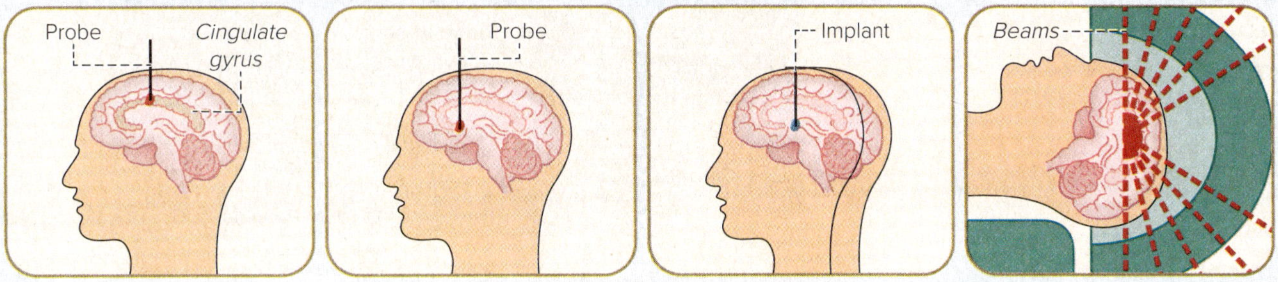

Cingulotomy
Probes are inserted into the brain to destroy a spot on the anterior cingulate gyrus, to disrupt a circuit that connects the emotional and conscious planning centers of the brain.

Capsulotomy
Probes are inserted deep into the brain and heated to destroy part of the anterior capsule, to disrupt a circuit thought to be overactive in people with severe OCD.

Deep brain stimulation
As an alternative to capsulotomy, an electrode is permanently implanted on one or both sides of the brain. A pacemaker-like device then delivers an adjustable current.

Gamma knife surgery
An MRI-like device focuses hundreds of small beams of radiation at a point within the brain, destroying small areas of tissue.

FIGURE 4 Forms of Psychosurgery for Treating Severe Obsessive-Compulsive Disorders That Are Beyond the Range of Standard Treatment

Even though ECT had largely fallen into disuse by the mid-1970s, psychiatrists continued to use it to treat patients who did not respond to other measures. A comprehensive review of controlled studies using ECT for treatment of major depressive disorder showed that, in the short term, ECT was more effective than medications in producing rapid improvement of symptoms (UK ECT Review Group, 2003). Clinicians working with older adults are concerned about its side effect of memory impairment. However, this effect appears to be transitory, even in older individuals who show structural brain aberrations (Wagenmakers et al., 2021). Nevertheless, researchers remain uncertain about how ECT's long-term risks, and whether any effects that it shows, can be attributed to the electricity, the seizure, or a combination of the two (Deng et al., 2023).

4.3 Trait Theory

Trait theory proposes that psychological disorders develop when the individual has maladaptive **personality traits**, which are enduring patterns of perceiving, relating to, and thinking about the environment and others. In the chapter "Assessment," you learned that some assessment methods focus on measuring these qualities of personality, which psychologists think of as stable, enduring dispositions that persist over time. For many personality trait theorists, these components of psychological functioning are more than long-standing qualities of personality that may even have some degree of heritability (Vukasović & Bratko, 2015).

personality trait
An enduring pattern of perceiving, relating to, and thinking about the environment and others.

It is easy for most people to relate to trait theory because it fits so closely with the use of the term *personality* in everyday life. When you think about how to describe the personality of someone you know, you will likely come up with a list of qualities that seem to fit the individual's typical way of behaving. These characteristics typically take the form of adjectives such as *friendly* or *calm*, or perhaps *anxious* and *shy*. Trait theories of personality propose that adjectives such as these capture the essence of the individual's psychological makeup. The fact that people use these adjectives in everyday life to describe themselves and others aligns with the basic principle of trait theory—namely, that personality is equivalent to a set of stable characteristic attributes.

FIGURE 5 Five Factor Model of Personality: Examples of Qualities Represented in Each of the Factors in the Five Factor Model

SOURCE: The Art of Passing a Personality Test. http://dandebat.dk/eng-person3.htm

Five Factor Model

		Low scorers	High scorers
1	Openness to experience	Conventional Down-to-earth Uncreative Uncurious	Original Imaginative Creative Curious
2	Conscientiousness	Negligent Lazy Disorganized Late	Conscientious Hard-working Well-organized Punctual
3	Extraversion	Loner Passive Quiet Reserved	Joiner Active Talkative Affectionate
4	Agreeableness	Critical Irritable Ruthless Suspicious	Lenient Good-natured Soft-hearted Trusting
5	Neuroticism	Calm Comfortable Even-tempered Unemotional	Worried Self-conscious Temperamental Emotional

Five Factor Model (or "Big Five")
Trait theory proposing that there are five basic dispositions in personality, each of which has six facets.

The predominant trait theory in the field of psychological disorders is the **Five Factor Model**, also called the FFM or "Big Five" (Figure 5) (McCrae & Costa, 1987). According to this theory, each of the basic five dispositions has six facets, which leads to a total of 30 personality components. The Five Factor Model includes the personality traits of neuroticism, extraversion, openness to experience, agreeableness, and conscientiousness (conveniently, their initials spell out "OCEAN" or "CANOE"). A complete characterization of an individual on the five factors consists of providing scores or ratings on each facet.

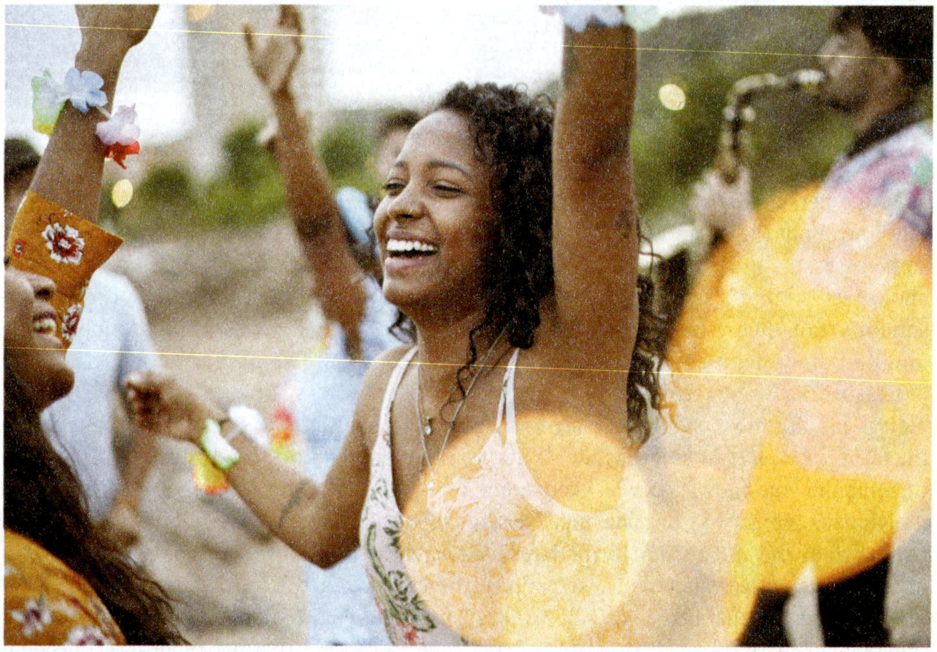

People high in extraversion thrive in social situations.

Carlos Barquero/Moment/Getty Images

HEXACO personality trait model
Trait-based approach that proposes personality traits fall into the six categories of honesty: humility, emotional stability, extraversion, agreeableness, and conscientiousness.

MINI CASE

Trait Theory Approaches to Treating Meera

Because trait theory does not have any direct clinical applications, there are no obvious ways in which a clinician would apply this perspective to Meera's depression. The information in Dr. Tobin's Case Report indicates that she was not diagnosed with a personality disorder. A clinician working with Meera from a trait theory approach could, however, order a more thorough assessment of Meera's personality traits that includes a personality trait–based measure to confirm these hypotheses and to determine whether she also has a comorbid personality disorder. Even if she does not have a personality disorder, it is possible that Meera's personality trait profile would be relevant to treatment. For example, she seems not to be overly introverted because she interacts frequently with friends. Her depressive symptoms appear not to be overlaid on personality traits that include high neuroticism. She seems to enjoy activities that include creativity and exploration of the outdoors, indicating a normative personality for her age in openness to experience. Prior to her depressive episode, she was at least average in conscientiousness, as her successful work history indicated, and there is no evidence to suggest that she is unusually low in agreeableness. The clinician can share feedback about these results to increase Meera's insight into her personality traits, which could be useful in helping select the most effective strategies for reducing her depression.

According to trait theory, where people fall on the 30 facets strongly influences the shape of their lives. People high on personality traits representing riskiness (thrill seeking) are more likely to get hurt because their personalities lead them into situations that can land them in trouble. Similarly, people high on the traits that define the less psychologically healthy end of each continuum may be more likely to experience negative life events, such as relationship problems, which contribute to life stress (Asselmann & Specht, 2020). Personality traits can also have important consequences for both health and cognitive functioning, particularly in later life (Pocnet, Popp, & Jopp, 2020).

An alternative to the Five Factor Model is the **HEXACO personality trait model** (Lee & Ashton, 2004) that includes the factors of extraversion, agreeableness, conscientiousness, and openness to experience from the FFM, but adds "honesty-humility" and "emotional stability" (the opposite of neuroticism) to the structure of personality. In part, the reason for adding honesty-humility as a personality dimension reflects the model's incorporation of psychopathological traits, including those that fall in the realm of antisocial behavior (e.g., Radević & Dinić, 2022).

What's in the *DSM-5-TR*

Theoretical Approaches

Versions of the *DSM* prior to *DSM-III* were based almost entirely on clinical judgments framed within the psychodynamic model of psychological disorders. The *DSM* used terms such as *neurosis* and *psychosis,* which had meaning in the psychodynamic world, to differentiate disorder categories. For example, anxiety disorders fell into the category of neurosis because their primary symptoms included irrational fears and worries. It labeled schizophrenia a psychotic disorder because its primary symptoms include lack of contact with reality and other cognitive distortions.

The *DSM-III* authors reconceptualized their approach along two major lines. First, they intended it to be atheoretical—meaning that there was no underlying theory, psychodynamic or otherwise. Second, they intended the diagnostic criteria to be ones that a variety of mental health professionals could reliably evaluate. The *DSM-III* task force therefore commissioned studies in which researchers could evaluate the reliability of the diagnostic criteria. Rather than use vague terminology (such as *neurosis*) that could be open to various interpretations, the *DSM-III* diagnostic spelled out criteria in exacting levels of detail. The *DSM-IV* and its later revision, the *DSM-IV-TR,* carried on this tradition of specifying diagnostic criteria in research-based, objective terms.

The *DSM-5-TR* continues this empirical tradition and remains atheoretical. Critics maintain that the *DSM-5-TR* should have represented disorders on spectrums or in larger grouping systems (Milinkovic & Tiliopoulos, 2020). Although the *DSM-5-TR* task force considered making this radical change, its members eventually decided to maintain the earlier categories, though with some alterations. The move away from categories and toward dimensions would have required not only a massive restructuring, but also retraining of clinicians who were trained on the earlier *DSMs*.

Whether future *DSM*s move away from the present system will depend largely on developments in the field of psychopathology. Section III of the *DSM-5-TR* contains a dimensional system that clinicians can use to supplement their formal diagnoses of the personality disorders. Diagnoses are now in groups or chapters according to their presumed underlying similarities or causes. Ultimately, the authors will make decisions on empirical grounds, which will maintain the intent of *DSM* to keep its atheoretical basis.

4.4 Psychodynamic Perspective

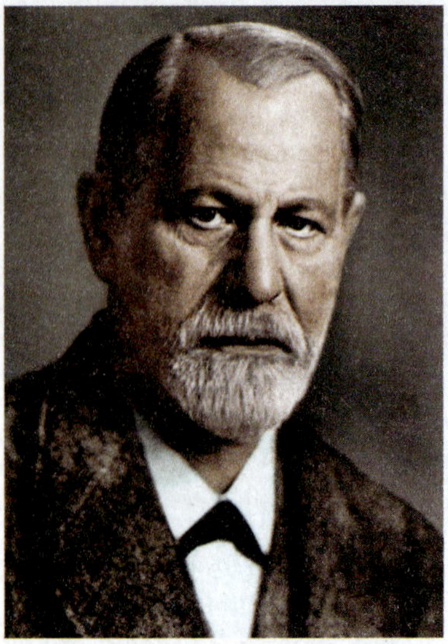

Sigmund Freud developed a theory that served as the foundation for the psychodynamic perspective.

Music-Images/Lebrecht Music & Arts/Alamy Stock Photo

psychodynamic perspective
The theoretical orientation in psychology that emphasizes unconscious determinants of behavior.

id
In psychoanalytic theory, the structure of personality hidden in the unconscious that contains instincts oriented toward fulfilling basic biological drives, including sexual and aggressive needs.

libido
An instinctual pressure that strives for gratification of sexual and aggressive desires.

pleasure principle
In psychoanalytic theory, a motivating force that seeks the immediate and total gratification of sensual needs and desires.

The **psychodynamic perspective** emphasizes unconscious determinants of behavior. Of all the psychological approaches, the psychodynamic gives greatest emphasis to the role of processes theorized to occur beneath the surface of awareness as influences on psychological disorders.

Freud's Theory

Starting in the late 1800s, Sigmund Freud began to explore the potential origins of psychological disorders through his own clinical work with patients having what seemed, at the time, to be unexplainable physical symptoms. By the time of his death in 1939, Freud had articulated a vision for cause and treatment of psychological disorders, with the basic tenet that most symptoms can be traced to roots buried deep within an individual's past.

According to Freud (1923), the mind has three structures: the id, the ego, and the superego. The **id** is the structure of personality hidden in the unconscious that contains instincts oriented toward fulfilling basic biological drives, including gratification of sexual and aggressive needs. The **libido** is the instinctual pressure that strives for gratification of sexual and aggressive desires.

The id follows the **pleasure principle**, a motivating force that seeks immediate and total gratification of sensual needs and desires. According to Freud, you can obtain pleasure only when you are able to reduce the tension of an unmet drive. The id, however, does not require tangible gratification of a need. Instead, it can use wish fulfillment to achieve its goals. Through wish fulfillment, the id conjures an image of whatever will satisfy the needs of the moment.

The center of conscious awareness in Freud's model of personality is the **ego**, the structure of personality that gives the individual the cognitive powers of judgment, memory, perception, and decision making. Freud (1911) described the ego as being governed by the **reality principle**, meaning that it tries to deal with real-life constraints to achieve its goals. For example, consider the following situation: You're hungry and a good friend walks by eating a donut. Your id might urge you to grab that donut for yourself, but your ego instead advises you to ask politely if you might have a bite.

The third part of the equation in psychodynamic theory is the **superego**, which is personality's seat of morality. The superego includes the conscience (sense of right and wrong) and the ego ideal, or aspirations. The superego would instruct you, for example, that to take someone else's donut constitutes theft and is therefore morally wrong.

In a healthy individual's personality, as described by Freud, the id achieves instinctual desires through the ego's ability to navigate in the external world within the confines the superego places on it. **Psychodynamics**, or the interplay among the structures of the mind, is thus the basis for both normal and pathological functioning.

Freud believed people were primarily sexual and aggressive in the content of their motives and therefore needed to be protected from knowing their own unconscious desires. They achieve this protection by using **defense mechanisms** (Table 3). According to Freud, everyone uses defense mechanisms on an ongoing basis to avoid recognizing the existence of their hidden desires. Although they can serve an adaptive function, defense mechanisms create problems when they prevent an individual from coming completely to terms with his or her true unconscious nature.

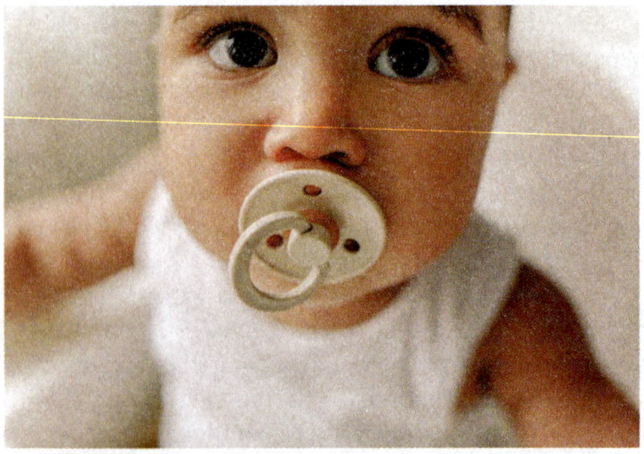

In Freudian psychodynamic theory, fixation on oral satisfaction is the main reason behind an infant's use of a pacifier.

Maskot/Getty Images

The topic of development forms an important piece of Freud's theory. In 1905, Freud proposed that normal development occurs through a series of what he called **psychosexual stages**, and that children go through these stages in accordance with the development of their libido. At each stage, the libido becomes fixated on a particular "erogenous" or sexually excitable zone of the body. For example, the "anal retentive" personality is overly rigid, controlled, and perfectionist. According to Freud, such an individual's personality would reflect the likelihood that the person had become fixated at the anal stage of development.

TABLE 3 **Categories and Examples of Defense Mechanisms**

Defense Mechanism	Definition
Displacement	Shifting unacceptable feelings or impulses from the target of those feelings to someone less threatening or to an object
Intellectualization	Resorting to excessive abstract thinking rather than focus on the upsetting aspects of response to issues that cause conflict or stress
Reaction formation	Transforming an unacceptable feeling or desire into its opposite in order to make it more acceptable
Repression	Unconsciously excluding disturbing wishes, thoughts, or experiences from awareness
Denial	Dealing with emotional conflict or stress by refusing to acknowledge a painful aspect of reality or experience that would be apparent to others
Projection	Attributing undesirable personal traits or feelings to someone else to protect one's ego from acknowledging distasteful personal attributes
Sublimation	Transferring an unacceptable impulse or desire into a socially appropriate activity or interest
Regression	Dealing with emotional conflict or stress by reverting to childish behaviors

Freud believed the adult personality reflects the way in which the individual resolves the psychosexual stages in early life, but that some reworking may occur at least up through middle adulthood. Freud also believed that the child's feelings toward the "opposite-sex" parent set the stage for later psychological adjustment. The outcome of what he called the **Oedipus complex** (named after a tragic character in ancient Greek myth who married his mother) determined whether the individual had a healthy ego or would spend a life marred by anxiety and repressed, conflicted feelings associated with wanting to engage in what society deems taboo behavior (incest). In the course of ordinary development, children's desire for the opposite-sex parent eventually submerges beneath the surface of conscious awareness, thus posing no further threat to their sense of self-acceptance.

Post-Freudian Psychodynamic Views

Freud developed his theory in the context of early 1900s Vienna, the location of his home and office. At the same time, he also encouraged like-minded neurologists and psychiatrists to work together with him to develop a new theory of the mind. Over a period of years, Freud and his followers spent many hours comparing notes about their clinical cases and trying to come to a joint understanding about normal and pathological functioning. Although they shared many of the same views when they began their discussions, several of his colleagues left his circle and went on to develop their own unique brands of psychodynamic theory. Each are now associated with their own schools of thought.

The most notable departure from Freud's school of thought came when Swiss psychiatrist Carl Jung (1875–1961) revamped the definition of the unconscious. According to Jung (1961), the unconscious is formed at its very root around a set of images common to all human experience, which he called **archetypes**. Jung believed that people respond to events in their daily lives on the basis of these archetypes, because they are part of one's genetic makeup. For example, Jung asserted that archetypal characters (such as today's Marvel Superheroes) are popular because they activate the "hero" archetype. For Jung, psychopathology resulted from an imbalance within related parts of the mind, especially when people fail to pay proper attention to their unconscious needs.

One group or category of post-Freudian theorists advocated for the study of **ego psychology**. These theorists believed that the ego, not the id, was the main driving force in personality. As a result, the post-Freudian theorists viewed personality and psychopathology

ego
In psychoanalytic theory, the structure of personality that gives the individual the mental powers of judgment, memory, perception, and decision making.

reality principle
In psychoanalyic theory, the motivational force that leads the individual to confront the constraints of the external world.

superego
In psychoanalytic theory, the structure of personality that includes the conscience and the ego ideal.

psychodynamics
Interplay among the structures of the mind.

defense mechanisms
Tactics that keep unacceptable thoughts, instincts, and feelings out of conscious awareness and thus protect the ego against anxiety.

psychosexual stages
According to psychoanalytic theory, the normal sequence of development through which each individual passes between infancy and adulthood.

Oedipus complex
According to Freud, the child's feelings toward the opposite-sex parent peak in early childhood.

archetypes
In Jung's theory, a set of images common to all human experience.

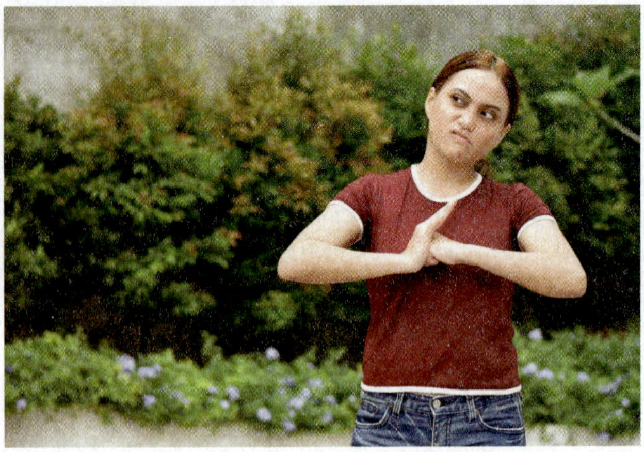

In Horney's theory, this woman would be said to demonstrate the antagonistic personality style of "moving against" people.

cheapbooks/Shutterstock

not as disturbances in id-like, primitive instincts, but as components of the individual's sense of self and relationships to other people.

Alfred Adler (1870–1937) focused on the "inferiority complex" as a cause of psychopathology. Neurotic individuals, he maintained, try to overcompensate for feelings of inferiority in their sense of self by constantly "striving for superiority." Karen Horney (1885–1952) proposed that neurotic individuals put up a false, idealized front to protect their very fragile true sense of self. Both Adler and Horney also emphasized social concerns and interpersonal relations in the development of personality. They saw close relationships with family and friends and an interest in the life of the community as gratifying in their own right, not because a sexual or an aggressive desire is indirectly satisfied in the process, as Freud might say. Although these theories date back to the mid-twentieth century, psychologists today continue to find their ideas to be relevant to the development of psychopathology, including certain forms of personality disorders (Calabrese et al., 2023).

ego psychology
Theoretical perspective based on psychodynamic theory emphasizing the ego as the main force in personality.

Perhaps the only psychodynamic theorist to give attention to the whole of life, not just childhood, was Erik Erikson (1902–1994). Like Adler and Horney, Erikson gave greatest attention to the ego in development. Erikson believed the ego goes through a series of transformations throughout life in which new strengths or abilities can mature. According to his theory, each stage builds on the one that precedes it and, in turn, influences all the stages that follow it. However, Erikson proposed that any stage could become a major focus at any age. Although identity issues are associated with adolescence, they can resurface at any point in adulthood, even after a person's identity has become relatively stabilized. For example, a middle-aged woman who is laid off from her job may once again question her occupational identity as she seeks to find a new position for herself in the workforce.

object relations
A psychodynamically oriented theory that focuses on the relationships people have with the others ("objects") in their lives.

attachment style
The way a person relates to a caregiver figure.

attachment figures
Caregivers or adults to whom the individual is attached.

Yet another group of psychodynamically oriented theorists focused on **object relations**, namely, the relationships people have with the others ("objects") in their lives. These theorists included John Bowlby (1907–1990), Melanie Klein (1882–1960), D. W. Winnicott (1896–1971), Heinz Kohut (1913–1981), and Margaret Mahler (1897–1995). Like the ego psychologists, the object relations theorists each have a particular model of therapy associated with their theories.

Despite the differences among them, all theorists in the object relations perspective believed the individual's relationship with the caregiver or caregivers become an inner framework or model for all close adult relationships. Themes of your adult relationships, in other words, reflect themes from your early childhood and the way your caregivers (parents, and other adults) treated you.

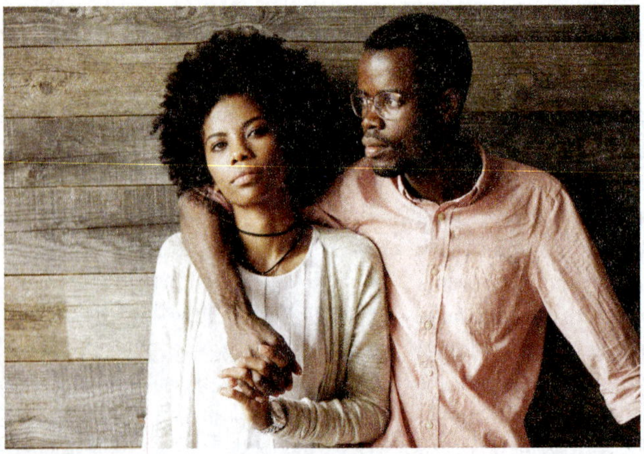

In object relations theory, adults who resist close relationships may have an insecure attachment style.

Cast Of Thousands/Shutterstock

Putting their theory to the test, Canadian psychologist Mary Salter Ainsworth (1913–1999) and her associates (1978) studied differences among infants in **attachment style**, or the ways they related to a caregiver figure. The caregivers or adults to whom the individual is attached are referred to as the **attachment figures**. Ainsworth developed the "Strange Situation," an experimental setting in which researchers separated infants from and then reunited them with their mothers. Children who accepted the mother's leaving and then her return were regarded as securely attached. Those who either became frantic, on the one hand, or seemed distant and remote, at the other extreme, were considered insecurely attached.

Although attachment style was designed as a theory of child development, later researchers have adapted it to apply to adult romantic relationships. Most children develop secure attachment styles, and later in life they relate to their close romantic partners without undue anxiety about whether their partners will care about them (Mohd Hasim, Hashim, & Mustafa, 2023). Those who are insecurely attached in childhood, however, may show a pattern of anxious attachment in adulthood in which they feel they cannot rely on their partner's love and support. Or they may show a dismissive or avoidant attachment style, in which they fear rejection from others and therefore try to protect themselves by remaining distant. Both these variations can, furthermore, become the basis for adult psychopathology (Smith & South, 2020), particularly personality disorders.

An individual's attachment style may also influence the way they respond to psychotherapy (Hill, Knox, & Duan, 2023). The therapeutic outcome can also be affected by interactions between the attachment styles of client and therapist (Shir & Thisby, 2023). As you will see shortly, psychodynamic therapy specifically takes such client-therapist relationships into account.

Treatment

The main goal of traditional psychoanalytic treatment as developed by Freud was to bring repressed, unconscious material into conscious awareness. To accomplish this task, Freud developed the therapeutic method of **free association**, in which the client literally says whatever comes to mind during the treatment session. Freud believed that clients needed to work through their unconscious conflicts, bringing these gradually into conscious awareness by speaking them aloud. Eventually they could gain insight into the forces that produced their thoughts and words.

free association
A method used in psychoanalysis in which the client speaks freely, saying whatever comes to mind.

Current psychodynamic treatment is focused on helping clients explore aspects of the self that are "unconscious" in the sense that the client does not recognize them. Therapists focus, in particular, on the way clients reveal and influence these aspects of the self in their relationship with the therapist. The key elements of psychodynamic therapy delve into the client's emotional experiences, use of defense mechanisms, close relationships with others, past experiences, and exploration of fantasy life in dreams, daydreams, and fantasies (Shedler, 2010).

Psychodynamic therapists also use **transference** to help inform their treatment by analyzing the feelings their clients seem to have toward them. The idea behind this step is that clients regard their therapists in a way similar to the way they felt about their parents, because they see their therapists as important figures in their lives. In the context of therapy, these feelings can be examined and put to valuable use.

transference
The carrying over of feelings that clients have from their parents to their therapists.

Unlike the stereotyped portrayal you might see in movies or on television, clinicians need not conduct psychodynamic therapy on a couch, for years at a time, or in total silence. However, given the impracticality of maintaining a long-term and intense form of treatment, psychotherapists began developing briefer and seemingly as effective forms of psychodynamic therapy. In keeping with principles of evidence-based practice, the effectiveness of psychodynamic therapy can be studied empirically, making it possible for those who work within this perspective to evaluate the effectiveness of shorter, more focused approaches (Keefe et al., 2020).

In one version of brief psychodynamic therapy, the clinician identifies the client's "Core Conflictual Relationship Theme" (CCRT). The clinician assesses the client's wishes, expected responses from others, and client responses either to the responses of others or to the wish itself. The client describes specific instances in relationships with others that allow the clinician to make the CCRT assessment. The clinician then works with the client in a supportive way to help him or her recognize and eventually work through these patterns (Grenyer & Marceau, 2022). For example, the therapist would induce individuals with obsessive-compulsive disorder to face the feared situation and use the aroused experiences to work on the underlying conflict (Leichsenring & Steinert, 2017). In another application, treatment consisted of helping clients with troubled relationships by examining the dynamics of their daily interactions (Day, Townsend, & Grenyer, 2022).

Clearly, the psychodynamic perspective has come a long way from traditional Freudian psychoanalysis, although it maintains its focus on helping clients understand and overcome interpersonal issues from their past that continue to create challenges in their present lives.

MINI CASE

Psychodynamic Approaches to Treating Meera

A clinician working with Meera from a psychodynamic perspective would assume that her difficulties stem from conflicts in early life. For example, the clinician would explore the resentment she feels toward her parents for favoring her sister, and her possible guilt over breaking away from the family when she established her own independent life. In treatment, the clinician would observe whether Meera reenacts her conflicted feelings about her parents in the relationship she establishes with the clinician. The Core Conflictual Relationship Theme (CCRT) approach would seem particularly appropriate for Meera, given the possible role of these difficult relationships in triggering her depressive disorder. Meera's depressive symptoms would warrant a time-limited approach focusing on her current episode, with the option for her to seek treatment in the future if her depression recurs.

4.5 Behavioral Perspective

behavioral perspective
A theoretical perspective in which it is assumed that psychological disorders are caused by faulty learning experiences.

According to the **behavioral perspective**, the individual acquires maladaptive behavior through learning. Consistent with its name, this perspective focuses on the individual's observable behavior, the factors that might precipitate it, and the consequences that maintain it over time.

Theories

Classical conditioning
The process in the behavioral perspective that accounts for the learning of emotional, automatic responses.

aversive conditioning
Classical conditioning in which the individual associates a maladaptive response with a stimulus that could not itself cause harm.

operant conditioning
A learning process in which an individual acquires a response by learning to pair a behavior with its consequences.

The two main approaches within the behavioral perspective of psychological disorders differ in focusing either on emotional, involuntary reactions such as fear, or on complex, voluntary actions such as engaging in an unwanted or undesirable habit.

Classical conditioning is the process in the behavioral perspective that accounts for the learning of emotional, automatic responses. As an extreme example, imagine someone tapped you hard on your knuckles whenever you reached for a piece of chocolate. If this continued, you would eventually come to dread that person, not to mention the scent or sight of chocolate. Much of the classical conditioning that behavioral clinicians attempt to help their clients overcome is this type of **aversive conditioning** in which the individual associates a maladaptive response with a stimulus that could not itself cause harm.

The learning of complex, voluntary behaviors occurs through **operant conditioning** in which an individual acquires a response by learning to pair a behavior with its consequences.

You Be the Judge

Evidence-Based Practice

As you learned in the chapter "Diagnosis and Treatment," APA adopted principles of evidence-based practice that provide guidelines for clinicians to follow in their provision of psychological treatment. In this chapter, you've learned about the wide range of theoretical models available to clinicians, ranging from psychosurgery at one extreme, to family therapy at another. Given the recommendation that psychologists provide the treatment best suited to the client's psychological disorder, the question is whether each clinician has the ability to provide treatment within each of these theoretical models. Is this a realistic expectation? Can we expect a clinician to be knowledgeable enough about each theoretical perspective to give clients the most effective interventions?

As research within clinical psychology and related fields continues to progress at an almost exponential rate, how can each clinician stay on top of all the latest developments well enough to be comfortable providing the most recent approaches to each client? According to the APA Ethical Guidelines, clinicians should work within their areas of expertise, and if they must extend outside this area, they should seek consultation from those who are knowledgeable in the area. Moreover, each state maintains strict licensing regulations to ensure that psychologists participate in continuing education. As a result, there are many safeguards to protect clients from outdated or inappropriate intervention methods.

Q: *You be the judge:* As a consumer of psychology, do you feel it is more important for potential clients to see a clinician whom they trust based on reputation, prior experience, or recommendations from other people, or should they instead find a specialist who, in the theoretical perspective, most closely adheres to evidence-based standards? Can a respected "generalist" provide care that is as high quality as another professional who is more narrowly trained? Ultimately, clients are protected against inadequate care by the standards that govern each profession (counseling, psychiatry, psychology, social work). However, it also benefits consumers to stay abreast of the latest developments so they can make the most informed choices possible.

The behavior's consequences are its **reinforcement**–the outcome that makes the individual more likely to repeat the behavior in the future.

Reinforcement can take many forms. For example, in positive reinforcement, your friends may laugh when you express outrageous opinions, making you more likely to express those opinions in the future. You might also learn through negative reinforcement to take an over-the-counter sleep medication if you find that it helps alleviate your insomnia. This is considered negative reinforcement because your behavior of taking the sleep medication increases by removing the aversive state of being sleepless. Both negative and positive reinforcement increase the frequency of the behaviors that precede them. In these examples, the behaviors that increase are speaking outrageous opinions (positive reinforcement) and taking sleep medication (negative reinforcement).

Derived from the behavioral perspective, **Applied Behavior Analysis (ABA)** uses principles of reinforcement both to understand and change behavior. ABA clinicians use positive reinforcements in the form of rewards help to establish and strengthen desired behaviors. They also base their work on an "A-B-C" model that identifies antecedents (precipitants) of behaviors, the resulting behavior, and the consequences that the behavior produces. Key to ABA is the importance of planning treatment specific to the individual's skills, needs, interests, and family situations. These considerations include cultural responsiveness, empathy, and assessments of the client's functional abilities (Gatzunis et al., 2023). ABA is often used in treating children with complicated symptoms related to Autism Spectrum Disorder, and other developmental disorders.

According to the behavioral perspective, you don't have to directly experience reinforcement in order for it to modify your behavior. Psychologists who study **social learning theory** believe that people can learn by watching others. Thus, **vicarious reinforcement** leads you to acquire a new behavior that you see reinforced in another person. Watching an advertisement for sleep medication showing how it helped the person in the ad could provide vicarious reinforcement for buying that same product.

You can also develop a perception of your own competence in various life situations, or **self-efficacy**, by watching the results of your own actions or those of other people with whom you identify. For example, you may wonder whether you have the ability to overcome your fear of public speaking, but if you see a fellow student give a successful presentation in class and feel you are not that different from this student, their success will build your feelings of self-efficacy, and you will be better prepared mentally to do well when it's your turn to get up and speak.

reinforcement
In operant conditioning, the outcome that makes the individual more likely to repeat the behavior in the future.

Applied Behavior Analysis (ABA)
Treatment approach within the behavioral perspective that uses principles of reinforcement both to understand and change behavior.

social learning theory
Perspective that focuses on understanding how people develop psychological disorders through their relationships with others and through observation of other people.

vicarious reinforcement
A form of learning in which a new behavior is acquired through the process of watching someone else receive reinforcement for the same behavior.

self-efficacy
The individual's perception of competence in various life situations.

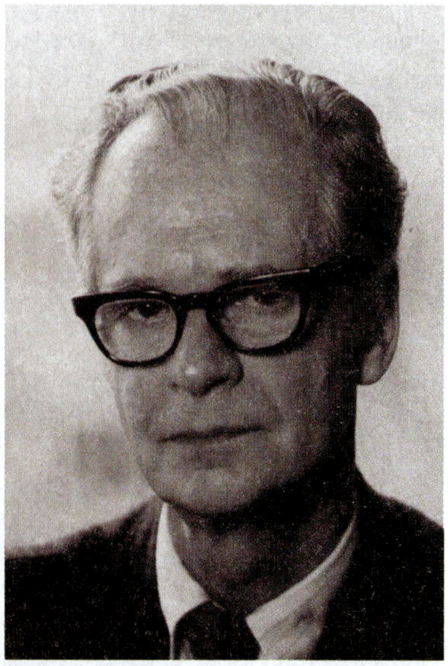

The American psychologist B.F. Skinner pioneered the behavioral perspective, showing how an individual's responses, both adaptive and maladaptive, can be acquired through the process of operant conditioning.

Science History Images/Alamy Stock Photo

MINI CASE

Behavioral Approaches to Treating Meera

Following from the behavioral assumption that clients experiencing major depressive episodes have developed maladaptive responses, a behaviorally oriented clinician would give Meera the opportunity to learn new, adaptive behaviors. As you will learn in the chapter "Depressive and Bipolar Disorders," behavioral approaches to major depressive disorder have clients increase the frequency of positively reinforcing events (known as "behavioral activation"). Meera would keep a diary of her interactions with friends, participation in exercise, and other enjoyable activities, which she would then show to her therapist. To increase the frequency of these behaviors, Meera and her clinician would identify a set of desirable rewards to occur with their completion. For the intervention to be most effective, the clinician would need to ensure that Meera can realistically obtain her goals so she continues to experience success in achieving them.

Treatment

counterconditioning The process of replacing an undesired response to a stimulus with an acceptable response.

systematic desensitization A variant of counterconditioning that involves presenting the client with progressively more anxiety-provoking images while in a relaxed state.

contingency management A form of behavioral therapy in which clinicians provide clients with positive reinforcement for performing desired behaviors.

Behavior therapists focus their therapeutic efforts on helping their clients unlearn maladaptive behaviors and replace them with healthy, adaptive behaviors. In **counterconditioning**, clients learn to pair a new response to a stimulus that formerly provoked the maladaptive response. In order for this process to work, incompatible with the old (undesirable) response. For example, it's more or less impossible to feel anxious and relaxed at the same time. In counterconditioning, as developed by physician Joseph Wolpe (1915–1997), clients learn to associate the response of relaxation with the stimulus that formerly caused them to feel anxious. Clinicians teach clients to relax through a series of progressive steps–for example, by first relaxing the head and neck muscles, then their hands and feet, and ultimately the rest of their bodies. They can then go through these steps when in the actual or virtual presence of the formerly feared stimulus.

Counterconditioning often occurs in gradual stages using the **systematic desensitization** method. The therapist breaks the maladaptive response into its smallest steps while pairing each step with relaxation, rather than exposing the client all at once to the feared stimulus.

To assist in the process of systematic desensitization, the client may begin by providing the therapist with a hierarchy, or list, of situations associated with the feared stimulus. Starting with the least fearful situation in the hierarchy, the clinician asks the client to imagine that situation and practice progressive relaxation at the same time. After the client has established the connection between that image and relaxation, the clinician then moves up the hierarchy to the next level. Eventually, the client can confront the feared situation while at the same time feeling entirely relaxed. At any point, though, if the client suffers a setback, the clinician moves back down the hierarchy to help the client relearn to associate relaxation with the image at the previous lower level.

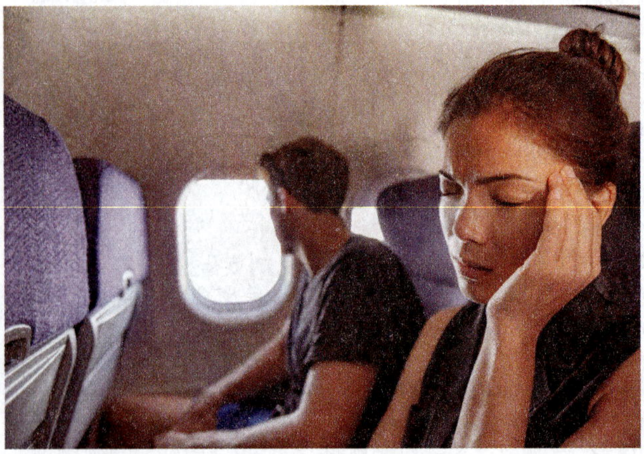

A behaviorally oriented psychologist would help a client overcome fear of flying by using such methods as breathing exercises, reducing physiological tensions, and overcoming automatic thoughts about the fear of flying.

Maridav/Alamy Stock Photo

Figure 6 shows an example of a fear hierarchy that a clinician might use in systematically desensitizing a person who fears spiders. Moving from the least-feared to the most-feared stimulus based on this hierarchy, the client should eventually be able to relax while holding the live spider. At each step of the hierarchy, the client would record, on a scale of 0–100, their levels of both fear and relaxation.

Based on principles of operant conditioning, **contingency management** is a form of behavioral therapy in which clinicians provide clients with positive reinforcement for performing desired behaviors. The client learns to connect the outcome of the behavior with the behavior itself, in order to establish a contingency or connection. The clinician works with the client to develop a list of positive reinforcements the client can receive only after performing the desired behavior.

For example, if the client is trying to quit smoking, the clinician suggests a schedule in which the client can receive the designated reinforcement after going without a cigarette for a specific amount of time (such as permission to play 10 minutes of video games). Gradually, the client extends the time period until they are able to cease smoking altogether. One contingency management form that residential settings use is the **token economy**, in which residents who perform desired activities earn tokens they can later exchange for tangible benefits. An advantage of token economies is that they can be readily taught to caregi vers who can use them in the home, as was done in Italy during the COVID-19 lockdowns in 2020 (degli Espinosa et al., 2020).

Behavioral treatments can also invoke the principle of vicarious reinforcement, in which clinicians show live or recorded models of people receiving rewards for demonstrating the desired behaviors (Bandura, 1971). For example, if a client is afraid of entering a small closet, the clinician treating them may show a video of a person reaching into a closet without fear to grab a shirt. The vicarious reinforcement in this situation is seeing the person in the video calmly looking for some clothes. The therapist might also use **participant modeling**, a form of therapy in which the therapist first shows the client a desired behavior and then guides the client gradually through the behavioral change. This could involve the therapist bringing the client into a cramped space while offering them guidance and support.

Clinicians working within the behavioral perspective often provide their clients with homework assignments. The clinician may ask the client to keep a detailed record of the behaviors he or she is trying to change, along with the situations in which the behaviors occur. The homework assignment might also include specific tasks the clinician asks the client to perform with instructions for observing the outcome of completing those tasks. Returning to the previous example, the client could be instructed to try entering a cramped space such as a closet at home while noting on paper their levels of fear.

Because these homework assignments can be completed in the client's own time, they can become an important adjunct to teletherapy and therefore useful for delivering treatment to underserved populations whose members may have limited access to in-person treatment (Trombello et al., 2020).

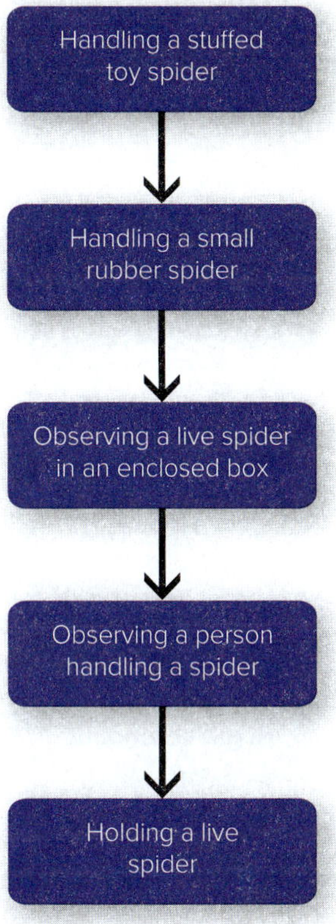

FIGURE 6 Fear Hierarchy in Systematic Desensitization

token economy
A form of contingency management in which a client who performs desired activities earns tokens that can later be exchanged for tangible benefits.

participant modeling
A form of therapy in which the therapist first shows the client a desired behavior and then guides the client through the behavioral change.

4.6 Cognitive and Cognitive Behavioral Perspectives

The **cognitive perspective** proposes that psychological disorders are the result of maladaptive thought processes that result in dysfunctional behaviors and emotions. If people can change these thoughts into ones that are more "rational" or logical, their behavior and emotions will become less dysfunctional and they can maintain their psychological health. The key to the cognitive perspective, then, is the "cognitive" or thought component of psychological functioning. When combined with the behavioral perspective, this approach becomes the **cognitive behavioral perspective**, which focuses on the role of both maladaptive thoughts and maladaptive behaviors in psychological disorders.

cognitive perspective
A theoretical perspective in which it is assumed that psychological disorders are the result of maladaptive thought processes that result in dysfunctional behaviors and emotions.

cognitive behavioral perspective
An approach that focuses on the role of both maladaptive thoughts and maladaptive behaviors in psychological disorders.

Theories

Theories in the cognitive perspective begin with the concept of **dysfunctional attitudes**, negative beliefs about the self that are also deeply ingrained and difficult to articulate. People with psychological disorders experience **automatic thoughts**, the product of dysfunctional attitudes so deeply entrenched the individual is not even aware they exist. Dysfunctional attitudes influence the ways that people with psychological disorders interpret their experiences.

Figure 7 illustrates this chain of events. Put yourself in the place of the person in the example shown here. You begin with the dysfunctional attitude that you will be the target of derision if you make a mistake. The fact that your self-esteem is based on this belief means that

dysfunctional attitudes
Negative beliefs about the self that are deeply ingrained.

automatic thoughts
Ideas that are the product of dysfunctional attitudes so deeply entrenched the individual is not even aware they exist.

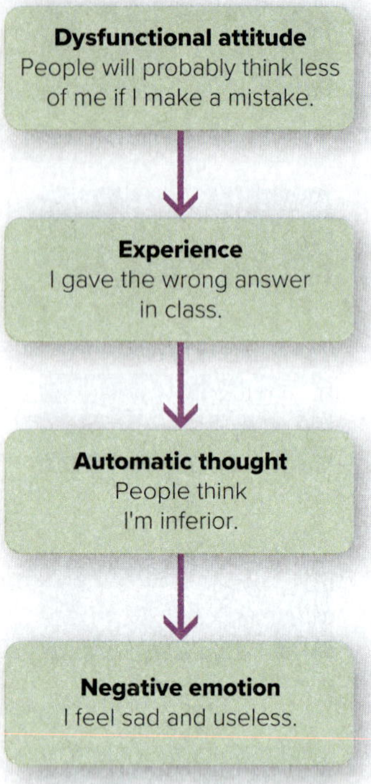

FIGURE 7 The Relationship Among Dysfunctional Attitude, Experience, Automatic Thought, and Negative Emotion

SOURCE: Adapted from Beck, A. T., Rush, A. J., Shaw, B. F., & Emery, G. (1987). *Cognitive therapy of depression*. Guilford Press.

should you actually make a mistake, such as giving the wrong answer in class, this will prompt the immediate, or automatic, thought that everyone will now judge you as inferior. Needless to say, this thought will trigger the negative emotion of feeling sad, and worse, useless.

As you imagine yourself in this situation, you can trace the way negative emotions evolve from a combination of dysfunctional attitudes, actual experiences, and automatic thoughts. Because so much of this process bypasses your ability to think critically about your own assumptions, your negative emotion will seem to be the only possible way you can feel under the circumstances.

Particularly problematic for people with psychological disorders, according to this perspective, are the unrealistic, extreme, and illogical ways in which they think about themselves and their behavior. Their irrational beliefs cause them to punish themselves because they fail to live up to the "musts" of being perfect (Ellis, 2005). When they invariably fail, they can become so despondent that they give up on the idea of ever getting better, and should they enter treatment, they take an unduly pessimistic approach about whether they will improve.

Treatment

Clinicians who adopt the cognitive perspective focus their attention on changing the thoughts, or dysfunctional attitudes, that ultimately produce the negative emotions. One key method used by cognitively oriented clinicians is **cognitive restructuring**, in which the clinician attempts to change the client's thoughts by questioning and challenging the client's dysfunctional attitudes and irrational beliefs. In this way, clients learn to reframe negative ideas into more positive ones. Returning to the example, you might decide that making a mistake is perfectly normal, meaning you won't jump to the extreme of feeling worthless because of one wrong answer.

In **cognitive behavioral therapy (CBT)**, as the term implies, clinicians focus on changing both maladaptive thoughts and maladaptive behaviors. Clinicians combine behavioral techniques, such as using homework and changing reinforcement patterns, with cognitive methods that challenge the logic of their dysfunctional thoughts. In working with their clinicians, clients can then try to identify situations, behavior, or people that help them counteract these emotions.

As an example, consider another type of situation. A client believes he is incapable of being liked by anyone but his close family members and therefore feels alone and isolated. He feels so incapacitated that he turns down invitations for casual get-togethers with his co-workers. The clinician seeks to break this cycle by assigning the homework of accepting one of those invitations and then reporting back in therapy on how the event actually went, focusing on the client's feelings at the time. This report can then become the basis for another assignment, with perhaps a slightly wider group of acquaintances, until the client has enough "data" to challenge her belief that no one could possibly like him.

Although known to have a solid backing in research demonstrating its efficacy, one criticism of CBT is that it is not tailored to a diverse range of clients. In **culturally adapted CBT (CA-CBT),** treatment aspects may be modified to take into account culturally relevant material, culturally matched clinicians, language, and session structure. In addition to being useful for populations within the United States from culturally diverse backgrounds, CA-CBT has also been successfully applied outside the continental United States (Silveus, Schmit, Oliveira, & Hughes, 2023).

The central aim of CBT, then, is to give clients greater control over their dysfunctional behaviors, thoughts, and emotions. Through this approach, CBT seeks to empower clients to find more adaptive ways to respond to life's challenges–thus not only improving their current symptoms but decreasing the likelihood they will reoccur in the future.

Like behavioral therapy, CBT also has the advantage of being readily adapted to teletherapy, as became evident in the early months of the COVID-19 pandemic in 2020 (Murphy, Calugi, Cooper, & Dalle Grave, 2020). Not only is CBT amenable to remote delivery, but it also proved to be useful for clients whose symptoms were exacerbated by social distancing and the fear of becoming infected by the virus.

cognitive restructuring
One of the fundamental techniques of cognitive behavioral therapy in which the clinician attempts to change the client's thoughts by questioning and challenging the client's dysfunctional attitudes and irrational beliefs.

cognitive behavioral therapy (CBT)
Treatment method in which clinicians focus on changing both maladaptive thoughts and maladaptive behaviors.

culturally adapted CBT (CA-CBT)
Cognitive behavioral approach in which treatment aspects may be modified to take into account culturally relevant material, culturally matched clinicians, language, and session structure.

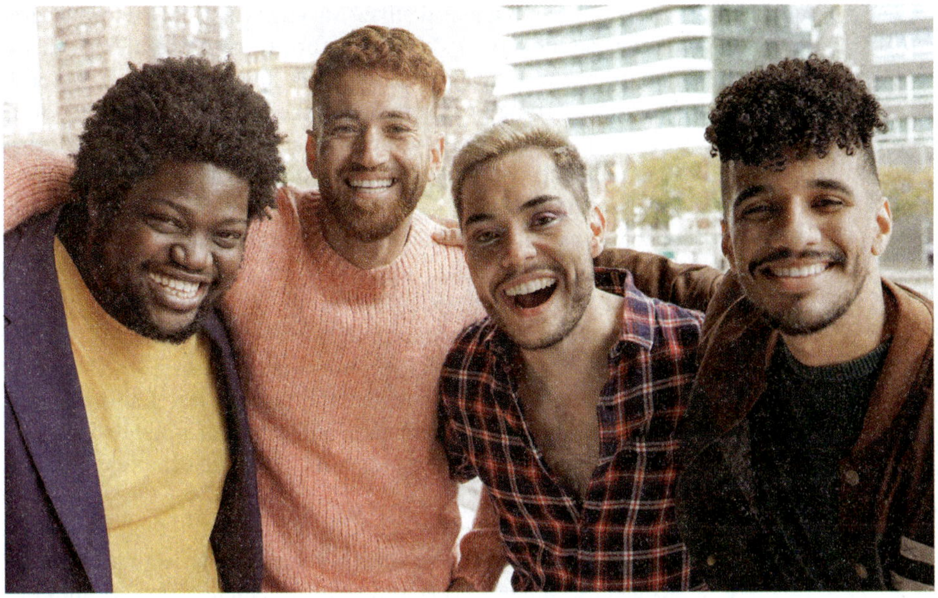

In cognitive behavioral therapy, a client may receive the homework assignment of accepting an invitation with friends to help challenge the belief that the client is unlikeable.

Sabrina Bracher/Shutterstock

MINI CASE

Cognitive Approach to Treating Meera

A clinician working within a cognitive perspective would treat Meera by helping her develop more adaptive thoughts. From a strictly cognitive point of view, the clinician would focus on Meera's beliefs that she has let down her family and friends and encourage her to challenge her conclusion, looking with her at the basis for her assumption about her family's feelings toward her.

Combining the cognitive and the behavioral approaches, the clinician would also ask Meera to keep a record of her behaviors, including her participation in positively rewarding activities. However, unlike the strict behaviorist, this clinician would also instruct Meera to keep a record of her dysfunctional thoughts, particularly those that exacerbate her negative emotions.

4.7 Humanistic Perspective

Psychologists who adhere to the **humanistic perspective** believe people are motivated to strive for self-fulfillment and meaning in life. The "human" in *humanistic* refers to the focus of this perspective on the qualities that make each individual unique. Furthermore, unlike the behavioral perspective, which translates principles from animal learning to the behavior of people, the humanistic perspective focuses specifically on the values, beliefs, and ability to reflect on our own experiences that separate humans from other species.

humanistic perspective
A theoretical view of personality and psychological disorder proposing that people are motivated to strive for self-fulfillment and meaning in life.

Theories

Humanistic theories gained prominence in the 1960s among psychologists who sought to break from the traditional focus of psychology, in which human behavior is viewed as the result of either outside (behavioral) or instinctive (psychodynamic) forces. These humanistic theorists joined together to form a "third force" in psychology, with the intention of challenging these established views. Psychologists working within this tradition also saw human behavior in much more positive terms and viewed psychological disorders as the result of restricted growth potential.

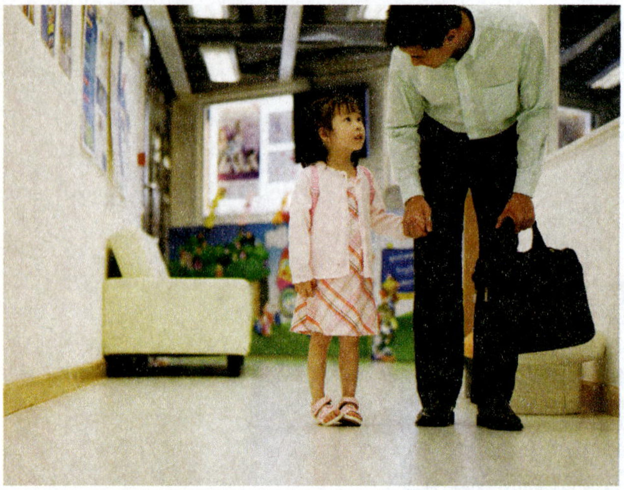

Psychologists from several theoretical perspectives believe that early childhood experiences with primary caregivers influence the way an individual behaves in interpersonal relationships throughout the life span.

©Michael Hall Photography Pty Ltd/Corbis

The work of humanistic theorists was heavily influenced by **existential psychology**, a theoretical position that emphasizes the importance of fully appreciating each moment as it occurs (May, 1983). According to existential psychology, if you are tuned in to the world around you and experience life as fully as possible in each moment, you will function at your maximum level of psychological health. Psychological disorders arise when people are unable to experience living in the moment due to restrictions modern society imposes on the ability to express one's inner self (Frankl, 1963; Laing, 1959).

The humanistic approach in clinical work is exemplified best by Carl Rogers's (1902–1987) **person-centered theory**, which focuses on each individual's uniqueness, the importance of allowing each individual to achieve maximum fulfillment of potential, and the need to confront honestly the reality of your experiences in the world.

In applying the person-centered theory to the therapy context, Rogers (1951) used the term **client-centered** to reflect his belief that people are innately good and that the potential for self-improvement lies within the individual rather than in the therapist or therapeutic techniques. This approach also applies to counseling, and it may be one you've encountered if a coach or guidance counselor encouraged you to find the best within yourself.

existential psychology
The theoretical position that emphasizes the importance of fully appreciating each moment as it occurs.

person-centered theory
The humanistic theory that focuses on the uniqueness of each individual, the importance of allowing each individual to achieve maximum fulfillment of potential, and the need for the individual to honestly confront the reality of his or her experiences in the world.

Rogers believed a well-adjusted person's self-image should be congruent with the person's experiences. In this state of congruence, a person is fully functioning–able to put their psychological resources to their maximal use. Conversely, a psychological disorder is the result of blocking the individual's potential for living to full capacity, resulting in a state of incongruence or mismatch between self-image and reality. Congruence is not a static state, however; to be fully functioning means the individual is constantly evolving and growing. Consider your own life; at times you may feel comfortable with who you are, only to question and challenge these feelings when situations change.

According to Rogers, psychological disorders have their origins in early life, when children are raised by parents who are harshly critical and demanding. Under such circumstances, children develop chronic anxiety about making mistakes that will cause their parents to disapprove of them even more. Rogers used the term **conditions of worth** to refer to the demands parents place upon children when they communicate the message that in order to be loved, they have to meet these criteria. As adults, children who were raised by these demanding parents are constantly trying to meet the expectations of others instead of feeling that others will value them for their true selves, flaws, and all.

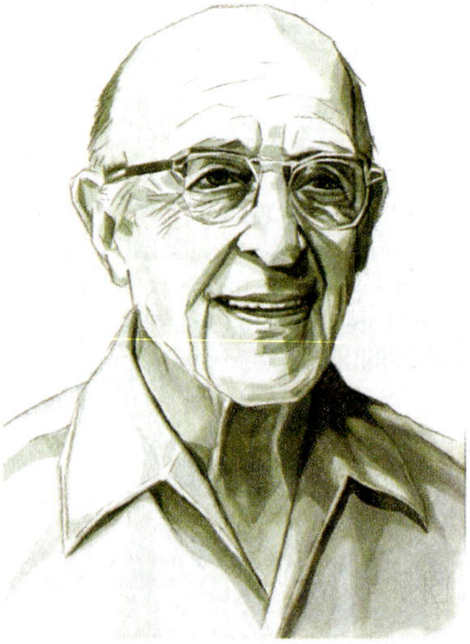

Psychologist Carl Rogers developed an approach to therapy based on humanistic principles known as the client-centered approach.

INTERFOTO/Personalities/Alamy Stock Photo

Less focused on therapy but also highly influential in the humanistic movement, Abraham Maslow's (1962) theory centers on the notion of **self-actualization**, the maximum realization of the individual's potential for psychological growth.

According to Maslow, self-actualized people have accurate self-perceptions and are able to find rich sources of enjoyment and stimulation in their everyday activities, a concept similar to the idea of the fully functioning person in the theory of Rogers. However, Maslow also proposed that self-actualization includes people's ability to have so-called "peak experiences," in which they feel a tremendous surge of inner happiness, as if they were totally in harmony with themselves and their world. Self-actualized people, furthermore, are not simply searching for sensual or spiritual pleasure. They also have a philosophy of life that is based on humanitarian and egalitarian values.

However, self-actualization is possible even when people are deprived of their basic needs. You may find yourself deriving inspiration from exactly these individuals who risk their own security in order to work toward a higher purpose. Maslow's view of self-actualization, unlike theories relevant only to psychological disorders, therefore, provides a unique perspective on the factors that can contribute to psychological health.

Common interpretations of Maslow's theory regard self-actualization as most likely to occur when people have first met their basic physical and psychological needs, or what he considered lower-order, survival motives.

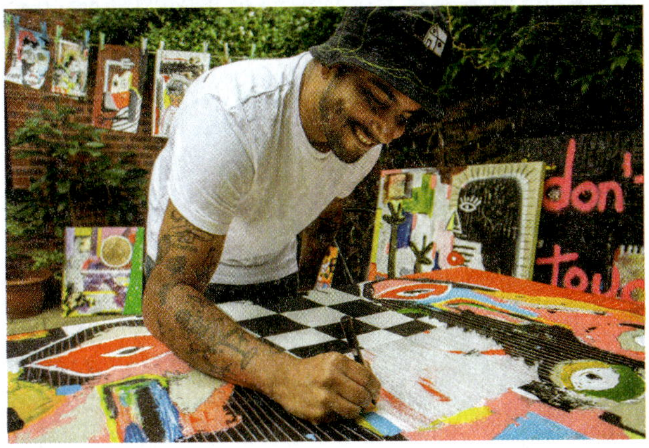

In Maslow's theory, people who are self-actualized are able to express their own true, unique feelings, motivations, and abilities.
horst friedrichs/Alamy Stock Photo

Treatment

A theory rich with implications for treatment, person-centered theory now forms the foundation of much of contemporary therapy and counseling. The client-centered model of therapy proposed specific guidelines for therapists to follow in order to ensure that clients are able to achieve full self-realization. According to Rogers, clinicians should focus on the client's needs, not on preconceived clinician notions about what is best for the client. In fact, reflecting this emphasis on the inherent strengths of people seeking treatment, Rogers originated the use of the term *clients* because it implies a partnership between the helper and the person being helped.

Rogers believed that a clinician's job is to help clients discover their inherent goodness and, in the process, to help each client achieve greater self-understanding. To counteract the problems caused by conditions of worth in childhood, Rogers recommended that therapists treat clients with **unconditional positive regard**, or total acceptance of what the client says, does, and feels. As clients begin to feel less self-critical, they become better able to tolerate the anxiety that comes with acknowledging their own weaknesses, because they no longer feel driven to see themselves as perfect. The clinician tries to be as compassionate as possible, and gradually the client feels increasingly confident about revealing their true, inner selves because they know the clinician will not reject or label them as inadequate.

Contemporary humanistic and experiential therapists emphasize that therapists can be most effective if they are empathic, or able to see the world from the eyes of their clients, as much as possible. Therapists working within the client-centered model are trained in the techniques of reflection and clarification in order to express empathic understanding. In reflection, the therapist mirrors back what the client has just said, perhaps rephrasing it slightly, and makes every attempt to see the client's situation as it appears to them. These techniques allow clients to feel that the clinician is listening empathically and not judging them.

Rogers also suggested that clinicians should provide a model of genuineness and willingness to disclose their personal weaknesses and limitations. Clients then realize they don't have to put up a false front, trying to appear as something they are not. Ideally, the client will see that it is acceptable and healthy to be honest in confronting personal experiences, even if those experiences have less than favorable implications. For example, the Rogerian clinician might admit to having experiences similar to those the client describes, such as feeling anxious about speaking before a group. This is the kind of self-disclosure a Freudian psychoanalyst would never engage in, because it takes away from the therapist's status as a completely neutral party. To a Rogerian clinician, the sharing of personal experiences (within bounds) helps the client feel more accepted and understood.

Motivational interviewing (MI) is another client-centered technique that uses empathic understanding as a means of promoting behavioral change in clients (Magill et al., 2018). Here the clinician collaborates with the client to strengthen the client's motivation to make changes by asking questions that elicit the individual's own arguments for change. MI, like the client-centered approach in general, emphasizes the client's autonomy.

The humanistic perspective permeates much of contemporary psychology, particularly informing the mission of positive psychology, which emphasizes growth and fulfillment rather than psychopathology and disorder. Maslow's theory is perhaps most heavily employed within a vocational and educational framework, and the principles of person-centered therapy developed by Rogers now are an implicit component of the focus in psychotherapy on empathy and the therapeutic alliance. Mindfulness and motivational interviewing now receive widespread attention, giving clinicians additional and accessible tools to use with clients in a range of ages with a range of disorders.

client-centered
An approach based on the belief held by Rogers that people are innately good and that the potential for self-improvement lies within the individual.

conditions of worth
The demands parents place on their children in which they communicate the message that to be loved, they have to meet certain criteria.

self-actualization
In humanistic theory, the maximum realization of the individual's potential for psychological growth.

unconditional positive regard
A method in client-centered therapy in which the clinician gives total acceptance of what the client says, does, and feels.

motivational interviewing (MI)
A technique that uses empathic understanding as a means of promoting behavioral change in clients.

MINI CASE

Humanistic Approaches to Treating Meera

In humanistic therapy, a clinician would work with Meera to establish a firm therapeutic alliance by empathically listening to her descriptions of her feelings. Consistent with Carl Rogers's emphasis on becoming more aware of our feelings, the clinician would encourage Meera to experience more fully her feelings about how she felt rejected by her family and her sadness as a result of her disconnectedness from them. In this process, the clinician would help Meera identify her feelings and accept them without undue self-criticism. The clinician might also focus on Meera's feelings of low self-worth by exploring how she felt her parents were negatively comparing her to her sister. Because she believed that she could only be accepted if she abided by their rules, Meera felt that people could not regard her as an individual on her own terms. To help increase authentic feelings of self-worth, the clinician would work with Meera to further her understanding of her own values and develop ways for her to build growth-enhancing experiences consistent with those values, rather than with those of her family.

4.8 Sociocultural Perspective

Theorists within the sociocultural perspective emphasize the ways that people, social institutions, and social forces influence individuals in the world around them. The sociocultural perspective reaches outside individuals to include the totality of factors that may contribute to their development of psychological disorders.

Theories

family perspective
A theoretical perspective in which it is assumed that psychological disorders are the result of disturbances in the pattern of interactions and relationships within the family.

social discrimination
Prejudicial treatment of a class of individuals, seen in the sociocultural perspective as a cause of psychological problems.

Proponents of the **family perspective** regard psychological disorders as caused by disturbances in the patterns of interactions and relationships that exist within the family. These disturbed patterns of relationships may create the "identified patient"—namely, the individual in treatment whose difficulties reflect strains within the family.

Researchers within the sociocultural perspective also focus on **social discrimination**, the prejudicial treatment of a class of individuals, as a cause of psychological problems. People are most likely to be identified as targets of social discrimination based on such factors as race or ethnicity, religion, immigration status, religion, age, and sexual orientation (Jackson et al., 2019). Discrimination against transgender people can be experienced as both traumatic and a cause for internalized transphobia, in which these individuals develop strong feelings of shame (Barr, Snyder, Adelson, & Budge, 2022). Social discrimination's effect on both mental and physical health reflects a combination of these sources of stress, inequities in access to health care, and the perception of discrimination (Hackett et al., 2020).

Natural and human-caused disasters, political oppression, poverty, violence, and war are further contributors to psychological disorders, according to the sociocultural perspective. The COVID-19 pandemic is proving to have significant effects on mental health with its global impacts on mortality, the economy, the trauma experienced by victims and survivors, and the need for quarantine (Fernández et al., 2020). Researchers continue to identify COVID-19's impact on specific populations including children and college students (Elharake et al., 2023) as well as older adults (Mushtaq & Khan, 2023). Climate change, with the associated increases in natural disasters, is also proving to have significant mental health effects (Lawrance et al., 2022).

Treatment

How do clinicians intervene to help people with mental health issues caused by or exacerbated by sociocultural factors? Clearly, it is not possible to change the world, but clinicians can play a crucial role in helping people come to grips with problems that have developed within a family system, the immediate environment, or extended society.

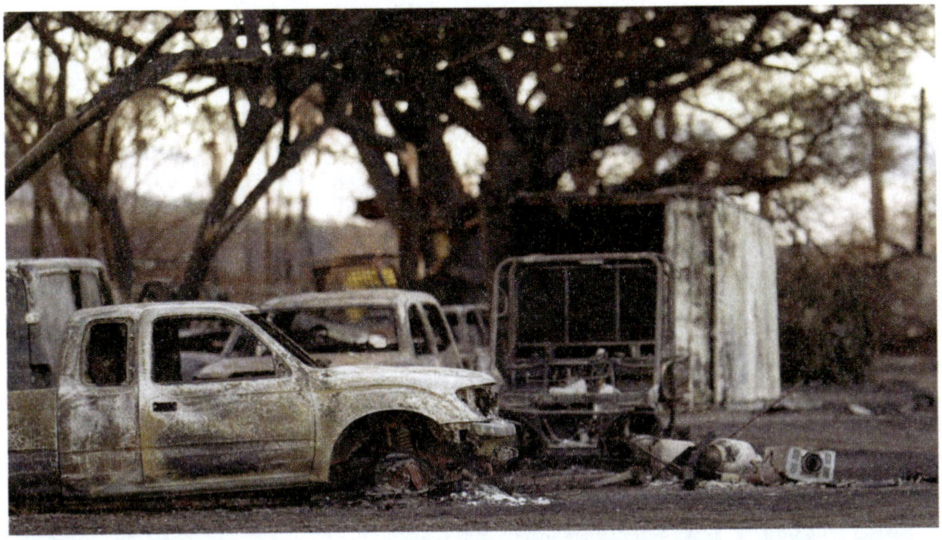

The destruction of Lahaina, Maui, in the August 2023 fire not only put individual's lives in danger but also presented a severe threat to the mental health of survivors.

American Photo Archive/Alamy Stock Photo

In the most immediate circle of the individual, namely the family, clinicians can intervene by encouraging all family members (however family is defined) to try new ways of relating to each other or thinking about their problems. The family therapist, sometimes working with a co-therapist, meets with as many family members as possible at one time. Rather than focusing on an individual's problems or concerns, family and couples therapists focus on the ways in which dysfunctional relational patterns maintain a particular problem or symptom. They also use a life-span perspective in which they consider the developmental issues, not only of each individual, but of the entire family or couple. Furthermore, family and couples therapists see the continuing relationships among the family members as potentially more healing than the relationship between clinicians and clients.

The particular techniques that clinicians use in family therapy depend greatly on the therapist's training and theoretical approach. An intergenerational family therapist might suggest drawing a diagram of all relatives in the recent past, in an effort to understand the history of family relationships and use this understanding to bring about change. A structural family therapist might suggest that a subset of the family members enact a disagreement as if they were characters in a play about the family. By doing so, the family members can step outside their current conflicts and see new ways of handling their recurring patterns of interaction. An experiential family therapist might work with the family members to develop insight into their relationships with each other by focusing on how they are feeling at the moment as they discuss their joint concerns.

In group therapy, people who share similar experiences share their stories with each other, aided by the facilitation of the therapist. According to Irvin Yalom (1931–2019), a founder of group therapy, clients can find relief and hope in the realization that their problems are not unique by hearing that others share their emotional experiences. In the group, they can also acquire valuable information and advice from people who share their concerns. Furthermore, in the process of giving to others, people generally find that they themselves derive benefit.

Due to the lockdowns and social distancing required by the COVID-19 pandemic, clinicians began to devise ways to deliver group therapy via telemental health. Clients appeared to respond favorably to remote interventions and, indeed appeared to find a number of benefits related to convenience and accessibility to mental health services (Maier, Riger, & Morgan-Sowada, 2021).

Clinicians use milieu therapy in treatment settings such as inpatient hospitals to promote positive functioning in clients by creating a therapeutic community. Community members participate in group activities, ranging from occupational therapy to training classes. Staff members encourage clients to work and spend time with other residents with the goal of increasing the positive bonds among them. Every staff person, whether a therapist, nurse, or paraprofessional, takes part in the overall mission of providing an environment that supports positive change and reinforces appropriate social behaviors. The underlying idea behind milieu therapy is that the pressure to conform to conventional social norms of

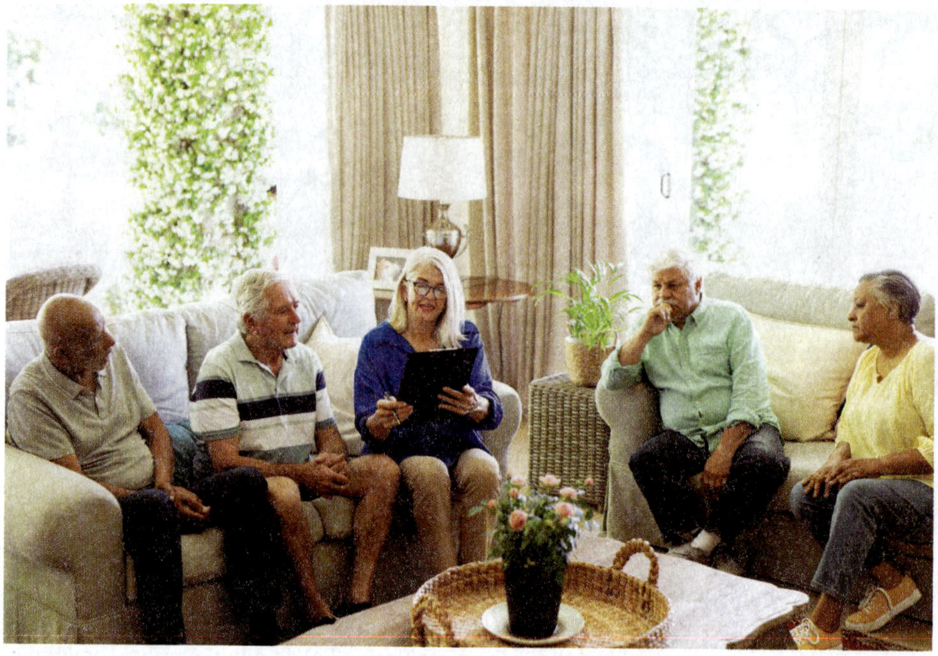

Group therapy provides a format for treatment in which clients can provide support to each other with the guidance of the therapist.
Wavebreak Media/Shutterstock

behavior fosters more adaptive behavior on the part of individual clients. In addition, the normalizing effects of a supportive environment are intended to help the individual make a smoother and more effective transition to life outside the therapeutic community.

multicultural approach
Therapy that relies on awareness, knowledge, and skills of the client's sociocultural context.

Although clinicians cannot reverse social discrimination, they can adopt a **multicultural approach** to therapy that relies on awareness, knowledge, and skills of the client's sociocultural context. In keeping with the principles of cultural formulations, therapy should be sensitive to the ways in which the client's cultural background interacts with his or her specific life experiences and family influences. Clinicians make a commitment to learning about the client's age, cultural, ethnic, and racial group and the way these factors play a role in assessment, diagnosis, and treatment. Multicultural skills include mastery of culture-specific therapy techniques that are responsive to a client's unique characteristics.

MINI CASE

Sociocultural Approach to Treating Meera

A clinician working within the sociocultural perspective would incorporate Meera's specific family issues within the context of her cultural background. Not only have Meera's symptoms likely emerged from her own construction of her family's attitude toward her work and relationship decisions, but they also reflect her Indian cultural background, which tends to place heavy emphasis on family obligations. By choosing a path different from that of her sister, Meera has perhaps, in reality or in her own perception, violated her familial and larger cultural expectations. In therapy, Meera should be encouraged to reflect on and develop her own sense of identity within both her family and the larger cultural context as a first-generation American, and to acknowledge how that affects her family dynamics and relates to her depressive symptoms. The clinician might suggest that Meera be seen with her family, if possible, to work through these cultural and relational conflicts. Or the clinician could help Meera develop a way to communicate her observations with her family and work toward managing their expectations of her. This could help to rebuild the relationship in a way that takes into account both Meera's framework and the family's own beliefs. Through the sociocultural lens, reworking the relationship in this way could help reduce Meera's depressive symptoms by allowing her to be herself within the family without feeling she is constantly violating their expectations.

REAL STORIES

Sylvia Plath (1932–1963)

At the age of 30, U.S. poet Sylvia Plath succumbed to her lifelong battle with depression. On the night of February 11, 1963, with her two infant children asleep, Plath carefully placed towels in the cracks under the doors to her children's bedroom and her kitchen, turned on the gas in her oven, and laid her head inside. She had left milk and bread in the children's room with the window open to the chilly London night so their breakfast would be fresh for the morning.

Only days before, she had begun a course of antidepressants, and experts believe her death by suicide occurred at a dangerous time in the course of treatment with such medications, when the individual—still depressed—becomes simultaneously more active, leading to an increased risk for suicide attempts. *Bitter Fame: A Life of Sylvia Plath*, by Anne Stevenson (1989) chronicles the life and writings of the notoriously tortured writer through her journal entries, personal letters, and interviews with those who were in her life. Born and raised around Boston, Massachusetts, Plath began writing at the age of 7. Throughout her childhood and adolescence, she produced an impressive number of poems and short stories that gave rise to her ultimate dream of being a professional writer.

Plath's experiences served to inspire her until the final days of her life. Perhaps the most influential was the sudden death of her father shortly after her 8th birthday, a loss that fueled her innermost fears and desires and became an ever-present theme in her work. It also left her incredibly sensitive to depression following abandonment from others in her life, particularly romantic partners.

Plath grew up in the prototypical New England town of Wellesley, Massachusetts, and attended Smith College in Northampton, Massachusetts, on an academic scholarship. Although the transition to college was initially difficult for her, her intelligence and diligent work ethic earned her high grades and a prominent reputation at Smith. As she grew into young adulthood, she began to experience heightened moodiness and bouts of depression. At age 19, she attempted suicide by swallowing her mother's sleeping pills and hiding in a crawlspace in her house. It was 2 days before anyone discovered her in a dazed and semiconscious state. Following the attempt, Plath entered a nearby psychiatric hospital for a 4-month period, where she received electroconvulsive therapy (ECT). This marked a major turning point in her life and in her writing.

"Attributable to her ECT," Stevenson writes in *Bitter Fame*, "is the unseen menace that haunts nearly everything she wrote, her conviction that the world, however benign in appearance, conceals dangerous animosity, directed particularly toward herself." We can observe Plath's deeply introspective nature in the personal journals she faithfully kept throughout her life. They served as an important source of self-expression into which she poured her every thought and feeling, particularly in times of distress, offering us an intimate view of her darkest moments.

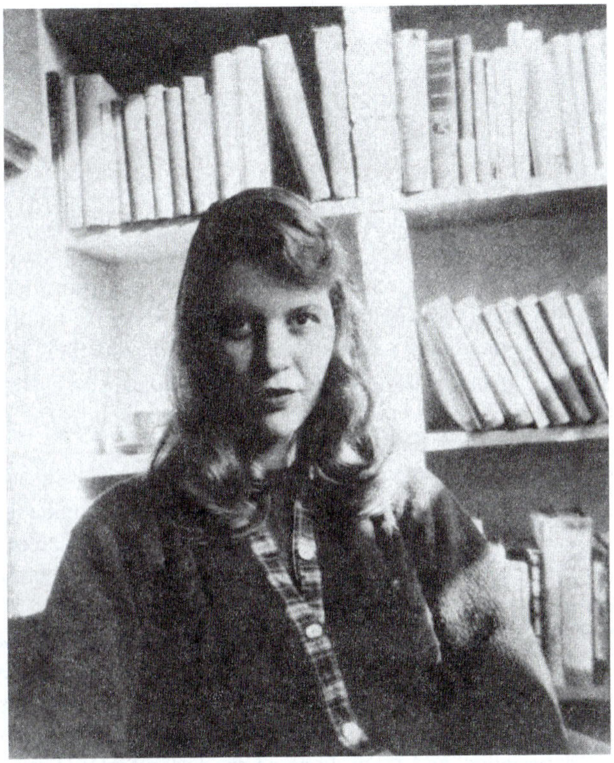

Sylvia Plath in 1957.

Bettmann/Getty Images

After her hospitalization, Plath returned to Smith, graduated summa cum laude in 1954, and went on to pursue graduate studies on a prestigious Fulbright scholarship in Cambridge, England. As she matured professionally while studying there, her romantic interests turned to a fellow poet whom she greatly admired, Ted Hughes. Upon meeting at a party, the two experienced an immediate attraction and, after a whirlwind romance, married in a secret ceremony in England. At the time, Plath was funded by a fellowship that she feared would be withdrawn should news of her marriage surface. Eventually their union became public, and the couple spent the first few months of their married life in Spain while Hughes was teaching.

In *Bitter Fame*, Stevenson describes how Plath's mood shifts became highly pronounced after the initial period of marital bliss faded. "Her moods seemed to soar and sink with alarming rapidity. Sylvia recorded in her journal her volatile and intense reactions to some unmentioned incident, possibly arising out of her husband's surprise at the rancor she displayed in a running tiff with the house owner, who wanted to raise the rent, or perhaps arising out of an evening when they had drinks with some English people who upset Sylvia. These moods, Ted found, were largely unaccountable: they began and ended like electric storms, and he came to learn simply to accept their occurrence."

The couple then moved to Plath's home state of Massachusetts, where she taught English courses at her alma mater, Smith College. Her initial excitement about the prestige of teaching at such a renowned institution quickly gave way to her anxiety about the amount of work it entailed, and particularly about the fact that it left no time for her to work on her own writing. She was further plagued by crippling periods of self-doubt that propelled her again into depression. She wrote, "Last night I felt . . . the sick, soul-annihilating flux of fear in my blood switching its current to defiant fight. I could not sleep, although tired, and lay feeling my nerves shaved to pain and the groaning inner voice: oh, you can't teach, can't do anything. Can't write, can't think. And I lay under the negative icy flood of denial, thinking that voice was all my own, a part of me, and it must somehow conquer me and leave me with my worst visions: having had the chance to battle it and win day by day, and having failed." Such thoughts of worthlessness are common to individuals suffering from major depression.

After a year of teaching, Plath and Hughes moved to Boston, where they became part of a closely knit community of poets and writers. At this point, Hughes had begun to gain considerable accolades for his writing, and the couple lived mainly off of his award money. This allowed Plath to spend the majority of her time developing her writing. When she was pregnant with the couple's first child, they moved to England, settling in an apartment in London and then in a home in the countryside prior to the birth of their second child.

Although by all accounts Hughes was a devoted husband and father, Plath was stricken by fears of his infidelity and often accused him of extramarital affairs. On one occasion, Hughes was late returning home from an interview with the BBC. Plath reacted by destroying a large portion of his writing materials, along with some of his most prized books. Eventually the two separated (although they never divorced), and after Hughes moved out of their home, Plath moved to a flat in London with their two children. Here, she experienced a surge of creative energy that produced many of her most famous poems. At this point she had completed her first and what was to be her only novel, *The Bell Jar*, a semi-autobiographical account of a young woman's journey through young adulthood, navigating the muddy waters of career, romance, and psychological distress. Much of the narrative of the book directly mirrors Plath's own experiences.

Her poetry, too, reflected her struggles as she continued to grapple with her deteriorating mental health. "As absorbed and intent as a cartographer," Stevenson writes in *Bitter Fame*, "Sylvia reported in her poems on the weather of her inner universe and delineated its two poles: 'stasis' and rage. At the depressed pole there was a turning in on herself, a longing for nonbeing. . . . It was as though she looked in a glass and a huge mirror image of her traumatized childhood self stared back."

Although she was experiencing a surge of creativity, Plath was falling into a deep depression. She began seeing a psychiatrist, who noted the severity of her condition. Unable to care for herself and her children, Plath stayed with friends while she tried to recuperate, too afraid to face another round of ECT in a psychiatric hospital. One day, she defiantly decided that she was ready to return to her flat with her children. Her friends, puzzled by her sudden determination, tried in vain to persuade her to stay in their care. The very evening she went home, finally away from watchful eyes, Plath ended her short but intense life.

In the years following her death, critics have come to regard Sylvia Plath as one of the most talented and influential poets of the twentieth century. Compiled by Ted Hughes, who went on to raise their two children with his second wife, *The Collected Poems*, a complete collection of the poems she wrote between adolescence and the end of her life, won the Pulitzer Prize in 1982.

4.9 Acceptance-Based Perspective

acceptance-based perspective
A theoretical perspective that is intended to promote psychological flexibility and reduce avoidance of experiences.

The **acceptance-based perspective** is based on the assumption that psychological health reflects psychological flexibility in adapting to, rather than avoiding, experiences and emotions. This perspective incorporates the underpinnings of behavioral and cognitive theories and is referred to as a "third-wave" or "contextual" behavior therapy. Therapists working in this perspective attempt to help their clients experience and accept their thoughts, feelings, memories, and emotions. The "acceptance" in this perspective refers to the individual's ability to acknowledge aspects of their experience without trying to challenge them or fight them off.

Underlying the acceptance-based perspective is the assumption that individuals can learn a set of skills to help change the way that they think about and cope with their experiences, thus leading to greater wellbeing. Consequently, each of the specific forms of therapy based on this perspective includes training intended to help clients continue to use these skills after therapy has ended.

Much like cognitive theories, acceptance-based approaches emphasize the importance of individuals examining the automatic interpretations they make about how they're thinking and feeling in the context of their experiences. The aim is not to change the experience itself when this is not possible. Instead, the focus is on acknowledging the importance of the experience, and then changing the individual's relationship to it in a way that increases psychological flexibility and helps the individual function more effectively and fluidly based on context, or the demands of the situation. Thus, the "acceptance" in this perspective refers to the individual's ability to acknowledge aspects of their experience, including negative thoughts and emotions, without trying to challenge them or fight them off.

Treatment within the acceptance-based perspective focuses on helping clients think differently about themselves and their experiences. Each method takes a slightly different approach, but they all help clients acquire a set of skills that will allow them to navigate their daily lives more successfully.

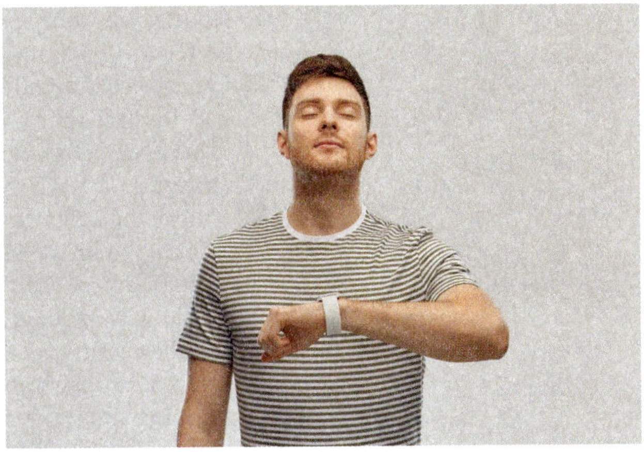

Mindfulness applications on smartwatches are making it easy for individuals to help refocus whenever they feel the need for a break.

Lev Dolgachov/Alamy Stock Photo

Mindfulness

Mindfulness is a mental state achieved by intentionally bringing one's awareness to the present moment without judgment of internal or external observations. Training in mindfulness is a core behavioral component of many of the acceptance-based approaches. You can practice mindfulness yourself by stopping for a moment and focusing your attention fully on your breathing, while noticing your other thoughts but refocusing attention to your breath.

Although mindfulness has its foundation in Buddhist meditation practice, there are important differences. Meditation often aims to focus awareness on a particular sensory experience. In contrast, mindfulness aims to expand awareness more broadly in order to increase psychological flexibility, or the ability to understand a situation or psychological state from multiple perspectives simultaneously. Secondly, mindfulness does not emphasize spirituality in the way that many meditation practices do (Kabat-Zinn, 2003).

mindfulness
A mental state achieved by intentionally bringing one's awareness to the present moment without judgment of internal or external observations.

Researchers have found that mindfulness has many therapeutic benefits, both on its own and through incorporation into psychological treatment. With the availability of mindfulness smartphone applications, it can also be possible for individuals to incorporate this important skill into their daily lives (Gál, Ștefan, & Cristea, 2021). Even smart watches are now equipped with "mindfulness" applications that individuals can consult at any point to take a minute (or longer) to refocus.

Acceptance and Commitment Therapy (ACT)

One of the more commonly known acceptance-based approaches used in psychotherapy is **acceptance and commitment therapy (ACT)** (Hayes et al., 2006) pronounced as one word. ACT is a behavior-based approach that incorporates the acceptance and adaptability of the general acceptance-based approach. Additionally, the "commitment" in the name implies that clinicians seek to help individuals commit to behaving in ways that are consistent with their values.

acceptance and commitment therapy (ACT)
A therapeutic approach that aims to indirectly reduce symptoms by focusing on improving psychological flexibility.

In ACT, values are framed as intangible, driving forces that are unique to each individual, and that change throughout the lifespan. Clinicians therefore aim to help individuals identify their own values and help them to prioritize their life goals and aspirations accordingly. For instance, an individual may value their health above all other aspects of life. An ACT-based clinician would then help the individual gear their actions and goals toward improving their overall health through making smaller, manageable goals such as exercising regularly and staying consistent with taking care of medical needs. The theory in ACT is that the more consistently you are able to make choices and commit to actions that are aligned with your values, the higher your sense of well-being, meaning, and purpose in life will be. Furthermore, ACT posits that aligning your actions with your values can reduce psychological suffering and symptoms such as anxiety and depression.

ACT also aims to help individuals understand how the use of language guides their understanding of themselves and the world around them. By putting thoughts and feelings into words, individuals can create their own realities to which they then, for better or worse, respond. These thoughts and feelings can include memories for past events. Perhaps the individual in the previous example recalls how much trouble they had the last time they tried to get on a regular exercise schedule. If they label this experience as showing they are a "total failure," they will feel that they can never change. In an ACT-based approach, you would look at the term *total failure* and work to remove the judgment. Working with the clinician, the individual would try to shift their thinking to understanding that not everyone is perfect, and that their inability to stick with an exercise plan earlier doesn't mean they are a failure as a person. Further, in ACT the individual may learn to connect the way the term *failure* automatically not only brings up negative feelings but also creates more painful feelings. By not using this term, then, they would be able to take a more neutral and ultimately productive way of thinking about the experience. A development of greater psychological flexibility may also help clients move away from labeling their psychological symptoms in stigmatizing ways (Kao, Li, Mak, & Cheung, 2023).

ACT hexaflex
In acceptance and commitment therapy (ACT), the six main psychological processes that can become the source of psychological disorders.

Moving onto the specifics of ACT, it is based on the proposal that six therapeutic processes allow for psychological well-being, a model referred to as the **ACT hexaflex**. The "hexa" refers to the six processes (which are situated at the outside points of a hexagon) and the "flex" to the idea that psychological health is based on the ideal state of mental flexibility. The six therapeutic processes are all interrelated within the hexaflex to symbolize the collective impact that they can have on each other. Psychological disorders arise when these processes become inflexible, so technically this becomes the "Inflexahex."

The first process in the hexaflex is *acceptance*, which refers to the process of attuning to thoughts and emotions as much as possible. *Inflexability* occurs when individuals engage in experiential avoidance, or ignoring painful thoughts and emotions. In order to improve attention to the present moment, clinicians help clients acknowledge and understand these negative thoughts and feelings without judgment or avoidance using specific exercises and tools such as mindfulness practice, where there is a deliberate focus on non-judgmental attunement to present thoughts and feelings. Take an example of an individual who is seeking treatment for support following a painful romantic breakup. An ACT clinician might help the individual to identify and describe the range of thoughts and feelings they are having, despite how difficult it is to sit with the discomfort these might bring. The thinking is that by openly embracing these emotions, the individual could better process them and effectively attend to their functional needs.

Next, *defusion*, or *cognitive defusion*, is a process that aims to provide psychological distance between internal experiences and language. For instance, in ACT theory, cognitive fusion occurs when individuals become overly attached to the language they use to label their thoughts and feelings. As a result, they find it impossible to think about their experiences in other, more adaptive, ways. For instance, an individual may have a thought after a romantic breakup, "I am never going to find love again." An ACT clinician would help the client to understand that this thought is not factual and further help them to gain more perspective on the thought using skills, for example changing the narrative to, "I am having the thought that I am never going to find love again" and through this process, find more opportunity to have a different perspective on their circumstances and feelings.

Self-as-context relates to the notion that rigid ways of thinking and behaving can come from an overly specific and rigid concept of yourself, based on past memories or narratives you have told yourself throughout your life. In the inhexaflex, this process is referred to as attachment to the conceptualized self. Thus, in ACT there is an effort by clinicians to help individuals view themselves through multiple perspectives, allowing them to see themselves as observers of their experiences instead of as being stuck within one particular narrative. In an ACT approach, the individual struggling through a romantic breakup might work on seeing their life as comprising more than just the recent breakup, seeing that event as just one of many in their lifespan.

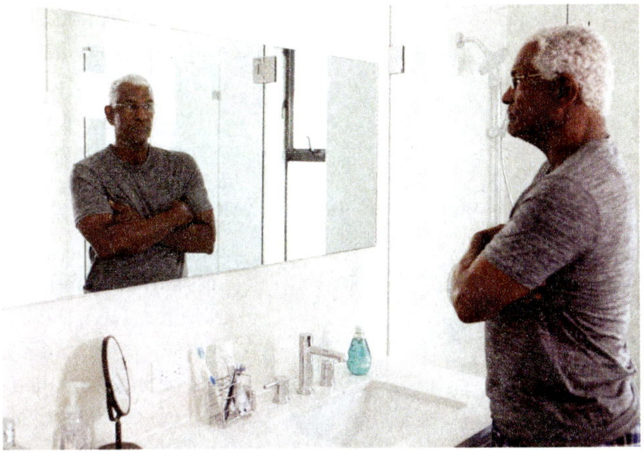

In acceptance-based approaches, clients are helped to adopt more flexible ways of thinking about themselves and their experiences.

Stockbroker/MBI/Alamy Stock Photo

Clinicians working in ACT regard *lack of values* as a barrier to developing ways to overcome psychological suffering, which can further perpetuate current maladaptive ways of thinking and feeling. Values are a key component of the hexaflex that aims to allow individuals to understand what drives and motivates them toward fulfillment. Think of a compass with multiple points—values represent points which guide an individual toward meaning and purpose. Importantly, values are multidetermined, meaning that many different kinds of goals may be connected to the same specific value. For instance, the individual who has lost a romantic partner may highly value romantic partnership, and so an ACT clinician would help this individual to view this loss in stride because they can seek out new romantic partners in the future. If the individual had a lack of values, they may not seek to find other relationships after the breakup, which may thus lead to less overall fulfillment and well-being.

Committed action is a process by which individuals can work on goals related to their larger values. In ACT, clinicians collaborate with clients to identify and then stay accountable to these goals, as inaction and impulsivity are seen as getting in the way of people's ability to live in ways that are consistent with their values.

Lastly, *contact with the present moment* allows individuals to be active and engaged with their current experiences openly and non-judgmentally. When individuals are not able to be engaged in the present, they can only think about the past and the future, making it difficult to stay grounded in the "here and now." The individual coping with a painful romantic breakup may stay stuck in the thoughts and feelings from the past, or ruminate about their future. An ACT clinician would help the client to acknowledge these feelings while also staying flexible and attending to other internal experiences while staying connected to their values. Over time this might help the client to get "un-stuck" from a mindset where they are overly focused on the emotions related to the breakup.

Dialectical Behavior Therapy (DBT)

Dialectical behavior therapy (DBT) is a skills-based approach originally developed by Marsha Linehan for the treatment of borderline personality disorder (Linehan, 1993). The term *dialectical* in DBT refers to what Linehan observed to be characteristic of individuals with BPD, whose experiences are often separated into opposite extremes. Since its inception, however, DBT has been used more broadly in therapy for treating a variety of psychological issues, including complex PTSD (Bohus et al., 2020) and depression (Gilbert et al., 2023) as examples. There is also evidence for long-term favorable effects of DBT on the quality of individuals' lives (Gillespie, Murphy, Kells, & Flynn, 2022).

dialectical behavior therapy (DBT)
Treatment approach for people with borderline personality disorder that integrates supportive and cognitive behavioral treatments to reduce the frequency of self-destructive acts and to improve the client's ability to handle disturbing emotions, such as anger and dependency.

Underlying DBT is the "biosocial theory," which hypothesizes that individuals who suffer from BPD, or similarly struggle with regulating their emotions, might be prone to these difficulties because of a combination of biological vulnerability and social environments that were either invalidating or ineffective in terms of teaching the individual how to cope with emotions. Such environments might include early life experiences with family or other caregivers where there was trauma involving emotional or physical abuse. These are referred to as "invalidating" environments through a DBT lens, due to the negative impact on coping skills that can come from avoidance or lack of acknowledgment of emotions or ability to navigate interpersonal conflict which are so vital to emotional health.

In its most recent version, the *DBT Skills Training Manual* comprises four main modules: Mindfulness, Emotion Regulation, Interpersonal Effectiveness, and Distress Tolerance. In treatment, these modules are covered step by step via structured worksheets and handouts that the therapist and client work through together (Linehan, 2014). The therapist helps the client to understand each concept, and then together they work through specific examples from the client's life to identify ways to make positive changes. For example, the Interpersonal Effectiveness module includes step-by-step instructions for navigating difficult situations that come up in relationships which individuals may have never learned during developmental years. Clients are encouraged to practice these tools outside of treatment in real time, and then work with their therapist to review their progress and develop the skills over time. The therapist is seen as a vital aspect of a successful outcome in DBT due to their unique ability to help clients stay accountable for practicing new skills as well as modeling healthy social dynamics. For instance, DBT therapists can use DBT skills and language in real time to help navigate grievances or other issues that might arise in the relationship. One specific example of this is the use of a technique called a "chain link analysis" that a clinician can utilize to help clients work through avoidance of practicing DBT skills in a non-judgmental and matter-of-fact approach.

Mindfulness-based cognitive therapy (MBCT)
Treatment that combines cognitive therapy with mindfulness skills.

Mindfulness-Based Cognitive Therapy (MBCT) **Mindfulness-based cognitive therapy (MBCT)** (Segal, Williams, & Teasdale, 2002) combines cognitive therapy with mindfulness skills to help individuals learn effective ways of managing their symptoms and preventing relapse. Through MBCT, clients learn "decentering" techniques, trying to build a more acceptance-based stance on painful thoughts and feelings, rather trying to change the thoughts themselves as in typical CBT. One advantage of MBCT is that it can be delivered in digital form, allowing clients to work through the program in a self-guided manner (Dimidjian et al., 2023).

MINI CASE

Acceptance-Based Approach to Treating Meera

A clinician working from an acceptance-based perspective would target Meera's experience of depression in the context of her stressors by focusing less on the content of her stress and more on her relationship to her thoughts and feelings. For instance, it might be that Meera has tried to "fight off" her depression, which, through an acceptance-based lens, would likely serve to exacerbate her feelings and make them more difficult to live with. The clinician could teach Meera mindfulness skills to help her become more aware of how she experiences her emotions in her body, so that she is able to process her feelings more fully rather than trying to suppress or avoid thinking about them. Often, mindfulness skills are taught as coping tools to help manage particular times of distress. This could be very helpful for Meera, who has struggled with ongoing suicidal ideation. Her clinician could also use materials from the DBT module on Distress Tolerance to teach her additional skills for adapting to acute feelings of sadness or hopelessness. A clinician working from an ACT-based perspective would help Meera identify her values and develop ways for her to act more consistently with the areas in her life that are important in order to promote feelings of well-being and agency.

4.10 The Biopsychosocial Perspective on Theories and Treatments: An Integrative Approach

Now that you have read about the major perspectives on psychological disorders , you can probably see value in each of them. Certain facets of various theories may seem particularly useful and interesting. In fact, you may have a hard time deciding which approach is the "best." Similarly, clinicians face many choices as they examine the range of potential theoretical approaches that inform their work with clients. A combination of factors, ranging from their prior training to their own philosophical preferences, are all important influences. However, with the emergence of evidence-based practice, multicultural guidelines, and guidelines based on principles of evidence-based practice, the ultimate decision about how to proceed with a client's treatment will rest on which approach will have the greatest potential value.

Return to the Case: Meera Krishnan

Following a more comprehensive psychological assessment as her treatment plan indicated, the clinician determined that Meera would benefit the most from a cognitive behavioral approach to psychotherapy in conjunction with medication. Meera followed up both these recommendations and saw a psychiatrist, who prescribed her an SSRI. She met with her psychiatrist once per week for the first month of her medication course and then once per month for a check-in. Meera also began seeing a therapist for weekly psychotherapy sessions. Using a cognitive behavioral perspective, the beginning of the work with her therapist focused on strategies such as behavioral activation that would help her cope with the depressive symptoms that were interfering with her functioning. Once Meera's depression remitted, the therapy began to focus on her maladaptive thought patterns regarding her interpersonal relationships. With help from her therapist, Meera recognized that she had created unachievable standards for herself, which she thought her friends and family were expressing. Looking more carefully at her relationships, she discovered that she was imposing these expectations upon herself and that her friends and family accepted her for who she was.

Dr. Tobin's Reflections: Given her response to treatment, Meera's depression appears to be a result of both a biological vulnerability and a maladaptive thought process that began to emerge as she grew into adulthood. Given that, it will be important for Meera to remain on the antidepressant medication to prevent future depressive episodes from occurring. Her therapist may also recommend that she stay in therapy, even after her initial symptoms have remitted, since it can take some time for her thought patterns to become more balanced and adaptive. The goal with therapy would be to ensure that she adapts to a more corrective way of coping with her environment and with stress. An additional area of focus in treatment will be exploring the impact of culture on Meera's development of beliefs around her place in her family. Through developing her own sense of identity, Meera can start to work on ways to resolve the tensions in her relationship with her family, which could help reduce the likelihood she may become symptomatic again in the future. Overall, Meera's strong commitment to recovery helped motivate her to receive the treatment that she needed, and as a result, her prognosis is quite positive.

SUMMARY

- Theoretical perspectives influence the ways in which clinicians and researchers interpret and organize their observations about behavior. In this chapter, you learned about the major theoretical perspectives: biological, trait theory, psychodynamic, behavioral, cognitive, cognitive behavioral, humanistic, sociocultural, and acceptance-based.
- Within the biological perspective, clinicians view disturbances in emotions, behavior, and cognitive processes as caused by alterations in the body's functioning. A person's genetic makeup can play an important role in precipitating certain disorders and also interacts with environmental factors. Treatments that clinicians base on the biological model involve a range of somatic therapies, the most common of which is medication. More extreme somatic interventions include psychosurgery and electroconvulsive treatment (ECT).
- Trait theory proposes that disordered behavior reflects maladaptive personality traits. The basic principle of trait theory is that personality is equivalent to a set of stable characteristics. In the study of psychological disorders, the predominant trait theory is the Five Factor Model, or "Big Five," which includes the personality traits of neuroticism, extraversion, openness to experience, agreeableness, and conscientiousness ("OCEAN" or "CANOE"). The HEXACO model adds "honesty-humility" as a sixth factor, applying primarily to personality disorders such as antisocial. Although these models do not necessarily provide a framework for psychotherapy, trait theory does provide a perspective for assessing for personality disorders and also for understanding the role between personality and physical health.
- The psychodynamic perspective is a theoretical orientation that emphasizes unconscious determinants of behavior and is derived from Freud's psychoanalytic approach. The term *psychodynamics* refers to the interaction among the id, the ego, and the superego. According to psychodynamic theorists, people use defense mechanisms to keep unacceptable thoughts, instincts, and feelings out of conscious awareness. Freud proposed that there is a normal sequence of development through a series of psychosexual stages.
- Post-Freudian theorists such as Jung, Adler, Horney, and Erikson departed from Freudian theory, contending that Freud overemphasized sexual and aggressive instincts. Object relations theorists proposed that interpersonal relationships, including attachment to caregivers, lie at the core of personality. Treatment within the traditional psychodynamic perspective may incorporate techniques such as free association, dream analysis, transference, and resistance. Newer approaches focus instead on relational themes, as in Core Confictual Relationships Theme.

- According to the behavioral perspective, faulty learning experiences cause psychological disorders. Behaviorists contend that individuals acquire many emotional reactions through classical conditioning. Operant conditioning, with Skinner's emphasis on reinforcement, involves the learning of behaviors that are not automatic. Social learning theorists emphasize the process of modeling, or acquiring new responses by observing and imitating the behavior of others. In interventions based on behavioral theory, clinicians focus on observable behaviors or may take advantage of principles of modeling.
- Cognitive theories emphasize disturbed ways of thinking. Clinicians adhering to a cognitive perspective work with clients to change maladaptive thought patterns. In the cognitive behavioral approach, clinicians devise treatments that involve changing thoughts and tracking the occurrence of maladaptive behaviors.
- At the core of the humanistic perspective is the belief that human motivation is based on an inherent tendency to strive for self-fulfillment and meaning in life, notions that are rooted in existential psychology. Person-centered theory focuses on the uniqueness of each individual, the importance of allowing the individual to achieve maximum fulfillment of potential, and the need for the individual to confront honestly the reality of his or her experiences in the world. Self-actualization theory focuses on the maximum realization of the individual's potential for psychological growth. In client-centered therapy, clinicians treat clients with unconditional positive regard and empathy, while providing a model of genuineness and a willingness to self-disclose.
- Theorists within the sociocultural perspective emphasize the ways that people, social institutions, and social forces influence individuals. Proponents of the family perspective see the individual as an integral component of the pattern of interactions and relationships that exists within the family. Psychological disturbance can also arise as a result of discrimination that occurs with attributes such as gender, race, or age or of pressures associated with economic hardships. General social forces such as fluid and inconsistent values in a society, and destructive historical events such as political revolution, natural disaster, or nationwide depression also can adversely affect people. Worldwide events, such as climate change and the COVID-19 pandemic, are proving as well to have significant effects on mental health. Treatments within the sociocultural perspective focus on the client's sociocultural context. In family therapy, clinicians encourage family members to try new ways of relating to each other and thinking about their problems. In group therapy, people share their stories and experiences with others in similar situations. Milieu therapy provides a context in which the intervention is the environment, rather than the individual, usually consisting of staff and clients in a therapeutic community.
- Acceptance-based approaches form part of the third wave of therapy, and share a focus on promoting flexible adaptation to the individual's experiences and social context. Acceptance and commitment therapy, referred to as ACT, aims to reduce psychological suffering by helping clients accept unwanted, difficult emotional experiences and modify behaviors to help increase time spent in valued activities. Other acceptance-based approaches include mindfulness, dialectical behavior therapy, and mindfulness-based cognitive therapy.

KEY TERMS

Acceptance and commitment therapy (ACT)
Acceptance-based perspective
ACT hexaflex
Allele
Applied Behavior Analysis (ABA)
Archetypes
Assortative mating
Attachment figures
Attachment style
Automatic thoughts
Aversive conditioning
Behavioral perspective
Biological perspective
Classical conditioning
Client-centered
Cognitive behavioral perspective
Cognitive behavioral therapy (CBT)
Cognitive perspective
Cognitive restructuring
Concordance rate
Conditions of worth
Contingency management
Counterconditioning
Cross-fostering study
Culturally adapted cognitive behavior therapy (CA-CBT)
Deep brain stimulation (DBS)
Defense mechanisms
Dialectical behavior therapy (DBT)
Default Mode Network (DMN)
Diathesis-stress model
DNA methylation
Dysfunctional attitudes
Ego
Ego psychology
Electroconvulsive therapy (ECT)
Endophenotypes
Epigenesis
Existential psychology
Family inheritance study
Family perspective
Five Factor Model (or "Big Five")
Free association
Genes
Genome-wide association studies (GWAS)
Genome-wide linkage study
Genotype
HEXACO personality trait model
Humanistic perspective
Id
Libido
Mindfulness

Mindfulness-based cognitive therapy (MBCT)
Motivational interviewing (MI)
Multicultural approach
Neuromodulation
Neurotransmitter
Niche-picking
Object relations
Oedipus complex
Operant conditioning
Participant modeling
Personality trait
Person-centered theory
Phenotype
Pleasure principle
Polygenic
Prefrontal lobotomy
Psychodynamic perspective
Psychodynamics
Psychosexual stages
Psychosurgery
Psychotropic medication
Reality principle
Reinforcement
Self-actualization
Self-efficacy
Single nucleotide polymorphism (SNP)
Social discrimination
Social learning theory
Superego
Systematic desensitization
Theoretical perspective
Token economy
Transference
Unconditional positive regard
Vicarious reinforcement

CHAPTER 5

Neurodevelopmental Disorders

OUTLINE

Learning Objectives

5.1 Explain the characteristics and causes of intellectual developmental disorder.

5.2 Explain characteristics, theories, and treatment of autism spectrum disorder.

5.3 Differentiate among learning, communication, and language disorders.

5.4 Explain characteristics, theories, and treatment of ADHD.

5.5 Describe motor disorders.

5.6 Analyze the biopsychosocial model of neurodevelopmental disorders.

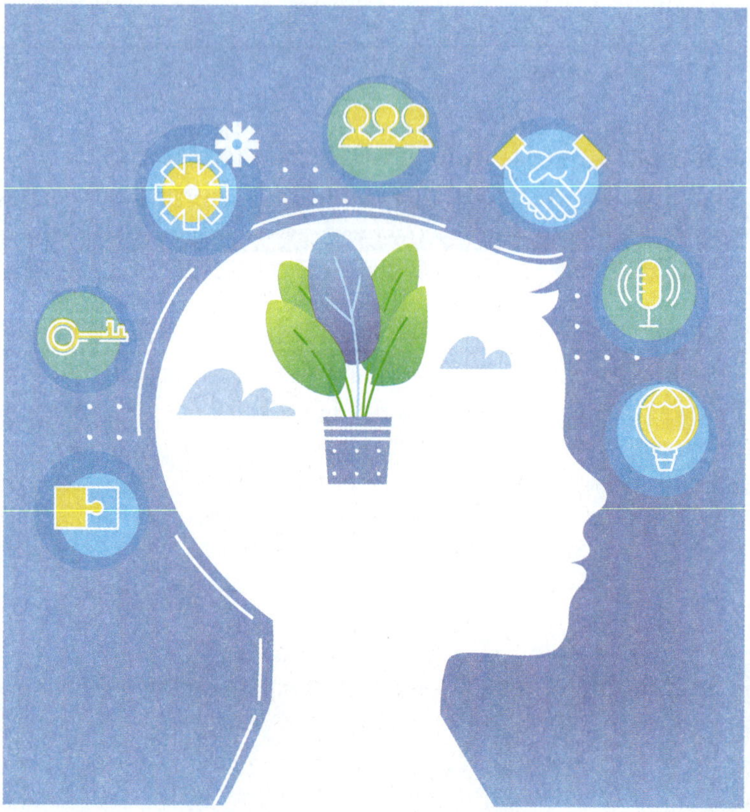

Batshevs/Shutterstock

Case Report

Jason Newman

Demographic information: 8-year-old White cisgender boy. Jason's pronouns are he/him/his.

History of present illness: Jason's third-grade teacher, Mrs. Brownstein, notes his increasingly hyperactive behavior and inability to pay attention in class from the first day of school. Because she does not wish to alarm his parents, she observes Jason's behavior over the first few weeks of the term to see whether settling into the classroom might decrease his rowdy behavior. However, Jason's behavior only deteriorates as the weeks go on, and Mrs. Brownstein decides to contact his parents, Pam and John Newman, and suggest a psychological evaluation for him. Though they had been advised by his earlier teachers to bring Jason to a psychologist, the Newmans' health insurance does not cover this expense, and they are unable to afford it on their own. However, it is becoming clear that treatment for Jason will be necessary in order for him to successfully complete his schooling. Mrs. Brownstein refers his parents to a local child psychologist with a private practice, Dr. Scott, who is able to work with the family on a sliding scale so that they can afford an evaluation.

Jason's mother, Pam, accompanies him to see Dr. Scott, who interviews her separately before seeing Jason. Pam explains that Jason has been a "very fidgety child" from infancy but that his disruptive and often inappropriate behavior in school has been getting notably worse over the past 3 years. Because he was their first child, Pam did not perceive that his apparent abundance of energy was unusual . The couple also has a 4-year-old child, Nicholas, whose behavior as an infant was much calmer in comparison, further alerting them that something was different about Jason. Pam further explains that outside the classroom environment, Jason is usually more restless than others in situations where he has to sustain attention for a long period of time. For instance, Pam notes that in church on Sundays, Jason typically starts to squirm in his seat after the first 5 minutes of the service. She remarks that this is quite embarrassing for her and her husband, who have difficulty getting Jason to sit still. As a result, they have stopped going to church altogether. She reports that it was often difficult to take care of Nicholas when he was an infant, because Jason would run into the nursery when Nicholas was being fed or changed and demand that Pam pay attention to him. On several occasions Jason grabbed the feeding bottle out of Pam's hand as she was feeding Nicholas.

Pam attempts to be very patient with Jason, but she reports that her husband, John, has more difficulty coping with their son's restless behavior. Pam describes instances in which Jason has been particularly "rowdy" in the home and has broken furniture and expensive items when he climbed on tabletops. She states that this has greatly strained the relationship between John and Jason and has been a source of tension between her and John as well, because they often disagree on how to discipline their son. Pam and John have tried, unsuccessfully, to implement a system of punishments and rewards based on his performance at school; however, this has only caused further frustration because they often disagree as to the appropriate amount of punishment.

Pam states that Jason's teachers have been describing the same patterns of behavior each year, though during this current school year his ability to pay attention has severely declined, perhaps, as Pam notes, because the material presented in the classroom is more complex and requires more attention and thought. During earlier years, the extent of Jason's inability to pay attention would manifest in his leaving classroom materials strewn about after he was finished, and he would never pick up after himself. Mrs. Brownstein has reported that during the current school year, when presented with difficult problems in the classroom, Jason bolts from his desk to another part of the room and begins playing with art supplies in the room even when she is giving a lesson. Pam is particularly concerned that Jason's behavior in school will continue to negatively affect the quality of his education throughout the years. Furthermore, it had been difficult for Jason to make friends at school, given his overly energetic demeanor and his propensity to be rude or impatient with other children. Pam states her fear that without good peer associations at school, Jason may become isolated and an object of ridicule to his schoolmates. She remarks that Jason and Nicholas do not get along very well either, because Jason tends to be bossy with his younger brother and is usually unwilling to play with him.

Case Report *continued*

When Dr. Scott calls Jason into his office after the interview with Pam, he finds that Jason has gone out into the hallway and is running up and down the staircase that leads to the office. Pam retrieves Jason and brings him back into the office, then waits outside while Dr. Scott interviews Jason individually. Once seated in the office, Jason sits still for several minutes but becomes increasingly restless, climbing out of his seat and trying to leave the office several times throughout the interview. His responses to Dr. Scott's questions are tangential and difficult to comprehend, and he repeatedly gets out of his chair while talking. When asked why it is so difficult for him to sit still, Jason responds, "I'm just bored all the time. I can't help it!"

In order to observe Jason's ability to maintain attention on a task, Dr. Scott presents him with colored markers and asks him to draw a house. Jason begins to draw the shape of a house but soon gives up the task and runs over to one corner of the room where he sees toy building blocks and begins playing with them. When Dr. Scott asks Jason to return to the task, Jason angrily states, "No! No! No! No! No! They make me draw in school all the time! Where is my mommy?" At this point, Jason begins to cry. Being careful not to cause undue distress, Dr. Scott calls Pam back into the office, and Jason immediately settles down and begins to smile.

Relevant history: Pam reports having no birth complications during her pregnancy, and Jason has had no health problems during his development. There is no family history of childhood or attention-deficit disorders.

Risk level: Low risk.

Case formulation: Based on his interview with Pam and his observation of Jason's behavior, Dr. Scott determines that Jason meets *DSM-5-TR* diagnostic criteria for attention-deficit/hyperactivity disorder, hyperactive-impulsive type. His symptoms have been present for longer than 6 months and were present before the age of 7. He displays predominantly hyperactive-impulsive symptoms, and though he has some symptoms of inattention, they are too few to distinguish him as having combined presentation.

Treatment plan: Jason will be referred to his pediatrician for a medication consultation. He will also be referred for behavior therapy at a low-cost clinic in the area.

Sarah Tobin, PhD

neurodevelopmental disorders
Conditions that begin in childhood and have a major impact on social and cognitive functioning.

Conditions that begin in childhood and have a major impact on social and cognitive functioning are known as **neurodevelopmental disorders**. These disorders typically become evident early in children's development, often before they reach school age. The associated deficits they experience include impairments in personal, social, academic, or occupational functioning. Some disorders have specifiers to indicate, for example, that the disorder is linked to a genetic variation or environmental factors affecting the individual during the prenatal period.

Because they strike so early, disorders that begin in childhood are particularly significant in affecting the lives of individuals with the disorders, their families, the schools, and society as a whole. Interventions at this time are particularly important because they can entirely reshape the direction of the individual's life. Yet, clinicians, parents, and teachers struggle with the decision whether to apply diagnoses of a particular disorder to children who show behavioral disturbances. Once given a diagnosis, these children may be treated differently by others and experience effects that go beyond their initial symptoms. For example, is it right to give a psychiatric diagnosis to a child who frequently loses his temper, argues with his parents, refuses to obey rules, acts in annoying ways, swears, and lies? How do these behaviors differ from those of the normal child going through phases such as the "terrible twos" or the rebellion of early adolescence? As you will learn, clinicians attempt to define these diagnoses as restrictively as possible to avoid confusing typical with atypical development. Invariably, however, cases arise in which a clinician considers a child's behavior as meeting the criteria for a psychological disorder.

One thing to keep in mind is that, by definition, neurodevelopmental disorders may show important changes over time. As individuals develop from childhood through adolescence and adulthood, they experience maturational changes that can alter the way their disorder manifests in particular behaviors. Fortunately, with appropriate interventions, clinicians can help children either learn to manage their symptoms or overcome the symptoms entirely.

5.1 Intellectual Developmental Disorder (Intellectual Disability)

The category of disorders marked by intellectual disability is used by clinicians to diagnose people who first began showing cognitive and adaptive deficits during childhood. The exact terminology used for these disorders varies across diagnostic systems, with the *ICD* using the term *disorders of intellectual development.* The *DSM-5-TR* uses the term **intellectual developmental disorder**, and in keeping with the American Association of Intellectual and Developmental Disabilities (AAIDD) recommendations, uses *intellectual disability* in parentheses.

intellectual developmental disorder (intellectual disability)
Diagnosis used to characterize individuals who have intellectual and adaptive deficits that first became evident when they were children.

To receive a diagnosis of intellectual developmental disorder, an individual's symptoms must meet criteria that fall into three sets. The first set includes deficits in the general intellectual abilities that an intelligence test might measure. These include problems in reasoning, problem solving, judgment, ability to learn from experience, and ability to learn in an academic context. The cutoff for meeting this criterion is a measured intelligence of approximately 70 or below on a test considered appropriate for the individual's cultural and linguistic background.

The second set of criteria for a diagnosis of intellectual disability includes impairments in adaptive functioning relative to a person's age and cultural group. These impairments occur in a variety of areas such as communicating, participating in social activities, and performing activities of daily living in an independent manner. People who show adaptive difficulties, for example, are unable to use money, cannot tell time, and relate inappropriately to others in social settings. As is true when they assess abilities with an intelligence test, clinicians should judge whether an individual's adaptive behavior is impaired using tests that are standardized, individualized, psychometrically sound, and culturally appropriate.

The third criterion refers to age, and specifies that age of onset must be under 18 years. It is most likely that individuals with this disorder would be brought to professional attention well before reaching adolescence. Therefore, this criterion is not relevant for a first diagnosis in adulthood, unless for some reason the disability was missed when the individual was a child.

Having established the diagnosis of intellectual developmental disorder, the clinician must next rate the degree of severity. In past versions of the *DSM*, level of severity was based entirely on an individual's intelligence test performance. In *DSM-5-TR*, the level of severity includes how well the individual is able to adapt in conceptual, social, and practical domains. Within each domain, clinicians rate their clients using four severity levels ranging from mild to profound. For example, in the conceptual domain, a mild level of severity would signify difficulties in learning academic skills, but the profound level would mean the individual is completely unable to think symbolically. Social skills similarly range from mild problems in emotional regulation to profound inability to engage in social interaction. Within the practical domain, the levels of severity range from the individual's needing support to carry out tasks such as shopping and money management to needing extensive training to perform even simple, everyday life tasks such as caring for all of their physical needs.

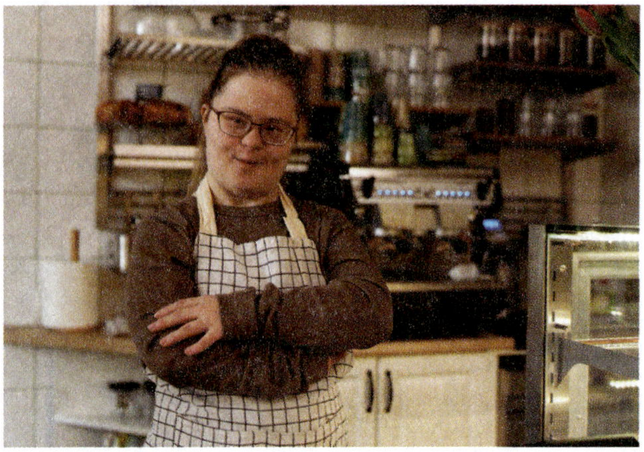

Individuals with developmental disabilities, such as this woman with Down syndrome, may have difficulty, but with training, can find productive employment.
Westend61 GmbH/Alamy Stock Photo

Compared to previous versions of the *DSM*, the combination in *DSM-5-TR* of improved specificity in adaptive behavior

MINI CASE

Intellectual Developmental Disorder

Juanita is a 5-year-old Latina cisgender girl with Down syndrome. Her mother was 43 when she and her husband decided to start their family. Because of her age, doctors advised Juanita's mother to have prenatal testing for any variations in the chromosomal makeup of the developing fetus. Juanita's parents were shocked and distressed when they learned the test results. When Juanita was born, her parents knew what to expect in terms of the child's appearance, behavior, and possible medical problems, but fortunately she needed no special medical attention. Very early in Juanita's life, her parents consulted with educational specialists, who recommended an enrichment program designed to maximize cognitive functioning. From age 6 months, Juanita attended a program each morning in which the staff made intensive efforts to facilitate her motor and intellectual development. Now that she is school age, Juanita will enter kindergarten at the local public school, where teachers will make efforts to bring her into the mainstream of education. Fortunately, Juanita lives in a school district where administrators recognize the importance of providing resources for pupils like Juanita so they will have the opportunity to learn and grow along with their peers.

criteria and inclusion of culturally sensitive tests can result in a more accurate basis for diagnosis and, ultimately, better treatment of individuals with intellectual developmental disorders.

Approximately 1.7 percent of children ages 3 to 17 years old in the United States meet the diagnosis of intellectual developmental disorder with higher rates among boys (2.3%) than girls (1.4%). Across racial and ethnic groups, the rates are highest among Black children (2.8%) compared to smaller rates in Hispanic (1.8%), White (1.8%) and Asian (0.07%) children (Zablotsky, Ng, Black, & Blumberg, 2023).

The World Health Organization regards the area of developmental disabilities as key to its Sustainable Development Goals, given the economic costs associated with these disorders. However, a meta-analysis of available evidence concluded that there are too many variations across countries in data quality and reporting to arrive at a reliable estimate of global prevalence (Olusanya et al., 2023).

Causes of Intellectual Developmental Disorder

Genetic Variations Genetic variations controlling prenatal development of the cortex are significant causes of intellectual developmental disorder. The three most important are **Down syndrome**, **phenylketonuria**, and **fragile X syndrome**. Down syndrome is estimated to occur in approximately 1 in every 700 births, affecting about 6,000 newborns per year (Mai et al., 2019). It is associated with older maternal age and can also reflect epigenetic factors (Iwase et al., 2017).

Down syndrome
Cause of intellectual developmental disorder in which individuals inherit an extra copy of chromosome 21 and therefore have 47 chromosomes instead of the typical 46.

phenylketonuria (PKU)
Condition in which children are born missing an enzyme called phenylalanine hydroxase.

fragile X syndrome
Cause of intellectual disability caused by a change in the gene *FMR1*.

The most common form of Down syndrome is caused by an extra copy of chromosome 21. In this form of Down syndrome, called trisomy 21, the extra chromosome causes changes in the brain and a set of characteristic physical features including a short neck, excess skin at the back of the neck, flattened facial profile and nose, upward slanting eyes, and small head, ears, and mouth.

The overall appearance of individuals with Down syndrome is affected further by the fact that they are short in stature, never reaching typical adult height. Physically, individuals with Down syndrome are at increased risk of heart defects, eye cataracts, hearing loss, hip problems, digestive distress, sleep apnea, underactive thyroid, and dental characteristics that can lead to difficulties in chewing. Individuals with Down syndrome also have a higher risk of developing Alzheimer's disease in adulthood, suggesting common genetic predispositions to both disorders (Boerwinkle et al., 2023).

Behaviorally, individuals with Down syndrome are more likely to act impulsively, experience difficulty with judgment and critical thinking, be easily distractible, and become frustrated and angry over their disability. The high levels of life stressors they face also make them vulnerable to developing major depressive disorder (Walton & Kerr, 2015).

Infants with phenylketonuria (PKU) are born missing an enzyme called phenylalanine hydroxylase, which breaks down phenylalanine, an amino acid found in foods that contain protein. Shortly after birth, as phenylalanine builds up in the body, the infant can suffer irreversible damage. Untreated, PKU leads to developmental delays, a smaller than typical head size, hyperactivity, jerking arm and leg movements, seizures, skin rashes, and tremors. Fortunately, a simple blood test administered to all babies shortly after birth can diagnose PKU.

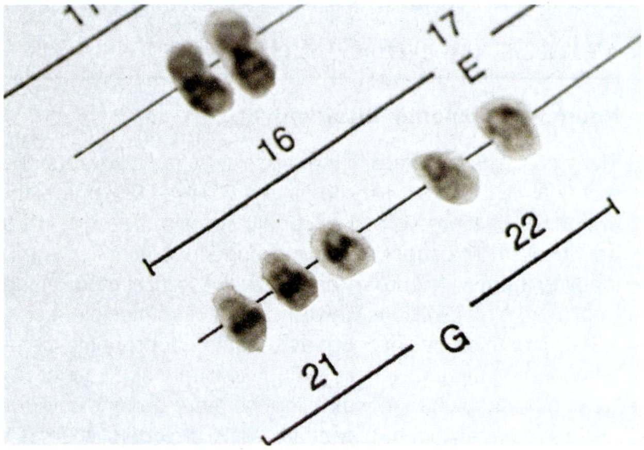

Down syndrome is caused by a condition known as trisomy 21, in which the individual has three instead of two copies of chromosome 21.

Jens Goepfert/Shutterstock

If they test positive, infants with PKU must be placed on a diet low in phenylalanine, particularly early in life. This means they must avoid eating milk, eggs, and other common foods high in protein, as well as the artificial sweetener aspartame. To compensate, they are advised to eat foods high in fish oil, iron, and carnitine (a food additive that promotes energy production in the cell). There is no cure for PKU, so individuals with this disorder must maintain a strict diet throughout life. Although there is no cure, adhering to this diet can potentially help mitigate some of the disorder's symptoms.

Children born with **Tay-Sachs disease** experience deficits in intellectual functioning due to a lack of hexosaminidase A, an enzyme that helps break down an otherwise toxic chemical in nervous tissue called ganglioside. The cause of Tay-Sachs disease is a defective gene on chromosome 15m, a recessively transmitted gene. For someone to develop the disease, both parents must have this genetic defect. If only one parent does, the child becomes a carrier and could transmit the disease to offspring if their partner also has the defective gene. The disease is known to be most common among the Ashkenazi Jews, who are of Eastern European descent. Increased risks have also been identified among individuals of French-Canadian descent living in Quebec (Sillon et al., 2020).

Tay-Sachs disease
An inherited disease that produces deficits in intellectual functioning due to a lack of hexosaminidase A, an enzyme that helps break down an otherwise toxic chemical in nervous tissue called ganglioside.

The symptoms of Tay-Sachs disease, in addition to developmental delays, include deafness, blindness, loss of muscle tone and motor skills, dementia, delayed reflexes, listlessness, paralysis, seizures, and slow growth. Although a milder form of Tay-Sachs disease can develop later in life, most individuals have the form that appears within the first 3 to 10 months after birth. The disease progresses rapidly, and most children with it do not live past the age of 4 or 5 years. There is no treatment for Tay-Sachs; however, prospective parents can receive genetic testing that may help prepare them for aspects of the disease before the child is born. Tay-Sachs screening may also be completed as part of premarital counseling, a situation that can create challenges for individuals who fear being stigmatized if they test positively (Rose et al., 2016).

The most common form of intellectual developmental disorder is fragile X syndrome, a genetic disorder caused by a change in the gene known as fragile X messenger ribonucleoprotein 1, or *FMR1*. A small part of the gene's code is repeated on a "fragile" area of the X chromosome, and the higher the number of repeats, the greater the deficit. This genetic condition is more likely to occur in people assigned male at birth, who have only one X chromosome.

Individuals assigned male at birth with fragile X syndrome can show some physical characteristics, including large head circumference and subtle changes in facial appearance, such as a large forehead and long face, flat feet, large body size, and large testicles after they start puberty. Individuals assigned female at birth with this disorder may show no symptoms other than premature menopause or difficulty conceiving a child.

The parents of children with fragile X syndrome notice delays in their children achieving benchmarks such as crawling or walking. These children can also show hyperactive or impulsive behavior, uncontrollable hand clapping or biting, speech and language delay, and a

What's in the *DSM-5-TR*

Neurodevelopmental Disorders

Many changes occurred in the organization of disorders of childhood when *DSM-5* was finalized, and are retained in the *DSM-5-TR*. Perhaps the most significant was the relabeling of a large group of conditions with the term *neurodevelopmental*. Although empirical studies supported this change in terminology, critics of *DSM-5* argue that labeling them as "neuro" presumes a theoretical model emphasizing biological causes that in the past clinicians viewed as reflecting multiple factors. Specifically, putting ADHD into this category suggests that the appropriate treatment would, in turn, focus on changing the individual's biology through medication.

Another key change was using the more generic category "specific learning disorder" to replace what had been separate disorders, such as mathematical skills disorder. The more generally accepted term *intellectual disability* replaced the term *mental retardation*. *Autistic spectrum disorder* replaced *autistic disorder*, and the term *Asperger's disorder* was completely eliminated. People who received the diagnosis of Asperger's disorder are now included in the autistic spectrum.

There were other major category shifts in the move to *DSM-5*. Separation anxiety disorder was included in disorders originating in childhood and is now included in the category of anxiety disorders. Oppositional defiant and conduct disorders moved to "disruptive, impulse control, and conduct disorders," a category you will read about in the chapter "Personality Disorders." Pica, rumination disorder, and feeding disorder of infancy and early childhood moved to the category "feeding and eating disorders."

By moving many of these childhood disorders to new or other existing categories, the *DSM-5* authors acknowledge the continuity of behavior from infancy through adulthood, a position consistent with life-span developmental principles. On the negative side, children may be more likely than they were in *DSM-IV-TR* to receive diagnoses that clinicians previously considered appropriate only for adults such as certain eating disorders.

tendency to avoid eye contact. As adolescents, boys with this disorder may also engage in a high degree of aggressive behavior (Britton, Wilkinson, & Hall, 2020).

Experts in the field stress the importance of early detection and diagnosis as well as greater understanding of the many complex factors that affect the lives of affected individuals and their families. Furthermore, much remains to be learned about subtypes of the disorder, genetics of the disorder itself, and possible genetically based treatments (Raspa et al., 2023).

Environmental Hazards

Environmental hazards that people experience while pregnant are the second category of causes of intellectual disability. These hazards, called **teratogens**, include drugs or toxic chemicals and maternal malnutrition. Pregnant people may develop infections that alter the neurological development of their unborn children, such as when they contract rubella (German measles) during the first 3 months of pregnancy. Infections, anoxia (oxygen deprivation) during birth, premature birth, and brain injury during delivery can also lead to intellectual deficits in the child. Diseases, head injuries caused by accidents or child abuse, and exposure to toxic substances such as lead or carbon monoxide can also cause loss of intellectual capacity.

teratogens
Environmental hazards mothers experience while pregnant that affect the developing child.

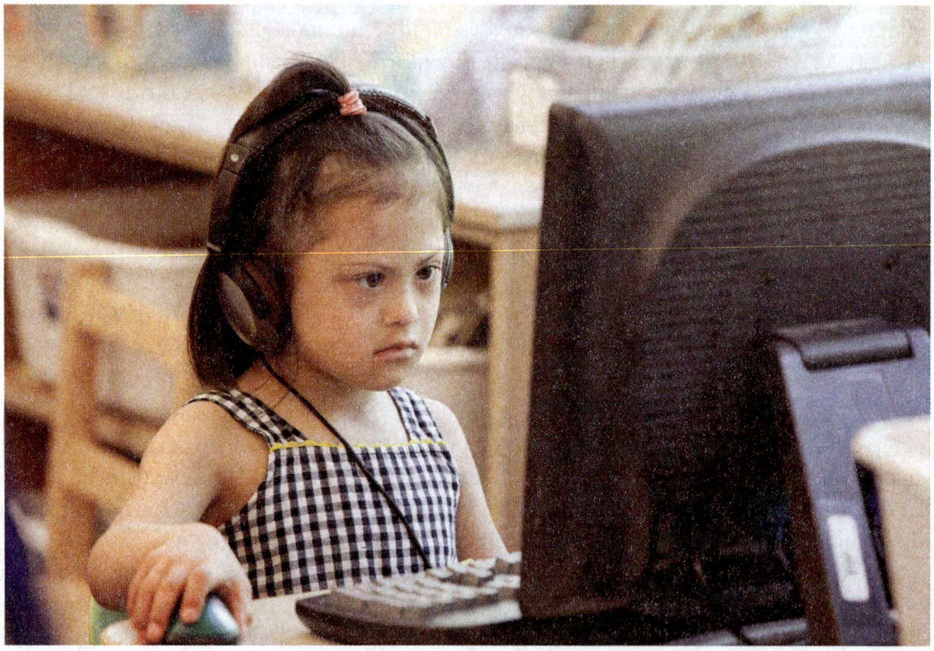

Children with Down syndrome can benefit from computer software and other forms of informational and computer technology that provide visual and auditory stimulation.
Robin Bartholick/Getty Images

Environmental hazards may also take the form of substance use on the part of the gestational parent during pregnancy. **Fetal alcohol syndrome (FAS)** is a condition associated with intellectual disability in a child whose gestational parent consumed large amounts of alcohol on a regular basis while pregnant. Children with FAS develop specific facial differences, slower than average growth patterns, and most importantly, nervous system delays that result in intellectual deficits. FAS falls along the more serious end of the set of disorders known as **fetal alcohol spectrum disorders (FASD)**.

fetal alcohol syndrome (FAS)
A condition associated with intellectual developmental disorder in a child whose mother consumed large amounts of alcohol on a regular basis while pregnant.

fetal alcohol spectrum disorders (FASD)
A group of conditions that can occur in a person whose mother drank alcohol during pregnancy.

Because of the high risks associated with alcohol intake during pregnancy, medical guidelines err on the side of conservatism by recommending complete abstinence from alcohol during pregnancy. Occasional studies may suggest that some alcohol use will not hurt the developing child, but for many gestational parents, it is simply easier to refrain from alcohol use altogether.

Table 1 shows recommended diagnostic guidelines for FASD, based on the consensus of expert panels commissioned by the German government to arrive at criteria for a development-based diagnosis of full-blown fetal alcohol syndrome in children and adolescents.

The cognitive deficits of children with FASD seem particularly pronounced in the area of executive functioning, meaning that they find it difficult to perform tasks that require them to regulate their attentional control and perform mental manipulations. Damage in the frontal areas of the brain associated with maternal alcohol use appears to contribute to these cognitive deficits (Kenton et al., 2020). Specifically, alcohol use throughout pregnancy appears to affect GABAgeric and glutamatergic systems, and affects the process of neuroplasticity that underlies memory and learning (Basavarajappa & Subbanna, 2023).

Epidemiologists estimate the prevalence of FASD at approximately 0.30 of every 1,000 children ages 7 to 9 in the United States (Centers for Disease Control and Prevention, 2023). Estimates based on the prevalence of alcohol use during pregnancy suggest that this number may be far higher, with a reported 14 percent of approximately 6 million pregnant women ages 18 to 49 reporting current and 5 percent binge drinking (Gosdin et al., 2022). Consequently, the actual rates of developmental delays and other problems during pregnancy that can affect the fetus may be underestimated.

Children with FASD are at risk for a variety of negative outcomes as they mature, including dropping out of school, committing criminal acts, and developing diagnoses of other mental health problems including substance use disorders. Their adaptive abilities are

TABLE 1 **Diagnosis of Fetal Alcohol Syndrome Disorders**

Area of Functioning	Criteria
Growth	Height, weight, or both at or below the 10th percentile (adjusted for age, sex, and race or ethnoracial factors)
Face	Smooth ridge between nose and lip, thin edge around the lip, and small separation between upper and lower eyelids (based on racial norms)
Central nervous system	Smaller head circumference and brain variations visible on imaging Performance on functional measures substantially below that expected for an individual's age, schooling, or circumstances in areas such as speech, fine motor skills, attention, arithmetic skills, and social skills or behavior
Maternal alcohol exposure	Confirmed prenatal alcohol exposure; if this information is not available, children who meet all three of the above criteria would be referred for further testing

SOURCE: Landgraf, M. N., Nothacker, M., Kopp, I. B., & Heinen, F. (2013). The diagnosis of fetal alcohol syndrome. *Deutsches Arzteblatt International, 110*(42), 703–710.

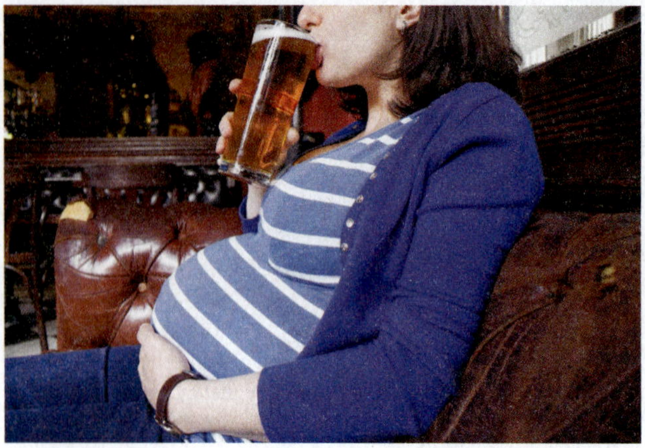

Drinking alcohol during pregnancy places the unborn child at higher risk of developing fetal alcohol syndrome.

Alex Segre/Alamy Stock Photo

challenged further as they enter into adult roles, particularly for those who have altered appearance and cognitive functioning (Lynch, Kable, & Coles, 2015). Families of individuals with FASD may also experience stress; these challenges affect not only parents but also other family members, including grandparents (Ilchena et al., 2023).

Treatment of Intellectual Developmental Disorder

People with intellectual developmental disorder can benefit from early intervention aimed at providing them with training in motor coordination, language use, and social skills. Early diagnosis is particularly important as a way to help educators place children in appropriate classes and get them the social services that can help them and their families.

mainstreaming
A governmental policy to integrate fully into society people with cognitive disabilities.

Educators can combine **mainstreaming**, which integrates children with intellectual disabilities into ordinary school classrooms, with special education that provides them with assistance geared to their particular needs. Peer training can also be beneficial in improving treatment toward children with intellectual disabilities (Nota, Ginevra, & Soresi, 2019).

Moving outside the classroom and into daily life, behavioral or social interventions can be useful for individuals, including coordinated care that integrates behavioral treatment, outreach, and multidisciplinary assessment. It may also be helpful to provide treatment of related conditions, as individuals with intellectual disabilities are at greater risk of developing psychological disorders over the course of their lifetimes (Lunsky, Langdon, Redquest, & Summers, 2021). Mindfulness interventions with staff can reduce their stress, allowing for both less need for restrictions as well as reduced aggressiveness among those they care for (Sturgeon, 2023).

Unfortunately, treatment for individuals with FASD seems to be lagging in the area of directly targeting mental health and substance use outcomes, particularly for adolescents and adults. Most interventions are aimed at children and focus on skills and strategies rather than family wellness. There is a need for these family wellness approaches (such as the "Circle of Security" program) that address both children with FASD and their caregivers, providing important support in the areas of attachment and positive child-caregiver interactions. Responding to risk and harm is the third component of successful treatment for those with FASD (Flannigan et al., 2020).

Ideally, rather than treating existing cases of FASD, it would be preferable to intervene so that no alcohol is consumed during pregnancy at all. In one promising approach, a program known as Multifaceted Case Management employed principles of motivational interviewing along with a "community reinforcement approach" intended to involve significant others in the birth parent's life to join in promoting positive changes in drinking and social behaviors. Five years after completion of the program, children in the treatment condition were less likely to develop FASD along with healthy neurobehavioral development (May et al., 2023).

5.2 Autism Spectrum Disorder

autism spectrum disorder
A neurodevelopmental disorder involving impairments in the domains of social communication and the performance of restricted, repetitive behaviors.

The neurodevelopmental disorder commonly called "autism" is titled **autism spectrum disorder** in *DSM-5-TR* and includes impairments in the domains of social communication and the performance of restricted, repetitive behaviors. This disorder incorporates a range of impairments in the ways that individuals interact with and communicate with others, as well as in the particular interests and activities they engage in. The constellation of diagnostic criteria associated with this disorder can persist throughout life, but depending on severity, it is possible for individuals to function independently, particularly if they receive appropriate help.

The *DSM-5-TR* diagnosis of autism spectrum disorder replaces the prior term *autistic disorder*, which had been placed in a separate category from other related disorders including Asperger's disorder, childhood disintegrative disorder, and pervasive developmental disorder not otherwise specified. The current term provides a more reliable and valid distinction between children who clearly show typical development and those who demonstrate a range of deficits in communication and social behaviors. Furthermore, this term puts those four disorders previously considered to be separate on a continuum with differing levels of severity (Pellecchia, Dickson, Vejnoska, & Stahmer, 2021).

To diagnose autism spectrum disorder, clinicians evaluate children along two core domains. Within each domain, clinicians specify one of three severity levels based on the amount of support required, ranging from some to substantial to very substantial.

The first domain includes disturbances in social relationships and communication Children with autism spectrum disorder may show developmental delays in the use of language. People with other disorders also show delayed language, so this quality is not unique to autism spectrum disorder. More typical of autism spectrum disorder are deficits in the social aspects of communication. Individuals with this disorder may avoid eye contact, and their facial expressions, gestures, and even posture may strike others as odd or unusual. For example, they may find it difficult to understand the body language of others, and their own body language may strike others as odd and extremely awkward.

The second domain incorporates the individual's interests and behaviors. In ASD, these interests occupy a narrow but intense range of hobbies or expertise. The behaviors exhibited by children with autism spectrum disorder are distinguished by extreme repetition and rigidity.

Unlike neurotypical children, those with autism spectrum disorder, or neurodivergent children, do not seem to enjoy playing with others, sharing experiences, or engaging in the usual give-and-take of social interactions. In extreme cases, they may completely avoid social interactions, or at least not attempt to initiate interactions with other people. Imaginative play, an essential component of typical development, presents these children with particular challenges. They may be unable to engage in the type of imitative play patterns that characterize the ordinary social interactions of young children who are able to copy each other as they share toys and play games.

Separate from the deficient communication and social patterns of neurodivergent people are disturbances in motor behavior in which they engage in restricted or repetitive behaviors, such as tapping their fingers incessantly or twisting their bodies around in unusual poses. The repetitive behaviors can also affect their speech, taking the form of **echolalia**, in

echolalia
Repetition of the same sounds over and over.

MINI CASE

Autism Spectrum Disorder

Jeong is a 6-year-old Chinese American cisgender boy currently receiving treatment at a residential school for children with intellectual disabilities. As an infant, Jeong did not respond well to his parents' efforts to play with and hold him. His mother noticed that his whole body seemed to stiffen when she picked him up from his crib. No matter how much she tried, she could not entice Jeong to smile. When she tried to play games by tickling his toes or touching his nose, he averted his eyes and looked out the window. Not until Jeong was 18 months old did his mother first realize that his behavior reflected more than just a quiet temperament—that he was, in fact, developing differently. Jeong never did develop an attachment to people; instead, he clung to a small piece of wood he carried with him everywhere. His mother often found him rocking his body in a corner, clinging to his piece of wood. Jeong's language, though, finally indicated serious disturbance. At an age when most children start to put together short sentences, Jeong was still babbling incoherently. His babbling did not sound like that of a typical infant. He said the same syllable over and over again—usually the last syllable of something that had just been said to him—in a high-pitched, monotone voice. Perhaps the most notable feature of Jeong's speech was that he did not direct it to the listener. Jeong seemed to be communicating in a world of his own.

which they repeat the same sounds over and over again. Repeating the same routines without permitting any changes may be another manifestation of their disorder. Although many children prefer certain routines, for neurodivergent children, any variation in such everyday activities as getting dressed or eating breakfast can become highly upsetting.

Particularly distressing to families are the disturbances that some individuals with autism spectrum disorder show in their altered sensitivity to sensory stimuli. They may seem almost impervious to pain, heat, or cold, and as a result they can easily place themselves at risk of significant injury. Conversely, these individuals may experience hypersensitivity to noise, light, or smell, leaving them unable to withstand ordinary atmospheric sights and sounds.

As they progress through adulthood, neurodivergent people may find challenges in maintaining their quality of life. These challenges include impaired relationships, poorer physical health, and lower overall levels of life satisfaction and sense of meaning (Graham Holmes et al., 2020). Additionally, these individuals are at higher risk of self-harm by the age of 16.

Some children with autism spectrum disorder appear to develop typically for the first 2 years but, at some point before age 10, start to lose language and motor skills as well as other adaptive functions, including bowel and bladder control. This rare condition was formerly called childhood disintegrative disorder, but the diagnosis was eliminated from *DSM-5* and is now incorporated into autism spectrum disorder.

One variant of autism spectrum disorder, called autistic savant syndrome, occurs when people possess an extraordinary skill such as the ability to perform extremely complicated numerical operations almost instantaneously or, as in the case of Derek Paravincini (see photo) can play an entire piece of music after hearing it only once.

Autistic savant syndrome typically appears at an early age, when a young child with the disorder appears to have exceptional musical skills, artistic talent, or the ability to solve extremely challenging puzzles. It is possible that the tendency to focus intensely on the physical attributes of objects gives people this uncanny set of abilities. Interestingly, their memory in areas outside their areas of expertise appears to be no better than that of people with autism spectrum disorder who do not have these special memory skills (Neumann et al., 2010).

Theories and Treatment of Autism Spectrum Disorder

Evidence pointing to patterns of familial inheritance supports the theory that autism spectrum disorder has a strong biological basis. Researchers estimate a heritability index of 0.98 (Tick et al., 2016). Identifying patterns of transmission is made highly complex by the fact that there are at least 60 genes, to date, involved in susceptibility to the disorder, as was discovered in sequencing studies involving over 42,000 U.S. cases (Zhou et al., 2022).

Advances in brain-scanning techniques, coupled with a movement to share data among teams of researchers, are helping to clarify possible neurological patterns in people with autism spectrum disorder. Some evidence suggests that altered brain activities in the default mode network (DMN) associated with ASD are thought to potentially underlie the social communication component of the disorder (Padmanabhan, Lynch, Schaer, M. & Menon, 2017).

Even as research on neurological variations in individuals with autism spectrum disorder is advancing, the behavioral perspective, specifically Applied Behavior Analysis, remains the most realistic and effective approach to treatment (Eckes, Buhlmann, Holling, & Möllmann, 2023). One method found to be useful for toddlers in inclusive classrooms relies on **naturalistic developmental behavioral interventions (NDBI)**, in which teachers or other interventionists can shape the child's behavior in the course of ordinary play or instruction. For example, the teacher can increase the frequency of a target behavior such as functional play by establishing predictable, repeatable, and clearly defined roles appropriate to a child's developmental level (Maye, Sanchez, Stone-MacDonald, & Carter, 2020).

naturalistic developmental behavioral interventions (NDBI)
A behavioral approach for autism spectrum disorders in which teachers or other interventionists can shape the child's behavior in the course of ordinary play or instruction.

Token economies are another behavioral intervention that may produce value for some children (Fiske et al., 2015). To be effective, the tokens themselves need to be carefully

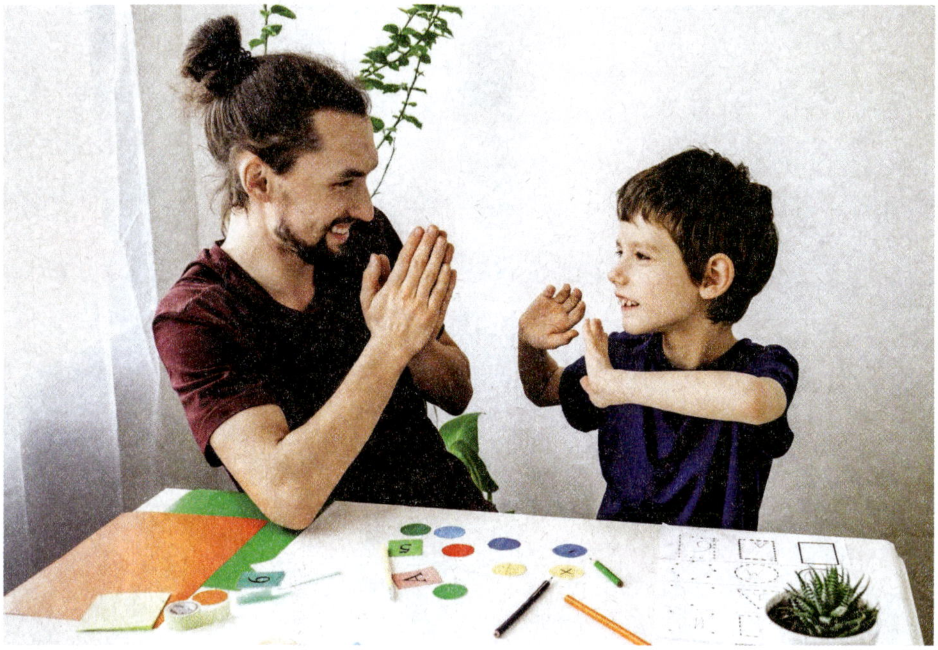

Therapy with children who have autism spectrum disorder may incorporate play and other enjoyable activities that help shape the child's behavior.

Alex and Maria photo/Shutterstock

chosen to be reinforcing to the child when linked to a tangible reinforcer (Fiske, Isenhower, Bamond, & Lauderdale-Littin, 2020).

Another approach to intervention is to have peers rather than adults interact with the child. This situation approximates a more typical type of social environment, in which children often serve a powerful role in modifying a peer's behavior. In contrast to interventions in which adults provide the reinforcement, peer-mediated interventions have the advantage of allowing children to carry on with their ordinary activities without adult interruption. In some cases, the peer interaction may take place with the exchange of pictures as the form of communication (Doherty, Bracken, & Gormley, 2018).

Rett syndrome
A rare genetic neurological disorder that develops within the first 18 months of life is more prevalent in girls and is characterized by such symptoms as nearly constant repetitive hand movements, loss of acquired spoken language, problems with gait, and partial or complete loss of acquired purposeful hand skills.

Taking advantage of new technologies, future treatments of children with autism spectrum disorder may be able to rely increasingly on virtual reality, in which individuals practice their social skills in a computer-generated environment. Another variant on this approach is augmented reality, which provides artificial information presented on the real-world environment. Although promising, studies evaluating the effectiveness of these treatments have only relatively few participants, and the samples are primarily male, meaning that further research is needed to establish their effectiveness (Dechsling et al., 2022).

Given that families are intimately involved in the planning of treatment for their children with autism spectrum disorder, it is important that their decisions take into account their own personal values. Apart from the need for evidence-based treatments, these value-based considerations become part of the clinician's planning and communication with parents (Saez, Davies, Kazemi, & Fields, 2023).

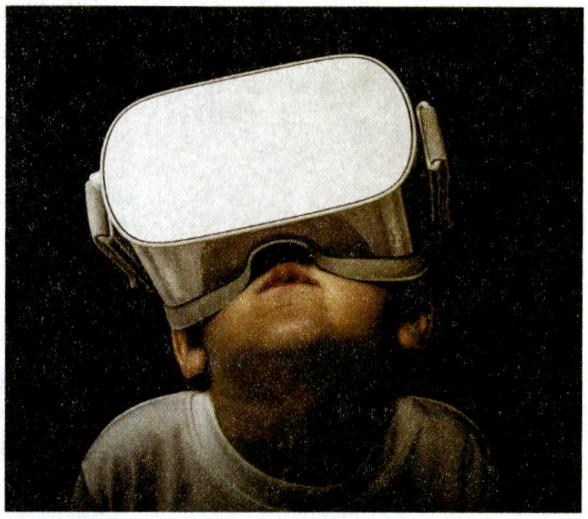

Virtual reality may provide a useful form of therapy for children with autism spectrum disorder in learning communication skills.

Neal Bryant/Shutterstock

Rett Syndrome

Rett syndrome is a rare genetic neurological disorder that develops within the first 18 months of life, is limited to girls, and is characterized by such symptoms as nearly constant repetitive hand movements, loss of acquired spoken language, an atypical gait, and partial or complete loss of acquired purposeful hand skills.

By the age of 4, disruption of social interaction only occurs in what is called the "regressive" phase of Rett syndrome. The *DSM-5-TR* therefore recommends that

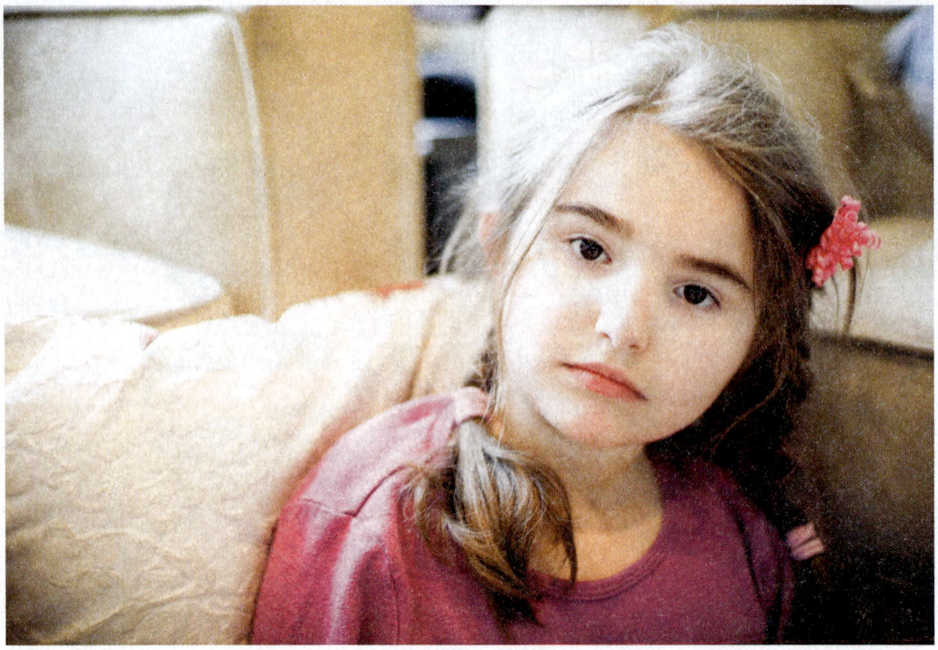

The symptoms of Rett syndrome begin to appear after about 5 years of age.
Megan Sorel Photography

Rett syndrome should be included in the differential diagnosis of autism spectrum disorder in children who are past that age.

Researchers identified the gene for Rett syndrome in 1999. Mutations in this gene, which is named MeCP2, lead to variations in the production of a specific protein important in the normal functioning of neurons. There is hope that studies involving genome editing to replace MeCP2 in mouse models will prove useful in the treatment of children with this disorder (Panayotis, Ehinger, Felix, & Roux, 2023). As of yet, although research is progressing on the use of psychotherapeutic medications, none have passed clinical trials (Gomathi, Padmapriya, & Balachandar, 2020). However, psychological approaches focusing on rehabilitation appear to have promise in treating symptoms of this disorder, including challenges in communication, motor skills, and cognition (Lim, Greenspoon, Hunt, & McAdam, 2020).

Asperger's Syndrome

Asperger's syndrome
A term once used to describe individuals with high-functioning autism spectrum disorder.

Asperger's syndrome is not in the *DSM-5-TR* but is a term used in prior *DSM*'s to define the high-functioning end of the autism spectrum. Although not part of the nomenclature, it is worth its own coverage here.

Asperger's syndrome is named after Hans Asperger, a Viennese physician. High-functioning people on the autism spectrum have less severe and more focused impairments than their lower-functioning counterparts, perhaps showing their symptoms only after they reach preschool age. At that point, when most children develop social and interactive skills, these children have difficulty reading the social cues of others and taking turns talking; additionally, they are unable to interpret language subtleties. Early in their lives, they tend to become preoccupied with a narrow set of interests about which they may talk extensively, not realizing that such one-sided conversations are not socially appropriate. Indeed, their parents are more likely to view the child as especially gifted rather than as having a disability. As the children get older, their challenges become more prominent, and it is then that parents and educators may seek to intervene.

There is some evidence that there is a neurological component to high-functioning autism spectrum disorder. In one large investigation comparing the executive functioning of individuals at the high end of the spectrum with typically developing adults, researchers

REAL STORIES

Greta Thunberg (2003–Present)

At 15, the Swedish activist Greta Thunberg started fighting inaction on climate change. She went on strike from school and took a handmade sign that read "School Strike for Climate" to the Swedish Parliament building, where she sat outside for days with the goal of convincing the Swedish government to make changes so the country would meet the carbon emissions target set forth by the international 2016 Paris Climate Agreement (BBC, 2020).

This small act turned into a worldwide movement in a matter of months, as Thunberg became an internationally recognized symbol of the movement for climate change, especially among young people. She inspired her generation to start taking part in weekly protests from school to continue protesting governments' relative inaction to reduce the existential threat of climate change. This culminated in the September 2019 global climate strike, which was the largest protest against climate change to date. That same year, Greta was named *Time Magazine*'s person of the year, the youngest recipient of the accolade.

Thunberg started participating in global forums on climate change, taking her message beyond Sweden to the rest of the world. Just prior to the global climate strike, she crossed the Atlantic as a passenger in a low-emissions boat to speak about climate change at a UN conference in New York City.

This remarkable journey began when Thunberg first learned about climate change in school. According to her TedX talk, she "could not understand why so little was being done about it" (Thunberg, 2019). In the documentary *I Am Greta* (Thunberg, 2020) she recalls that this realization led to a long period of depression lasting several years in which she recalls she stopped eating and stopped speaking.

Thunberg attributes this response in part to her autism spectrum disorder. More specifically, she meets criteria for the former diagnosis of Asperger's disorder. She has also been open about her diagnosis of selective mutism. In *I Am Greta,* Thunberg describes some of the ways she is especially affected by her diagnosis: "I don't like making small talk with people or socializing. Sometimes I go quiet and can stay so for hours because I simply can't talk. . . . I like to have routines and I notice details. Once I get interested in something, I can get laser focused on it for hours without getting bored." In the documentary, her father adds that she has an "almost photographic memory for things she is interested in."

In her TedX talk, Thunberg elaborates further on how her ASD has influenced her approach to climate change: "For those of us who are on the spectrum, almost everything is black or white. . . . Especially when it comes to the sustainability crisis, where everyone keeps saying that climate change is an existential threat, and the most important issue for all. And yet they just carry on like before. I don't understand that, and we have to stop the emissions. To me that is black or white. To me there is no gray area when it comes to survival."

Because of her specific traits and perspective, Thunberg seems uniquely poised to be one of the fiercest advocates for climate change. In fact, she considers her ASD diagnosis to be her "superpower" (Applied Behavior Analysis, 2020) and has approached her view with humor, noting, "I think in many ways that we autistic are the normal ones, and the rest of the people pretty strange" (Thunberg, 2019).

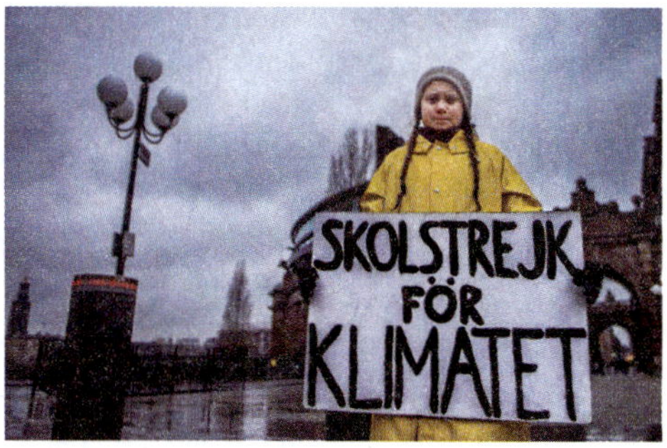

16-year-old Greta Thunberg as she demands action on the world's climate crisis.

Jasper Chamber/Alamy Stock Photo

For instance, Thunberg is straightforward when she speaks and is able to express her passion for the issue of climate change in clear, unmistakable terms. Though she has spoken in front of worldwide audiences, she seems unfazed by this level of exposure and has remained true to herself and her vision despite sudden global fame.

Thunberg's work and public persona have also drawn a good deal of criticism and judgment from around the world, a fact that does not seem to trouble her or slow her down in recent years. Her response has been to take the high road. In a Tweet from early 2020, in response to a defamatory bumper sticker that depicted her being sexually assaulted, she states, "They are starting to get more and more desperate.... This shows that we're winning" (Thunberg, 2020).

Looking back at her intense journey from first learning about climate change to her depression and then her meteoric rise as the world's most recognizable activist for climate change, in *I Am Greta* Thunberg reflects, "It took years, but slowly I started to feel better. I felt that why should I give up, when there are so many different things you can do to make a difference?"

reported deficits primarily in the areas of flexibility and planning. These deficits emerge early in life and continue throughout adulthood, and may play an important role in the stereotyped and persistent behavior patterns that individuals with high-functioning autism disorder display. From a treatment standpoint, it therefore would be important for these individuals to receive support in navigating tasks of daily life that require cognitive flexibility and planning (Xie, Sun, Yang, & Guo, 2020).

5.3 Learning and Communication Disorders

Specific Learning Disorder

specific learning disorder
A delay or deficit in an academic skill that is evident when an individual's achievement and skills are substantially below what would be expected for others of comparable age, education, and level of intelligence.

Children who have a **specific learning disorder** experience a delay or deficit in their ability to acquire a basic academic skill. These difficulties become evident when their achievement and skills are substantially below the level of performance based on their age, education, and measured intelligence. Within this general category, clinicians also specify which academic domain the disorder affects and its level of severity (mild, moderate, or severe).

In the United States, researchers estimate that approximately 7.7 percent of children have a diagnosed learning disorder (Zablotsky & Black, 2020).

The factors that can increase a child's risk of developing a learning disorder include a range of sociocultural factors including poverty, bullying, neglect, parental depression, permissive or overly harsh parenting, and lack of support systems for the family. Additionally, challenges related to having a child with a learning disorder can add stress to the parents, leading them to feel lonely, isolated, and confused, further affecting their parenting style (Gyereh & Shukla, 2023).

One area in which children with learning disorders experience difficulty includes typing on computers, which requires language processing as well as overall technique. Their academic performance will invariably be affected, particularly when they enter higher education, where advanced computer skills are required (Abecassis. Magen, & Weintraub, 2023).

specific learning disorder with impairment in mathematics
A learning disorder in which the individual has difficulty with tasks and concepts involving numbers and numerical reasoning.

dyscalculia
A pattern of difficulties in number sense, ability to learn arithmetic facts, and calculations.

Individuals with **specific learning disorder with impairment in mathematics** have difficulty with tasks and concepts relying on numbers and numerical reasoning; they may be unable to understand mathematical terms, symbols, or concepts. Some may have **dyscalculia**, a pattern of difficulties in number sense, ability to learn arithmetic facts, and calculations. A school-age child with this disorder may have problems completing homework. An adult may be challenged in paying bills and taking care of finances.

Children with this disorder may have other learning disabilities, involving reading and writing, as well as poorer memory, and lower scores on nonverbal intelligence tests (Louni et al., 2023). Additionally, there are serious long-term consequences of having a specific learning disorder with impairment in mathematics. Apart from the impact on school performance, individuals with this disorder will face greater challenges in the job market and as adults may have lower income, higher risk of being sick, and even a higher risk of mortgage default (Kuhn, 2015).

specific learning disorder with impairment in written expression
A learning disorder in which the individual's writing is characterized by poor spelling, grammatical or punctuation errors, and disorganization of paragraphs.

In **specific learning disorder with impairment in written expression**, individuals have difficulty spelling, properly using grammatical or punctuation rules, and organizing paragraphs. Such challenges lead children to have serious problems in many academic subjects. For adults, the disorder of written expression can create numerous interpersonal and practical problems. Fewer job opportunities will be open to them, particularly if their symptoms place them in the severe level of functioning.

specific learning disorder with impairment in reading (dyslexia)
A learning disorder in which the individual omits, distorts, or substitutes words when reading and reads in a slow, halting fashion.

Individuals with **specific learning disorder with impairment in reading**, commonly called **dyslexia**, omit, distort, or substitute words when they read. Consequently, they read in a slow, halting fashion. Their disorder can cause children to fail to show adequate progress in a variety of school subjects. Like other individuals with specific learning disorders, as adults these individuals also experience lower educational attainment and occupational success (Smart et al., 2017).

Practitioners believe the best way to identify children with learning disorders is the response to intervention (RTI) approach, a multi-tiered evidence-based procedure that consists of a monitoring model of how students respond to interventions gradually increasing in intensity. In the first tier, all students are given ordinary instruction. Progressing to the second tier, teachers provide additional support to those students identified as being at risk, preferably in a small group. In subsequent tiers, if children do not progress, teachers either repeat Tier 2 or move on to an even more intensely focused level of instruction. The benefit of RTI is that it is a proactive approach, providing intervention early rather than waiting for children to fail academically (Roos et al., 2023).

Educating children with learning disabilities not only in academic skills but also in emotional and social spheres can be an important component of treatment. Such an approach can mitigate against the child experiencing low self-esteem and loneliness, and the desire to keep the disorder a secret from peers (Musetti, Eboli, Cavallini, & Corsano, 2019).

As adults, individuals with learning disorders can benefit from vocational rehabilitation programs designed specifically for their needs. Partnering with employers, such approaches identify areas in which new employees are in need of training while they learn the skills required for their particular jobs (Müller & VanGilder, 2014). Vocational training can also include virtual environments, allowing these individuals to learn transferable skills to the workplace in an affordable and accessible manner (Michalski, Ellison, Szpak, & Loetscher, 2021).

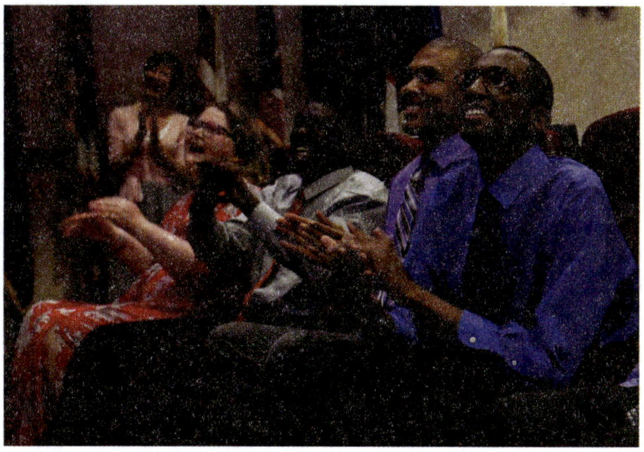

Project SEARCH graduates laugh during a presentation in Fort Eustis' Wylie Theater at Joint Base Langley-Eustis, Virginia, June 7, 2018. They spent their senior year of high school learning job skills while interning at various locations on Fort Eustis.

Airman 1st Class Monica Roybal/NARA

Project SEARCH, a business-led transition program for high school students, is intended to provide on-the-job training for young adults. A main principle of Project SEARCH is that of "supported employment"–namely that trainees become integrated with other workers in the workplace in an inclusive manner (Almalki, 2021). In one test of its effectiveness (Müller & VanGilder, 2014), the program successfully improved job readiness by focusing on both specific job skills and overall "soft skills" in the areas outlined in Table 2. Although developed in the United States, it appears to be transportable to international contexts, with Project SEARCH UK showing an average employment rate of its participant of 50 percent (Kaehne, 2016). In addition to having beneficial effects on young people with learning disorders, researchers report that Project SEARCH has a variety of positive outcomes for those with autism spectrum disorder, including improved social and occupational skills as well as a better quality of life (Syriopoulou-Delli & Sarri, 2023).

communication disorders
Neurodevelopmental disorders involving impairment in language, speech, and communication.

language disorder
A communication disorder characterized by having a limited and faulty vocabulary, speaking in short sentences with simplified grammatical structures, omitting critical words or phrases, and putting words together in peculiar order.

Communication Disorders

Communication disorders are conditions characterized by impairment in language, speech, and communication. Children with **language disorder** lack the ability to express themselves in ways appropriate to their age and developmental level. They use limited and faulty vocabulary and speak in short sentences with simplified grammatical structures, omitting critical words

TABLE 2 **Hard and Soft Job Skills Focused on in Project SEARCH**

Job Skills Overall	Soft Skills
Copying	Work ethic
Organizing supplies	Self-esteem
Assembly/collating/labeling	Remaining on task
E-mailing	Meeting deadlines
Using Microsoft Word and Excel	Flexibility in handling change
Delivering	Interacting with supervisors and co-workers
Lifting	Calling in when sick or late
	Traveling to and from work
	Navigating the workplace

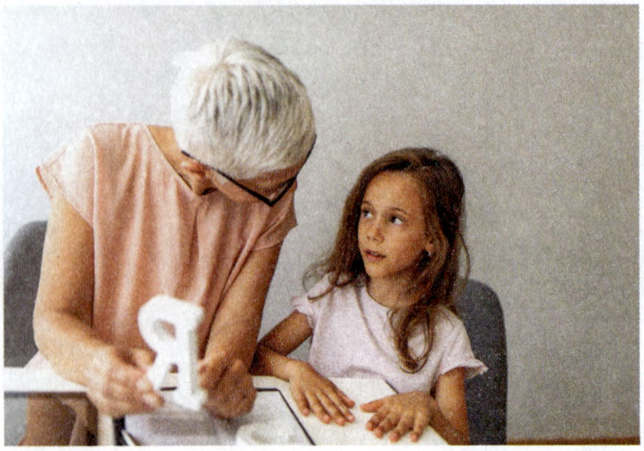

Treatment for stuttering includes speech therapy which can also have the beneficial effect of helping children develop resilience.
Dragana Gordic/Shutterstock

or phrases. They may also put words together in a peculiar order. A person with this disorder may, for example, always use the present tense, saying, "I have a good time yesterday" instead of "I had." Developmental delays may cause expressive language disorders, but similar symptoms can arise from a medical illness or head injury.

The expressive difficulties of some people with communication disorders are characterized not by their inability to understand or express language, but by difficulties in using correct pronunciation. A person with **speech sound disorder** substitutes, omits, or incorrectly articulates speech sounds. For example, a child may use a *t* sound for the letter *k*, saying "tiss" rather than "kiss." People often regard the mispronunciations of children as cute; however, these childhood speech patterns are likely to cause problems in school as the child grows older.

Children who experience **childhood-onset fluency disorder or stuttering** are unable to produce fluent speech. They may emit verbalizations such as sound repetitions and prolongations, use broken words, block out sounds entirely, avoid words they have problems producing, and excessively tense up when expressing certain words. Stuttering is known to have an adverse effect on children due both to the negative thoughts, feelings, and behaviors they develop in reaction to the behavior, and challenges they can experience in the real world caused by their speech difficulties. However, individuals nevertheless can develop resilience, allowing them to protect their self-esteem and overall well-being (Walsh et al., 2023).

speech sound disorder
A communication disorder in which the individual substitutes, omits, or misarticulates speech sounds.

childhood-onset fluency disorder (stuttering)
A communication disorder that involves a disturbance in the normal fluency and patterning of speech characterized by such verbalizations as sound repetitions or prolongations, broken words, the blocking out of sounds, word substitutions to avoid problematic words, or words expressed with an excess of tension.

social (pragmatic) communication disorder (SPCD)
Disorder involving deficits in the ability to use verbal and nonverbal communication in relating to others.

Treatment for stuttering that incorporates not only speech therapy but training in the kind of resilience that may mitigate against the potentially negative consequences of the disorder, particularly if the parents are active in the process. Parents can engage in activities as simple as rewarding the child for independent dressing, allowing the child to explore solving puzzles or building with plastic blocks, and having children ask for help without whining when they have a problem (Druker, Mazzucchelli, & Beilby, 2019).

Children who have **social or pragmatic communication disorder** experience deficits in their ability to use verbal and nonverbal communication in relating to others. They have problems adjusting their behavior to the social context, such as by knowing how to greet people or interpret the way others greet them. In addition, they are unable to match their communication with the needs of the listener, such as by talking in different ways to children and adults. In a conversation, they have difficulties following the ordinary conventions of taking turns when speaking. Finally, they have trouble understanding implicit or ambiguous meanings such as expressions used in humor and metaphors. These deficits can make it difficult for individuals not only to communicate effectively, but also to perform on the job and participate in ordinary social interactions.

Rarely seen in isolation (with an estimated prevalence of less than 1% of children), SPCD appears to co-occur with symptoms of language and behavioral deficits in children, as well as symptoms of autism spectrum disorder. Together, the combination of these attributes can negatively impact a child's academic attainment early in the school years as well as other behavioral outcomes (Saul, Griffiths, & Norbury, 2023).

5.4 Attention-Deficit/Hyperactivity Disorder (ADHD)

attention-deficit/hyperactivity disorder (ADHD)
A neurodevelopmental disorder involving a persistent pattern of inattention and/or hyperactivity.

Individuals with **attention-deficit/hyperactivity disorder (ADHD)** show persistent and heightened patterns of inattention and/or hyperactivity. The "slash" in the name of this disorder implies that individuals can be diagnosed with primarily an attentional disorder, primarily a hyperactivity disorder, or a combination of both. As with other psychological disorders, the individual's symptoms must be severe enough that they interfere with daily functioning; for children, these symptoms can negatively impact their development. Although the symptoms can vary for children and adults in their specific manifestation, these disturbances remain at the core of the disorder regardless of the individual's age.

The first set of criteria for ADHD includes noticeable disturbances in attention, including failing to track details, making careless mistakes, having difficulty staying focused on tasks at school or play, appearing not to listen when others are speaking, failing to follow through on projects, taking disorganized approaches to tasks, being distractible, showing forgetfulness, having a tendency to lose things, and being reluctant to engage in tasks requiring sustained mental effort.

The second set of ADHD criteria includes signs of hyperactivity such as fidgeting, being unable to sit in one place, showing extreme restlessness, being unable to engage in quiet activities, talking excessively, finding it difficult to wait for a turn when speaking or taking part in group activities, and interrupting while in conversation.

For both sets of criteria, individuals need to exhibit at least six symptoms for at least 6 months. Children who show these symptoms must do so more than would be expected for their developmental level. Furthermore, the symptoms must have a direct negative impact on the individual's life.

Clinicians diagnose people with ADHD "combined type" who meet both sets of criteria for at least 6 months. ADHD "predominantly inattentive type" is diagnosed if the client meets the criteria for inattentiveness but not hyperactivity-impulsivity for the past 6 months. Finally, clinicians can diagnose clients as "predominantly hyperactive-impulsive" if they meet the second set of criteria but have not shown inattentiveness for the previous 6 months. The fact that ADHD is considered a neurodevelopmental disorder implies that it begins early in life, no later than the age of 12. If an adult shows these symptoms, the *DSM-5-TR* authors assume the disorder was present in childhood but simply not diagnosed at that time.

The estimated lifetime prevalence of ADHD in the United States for children ages 3 to 17, based on survey reporting, varies somewhat by source, but averages 10 percent. These rates rise from a low of about 2 percent in children ages 3 to 5 to 13 percent in teens 12 to 17. Boys are nearly twice as likely as girls to have ADHD, and among racial/ethnic groups, the highest prevalence is in Black non-Hispanic children, followed by White non-Hispanic, Hispanic, and Asian non-Hispanic children (categories based in the Centers for Disease Control reporting system) (Bitsko et al., 2022).

Researchers estimate the mean prevalence of ADHD in individual 18 and older around the world at 6.8 percent, with persistent ADHD at 2.6 percent (Song et al., 2021), but prevalence rates vary widely by country and region of the world. Additionally, prevalence rates of both lifetime and currently symptomatic are lower in increasingly older age groups of adults (see Figure 1) (Song et al., 2021).

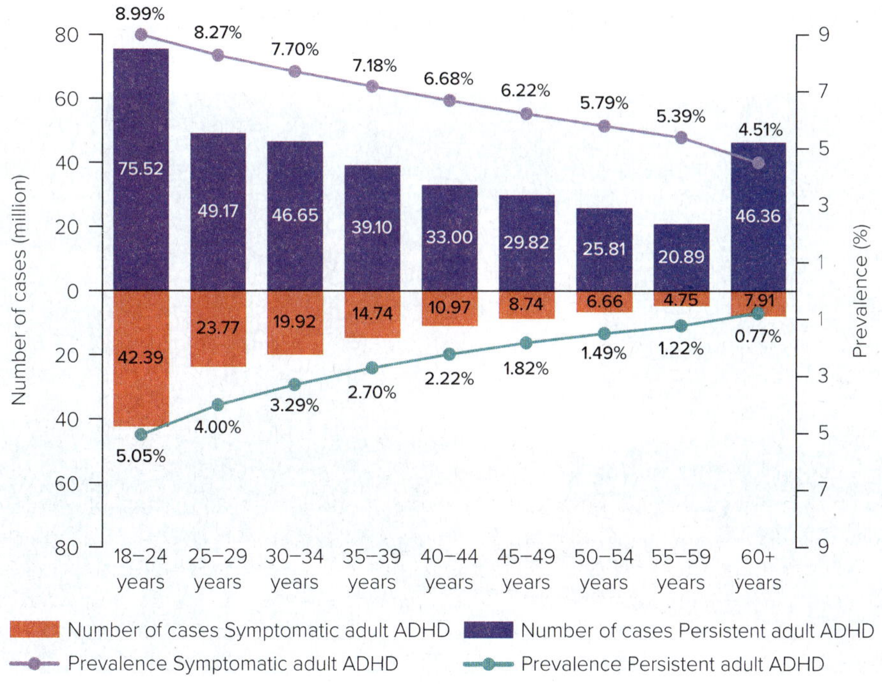

FIGURE 1 Prevalence of lifetime and currently symptomatic cases of adult ADHD.

MINI CASE

Attention-Deficit/Hyperactivity Disorder

Zaman's mother has just had a conference with her son's teacher, who related that Zaman, a 7-year-old Iranian boy, has been extremely restless and distractible in class. Every few minutes, he is up from his desk, exploring something on a bookshelf or looking out the window. When he is in his seat, he kicks his feet back and forth, drums his fingers on the table, shifts around, and generally keeps up a constant high level of movement. He may ask to go to the bathroom three times in an hour. He speaks very quickly, and his ideas are poorly organized. During recess, Zaman is aggressive and violates many of the playground rules. His mother corroborates the teacher's description of Zaman with similar stories about his behavior at home. Although Zaman is of average intelligence, he is unable to sustain concentrated attention on any one activity for more than a few minutes.

Turning now to understanding what life is like for those diagnosed with ADHD, it is clear that individuals who experience this disorder can face many challenges that persist throughout their adult lives, manifesting in poorer academic performances as schoolchildren (Voigt et al., 2017). They are likely to have trouble organizing tasks, make careless mistakes, lose things, and struggle with tasks that require them to prioritize activities on the basis of importance associated with deficits in executive functioning (Roselló et al., 2020). Men who are diagnosed with ADHD in young adulthood often remain in the so-called "peripheral" labor market, meaning that they are not able to experience stable career paths. Women also are at risk for occupational instability but in addition have greater difficulty maintaining stable relationships (Ahlberg et al., 2023). A large-scale meta-analysis also revealed that adults with ADHD have higher prevalence rates of major depressive disorder, bipolar disorder, and substance use disorder (Hartman et al., 2023).

Unfortunately, educators and clinicians are likely to miss a diagnosis of ADHD in girls, whose symptoms tend to be less overt than those of boys and may include unusual forgetfulness, disorganization, low self-esteem, and demoralization. Unlike boys, girls with ADHD tend to internalize their symptoms and show symptoms of anxiety (Tung et al., 2016). Similarly, women with ADHD are likely to show more subtle symptoms of the disorder than do men (Young et al., 2020). Therefore, girls and women who show these symptoms of ADHD may be misdiagnosed and not receive appropriate treatment.

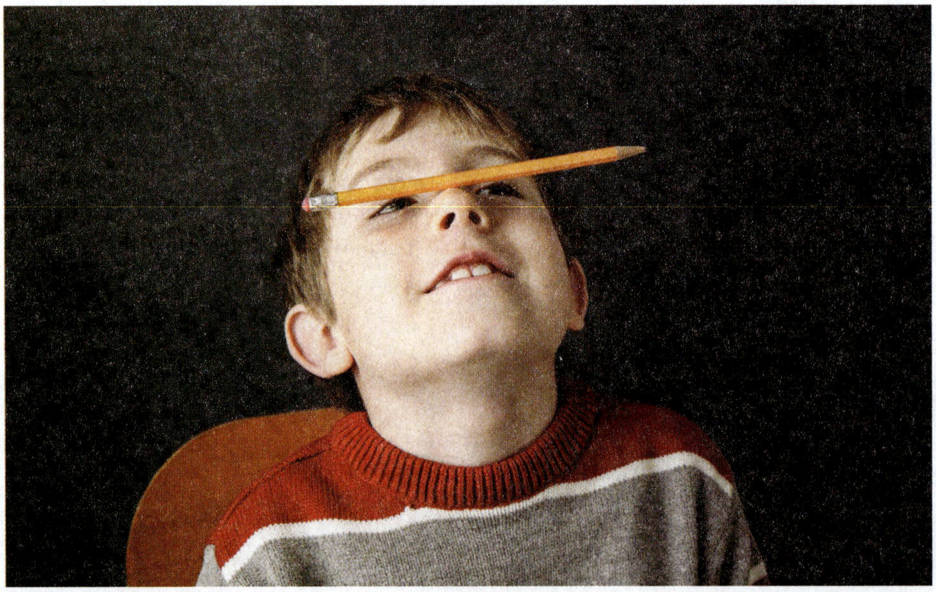

Children and adolescents with ADHD experience significant difficulties in keeping up with their schoolwork due to symptoms such as inattention and extreme restlessness.

Suzanne Tucker/Shutterstock

Theories and Treatment of ADHD

The biological determinants of ADHD have been well established by family, twin, adoption, and molecular genetic studies. A large long-term Swedish study of twins diagnosed with ADHD placed heritability at 64 to 65 percent, meaning that there remains a strong environmental component (Taylor et al., 2023). There may be as many as 27 separate gene variations responsible for this disorder, and researchers also estimate that some of these genetic vulnerabilities are due to methylation via stressful life events, poor nutrition, and toxins during fetal development (Hubers et al., 2023). Researchers using genetic association studies have also showed that a certain pattern of cognitive performance involving impaired executive control appeared in biological relatives with attention-deficit hyperactivity disorders, providing support for a possible endophenotype (Saraçaydın et al., 2023).

You Be the Judge

Prescribing Psychiatric Medications to Children

Research on human participants of any age requires that investigators adhere strictly to the APA Ethical Principles of Psychologists and Code of Conduct. In the case of children, however, the issues shift considerably given that they are vulnerable populations. This means they may be at increased risk for abuse and exploitation. Consequently, for decades, researchers avoided conducting studies to test the efficacy of psychotherapeutic medications on children, to avoid exposing them to unnecessary harm during research trials. With no conclusive data about effectiveness, safety, or pharmacological action on which to base treatment recommendations, psychiatrists treated their pediatric patients using so-called "off-label" prescriptions that had not received U.S. Food and Drug Administration (FDA) approval.

The practice of prescribing off-label medications for disorders is widespread in the United States, but because of the problems of conducting research on children, these prescriptions are often targeted toward this population. The FDA has no authority to regulate the way in which physicians practice medicine, so doctors must make their own decisions about whether to prescribe an off-label medication to a child. In the process, they must balance the potential benefits with the risks of the medication. With few studies on the safety and efficacy of the medications, physicians rely on their own experience (Spetie & Arnold, 2007).

Children may therefore be at greater risk of side effects than other populations about whom extensive data exists. This situation was brought to light in a dramatic manner in 2003 when the FDA received reports showing an association between SSRI use in adolescents and a heightened risk of self-harm and suicidal thoughts. By 2007, these medications had received "black box" warnings from the FDA: warnings that appear on the package insert for certain prescription drugs to call attention to serious risks. These new warnings applied not only to children and adolescents, but also to young adults. Because the FDA did not have extensive data on the use of these medications for young people, its administrations used the information they had at their disposal to make this ruling. Considerably more information about these medications is now available, suggesting that antidepressants may, in fact, reduce suicide risks in this population over the course of continued treatment (Dudley, Goldney, & Hadzi-Pavlovic, 2010).

Q: *You be the judge:* Should researchers conduct more studies on psychotherapeutic medication with children? Do the risks of side effects that may occur during this research justify such investigations? Furthermore, if researchers discover that a medication has harmful side effects, how should prescribing health professionals weigh these against the possible benefits?

Although deficits in executive functioning may reflect underlying brain variations, it is still possible for individuals to live with these symptoms, as indicated by research showing that, as they get older, some individuals with ADHD are able to compensate for these symptoms by engaging their frontal lobes while carrying out cognitive activities (Yap, Abdul Manan, & Sharip, 2021).

Individuals with ADHD who are treated from the biological perspective receive medications intended to control their symptoms. Although there are more than a dozen brand names under which such prescriptions are written, most medications are based on methylphenidate (Ritalin). Although effective for brief durations (3 to 5 hours), these require multiple well-timed doses throughout the day.

Methylphenidate continues to receive empirical support as a treatment for children with ADHD. Supporting its role in altering brain circuits, one randomized trial showed improvements through the medication's ability to reduce the activity of the default mode network, which would have the effect of increasing the child's ability to concentrate on a task (Cai, Mizuno, Tomoda, & Menon, 2023).

As an alternative to short-term forms of methylphenidate, extended-release formulations work in one of two ways: via so-called "back-loaded" delivery systems that work later in the dosage interval, and through beaded 50–50 delivery systems that divide delivery up equally early and late. One advantage of long-acting medications is that they are less likely to be abused (Mao, Babcock, & Brams, 2011). The individual is also less likely to forget to take the medication because there is a longer time frame between doses.

Concerta is a form of extended-release medication known as a "back-loaded product," meaning that only 22 percent of the dose is in the immediate release overcoat, and 78 percent is delivered approximately 4 hours after ingestion. Adderall XR is a delayed release medication that mimics the effect of taking two equal doses. The duration of action is 7 to 9 hours in adults.

Nonstimulant medications for ADHD have been available since the approval by the FDA of atomoxetine and extended-release versions of guanfacine and clonidine (2009 and 2010) and viloxazine extended-release in 2021; of these only guanfacine and clonidine (extended release) are approved only in children. These medications reduce ADHD symptoms by modulating adrenergic and/or dopamine neurotransmitter mechanisms. A meta-analysis on controlled interventions with adults demonstrated that all were equally effective, suggesting that these medications could be used alone or as an adjunct to treatment with stimulants (Radonjić et al., 2023). Stimulant medications continue to be recommended as a first-line treatment for children, but nonstimulants and so-called "off-label" ADHD medications (such as those used for treating depression) are also recommended, particularly in those children who do not respond or cannot tolerate stimulants (Newcorn, Krone, & Dittmann, 2022).

Behavioral methods of reducing ADHD symptoms in children are an important component to treatment, particularly as these can be implemented in the classroom environment. In self-management (or self-regulation), children are encouraged to gain self-awareness as a means of controlling and overseeing their own changes in behavior rather than relying on monitoring by their teachers. This approach can include self-monitoring, in which they observe and record their own behavior, and goal-setting, which allows them to develop their own plan for change. In goal-setting, children can take ownership over their behavior and learn to see the connection between their current and desired levels of performance. Shown to have effectiveness in numerous studies, one group of researchers, using a multiple-baseline approach, established the efficacy of their combined use for elementary children (McKenna et al., 2023).

Interventions from a cognitive behavioral perspective (CBT) are another alternative to medication that are shown to be efficacious for adults with ADHD. Such interventions have a long-term advantage over medication, which become less effective over time. In CBT, individuals learn to understand the nature of ADHD, regulate their emotions, manage their

TABLE 3 Sample Items from ADHD Tracking Scale

Rate each symptom from 0 (never or rarely) to 3 (very often)
Poor attention to details or careless in my work
Fidgety or squirm when seated
Don't listen when others speak to me
Poorly organized in tasks
Procrastinate work that requires prolonged effort
Talk too much
Interrupt what others may be doing
Rate the extent to which the above problems interfere with your ability to function in each area of these life activities
In my home life with immediate family
In social relations with others
In school or other learning environments (if involved in an educational setting)
In managing my money and finances
In dating or marital relationships
In my handling of daily chores or other activities

time more effectively, undergo cognitive training, and reduce the so-called "internalizing" symptoms that can hinder their ability to improve. A meta-analysis of CBT-based interventions on 28 studies demonstrated its effectiveness in reducing core ADHD symptoms, depression, and anxiety as well as improving self-esteem and overall quality of life (Liu, Hua, Lu, & Goh, 2023).

As an adjunct to behavioral interventions, clinicians and parents (or adult clients) can benefit from specific methods of symptom tracking. The ADHD Symptom Tracking Scale (Barkley & Benton, 2021), shown in Table 3, provides a highly accessible tool which can be used both as a self-assessment and as a guide through treatment.

5.5 Motor Disorders

Developmental Coordination Disorder

Children with **developmental coordination disorder** experience marked impairment in their abilities to coordinate the movements of their hands and feet. With its estimated prevalence in 5 to 6 percent of children cross-nationally (Zwicker, Missiuna, Harris, & Boyd, 2012), developmental coordination disorder can lead to problems in academic achievement and ability to engage in ordinary tasks of daily life . Developmental coordination disorder often occurs with the comorbid disorders of ADHD and autism spectrum disorder, language disorders, dyslexia, and anxiety as well as being associated with low self-esteem. Bullying by other children and stress in the family can also affect negatively the children with this disorder (Lino & Chieffo, 2022).

developmental coordination disorder
A motor disorder characterized by marked impairment in the development of motor coordination.

In infancy and early childhood, children with developmental coordination disorder have trouble crawling, walking, and sitting. As they develop, their performance on other age-related tasks also is below average. They may be unable to tie their shoelaces, play ball, complete a puzzle, or even write legibly. Consequently, they may experience problems of low self-esteem. In addition, their lack of coordination may make them less able to participate in sports and exercise programs, leading them to become overweight.

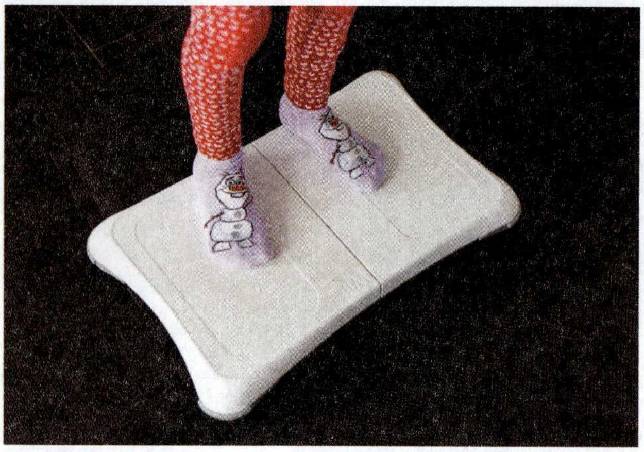

Children with developmental coordination disorder can benefit from the training provided by Wii-fit technology.
Jose Ivan/Shutterstock

There may be subtypes of developmental coordination disorder, with one subtype limiting hand-eye coordination and the other causing visual-spatial difficulties. Children whose coordination disorder represents deficits in executive function, meaning they cannot gain control over their motor functions, represent another important subtype (Michel, Molitor, & Schneider, 2018). In addition to type of disorder, children differ in the severity of their motor symptoms. Those with moderate motor coordination difficulties are able to catch up to their non-impaired peers over time. Children whose disorder is severe do progress but are not able to reach the levels of performance of their age peers (McQuillan et al., 2021).

Given the complexity of their symptoms, children with motor disorder seem to benefit from an integrated approach that identifies their needs and the needs of families in the early stages, when symptoms first begin to emerge. An integrated approach to assessment can then proceed in which children, families, and professionals share their perspectives on the child's symptoms and start to formulate therapeutic goals. Next, professionals, parents, and children plan how intervention will proceed, taking advantage of community resources. Here again, all must collaborate in setting goals for the child. They should base their planned interventions on evidence-supported treatments. Finally, the intervention team should develop strategies that will continue to support the children and their families as they transition to self-management within the home, school, and the community (Forsyth et al., 2008).

In addition to more traditional methods of intervention, videogame training can also benefit children with developmental coordination disorder. These include Nintendo Wii-Fit and Xbox Kinect. An advantage of these methods is that they are also highly motivating and easily delivered in remote formats (Jelsma et al., 2023).

Early identification of these disorders also appears to be key, with interventions that happen before a child enters school regarded as particularly beneficial. Such interventions can also help prevent secondary consequences of the disorder including of poor self-esteem and increased risk of depression, anxiety, and obesity (Lee & Zwicker, 2021).

Tic Disorders

tic
A rapid, recurring, nonrhythmic, and involuntary movement or vocalization.

Tourette's disorder
A disorder involving a combination of chronic motor and vocal tics.

A **tic** is a rapid, recurring, nonrhythmic, and involuntary movement or vocalization. There are several kinds of tic disorders. Examples of motor tics are eye blinking, facial twitches, and shoulder shrugging. Vocal tics include coughing, grunting, snorting, coprolalia (the uttering of obscenities), and tongue clicking.

Tourette's disorder is perhaps the best known of the tic disorders, affecting approximately 0.6 percent of children, the majority of whom are boys. People with this disorder experience a combination of chronic motor and vocal tics. Their disorder begins gradually, often with a single tic, such as eye blinking, which over time grows into more complex behaviors. The tics can include uncontrollable movements of the head and sometimes parts of the upper body. In some cases, individuals engage in complex bodily movements involving touching, squatting, twirling, or retracing steps. At the same time, they utter vocalizations that sound odd to others; for example, an individual may have a complex tic behavior in which he rolls his head around his neck while making sniffing and barking noises. In only a small percentage of cases do people with Tourette's disorder utter obscenities.

This is not a passing condition but one that can be lifelong, with onset in childhood or adolescence. Individuals with this disorder also have other psychological symptoms, the most common of which are obsessive-compulsive symptoms, speech difficulties, and attentional problems. They have an increased risk of suicide or suicide attempts, especially into adulthood if the symptoms do not resolve. Deficits in brain inhibitory mechanisms in the prefrontal cortex may be involved in Tourette's disorder, a feature that is shared with obsessive-compulsive disorder and ADHD (Aliane et al., 2011). The condition may resolve itself by adulthood, as the brain structures that inhibit the tics mature; however, women and those with more severe tics are likely to show less improvement (Ricketts et al., 2022).

Children with Tourette's can benefit from educational interventions that help bolster self-esteem and provide supportive counseling. However, if the tics are painful, self-injurious (such as scratching), and cause significant disability or risk of suicide, clinicians need to intervene more systematically. Individuals with these symptoms can benefit from a form of cognitive behavioral therapy that uses habit reversal. In this approach, the professional trains clients to monitor their tics and the sensations that precede them and then respond to them with a voluntary behavior that is physically incompatible with the tics.

Cognitive behavioral treatment is the first line of treatment (Martino & Pringsheim, 2018), delivered individually or in group form (Bekk et al., 2023). If this proves to be ineffective, clinicians may place the individual on pharmacological therapy, which can include SSRIs, atypical antipsychotic agents, and, in extreme cases, deep brain stimulation (Budman et al., 2018).

Stereotypic Movement Disorder

Children with **stereotypic movement disorder** engage in repetitive, seemingly driven nonfunctional behaviors. These can include waving their hands, rocking their bodies, banging their heads, and biting and picking at their skin. This disorder appears before the age of 3 years and can continue into adulthood (Mackenzie, 2018).

stereotypic movement disorder
A disorder in which the individual engages in repetitive, seemingly driven nonfunctional behaviors.

As you can imagine, these behaviors can interfere with their normal functioning and cause them to injure themselves. It is important to distinguish stereotypic movement disorder from the developmentally normal repetitive movements estimated to occur in as many as 60 percent of children between the ages of 2 and 5 years old. Subgroups of children are particularly likely to engage in stereotyped motor disorders, including children who are blind and those who have developmental delays.

For children who are truly impaired, or who risk serious injury as a result of their behavior, behavior modification appears to be the most efficacious way to help them stop engaging in the behavior. Parents can be taught how to use behavior therapy in the home, an effective method particularly for children between the ages of 7 and 8 years old (Specht et al., 2017).

5.6 Neurodevelopmental Disorders: The Biopsychosocial Perspective

The disorders that you read about in this chapter include a range of conditions that reflect, to differing degrees, combinations of biological, psychological, and sociocultural influences. Genetic influences on many of these disorders are clearly evident, but even so, interactions with social context play an important role. Moreover, because these disorders begin early in life, they have the potential to exert profound psychological effects on an individual. Family factors also play a critical role, given the importance of early childhood experiences as contributors to psychological outcomes.

Just as the disorders reflect multiple influences, so do treatments. In providing interventions to children, clinicians are becoming justifiably concerned about the use of medication. Treatment from the behavioral perspective seems to have a number of advantages, because children's symptoms may be particularly receptive to treatments that focus on principles of reinforcement.

The tremendous growth of interest within the past few decades in the conditions that can affect children means that considerably more information about causes and interventions is available than was true even a few years ago. Although interventions can be effective for people of any age, targeting children as soon as possible can help them achieve favorable outcomes that can influence their lives for decades to follow.

Return to the Case: Jason Newman

Jason was started on a stimulant medication, and both his parents and Mrs. Brownstein noted an improvement in his ability to pay attention and to sit still for longer periods of time. Though he continued to feel restless, Jason's behavioral work with a therapist at the clinic began to help decrease his disruptive behavior at school. The therapist also worked with Pam and John to create a consistent system of rewards and punishment for Jason's behavior. Together they realized that due to their differing opinions on how strict to be with Jason, Pam and John had been sending him diverging reinforcement messages. In order to facilitate an agreement on how to punish or reward Jason, Pam and John worked on creating a set system of reinforcement that they then shared with him, so that he was better informed about what to expect should he misbehave. After several months of medication and therapy, and with his parents' improved ability to discipline him, Jason became less hyperactive while in school, and his grades began to improve. He started getting along better with his classmates and joined a basketball league, which allowed him to make friends and channel his energy appropriately.

Dr. Tobin's Reflections: It can be difficult to differentiate normal overactivity in young children from the more severe symptomatology indicative of ADHD. Dr. Scott made careful consideration of this when diagnosing Jason, based on Pam's description of his behavior over the years. It was clear that Jason's behavioral problems were severely interfering with his ability to lead a normal childhood and attain an education. Especially compared with his brother Nicholas, Jason was visibly struggling with symptoms that went beyond normative childhood behavior.

ADHD is typically diagnosed during the elementary school years, and though the disorder can last through adolescence, with appropriate treatment such as the kind Jason is receiving, the symptoms can begin to diminish toward adulthood. It can be a difficult ethical decision to place children on stimulant medication. In Jason's case, however, medication was important in helping decrease the hyperactive symptoms that were causing him problems at school and that would have made behavior therapy difficult to conduct. With continued therapy and behavioral strategies implemented by his parents, it is hoped that he will be able to discontinue medication in the near future.

SUMMARY

- Neurodevelopmental disorders include disorders that strike children early in life and appear to affect their behavioral functioning by creating brain variations.
- Intellectual developmental disorder refers to intellectual and adaptive deficits that are first evident in childhood. Genetic variations are a significant cause. The three most important genetic causes are Down syndrome, phenylketonuria, and fragile X syndrome. Another genetic disorder is Tay-Sachs disease.
- Environmental hazards during prenatal development are the second category of causes of intellectual disability. These hazards, called teratogens, include drugs and toxic chemicals, maternal malnutrition, and infections in pregnant people during critical phases of fetal development. Consumption of alcohol during pregnancy can lead to fetal alcohol syndrome (FAS).
- People with intellectual disability can benefit from early intervention aimed at providing them with training in motor coordination, language use, and social skills. Educators can combine mainstreaming, which integrates them into ordinary school classrooms, with special education that provides them with assistance geared to their particular needs.
- The *DSM-5* authors created the category of autism spectrum disorder to provide a more reliable and valid distinction between children who clearly show typical development and those who demonstrate the range of deficits in communication and social behavior that *DSM-IV-TR* attempted to differentiate. These changes were retained in the *DSM-5-TR*. The new spectrum format for this category underscores the commonalities between disorders previously considered discrete. Disorders such as Asperger's, autism, childhood disintegrative disorder, and pervasive developmental disorder are included in autism spectrum disorder. Symptoms that formerly differentiated these disorders from one another now are indicated by diagnostic specifiers. Rett syndrome is considered as part of differential diagnosis.
- Evidence pointing to patterns of familial inheritance supports the theory that autism spectrum disorder is biologically caused. Although it is evident that neurological differences exist between people with and without this autism spectrum disorder, the basis for these differences and their implications are not clear.
- The behavioral perspective is the most relevant to treatment of autism spectrum disorder, particularly interventions that rest

on principles of operant conditioning practiced by student therapists and parents. Disruptive and self-stimulatory behaviors will decrease if children with autism spectrum disorder receive reinforcement for appropriate behaviors, such as asking for help or feedback. In such instances, they are less likely to engage in self-injurious or aggressive behaviors.

- The specific learning disorders include impairment in mathematics, written expression, reading, and communication. Communication disorders include speech sound disorder, childhood-onset fluency disorder, and social communication disorder. For the majority of children with specific developmental disorders, schools are the primary intervention site.
- Attention-deficit/hyperactivity disorder (ADHD) is characterized by inattentiveness or hyperactivity and impulsivity. Although researchers have found fundamental and structural variations in the brains of people with ADHD, most agree that genetic vulnerability interacts with environmental exposure. Treatment takes a multipronged approach.
- Developmental coordination disorders are characterized by tics, recurring involuntary movements or vocalizations. This type of disorder includes Tourette's and stereotypic movement disorder.
- The disorders covered in this chapter include a range of conditions that reflect, to differing degrees, combinations of biological, psychological, and sociocultural influences. Genetic influences on the development of many of these disorders are clearly evident, but even so, interactions with social context play an important role. Moreover, because these disorders begin early in life, they have the potential to exert profound psychological effects on an individual, making early intervention particularly crucial.

KEY TERMS

Asperger's syndrome
Attention-deficit/hyperactivity disorder (ADHD)
Autism spectrum disorder
Childhood-onset fluency disorder (stuttering)
Communication disorders
Developmental coordination disorder
Down syndrome
Dyscalculia
Echolalia
Fetal alcohol spectrum disorder (FASD)
Fetal alcohol syndrome (FAS)
Fragile X syndrome
Intellectual developmental disorder (intellectual disability)
Language disorder
Mainstreaming
Naturalistic developmental behavioral interventions (NDBI)
Neurodevelopmental disorders
Phenylketonuria (PKU)
Rett syndrome
Social (pragmatic) communication disorder
Specific learning disorder
Specific learning disorder with impairment in mathematics
Specific learning disorder with impairment in reading (dyslexia)
Specific learning disorder with impairment in written expression
Speech sound disorder
Stereotypic movement disorder
Tay-Sachs disease
Teratogens
Tic
Tourette's disorder

CHAPTER 6

Schizophrenia Spectrum and Other Psychotic Disorders

OUTLINE

Learning Objectives

6.1 Identify the characteristics of schizophrenia.

6.2 Identify the characteristics of brief psychotic disorder.

6.3 Identify the characteristics of schizophreniform disorder.

6.4 Identify the characteristics of schizoaffective disorder.

6.5 Identify the characteristics of delusional disorders.

6.6 Explain the theories and treatments of schizophrenia.

6.7 Analyze the biopsychosocial model of schizophrenia.

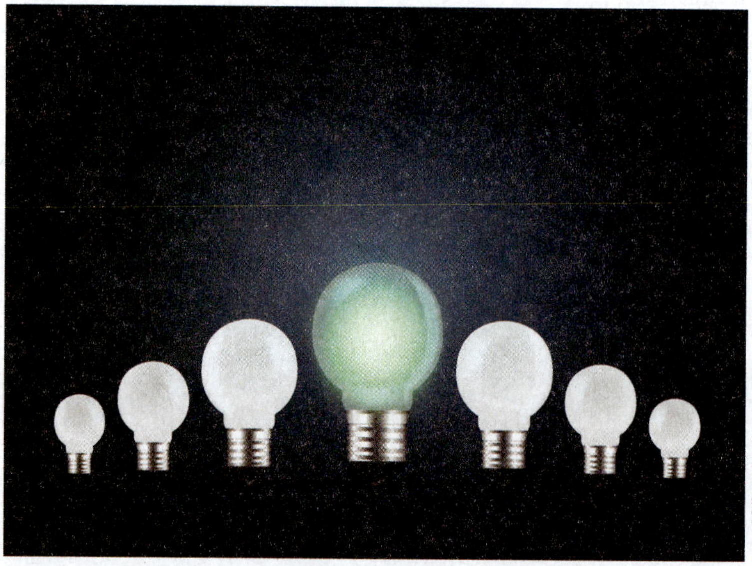

solar22/Shutterstock

Case Report

David Chen

Demographic information: 19-year-old Chinese American, non-binary person who identifies as queer. David's pronouns are they/them/theirs.

History of present illness: David was evaluated at an inpatient psychiatric facility following their second psychotic episode within a 1-year period. They were brought to the hospital by their mother, Ann, who had noticed that David's behavior had become increasingly bizarre over the past year. David's mother was the main source of information during the interview. David was unable to give an accurate personal history.

David is a college sophomore attending a university in their hometown. Though they lived at home during their first year (Ann has raised them since getting a divorce when David was 5), David and Ann decided it would be beneficial for them to move into the dormitories to gain a sense of independence. Ann reported that David was doing well for the first 2 weeks of living in the dormitories. She and David typically spoke on the phone a few times per week, and they had been coming home for dinner on Sunday evenings.

One Sunday evening in mid-October, Ann reported that David failed to show up for dinner as planned. She called David's best friend Mark, who had not heard from them for a few days and was himself worried about David. Mark has known David since high school and lives in the same town. He noted to Ann that David didn't "quite seem to be themself lately," as they had been acting particularly aloof. Mark had been concerned that he hadn't heard from David, so he went to search for them in different parts of town where he knew David liked to spend time and eventually found them outside a coffee shop.

When Mark approached them, David stated that they wished to be referred to as "Joey." Mark noted that David appeared particularly unkempt, which was unusual because they normally took very good care of themself. Mark also noticed that David was smiling and laughing to themself. Mark assumed that they were doing so because they were in a particularly good mood, though David's tone became more serious when Mark offered to drive them back to their dorm room. David refused, stating, "I have a lot of writing to do. My poems are going to be published and they want me to write 20 more so they can publish a book of my poems." Writing had always been one of David's hobbies, and David and Mark often discussed their respective creative endeavors. Mark was alarmed when he looked down at David's notebook, which was open in their lap while they were talking, and noticed only illegible scribbling. Mark also noticed that throughout their conversation, David's left arm repeatedly and seemingly involuntarily extended with a jerking motion every few minutes. Mark was unable to convince David to go back to campus with him, and he reluctantly left the coffee shop. After hearing these details Ann was shocked about David's behavior, remarking that she had never seen David acting so oddly. Unsure what to do, Ann decided to wait until she heard from them.

David eventually returned to their dorm room and called Ann around 3 a.m., stating, "I'm in New York City . . . I can't stay here because there are no poets here. They need me there. Meeting, meeting, bus, poems. I need poems for a money to go to meet. A meeting. I have to get there. I have got there. I have to go there." They repeated this last part several times. Confused, Ann asked David what they meant, at which point David hung up the phone. After that, Ann reported, she didn't hear from them for about a week.

David was returned to Ann's house by the police, who had found them on campus causing a disturbance by yelling at some other students who were waiting for a bus nearby. Ann was unsure whether David had actually gone to New York—which was about 3 hours away by train—or had been on campus the whole time. She was able to extract from them that they had not been attending their classes. She decided to write to David's professors and ask for an incomplete grade, since it was clear they were unable to successfully complete their classes in their current state.

David stayed with Ann for the next 3 weeks, during which time they continued to display bizarre behavior. Ann hoped they were going to recover at any moment, but it was becoming clear that they were not improving. When Ann returned home from work, she would find dirty laundry, dishes, pizza boxes, and cigarette ashes all around

Case Report *continued*

the house. Often David would stay in their room all day, coming out only to use the bathroom or eat a meal. When Ann did see them, she noticed that they appeared rather sad and withdrawn, barely speaking to her. Normally they had a very close relationship and enjoyed spending time together around the house. Though she worried about them, she wasn't sure what she could do to help. They decided it would be best for David to take the next semester off, since Ann didn't feel they would be able to focus enough on their school work and wanted to make sure they could handle the stress of going back to school.

By the end of the summer, Ann felt that David seemed to have made a great improvement—they were engaging more with her at home and were less messy, and the content of their speech was less bizarre. They did seem much more withdrawn in general than they once had been, engaging in minimal activities and rarely leaving the house. In the spring they were able to hold a part-time job at a gas station for a month before being fired for showing up late too many times. Otherwise, they mostly stayed in their room listening to music and writing. They spent time with Mark occasionally, though David often cancelled their plans, stating that they simply didn't feel like being around people. Ann took David to China to visit relatives for a few weeks, and she remembers their behavior there as normal for the most part.

David and Ann eventually decided that they should reenroll at the university to resume their degree in the fall, and at David's request, they left home to live in the dorm again. Two weeks later, David once more disappeared. As before, Ann got a phone call from them one evening, during which they said they had been living in Manhattan. She reported that David said they had owed their landlord some money for a new set of keys. Ann had been unaware that David even went to New York or that they were living there. David asked for her credit card information and said that if they didn't come up with the money the landlord was threatening violence against them. When Ann asked where they were exactly, David hung up the phone. She did not hear from them until they showed up at her house 3 days later, completely disheveled and visibly filthy. They told Ann that they were afraid their roommate was going to burn all of their belongings. While they were telling the story, they were laughing and smiling. It appeared to Ann that David was once again acting bizarrely, and after the previous experience she knew that this time something had to be done, because she felt very worried about their safety. Unsure where to turn, Ann brought David to the closest emergency room. The doctors in the ER sent them to a nearby hospital, where they were admitted to the psychiatric inpatient unit.

Psychiatric history: David has no previous history of psychiatric treatment. Their mother reported that they had experienced some mild depression earlier in their teenage years. They recalled that David had always been "somewhat different" from their peers, noting that they had only a few close friends throughout their childhood and adolescence.

In terms of family history, Ann reported that David's paternal grandfather had been diagnosed with schizophrenia, though there was no other known family history of mental illness.

Case formulation: It is clear from the presenting story that David had experienced two psychotic episodes over the past year. The first occurred after a major stressor—moving away from home for the first time. This change came around the developmental period when psychotic symptoms may begin to fully emerge, due to the high base rate of major life events that occur during this time. By Ann's report, David may have displayed some prodromal symptoms as an adolescent, which is typical in the case of individuals with schizophrenia.

David meets *DSM-5-TR* diagnostic criteria for schizophrenia because they displayed delusions, disorganized speech, grossly disorganized behavior, and negative symptoms (constricted affective expression) for over 1 month. There were signs of the disturbance for at least 6 months, including more than 1 month of active symptoms, and a period of negative symptoms. Further, David's general level of functioning was greatly reduced following the first psychotic episode; they were unable to hold a job and remained withdrawn from their interpersonal relationships. Lastly, they were not taking any substances, nor did they have a medical condition that would contribute to their symptoms.

Risk level: High, due to David's current psychotic state, they are unable to exercise appropriate judgment and have reduced decision-making capacity, and currently pose a risk to their own safety and well-being.

Case Report *continued*

Treatment plan: David will be stabilized on antipsychotic medication while in the hospital, and their psychiatrists will aim to find a suitable maintenance dose for the point at which they are discharged to go home. They will be set up with an outpatient psychiatric facility to provide them medication and weekly psychotherapy. It is also recommended that David find a case manager to help them with vocational activities and to decide whether continuing to pursue a higher educational degree is a possibility, given their past vulnerabilities when enrolled in college.

Sarah Tobin, PhD

6.1 Schizophrenia

The broad category of **schizophrenia** includes a set of disorders in which individuals experience distorted perception of reality and impairment in thinking, behavior, affect, and motivation. Schizophrenia is a serious mental illness, given its potential impact on an individual's ability to live a productive and fulfilling life. Although a significant number of people with schizophrenia eventually manage to live symptom-free lives, in some ways, all must adapt their lives to the reality of the illness.

schizophrenia
A disorder with a range of symptoms involving disturbances in content of thought, form of thought, perception, affect, sense of self, motivation, behavior, and interpersonal functioning.

Schizophrenia is one of the top 15 leading causes of disability on a worldwide basis (Global Burden of Disease, 2017). In the United States, it is estimated to cause an average of 28.5 years of potential life lost for an individual with the disorder (Olfson et al., 2015).

General Features of Schizophrenia

A key symptom of schizophrenia is the presence of a **delusion**, a deeply entrenched false belief not consistent with the client's intelligence or cultural background. You can read examples of delusions in Table 1. The *DSM-5-TR* authors note the importance of cultural considerations in diagnosing delusions, and recommend use of a cultural formulation interview and the need to consider language to avoid misunderstanding unfamiliar metaphors as delusions.

delusion
Deeply entrenched false belief not consistent with the client's intelligence or cultural background.

A second major symptom of schizophrenia is **hallucinations**, which are false perceptions not corresponding to the objective stimuli present in the environment. People may suffer from hallucinations in several sensory modalities, including vision, hearing, smell, and touch. Individuals who experience both visual and auditory hallucinations appear to have more significant cognitive deficits than those who experience hallucinations in one sensory modality, who in turn are more significantly impaired than individuals with no hallucinations (Mahfoud et al., 2023).

hallucination
A false perception not corresponding to the objective stimuli present in the environment.

Associated with delusions or auditory hallucinations related to a theme of persecution may be **paranoia**, the irrational belief or perception that others wish to cause you harm. People who experience paranoia become unable to trust others, feeling convinced that they will be mistreated or even threatened with bodily injury.

paranoia
The irrational belief or perception that others wish to cause you harm.

Language that is incomprehensible and incoherent is referred to as **disorganized speech**. The thought process underlying this type of speech reflects **loosening of associations**–that is, a flow of thoughts that is vague, unfocused, and illogical. The speech of individuals with schizophrenia may contain **neologisms**, which are words not contained in language. Unlike words that eventually may become accepted words in a particular language (such as *google*), these words have highly idiosyncratic meanings that are used only by the individual.

disorganized speech
Language that is incomprehensible and incoherent.

loosening of associations
Flow of thoughts that is vague, unfocused, and illogical.

neologisms
Invented ("new") words.

Another characteristic symptom that people with schizophrenia may show is **inappropriate affect**, meaning that the person's emotional response does not match the social cues present in a situation or the content of what is being discussed. The individual may, for example, burst into laughter during a sad situation or when hearing someone express discontent or unhappiness. You saw this in the case of David, who was laughing and smiling

inappropriate affect
The extent to which a person's emotional expressiveness fails to correspond either to the social cues present in a situation or to the content of what is being discussed.

TABLE 1 **Types and Examples of Delusions**

Grandeur A grossly exaggerated conception of the individual's own importance. Such delusions range from beliefs that the person has an important role in society to the belief that the person is actually Christ, Napoleon, or a famous celebrity.
Control The feeling that one is being controlled by others, or even by machines or appliances. For example, a man may believe that his actions are being controlled by information on a social media website, which is "forcing" him to perform certain actions against his will.
Reference The belief that the behavior of others or certain objects or events are personally referring to oneself. For example, a woman believes that an action movie is really telling the story of her life, or a man believes that the sale items at a local food market are targeted at his own particular dietary deficiencies.
Persecution The belief that another person or persons are trying to inflict harm on the individual or on that individual's family or social group. For example, a woman feels that a neighbor is planning to have her evicted.
Self-blame Feelings of remorse without justification. A man holds himself responsible for an earthquake on the other side of the world because of certain unkind or sinful actions that he believes he has committed.
Somatic Inappropriate concerns about one's body, typically related to a disease. For example, without any justification, a woman believes she has brain cancer and that ants have invaded her head and are eating away at her brain.
Infidelity A false belief usually associated with pathological jealousy involving the notion that one's lover is being unfaithful. A man lashes out in violent rage at his wife, insisting that she is having an affair with the mail carrier because of her eagerness for the mail to arrive each day.
Thought broadcasting The idea that one's thoughts are being broadcast to others. A man believes that everyone else in the room can hear what he is thinking, or possibly that his thoughts are actually being carried over onto a stranger's social media feed.
Thought insertion The belief that outside forces are inserting thoughts into one's mind. For example, a woman is certain that her co-worker is placing ideas into her head in order to control her or upset her.

while telling their mother that they believed their roommate was going to burn their belongings.

Table 2 contains the six criteria associated with a diagnosis of schizophrenia. The symptoms in Criterion A refer to the **active phase** of the disorder, that is, the period during which the individual's symptoms are most prominent. The symptoms the individual experiences during the active phase fall into two categories based on their nature. In the first category are **positive symptoms**, exaggerations or distortions of normal thoughts, emotions, and behavior. In Table 2, the disturbances numbered 1 through 4 under Criterion A fit into the category of positive symptoms.

The symptoms in Criterion A-5 are **negative symptoms**, which relate to functioning that is below the normal level of behavior or feeling. **Restricted affect** refers to a narrowing of the range of outward expressions of emotions. **Avolition** is a lack of initiative, either not wanting to take any action or lacking the energy and will to take action. **Asociality** refers to a lack of interest in social relationships, including an inability to empathize and form close relationships with others.

active phase
A period in the course of schizophrenia in which psychotic symptoms are present.

positive symptoms
The symptoms of schizophrenia that represent exaggerations or distortions of normal thoughts, emotions, and behavior.

negative symptoms
The symptoms of schizophrenia that involve functioning below the level of normal behavior.

restricted affect
Narrowing of the range of outward expressions of emotions.

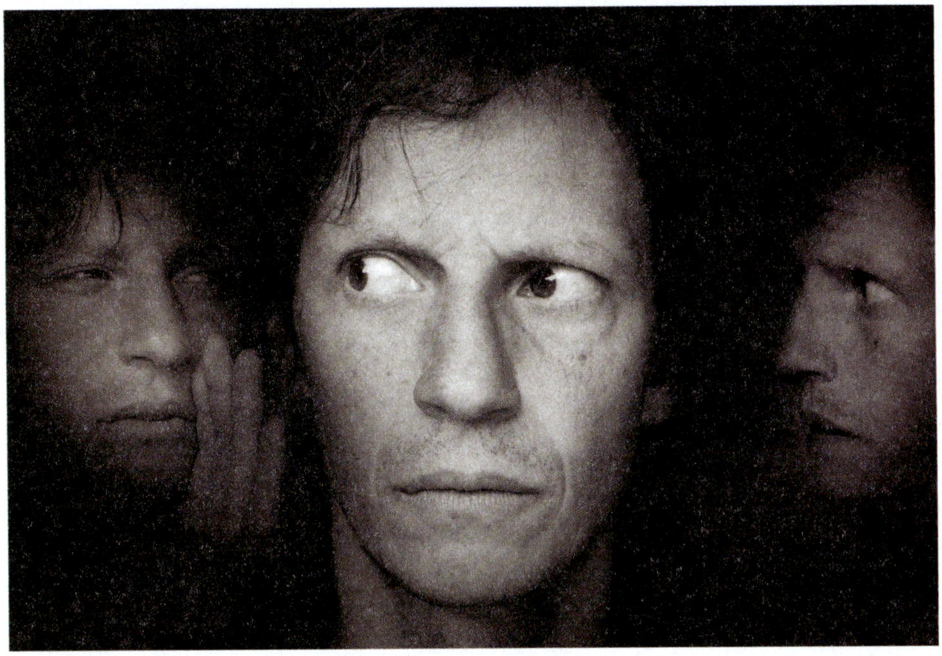

People with schizophrenia may experience thought insertion in which they hear voices which they believe come from others.

Javier ki/Shutterstock

avolition
A lack of initiative, either not wanting to take any action or lacking the energy and will to take action.

asociality
Lack of interest in social relationships.

TABLE 2 **Diagnostic Features of Schizophrenia**

To be diagnosed with schizophrenia, an individual must meet all the criteria listed in A–F.	
A.	Two (or more) of the following symptoms must be present for a significant portion of time during a 1-month period (although this can be less if the individual is successfully treated). At least one symptom must be from the first three categories. 1. Delusions 2. Hallucinations 3. Disorganized speech 4. Grossly disorganized or catatonic behavior 5. Negative symptoms such as restricted affect, avolition, and asociality
B.	Social role dysfunction:
	For a significant portion of the time since the onset of the disturbance, one or more major areas of functioning such as work, interpersonal relations, or self-care are markedly below the level achieved prior to the onset (or when the onset is in childhood or adolescence, the person fails to achieve expected level of interpersonal, academic, or occupational achievement).
C.	Duration of at least 6 months:
	Continuous signs of the disturbance must persist for at least 6 months. During at least 1 of these 6 months, the person must show the active-phase symptoms from Criterion A (or less if the person was successfully treated). The 6 months may include periods during which the individual had symptoms leading up to (prodromal) or following (residual) an active phase. During these periods, the person must show only negative symptoms or two or more of the active-phase symptoms but in attenuated form.
D.	No evidence of schizoaffective, depressive, or bipolar disorder.
E.	Symptoms are not due to substance use disorder or general medical condition.
F.	If there is a history of autism spectrum disorder or a communication disorder of childhood onset, the additional diagnosis of schizophrenia is made only if prominent delusions or hallucinations are also present for at least a month (or less if successfully treated).

MINI CASE

Schizophrenia, Continuous

Joshua is a single 43-year-old biracial heterosexual cisgender man. Most days, he stands near the steps of a local bank on a busy street corner, wearing a Red Sox baseball cap, a yellow T-shirt, worn-out hiking shorts, and orange sneakers. Rain or shine, day in and day out, Joshua maintains his post at the bank. Sometimes he converses with imaginary people. Sometimes he explodes in shrieks of laughter. Without provocation, he sobs miserably. Police and social workers keep taking him to shelters for people experiencing homelessness, but Joshua manages to get back on the street before he can receive treatment. He has repeatedly insisted that these people have no right to keep bothering him.

Criterion B is consistent with other, general *DSM* criteria for psychological disorders, in that it stipulates that there must be significant impairment. The degree of impairment in schizophrenia, however, implies a particularly serious and far-reaching impact in the individual's life. Criterion C, indicating the period of disturbance, is also carefully delineated to ensure that individuals receive this diagnosis only if they show a substantial duration of symptoms.

Criteria D and E refer to other disorders that should not be present in people diagnosed with schizophrenia. It is particularly important for clinicians to rule out Criterion D, schizoaffective disorder, when making their diagnosis (discussed later in the chapter. Similarly, in the interests of differentiating schizophrenia from other disorders, Criterion F makes it clear that the symptoms of schizophrenia involving, for example, communication must not overlap with symptoms of an autism spectrum disorder.

Before publication of *DSM-5*, the diagnostic criteria for schizophrenia included five subtypes based on which symptoms were most prominent in the individual. These subtypes were labeled catatonic, disorganized, paranoid, undifferentiated, and residual. They were dropped from *DSM-5*, since researchers studying schizophrenia now believe they represent fine-grained distinctions not supported by empirical evidence. The *DSM-5-TR* retained these changes.

catatonia
A condition in which the individual shows marked psychomotor disturbances.

Additionally, **catatonia**, which was once a subtype of schizophrenia, is included in the *DSM-5-TR* as a set of symptoms that can occur in the context of other disorders. It is defined as a condition involving marked psychomotor disturbances. These disturbances may consist of decreased, excessive, or peculiar motor activity that is not in response to what is occurring in the individual's environment. For example, with no apparent provocation, the individual may hold odd, rigid poses for long periods of time as well as being unable to speak or move. Catatonia may be diagnosed in association with another psychological disorder, a medical condition, or a cause the clinician cannot identify.

History of Schizophrenia

Schizophrenia has a long and fascinating history. French physician Benedict Morel (1809–1873) first identified it as a disease that he named *démence precocé* (brain dementia of the young). The next major point in schizophrenia's history is associated with the German psychiatrist Emil Kraepelin (1856–1926), who used Latin to refer to the condition, which then became known as *dementia praecox*. At the root of its symptoms, Kraepelin believed, was one underlying and progressively degenerating disease process that caused, in his terms, the "weakening" of mental processes.

In 1911, Swiss psychologist Eugen Bleuler (1857–1939) revised the concept of schizophrenia once again to reflect his belief that the disorder was actually a set of diseases. He coined the term *schizophrenia* to signify that the underlying cause was a splitting ("schiz") among the functions of the mind. Unlike Kraepelin, Bleuler thought it was possible for people with schizophrenia to recover from the disorder.

MINI CASE

Catatonia, Unspecified

Maria is a single 21-year-old Latina heterosexual cisgender woman. She is a junior in college who has been psychiatrically hospitalized for a month. The resident assistant in Maria's dormitory notified the campus police because she had grown increasingly concerned about Maria's deteriorating behavior over the course of the semester. When Maria returned to college in September, her roommate told others, including the resident assistant, that Maria's behavior seemed odd. For example, she had a habit of repeating other people's words, she stared listlessly out the window, and she ignored her personal hygiene. As the semester's end approached, Maria retreated more and more into her own world, until her behavior reached a point at which she was completely unresponsive to others and had not left her room for about a week. Eventually, her resident assistant performed a wellness check, at which point she determined she had to call the campus police to intervene.

The police found Maria in a trancelike state, unable to respond to any of their questions or attempts to engage with her. She was sent to the hospital for a psychiatric evaluation and was admitted because she was deemed unable to take care of herself. In the hospital, Maria maintains rigid posturing of her body, while staring blankly most of the time. The staff members treating her are in a quandary about what intervention to use because of her hypersensitivity to most medications. At present, the clinicians are attempting to determine whether she has another medical condition or a psychological disorder, but because they cannot identify any, for the moment they have diagnosed her as having unspecified catatonia.

Reflecting the importance of Bleuler's contributions, clinicians still refer to the fundamental features of the disorder as **Bleuler's "Four A's"**. Briefly, the four A's are:

Bleuler's "Four A's"
According to Swiss psychologist Eugen Bleuler, the four fundamental features of schizophrenia include disorders in association and affect, ambivalence, and autism.

1. *Association*–thought disorder, as might be evident through rambling and incoherent speech
2. *Affect*–disorder of the experience and expression of emotion
3. *Ambivalence*–inability to make or follow through on decisions
4. *Autism*–withdrawal from reality

Note that Bleuler did not intend for the "splitting" to be a splitting of personalities, as is often mistakenly thought (as in "split personality"). Instead, the splitting refers to a division, or dissociation, between the individual's experience of an emotion and the way the emotion is expressed.

In the decades following Bleuler's work, clinicians in Europe and the United States proposed further distinctions among the forms of schizophrenia. One notable contributor to the debate was the German psychiatrist Kurt Schneider (1887–1967), who believed clinicians should diagnose schizophrenia only when an individual displays what he called **first-rank symptoms (FRS)**. These are the symptoms that are truly key, defining features of the disorder. They include audible thoughts (voices heard arguing), the experience of outside influences on the body, the belief that others are taking thoughts out of one's head, and diffuse or vague thoughts, delusions, and acts or behaviors seen as reflecting the influence of other people on the individual.

first-rank symptom (FRS)
Symptom that is truly defining, or key, in the diagnosis of schizophrenia.

First-rank symptoms retain a special meaning even today (e.g., Crump et al., 2017). *DSM-III* and the *ICD-10* included them as an advance on the less precise set of criteria included in earlier diagnostic manuals. However, researchers disagree on whether FRS represent valid criteria, and can provide worthwhile information above and beyond the presence of other delusions and hallucinations (Peralta & Cuesta, 2020).

As debate continues on the FRS, researchers are also rethinking whether schizophrenia is best thought of as a spectrum rather than a single disease entity. The **schizophrenia spectrum** refers to a range of disorders that reflect a similar underlying disease process. To this end, a provisional section of the *DSM-5-TR* (Section III) includes a set of symptom severity ratings (see Table 3). Although not formal diagnostic categories, they can inform the assessment process as

schizophrenia spectrum
Range of disorders that reflect a similar underlying disease process as that involved in schizophrenia.

TABLE 3 Dimensions of Psychosis Symptom Severity in Section III of *DSM-5-TR*

	0	1	2	3	4
Hallucinations	Not present	Equivocal (severity or duration not sufficient to be considered psychosis)	Present, but mild (little pressure to act upon voices, not very bothered by voices)	Present and moderate (some pressure to respond to voices, or is somewhat bothered by voices)	Present and severe (severe pressure to respond to voices, or is very bothered by voices)
Delusions	Not present	Equivocal (severity or duration not sufficient to be considered psychosis)	Present, but mild (delusions are not bizarre, or little pressure to act upon delusional beliefs, not very bothered by beliefs)	Present and moderate (some pressure to act upon beliefs, or is somewhat bothered by beliefs)	Present and severe (severe pressure to act upon beliefs, or is very bothered by beliefs)
Disorganized speech	Not present	Equivocal (severity or duration not sufficient to be considered disorganization)	Present, but mild (some difficulty following speech and/or occasional bizarre behavior)	Present and moderate (speech often difficult to follow and/or frequent bizarre behavior)	Present and severe (speech almost impossible to follow and/or behavior almost always bizarre)
Atypical psychomotor behavior	Not present	Equivocal (severity or duration not sufficient to be considered atypical psychomotor behavior)	Present, but mild (occasional atypical motor behavior)	Present and moderate (frequent atypical motor behavior)	Present and severe (atypical motor behavior almost constant)
Negative symptoms (restricted emotional expression or avolition)	Not present	Equivocal (decrease in facial expressivity, prosody, gestures, or self-initiated behavior)	Present, but mild (decrease in facial expressivity, prosody, gestures, or self-initiated behavior)	Present and moderate (decrease in facial expressivity, prosody, gestures, or self-initiated behavior)	Present and severe (decrease in facial expressivity, prosody, gestures, or self-initiated behavior)
Impaired cognition	Not present	Equivocal (cognitive function not clearly outside the range expected for age or SES, i.e., within 0.5 SD of mean)	Present, but mild (some reduction in cognitive function below expected for age and SES, 0.5–1 SD from mean)	Present and moderate (clear reduction in cognitive function below expected for age and SES, 1–2 SD from mean)	Present and severe (severe reduction in cognitive function below expected for age and SES, >2 SD from mean)
Depression	Not present	Equivocal (some depressed mood, but insufficient symptoms, duration, or severity to meet diagnostic criteria)	Present, but mild (meets criteria for major depression, with minimum number of symptoms, duration, and severity)	Present and moderate (meets criteria for major depression with somewhat more than the minimum number of symptoms, duration, and/or severity)	Present and severe (meets criteria for major depression with many more than the minimum number of symptoms and/or severity)
Mania	Not present	Equivocal (some inflated or irritable mood, but insufficient symptoms, duration, or severity to meet diagnostic criteria)	Present, but mild (meets criteria for mania with minimum number of symptoms, duration, and severity)	Present and moderate (meets criteria for mania with somewhat more than the minimum number of symptoms, duration, and/or severity)	Present and severe (meets criteria for mania with many more than the minimum number of symptoms and/or severity)

Note: SD = standard deviation; SES = socioeconomic status

well as allow clinicians to track changes in a client's symptoms across time and over the course of treatment.

Estimates from the United States place the lifetime prevalence of schizophrenia at under 1 percent with a range of between 0.25 and 0.64 percent of the population; globally, prevalence estimates range from 0.33 to 0.75 percent (National Institute of Mental Health, 2023). People of all genders are equally likely to develop the disorder over the course of their lifetimes, although females typically do so later in life (Falkenburg & Tracy, 2014).

The prevalence of schizophrenia is relatively low compared to other psychological disorders, but a surprisingly high percentage of adults report experiencing minor psychotic symptoms. Reviewing a large number of studies on psychotic symptoms, one group of researchers estimate the lifetime prevalence at approximately 5.8 percent. These symptoms, although short of being diagnosable, can be associated with cognitive impairment, higher rates of substance use, disability, suicidality, and atypical brain structures and functions (Mennigen & Bearden, 2020).

What's in the *DSM-5-TR*

Schizophrenia Subtypes and Dimensional Ratings

The *DSM-5* authors implemented major changes in their approach to diagnosing schizophrenia. As you read about it at the beginning of the chapter, they eliminated the subtypes of schizophrenia. Instead, using a scale that is in Section III of the *DSM-5*, clinicians assign a diagnosis of schizophrenia to which they can add a rating of the individual's symptoms along a set of dimensions, as Table 3 shows.

By eliminating the subtypes of schizophrenia, the *DSM-5* authors sought to improve both the diagnostic reliability and the validity of the system. They also sought to establish a more quantifiable basis for research into the disorder's causes and for treatment planning. For example, a clinician evaluating the results of cognitive behavioral therapy could use the ratings of hallucination and delusion severity to determine whether the intervention is reducing the specific symptoms toward which they are targeting treatment.

The *DSM-5* authors also decided to include cognitive impairment as a dimension in the Section III severity ratings, given the importance of cognitive deficits in current understandings of the individual's ability to carry out social and occupational activities and the tasks of everyday living.

The current system in the *DSM-5*, now the *DSM-5-TR*, represents a step away from the old categorization system and toward the dimensional approach. Including severity ratings rather than subtypes in Section III makes it possible for clinicians and researchers to track individuals over time in a quantifiable fashion.

The *DSM-5* authors also considered eliminating schizoaffective disorder as a separate entity but decided not to. They believe clinicians will eventually diagnose schizophrenia as a spectrum disorder. This would mean that even diagnoses long in use in psychiatry would disappear, including schizophreniform disorder, schizoaffective disorder, and two of the personality disorders associated with schizophrenia-like symptoms, which you will read about in the chapter "Personality Disorders."

Course of Schizophrenia

The course of schizophrenia, as mentioned, was once thought to be lifelong. This situation began to change during the 1970s as researchers and clinicians developed a better diagnostic system and understanding of the nature of psychotic disorders. Researchers now know that schizophrenia may take one of several courses.

Researchers who follow people with schizophrenia for extended periods of time suggest that as many as 25 to 35 percent show chronic psychotic symptoms throughout their lives. Among the remainder, 40 percent show significant improvement if they receive current treatment during their acute phase. Recovery is least likely for individuals who have negative symptoms and have longdurations of their untreated episodes (Mennigen & Bearden, 2020). Both positive and negative symptoms can become exacerbated, furthermore, in those who

MINI CASE

Schizophrenia, Multiple Episodes, Currently in Full Remission

Esther is a single 36-year-old White heterosexual cisgender woman. She lives with her mother, and for the past 10 years she has worked as a clerical assistant in an insurance company and no longer shows the delusions, disorganized speech, and lack of emotional expression that originally led to her two prior hospitalizations within a 2-year period. At the moment, she is able to hold her job and maintain a relationship with her mother and a few friends.

You Be the Judge

Schizophrenia Diagnosis

As you read in the chapter, schizophrenia is a complex and debilitating disorder which has a significant impact on those who experience it. Although many people do achieve recovery, particularly if they are treated early in the course of the disorder, people with schizophrenia nevertheless face substantial risks of relapse over the rest of their lives. Therefore, when a mental health professional delivers a diagnosis of schizophrenia, it is serious news that could lead the individual to experience great distress.

Practitioners thus face some ethical issues when working with people diagnosed with schizophrenia (Howe, 2008). Not only must they attempt to determine whether to provide a diagnosis of this serious disorder; they must also address specific questions relevant to the individual's particular symptoms. For example, the clinician may consider it more acceptable to inform clients with delusional disorder that they are receiving medication for anxiety, stress, or dysphoria rather than for delusions. To inform the client about the actual nature of their symptoms might interfere with the ability to form a therapeutic alliance, which could in turn interfere with the ultimate success of the treatment.

To overcome this obstacle, a clinician may decide to share a partial truth. Specifically, the clinician may reframe a client's symptoms as strengths. Rather than seeing a client's attachments to inanimate objects as a symptom, for example, the clinician may reframe the behavior as proving the client's exceptional capacity for caring.

A second ethical dilemma arises in balancing a client's desire to succeed in life with the reality that, due to the disorder, they may be unable to realize these ambitions. The stress of a competitive career, for example, might push the client over the edge into a relapse. Should the clinician try to protect the client from undertaking this venture, or respect the client's autonomy to make his or her own decisions?

As if these two challenges were not enough, consider the situation in which a clinician wishes to involve the client's family in treatment. As you will see later in the chapter, overinvolved and critical family members can exacerbate a client's symptoms. Should the clinician try to persuade the client to make the family part of the treatment, knowing this could improve the client's chances of recovery? Or would such persuasion be unethical, a violation of the client's autonomy?

Finally, given that people with a family history of schizophrenia have increased risk of developing the disorder, how much should clinicians warn high-risk adolescents or young adults? On the one hand, telling people who are asymptomatic that they may develop this serious illness could itself provoke an episode. On the other hand, not telling those at genetic risk about the possibility of their developing schizophrenia may mean they don't take preventive steps.

Howe (2008) suggests that mental health professionals can navigate these ethical dilemmas by using an "ethical sliding scale." In other words, they can make their ethical decisions by taking into account the client's ability to achieve insight, the strength of their own relationship with the client, and the nature and strength of the client's relationship with family. Although respecting the client's autonomy should be the primary guiding principle, clinicians should balance it against the client's decision-making abilities.

Q: *You be the judge:* Do you agree with the idea of using an ethical sliding scale?

experience negative life events, such as job loss, poor wages, relationship endings, and miscarriages (Donaldson et al., 2022).

Understanding the life course of schizophrenia is made more complicated by the fact that people with schizophrenia are two to three times more likely to die than others in their age group, leading to a reduction in life expectancy of 15 to 20 years (Gatov, Rosella, Chiu, & Kurdyak, 2017). This higher mortality reflects, in part, the economic and social challenges these individuals face in their daily lives. The use of antipsychotic medications may improve mortality by reducing suicide rates, but alternatively may increase mortality due to negative effects on cardiovascular health (Vermeulen et al., 2017).

6.2 Brief Psychotic Disorder

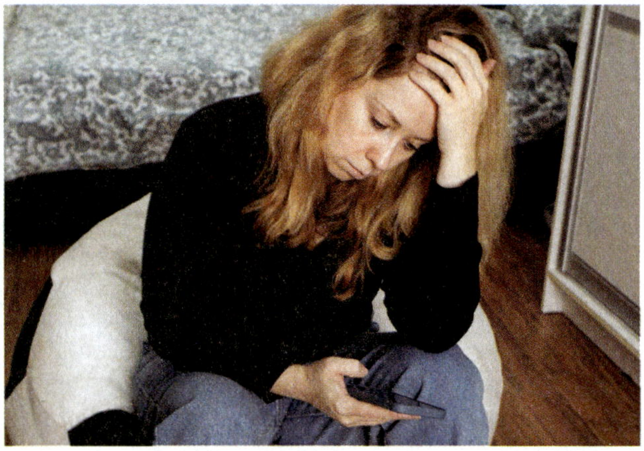

Individuals who are experiencing symptoms such as delusions and hallucinations for a short period of time may have brief psychotic disorder.

Yta23/Shutterstock

As the term implies, **brief psychotic disorder** is a diagnosis that clinicians use when an individual develops symptoms of psychosis for a short period of time, specifically, more than a day but less than a month. To receive this diagnosis, the individual must experience one of four symptoms, which are delusions, hallucinations, disorganized speech, and grossly disorganized or catatonic behavior.

Clinicians assigning this particular diagnosis need to note the context in which individuals display the psychotic symptoms. Has the client experienced a recent stressor, such as a natural disaster, the loss of a close relative, or an accident? Another possibility is that a woman develops this disorder soon after giving birth. In such cases, the clinician adds a specification to indicate that the symptoms are associated with a stressor. A woman who develops this disorder during pregnancy or within 4 weeks of giving birth would receive a separate specification as having brief psychotic disorder, postpartum onset.

The COVID-19 pandemic, with its associated stressors involving loss of life, social distancing, and general disruptions of people's ordinary existence contributed to a rise in cases of brief psychotic disorder reported around the world. Individuals prone to developing this disorder appeared to be responding to such stressors as contamination phobia, death anxiety, grief, economic stress, and loss of cultural traditions and their personal meanings, among other concerns. Those at particular risk for then developing a more longstanding disorder were young adult men, those with poor adjustment prior to COVID-19, and individuals experiencing hallucinations and other first-rank symptoms (Valdés-Florido et al., 2022).

brief psychotic disorder
A diagnosis clinicians use when an individual develops symptoms of psychosis for more than a day but less than a month.

6.3 Schizophreniform Disorder

People receive a diagnosis of **schizophreniform disorder** if they experience symptoms of schizophrenia for a period of 1 to 6 months. If symptoms persist for longer than 6 months, the clinician conducts an evaluation to determine whether a diagnosis of schizophrenia is appropriate.

schizophreniform disorder
A disorder characterized by psychotic symptoms that are essentially the same as those found in schizophrenia, except for their duration; specifically, symptoms usually last from 1 to 6 months.

MINI CASE

Brief Psychotic Disorder, with Marked Stressors

Anthony is a 22-year-old White heterosexual cisgender man. He is a senior at a prestigious small college. His family has traditionally held high standards for Anthony, and his father had every expectation that his son would go on to study at Harvard Law School. Anthony often felt intensely pressured as he worked day and night to maintain a high grade-point average, while diligently preparing for the national examination for admission to law school. His social life became devoid of any meaningful contact. He even began skipping meals, because he did not want to take time away from studying. When Anthony received his scores on the law school admission exam, he was devastated, because he knew they were too low to allow him to get into any of the better law schools. He began crying uncontrollably, wandering around the dormitory hallways, screaming obscenities, and telling people there was a plot on the part of the college dean to keep him from getting into law school. After 2 days of this behavior, Anthony's resident advisor convinced him to go to the infirmary, where clinicians diagnosed and treated his condition. After a week of rest and medication, Anthony returned to normal functioning and was able to assess his academic situation more rationally.

MINI CASE

Schizophreniform Disorder, with Good Prognostic Features

When Deion, Black heterosexual cisgender man, developed a psychological disorder, he was 26 years old and worked for a convenience store chain. Although family and friends always regarded Deion as unusual, he had not experienced psychotic symptoms. This all changed as he grew more and more disturbed over the course of several months. His mother thought that he was just "stressed out" because of his financial problems, but Deion did not seem concerned about such matters. He gradually developed paranoid delusions and became preoccupied with reading the Bible, though he did not actively practice any religion. What brought his disturbance to the attention of his supervisors was the fact that he had submitted an order to the district office for 6,000 loaves of bread. He had scribbled at the bottom of the order form, "Jesus will multiply the loaves." When his supervisors questioned this inappropriate order, Deion became enraged and insisted that they were plotting to prevent him from fighting world hunger. Paranoid themes and bizarre behaviors also surfaced in Deion's interactions with his wife and children. Following 2 months of increasingly disturbed behavior, Deion's boss urged him to see a psychiatrist. With rest and relatively low doses of antipsychotic medication, Deion returned to normal functioning after a few weeks.

Those clients who show a rapid development of symptoms (within a span of 4 weeks), seem confused or perplexed while in the peak of the episode, and have otherwise good social and personal functioning prior to the episode have a better chance of not developing schizophrenia. They are also likely to have a good prognosis if they do not show the negative symptoms of apathy, withdrawal, and asociality or lack of interest in being with other people.

schizoaffective disorder
A disorder involving the experience of a major depressive episode, a manic episode, or a mixed episode while also meeting the diagnostic criteria for schizophrenia.

delusional disorder
Disorder in which the only symptoms are delusions that have lasted for at least 1 month.

erotomanic type of delusional disorder
Delusional disorder in which individuals falsely believe that another person is in love with them.

6.4 Schizoaffective Disorder

In **schizoaffective disorder**, individuals with a mood disorder (depressive or bipolar) also experience delusions and/or hallucinations. However, the diagnosis can be made only if, during a 2-week period, clients have psychotic but not mood disorder symptoms. For most of the duration of their illness, they must have a major mood episode (depressive or manic) as well as show symptoms of schizophrenia. In other words, they must have both a mood episode and a psychotic disorder, and at least 2 weeks during which delusions and/or hallucinations are the only symptoms they show.

MINI CASE

Schizoaffective Disorder, Bipolar Type

At the time of her admission to a psychiatric hospital, Hazel, a married White heterosexual cisgender woman originally from Canada, was a 52-year-old mother of three children. She had a 20-year history of schizophrenia-like symptoms, and she experienced periodic episodes of mania. Her schizophrenia-like symptoms included delusions, hallucinations, and thought disorder. These symptoms were fairly well controlled by antipsychotic medications, which she received by injection every 2 weeks. She was also treated with lithium to control her manic episodes; however, she often skipped her daily dose because she liked "feeling high." On several occasions following extended periods of abstinence from lithium, Hazel became manic. Accelerated speech and bodily activity, sleepless nights, and erratic behavior characterized these episodes. At the insistence of her husband and her therapist, Hazel would resume taking her lithium, and shortly thereafter her manic symptoms would subside, although her schizophrenia-like symptoms were still somewhat evident.

6.5 Delusional Disorders

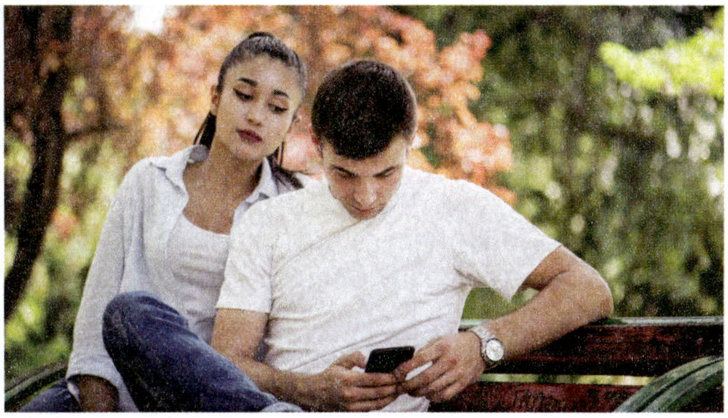

People with jealous delusional disorder believe that their romantic partners are being unfaithful to them.

Emilija Manevska/Moment/Getty Images

People with **delusional disorders** have delusions that have lasted for at least 1 month as their only symptom. Furthermore, this diagnoses requires they must have no other symptoms of schizophrenia and must never have met the criteria for schizophrenia. In fact, these individuals can function very well and do not seem odd to others except when they talk about their particular delusion.

Based on which delusional theme is prominent, clinicians diagnose these individuals with one of five major types of disorder, or with mixed or unspecified types that include people who do not have a single prominent delusion. A delusion is diagnosed as "with bizarre content" if it is clearly implausible, not understandable, and not derived from ordinary life experiences.

People with the **erotomanic type of delusional disorder** falsely believe that another person is in love with them. Often, the target of their delusion is usually a person of higher status than they are. For example, a person may be certain that a famous singer is in love with them and that the singer's songs contain secret love messages to them.

The conviction that they possess special and extremely favorable personal qualities and abilities characterizes people who have the **grandiose type of delusional disorder**. A person may believe that they are the Messiah waiting for a sign from heaven to begin their active ministry.

In the **jealous type of delusional disorder**, individuals are certain their romantic partner is unfaithful to them. They may even construct a plan to entrap their partner to prove their infidelity.

People with the **persecutory type of delusional disorder** believe that someone close to them is treating them in a malevolent manner. They may, for example, become convinced that their neighbors are deliberately poisoning their water.

People with the **somatic type of delusional disorder** believe they have a medical condition causing a bodily reaction that does not actually exist. For example, a person may be convinced that they have lesions on their skin that have spread to their internal organs.

Shared psychotic disorder is a diagnosis applied when one or more people develop a delusional system as a result of a close relationship with a psychotic person who is delusional. You may have heard this disorder referred to as *folie à deux* (folly of two) when two people are involved. Occasionally, three or more people or the members of an entire family are affected.

Children may develop this disorder, particularly if they are socially isolated, perhaps because they are less exposed to the outside world. Those who spread the delusions are themselves more likely to develop a psychotic illness as they get older (Vigo et al., 2019).

grandiose type of delusional disorder
An exaggerated view of oneself as possessing special and extremely favorable personal qualities and abilities.

jealous type of delusional disorder
Delusional disorder in which individuals falsely believe that their romantic partner is unfaithful to them.

persecutory type of delusional disorder
Delusional disorder in which individuals falsely believe that someone close to them is treating them in a malevolent manner.

somatic type of delusional disorder
Delusional disorder in which individuals falsely believe that they have a medical condition.

shared psychotic disorder
Delusional disorder in which one or more people develop a delusional system as a result of a close relationship with a psychotic person who is delusional.

MINI CASE

Delusional Disorder, Jealous Type

Paul is a 32-year-old Black heterosexual cisgender man who has recently experienced tremendous stress at his job of 5 years. Although he has avoided dwelling on his work problems, he has begun to develop irrational beliefs about his girlfriend, Elizabeth. Despite Elizabeth's repeated vows that she is consistently faithful in the relationship, Paul has become obsessed with the belief that she is sexually involved with another person. He is suspicious of everyone with whom Elizabeth interacts and questions her about every insignificant encounter. He searches her closet and drawers for mysterious items, looks for unexplained charges on credit card bills, listens in on Elizabeth's phone calls, and has contacted a private investigator to follow her. Paul is now insisting that they move to another state.

MINI CASE

Delusional Disorder, Persecutory Type

Julio is a 25-year-old Latino cisgender man who identifies as pansexual. Recently Julio met with his co-worker Ernesto in the company cafeteria of the accounting firm where they both work. After a brief and very casual conversation, Julio began to develop the belief that Ernesto was secretly trying to break into his workstation to plant faulty reports. Soon Julio became convinced that Ernesto was conspiring with three others in their unit to make it appear that he was incompetent. He requested a reassignment so his job would, in his opinion, no longer be jeopardized by the behavior of his co-workers.

6.6 Theories and Treatment of Schizophrenia

Schizophrenia reflects a complex interplay of biological, psychological, and sociocultural forces. As a result, researchers are well aware of the need to approach the disorder from an interactive perspective.

vulnerability
The idea that individuals have a biologically determined predisposition to developing schizophrenia but that the disorder develops only when certain environmental conditions are in place.

A key concept in understanding schizophrenia's causes is **vulnerability**, the idea that individuals have a biologically determined predisposition to developing schizophrenia but that the disorder develops only when certain environmental conditions are in place. As you read about each of the contributions to a vulnerability model, keep in mind that no single theory contains the entire explanation.

Biological Perspective

Theories Biological explanations of schizophrenia have their origins in the writings of Emil Kraepelin, who thought of schizophrenia as a disease caused by degenerative processes in the brain. Although scientists following Kraepelin's work became interested in possible brain variations in people with schizophrenia, nineteenth-century technology was not up to the kind of research needed to identify those variations.

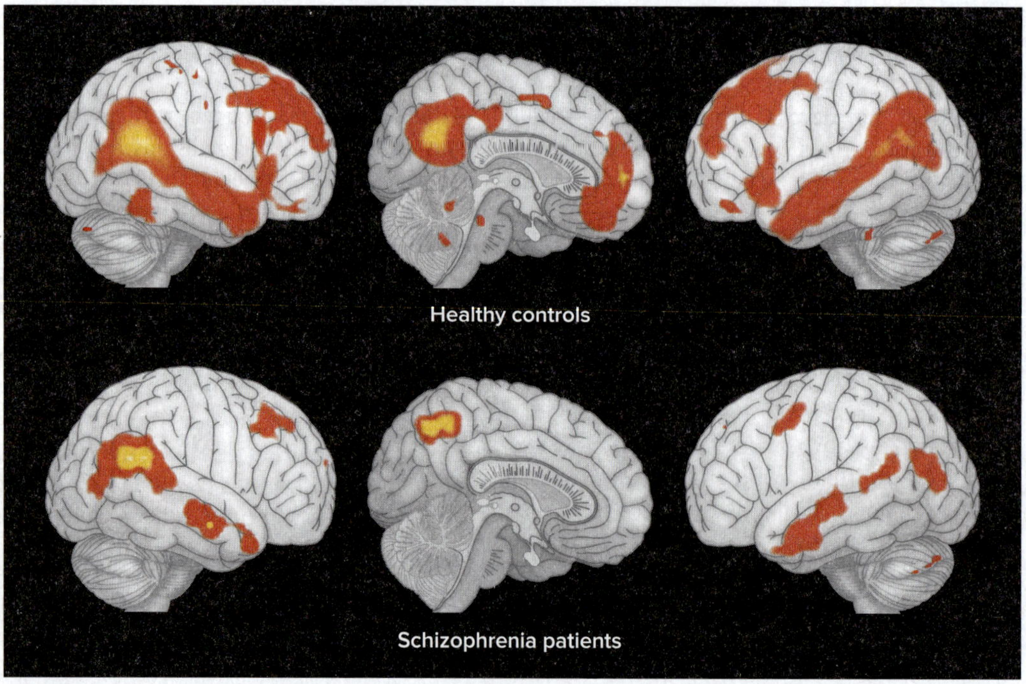

FIGURE 1 fMRI Scans Comparing Healthy Controls with Schizophrenia Patients

As is seen in comparing the top and bottom rows, the brains of patients with schizophrenia show reduced activation in the frontal and temporal lobes involved in social judgment.

SOURCE: Walter, H., et al. (2009) Dysfunction of the social brain in schizophrenia is modulated by intention type: An fMRI study. *Social Cognitive and Affective Neuroscience*, 4(2): 166–176. Oxford University.

Contemporary neuroimaging methods are making it possible for researchers to look for alterations in the brain activity of people with schizophrenia compared to healthy controls. You can see in Figure 1 the types of variations researchers can identify using such methods. In this case, researchers compared the fMRIs of individuals with schizophrenia with healthy controls while the participants completed the task of guessing the intentions of fictional characters depicted in comic strips. Such a task involves the frontal and temporal lobes of the brain. Yellow and red colorations indicate greater activation and, as you can see, there are fewer of these areas of activation in the brains of those with schizophrenia (Walter et al., 2009).

These alterations could have important implications for the functioning of people with schizophrenia. Altered activity in the frontal and temporal lobes of the brain seems related both to negative symptoms and to cognitive deficits (Abram et al., 2017). Decreased activity in the frontal lobe also has been shown to be linked to poorer social functioning (Watanabe, Urakami, Hongo, & Ohtsubo, 2015), due to the loss of inhibitory control over behavior that this area of the brain ordinarily provides in mature adults.

Changes also appear to occur in individuals with schizophrenia that affect the ability of parts of the brain to communicate with each other during cognitive tasks, including the ability to focus on stimuli requiring attention (Huang et al., 2020). People with schizophrenia also show alterations in the connections among parts of the brain that support coordinated cognitive operations (Lei et al., 2020).

Positive and negative symptom patterns are also related to structural variations in the brain. The brains of individuals with deficit symptoms are more likely to be characterized by widespread thinning of the cortex compared to healthy controls. The brain scans of individuals with positive schizophrenia symptoms show, in contrast, smaller overall surface area (Banaj et al., 2023).

As important as they may be, structural changes alone cannot entirely explain what happens to the brain to increase the individual's vulnerability to developing schizophrenia. Instead, researchers believe that additional clues to schizophrenia's causes exist in the neurotransmitters responsible for communicating information in the nervous system. An early candidate for such altered neurotransmitter functioning is dopamine. Specifically, alterations in dopamine receptors mean that they do not bind properly when dopamine is released from presynaptic neurons. Such alterations, in turn, lead to excess amounts of dopamine in the brain that contribute to schizophrenia's effects on cognition and goal-directed behavior (Vyas et al., 2017).

Gamma-aminobutyric acid (GABA), an inhibitory neurotransmitter, also appears to play a role in schizophrenia due to changes the disorder may produce in the N-methyl-D-aspartate (NMDA) receptors. Evidence supporting this possibility is based on the fact that the drug ketamine reduces the activity of NMDA receptors, and is associated with memory losses comparable to those associated with negative symptoms (Suárez Santiago, Roldán, & Picazo, 2023).

Research on patterns of family inheritance has long supported the idea that schizophrenia is, in part, a genetically caused disorder, with heritability estimates at 80 percent (Ji et al., 2021). Genome-wide association studies (GWAS) are providing information about which genes may contribute to this high heritability. Recognizing that much of this research is conducted on populations of European descent, investigators are expanding their work to include populations of African and Latino ancestry, leading to the identification of more chromosomes as involved in schizophrenia than previously reported (Bigdeli et al., 2020). The search for the specific genetic loci associated with schizophrenia remains challenging, because literally hundreds are potential candidates (Chang et al., 2020).

According to the **neurodevelopmental hypothesis** (Andreasen, 2010), schizophrenia is a disorder of development that arises during adolescence or early adulthood due to alterations in the genetic control of brain maturation. The genetic vulnerability some individuals inherit becomes evident if they are exposed to certain risks during early brain development. These risks can occur during the prenatal period in the form of viral infections, malnutrition, or exposure to toxins. Thus, schizophrenia may reflect not only atypical genetic inheritance but also deficits associated with epigenetic processes. As their illness progresses over time,

neurodevelopmental hypothesis
Theory proposing that schizophrenia is a disorder of development that arises during adolescence or early adulthood due to alterations in the genetic control of brain maturation.

REAL STORIES

Elyn Saks (1956-Present)

In her memoir, *The Center Cannot Hold: My Journey Through Madness* (Saks, 2007), UCLA professor Elyn Saks tells the moving story of her lifelong struggle with schizophrenia. Her story provides a unique perspective on one of the most debilitating psychological disorders and a first-hand account of the experience of psychosis.

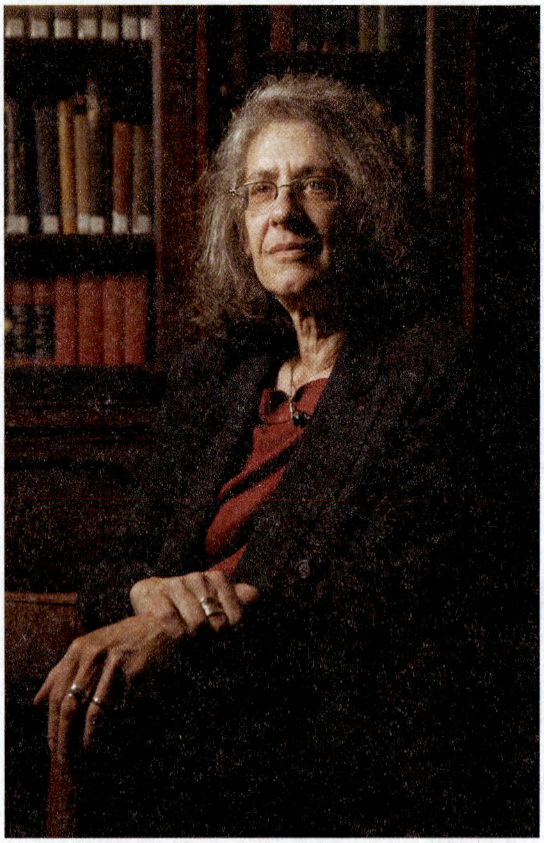

Elyn Saks has enjoyed a successful law career despite being diagnosed with schizophrenia.

Damian Dovarganes/AP Images

Saks begins the book by describing the first signs of her illness when she was a child growing up in an upper-middle-class family in Miami, Florida. These included idiosyncratic behaviors like organizing and lining up her possessions in her room, and frightening dissociative experiences when she was only 8 years old. Saks recalls feeling fearful of these experiences, partly because she was unable to express what was happening to her even though her family was otherwise supportive and caring.

Throughout her formative years, Saks continued to experience what she now recognizes as prodromal symptoms of schizophrenia. At the time her experiences caused her to feel paranoid around others, afraid they would find out her secret. She attended Vanderbilt University and at first greatly enjoyed her newfound independence. However, within the first 2 weeks of school, away from the protective clutches of her family and all the comforts that came with being taken care of, everything, as she puts it, "slowly began to unravel." Her inability to perform self-care activities such as bathing signaled the start of her illness, and Elyn had several brief psychotic episodes that resolved without intervention. In the book, she describes the insidious nature of her illness when it began to manifest itself.

After returning home from her freshman year of college, Saks continued to experience paranoia and occasional hallucinations. In addition to those symptoms, she was feeling depressed and lethargic. Her parents took her to see a psychiatrist, whose only insight into her condition was that she "needed help." Once Saks returned to Vanderbilt for her sophomore year, her symptoms subsided as she found comfort in her studies and a close-knit group of friends. With strong social support, Saks was able to remain in a relatively stable condition for the rest of her time in college. However, that comfort quickly turned to fear as graduation approached and she felt the fragile structure that kept her content was about to be shaken.

Saks won a highly prestigious Marshall scholarship to study philosophy at Oxford University in England. She was terrified of living in a new country, so far away from everything she knew, and particularly of being away from her routine and friends at college. Indeed, after just a few weeks at Oxford, Saks's still unnamed illness again began to take hold, and her fear of her illness turned into suicidal ideation. At the urging of a friend, she saw a psychiatrist and admitted that she had thoughts of ending her life. She entered a day treatment program at a psychiatric hospital, though she had no idea just how ill she was. Her perspective on her symptoms at the time was that they were simply a problem that needed to be solved and could be easily fixed, a view that grossly underestimated the complexity of her illness.

During her hospitalization, Saks received intensive psychotherapy and spent the rest of her time working on her studies. Her academic program did not require her to attend classes, so she was able to isolate herself in her apartment while she worked, which made it difficult for her to realize the extent of her psychological difficulties. She was not taking any medication at the time, and her ability to attain a firm grasp on reality slowly deteriorated. When she reported to her psychiatrist that her suicidal ideation had worsened, she was urged to become a full-time patient at the hospital, where she remained for 2 weeks. After beginning a course of psychotherapeutic medication, Saks eventually felt well enough to return to her studies, although she soon began to deteriorate psychologically. She returned to the hospital, where she languished in psychosis and depression for several months. Once she was stabilized, her psychiatrist recommended that she enter psychoanalysis. Determined to complete her degree at Oxford, Saks continued her studies while seeing a psychoanalyst 5 days a week. Even after finishing her studies, which ended up taking 4 years instead of 2, Saks felt that her relationship with her analyst was helping her so much that she decided to stay in England to continue their work together for 2 more years.

In the book, Saks describes her experience of living with her illness during this time in her life. "Completely delusional, I still understood essential aspects of how the world worked. For example, I was getting my schoolwork done, and I vaguely understood the rule that in a social setting, even with the people I most trusted, I could not ramble on about my psychotic thoughts. To talk about killing children, or burning whole worlds, or being able to destroy cities with my mind was not part of polite conversation. . . . At times, though, I was so psychotic that I could barely contain myself. The delusions expanded into full-blown hallucinations, in which I could clearly hear people whispering. I could hear my name being called when no one was physically around–in a corner of the library, or late at night, in my bedroom where I slept alone. Sometimes, the noise I heard was so overwhelming it drowned out almost all other sound."

After leaving England, Saks decided to attend law school at Yale University, where she continued to struggle with psychotic episodes that resulted in several lengthy hospitalizations, although she was eventually able to finish her degree. After working in a mental health law clinic, she had discovered a passion for helping psychiatric patients, fueled by her intimate understanding of the experience of being a psychiatric patient. Throughout her career she has worked toward creating a high legal standard of care for psychiatric patients in the United States.

Saks eventually took a position at the law school at UCLA, where she continues to work as a tenured faculty member. Over the years she has worked hard to keep her psychotic symptoms at bay with help from a combination of talk therapy, medication, and social support from her husband and close friends. Though Saks struggled for many years to accept the reality of her illness, she now accepts her diagnosis and all that it entails. At the end of the book, Saks writes that she feels grateful to be one of the lucky few able to successfully live with schizophrenia. She dispels the idea that she has had a better life because of schizophrenia but instead states that she has been able to live her life despite it.

Throughout her career, when discussing legal aspects of mental health treatment, she often noticed others stigmatizing those with mental illness, not believing they could lead normal lives or even be trusted to not be violent. When describing why she decided to write the book and "out" herself as someone with mental illness, she explains, "I want to bring hope to those who suffer from schizophrenia, and understanding to those who do not."

individuals may show continued deleterious changes through a process of neuroprogression, in which the effects of schizophrenia interact with brain changes caused by normal aging.

Somewhat related to the neurodevelopmental hypothesis is the idea that cognitive deficits of people with schizophrenia reflect deficits in **neuroplasticity**, adaptive changes in the brain that occur in response to experience. Deficits in neuroplasticity could result, for example, in changes in the ability to learn and remember and distortions in the perception of experiences. Structural changes could also occur with loss of neuroplasticity, leading to interference in neuronal circuits that communicate throughout the brain (Fišar, 2023).

neuroplasticity
Adaptive changes in the brain in response to experience.

Treatments

The primary biological treatment for schizophrenia is antipsychotic medication. As you learned in the chapter "Theoretical Perspectives," there are three categories of antipsychotic medications: the so-called typical or first-generation antipsychotics, the atypical or second-generation antipsychotics, and the third-generation, also considered atypical.

Chlorpromazine (Thorazine) and haloperidol (Haldol) are two of the typical antipsychotic medications. They are intended to reduce symptoms by acting on the dopamine receptor system in areas of the brain associated with delusions, hallucinations, and other positive symptoms.

In addition to being highly sedating, causing a person to feel fatigued and listless, the typical antipsychotics also have serious undesirable consequences. These include **extrapyramidal symptoms (EPS)**, which are motor disorders like rigid muscles, tremors, shuffling movement, restlessness, and muscle spasms affecting posture. After several years, people being treated with the typical antipsychotics can also develop **tardive dyskinesia**, another motor disorder, which consists of involuntary movements of the mouth, arms, and trunk of the body.

extrapyramidal symptoms (EPS)
Motor disorders involving rigid muscles, tremors, shuffling movement, restlessness, and muscle spasms affecting posture.

tardive dyskinesia
Motor disorder that consists of involuntary movements of the mouth, arms, and trunk of the body.

The distressing side effects and failure of typical antipsychotics to treat negative symptoms of schizophrenia led researchers several decades ago to embark on a search for alternatives that would both be more effective and have fewer motor symptoms. These medications, called atypical antipsychotics, include clozapine (Clozaril) and resperidone (Risperdal), olanzapine (Zyprexa), and quetiapine (Seroquel). Also called serotonin-dopamine antagonists, the atypical antipsychotics operate against both serotonin and dopamine neurotransmitters. The third generation of antipsychotic medications includes caraprazine (Vraylar), which acts on other dopamine receptors than those targeted by the typical antipsychotics to reduce both positive and negative symptoms, and with fewer side effects. It also appears to be useful in reducing episodes of aggressive and hostile behavior (Citrone & Valavka, 2021).

Despite initial hopes that the atypical antipsychotic medications would result in fewer side effects, one of the first, clozapine, unfortunately was found to have potentially lethal side effects. These side effects include agranulocytosis, a condition that affects the functioning of the white blood cells. Even medications in the newer group of atypical

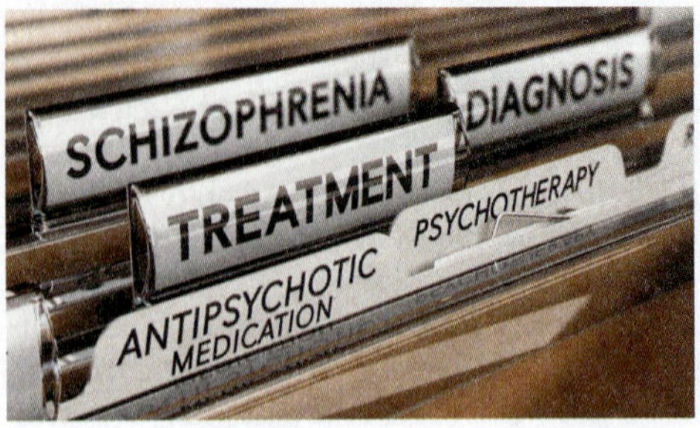

Treatment of schizophrenia involves a complex mixture of medications and psychotherapy.

Olivier Le Moal/Shutterstock

antipsychotics are not without potentially serious side effects, however. These include weight gain, increases in blood cholesterol, and greater insulin resistance, placing clients at greater risk of diabetes and cardiovascular disease (Ringen et al., 2014). For treatment-resistant clients, though, clozapine is the only approach that has empirical support, preferably if administered early in the course of the disorder (Correll et al., 2022).

Because of the many complexities in the biological treatment of individuals with schizophrenia, researchers and clinicians increasingly recognize the need to take the individual's medical and psychiatric profile into account. Toward this end, clinicians may attempt to find either a combination of antipsychotics or a combination of antipsychotics and other classes of medications.

Psychological Perspective

Theories

Although evidence continues to accumulate regarding the role of genetics and neurobiology in schizophrenia, researchers nevertheless believe that psychological theories can provide important insights.

social cognition
The ability to read the emotions and thoughts of other people.

In addition to having cognitive functioning deficits in areas such as attention and memory, people with schizophrenia show impairment in **social cognition**, meaning the ability to accurately read the emotions and thoughts of others. One component of social cognition is called "Theory of Mind," or the ability to formulate ideas about how other people are thinking and feeling. A second component of social cognition is empathy, or the ability to pay attention to the inner experiences of other people. Deficits in these areas can contribute, above and beyond the negative cognitive symptoms of schizophrenia, and contribute to the poorer social functioning of adults with the disorder (Canty, Cao, Neumann, & Shum, 2021).

These impairments in cognitive and social functioning can set up a vicious cycle that leads to a worsening of the individual's everyday life and relationships. Problems in memory, planning, and processing speed, for example, interfere with the ability to hold mentally challenging jobs. The limitations people with schizophrenia have in social cognition and communication make it particularly difficult for them to work in people-oriented jobs. Unable to maintain consistent employment, they can slip into poverty, which creates additional stress and practical challenges as well as creating inequities in their ability to access health and mental health care resources (Aldridge et al., 2018).

One implication of these changes is that clinicians consider incorporating assessments of Theory of Mind and empathy along with more traditional diagnostic measures. These can include asking the individual to describe what another person is thinking or feeling during an imaginary social interaction. Researchers believe that such instruments could be helpful in understanding how well a person with schizophrenia can adapt to daily life (Pijnenborg et al., 2009).

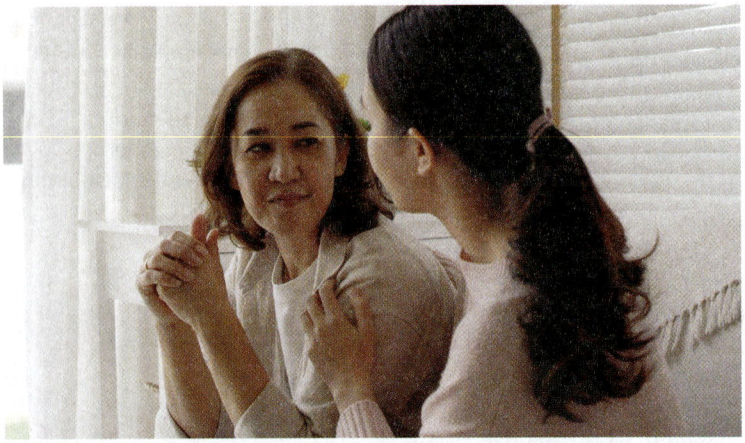

People with schizophrenia may have difficulty understanding what other people are thinking and feeling.

Chay_Tee/Shutterstock

Treatments

For many years, the most common psychological interventions for people with schizophrenia were behavioral treatments intended to lower the frequency of the kind of maladaptive behaviors that interfere with social adjustment and functioning. These interventions typically employed the token economy method of contingency management (see the chapter "Theoretical Perspectives") in which individuals receive rewards for acting in socially appropriate ways. The expectation was that, over time, the new behaviors would become habitual and the person would not depend on reinforcement in order to engage in them.

However, given that a token economy depends in large part on the individual's living or being treated in a controlled environment, this approach is no longer considered practical. In addition, there is little data on its effectiveness, and with clinicians focusing on evidence-based treatment, the profession cannot justify its use (Dickerson, Tenhula, & Green-Paden, 2005).

More promising is **cognitive behavioral therapy for psychosis (CBTp)** in which clinicians do not try to change clients' delusions or eliminate their hallucinations but instead try to reduce their distress and preoccupation with these symptoms. In addition, they attempt to teach their clients coping skills to improve their ability to live independently. They might assign their clients the homework of keeping a diary of their experiences of hearing voices or making a "reality check" of their delusional beliefs.

cognitive behavioral therapy for psychosis (CBTp)
Method of treating symptoms of psychosis in which clinicians do not try to change clients' delusions or eliminate their hallucinations but instead try to reduce their distress and preoccupation with these symptoms.

CBTp was initially developed in the United Kingdom, perhaps because service providers were more interested in finding nonmedical approaches to treating the symptoms of psychosis than is true in the United States. However, the method is gaining more widespread acceptance in the United States based on studies showing its effectiveness, particularly in conjunction with atypical antipsychotics (Li et al., 2015). CBTp can be administered in a milieu therapy format that would make access possible for a larger number of individuals in a variety of treatment settings (Riggs & Creed, 2017).

A large-scale meta-analysis of treatments based on the cognitive behavior perspective provided support for the value of this approach. Additionally, the analysis revealed the potential of the "third wave" forms of cognitive behavior therapy in schizophrenia that include acceptance and commitment therapy along with mindfulness training (Bighelli et al., 2023).

Researchers are also finding success with interventions designed to improve social cognition. In the 12-session Social Cognition Training Program, individuals learn about the concept of social cognition and complete a set of practical exercises simulating real-life situations. They learn how to recognize emotions in the faces of others, understand how to interpret language and avoid jumping to conclusions, and gain familiarity with social norms and appropriate behavior in social settings. This approach appears to have value in helping people with schizophrenia become more adept in these key aspects of social interaction (Fernández-Modamio et al., 2020).

Sociocultural Perspective

Theories

Family Perspective In some of the earliest formulations of the causes of schizophrenia, psychological theorists proposed that disturbed patterns of communication in a child's family environment could precipitate the development of the disorder. In studies of modes of communication and behavior within families with a schizophrenic member, researchers defined these deviant patterns as **expressed emotion (EE)**; they include interactions with the individual that reflect criticism, hostile feelings, and emotional overinvolvement or overconcern. Clinicians thought these disturbances in family relationships led to the development of defective emotional responsiveness and cognitive distortions fundamental to the psychological symptoms of schizophrenia.

expressed emotion (EE)
Family interactions with the individual that reflect criticism, hostile feelings, and emotional overinvolvement or overconcern.

Contemporary researchers have changed their approach to understanding how family dynamics contribute to the maintenance of an individual's symptoms. Rather than regarding a disturbed family as the cause of schizophrenia, they view it as a potential source of stress in the environment of the person trying to recover from a schizophrenic episode. Treatment based on this revised understanding focuses on reducing problematic day-to-day interactions between the client and the caregiver by applying principles of cognitive behavioral therapy to improve communication and coping strategies. As demonstrated in a large analysis of existing intervention studies using this modality, there is extensive empirical support although a lag exists in implementation of family-based cognitive behavioral therapy (Jolley and Grice, 2023).

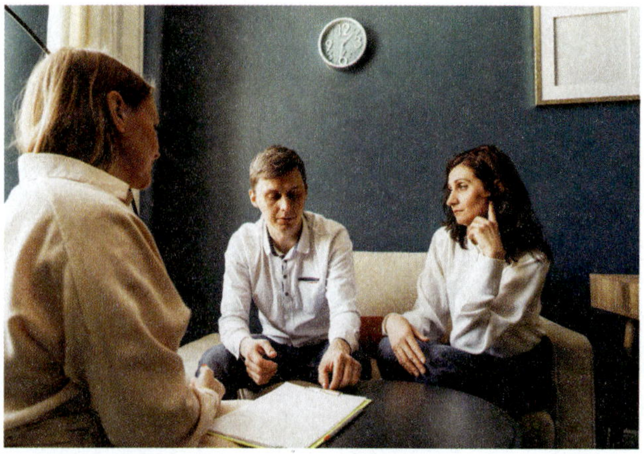

Family interventions incorporating cognitive behavior therapy are designed to involve caregivers in helping individuals with schizophrenia improve their patterns of coping and communication.
Fiordaliso/Moment/Getty Images

Social Factors Moving beyond the family environment, researchers have also studied broader social factors such as social class and income in relationship to schizophrenia. In perhaps the first epidemiological study of mental illness in the United States, Hollingshead and Redlich (1958) observed that schizophrenia was far more prevalent among people living in low income areas inhabited by people with less education who were employed in occupations with lower social status or prestige. These findings continue to be supported by more recent large-scale statistical analyses (Gallagher, 2018).

One possible cause of the social class–schizophrenia link is that people with schizophrenia experience **downward drift**, meaning that their disorder drives them into poverty, which interferes with their ability to work and earn a living. The other possibility is that the stress of living in isolation and poverty in urban areas contributes to the risk of developing schizophrenia (Hudson, 2012).

Higher rates of schizophrenia are also found in **migrants**, people who live in a different place than their usual residence. Contributing to this higher vulnerability are discrimination, exclusion, and language differences when the migration is to another country. At the same time, however, migrants who live near other migrants may provide a buffer in the form of social support (Henssler et al., 2020).

Other sociocultural risk factors for schizophrenia, or at least for symptoms of psychosis, include adversity suffered in childhood, such as parental loss or separation, abuse, and bullying. Living in quarantine or lockdown associated with the COVID-19 pandemic could be seen as a risk that exacerbated the symptoms of people with schizophrenia as well as other psychiatric disorders (Solé et al., 2021).

Recognizing that the causes of schizophrenia are multifaceted and develop over time, Stilo and Murray (2010) proposed a **developmental cascade hypothesis** that integrates genetic vulnerabilities, damage occurring in the prenatal and early childhood periods, adversity, and drug abuse as ultimately leading to changes in dopamine expressed in psychosis.

More recently, the **developmental risk factor model** regards schizophrenia on a continuum, developing in people with a liability to a spectrum of disorders involving psychotic symptoms (Murray, Bhavsar, Tripoli, & Howes, 2017). Life stresses that continue throughout adulthood become additional contributions to the likelihood of an individual experiencing psychotic symptoms through a combination of emotional responses, anticipation of threat from their stressful environment, and misinterpretations of otherwise innocuous stimuli (Klippel et al., 2017).

downward drift
A progression observed in people with schizophrenia in which their disorder drives them into poverty, which interferes with their ability to work and earn a living.

migrants
People who move away from their place of usual residence.

developmental cascade hypothesis
A proposal for the cause of schizophrenia that integrates genetic vulnerabilities, damage occurring in the prenatal and early childhood periods, adversity, and drug abuse as causes of changes in dopamine expressed in psychosis.

developmental risk factor model
Regards schizophrenia on a continuum, developing in people with a liability to a spectrum of disorders involving psychotic symptoms.

assertive community treatment (ACT)
Treatment modality in which a team of professionals from psychiatry, psychology, nursing, and social work reach out to clients in their homes and workplaces.

Treatments

The coordination of services is especially important in programs geared toward helping people with schizophrenia. One approach to integrating various services is **assertive community treatment (ACT)**, in which an interprofessional team representing psychiatry, psychology, nursing, and social work reaches out to clients in their homes and workplaces. An important component of ACT is rehabilitation, building in the opportunities for individuals to gain skills needed to maintain their quality of life (Siskind et al., 2021).

ACT's focus on engendering empowerment and self-determination is reflected in its use of the term *consumers*, to refer to their clients. Typically, a team of about a dozen professionals work together to help approximately 100 consumers with issues such as complying with medical recommendations, managing their finances, obtaining adequate health care, and dealing with crises when they arise. This approach brings care to the individuals in treatment, rather than waiting for them to come to a facility for help, a journey that may be too overwhelming for seriously impaired people.

Although research using randomized controlled trials supports the effectiveness of ACT in some countries such as the United States and Australia, in the United Kingdom and other European countries ACT was less effective in reducing hospitalizations and improving overall client functioning. Based on research carried out in mainland China, where the role of family in providing services to individuals with serious mental illness was taken into account, ACT's approach may need to be tailored both to the culture and to the mental health resources available in the community (Luo et al., 2019).

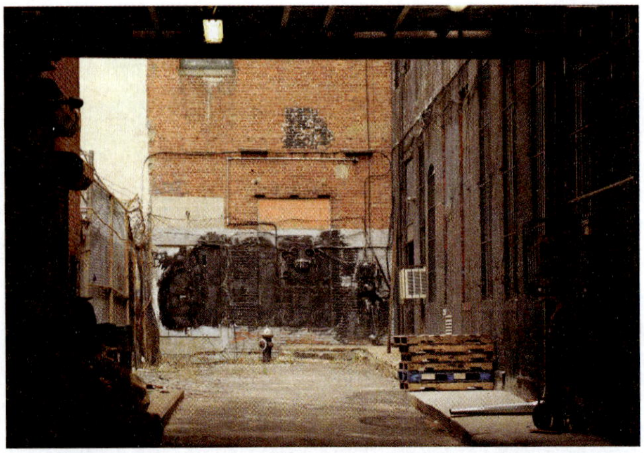

Living in an impoverished neighborhood creates adverse, stressful contexts and experiences that can contribute to psychotic symptoms in predisposed individuals.

Busà Photography/Moment/Getty Images

6.7 Schizophrenia: The Biopsychosocial Perspective

Definitions and diagnostic approaches to schizophrenia have changed over the past several decades even while researchers have gained a great deal of understanding about its many possible causes. Perhaps most exciting is the evolution of an integrated approach to theories that focus on underlying brain mechanisms as expressed in cognitive deficits and in response to social contextual influences. Treatment is moving beyond the provision of medication to greater use of evidence-based psychological interventions. Together, these advances are increasing the chances that individuals with these disorders will receive integrated care, maximizing their chances of recovery (Kerkemeyer et al., 2018).

Clinicians also increasingly understand schizophrenia from a life-span perspective. The needs and concerns of individuals with this disorder vary over the years of adulthood, and many recover. Thus, researchers and mental health practitioners are recognizing that part of their job is to provide ways to help people with long-term schizophrenia adapt to changes in both the aging process and the evolution of the disease. The idea that schizophrenia is a disorder with neurodevelopmental underpinnings highlights this important focus and provides a basis for interventions that take into account individual changes over time.

Return to the Case: David CHEN

David was eventually able to return to school part-time, living at home with Ann. Though they struggled with the change in their level of functioning, they were able to use therapy and case management to understand their limitations. The aim was to prevent future stressors from occurring and triggering psychotic episodes. It is difficult to completely avoid all symptoms of psychosis with a disorder as severe as schizophrenia. However, with the proper contingencies and social support, David will be better able to tolerate their symptoms and live a meaningful life.

Dr. Tobin's Reflections: David's move into the dorms presented them with their first major life stressor. Although they had previously been living on campus at school, living with their mother after their first hospitalization seemed to have provided a feeling of safety that was shattered once they moved back to school. It was difficult, though, because David certainly wished they could attain independence successfully. Though they were not at their same level of functioning as before, David and Ann had assumed that whatever they had been going through was finished. Returning to the dormitories, however, proved too great a stressor and so David's symptoms resurfaced once again.

Luckily for David, Ann was able to take action to help them after it became clear that they were suffering from something very serious that neither of them had quite understood. With the disorder identified early on, entering a treatment program was beneficial in decreasing the likelihood that David's life will be complicated by the fallout from future psychotic episodes. However, prevention of future episodes is contingent upon their participation in therapy and their medication compliance.

SUMMARY

- Schizophrenia is a serious mental illness, given its potentially broad impact on an individual's ability to live a productive and fulfilling life. Although a significant number of people with schizophrenia eventually manage to live symptom-free lives, many must find ways to adapt their lives to the reality of the illness.
- There are six diagnostic criteria for schizophrenia (see Table 2). In addition to the diagnostic criteria for schizophrenia and related psychotic disorders, the *DSM-5-TR* authors provide a set of severity rating criteria in several spheres of functioning. In diagnosing delusions, it is important to take cultural and language considerations into account.
- Using the *DSM-IV-TR*, clinicians could make subtype diagnoses to provide more information about the presenting symptoms. With *DSM-5*, these same subtypes (disorganized, paranoid, undifferentiated, and residual) became specifiers and are still in *DSM-5-TR*. Specifiers serve the same purpose of providing more diagnostic information, without standing alone as discrete disorders. The exception to this change is catatonia, which has become its own disorder.

- Schizophrenia may take one of several courses. The course and outcome are poorer for people with schizophrenia than for people with other psychological disorders.
- Other disorders on the schizophrenia spectrum include brief psychotic disorder, schizophreniform disorder, schizoaffective disorder, and several specific types of delusional disorders including erotomanic type, grandiose type, jealous type, persecutory type, and somatic type. Delusions that are clearly implausible, not understandable, and not derived from ordinary life experiences are specified as "with bizarre content."
- Theories accounting for the origin of schizophrenia have traditionally fallen into two categories: biological and psychological. The developmental risk hypothesis states that schizophrenia is a disorder of development that arises during the years of adolescence or early adulthood due to alterations in the genetic control of brain maturation and responds throughout life to external stressors.
- The primary biological treatment for schizophrenia is antipsychotic medication. The two main categories of these medications are the "typical" or "first- generation" and "atypical" or "second-generation" and "third-generation" antipsychotics. The distressing side effects and failure of typical antipsychotics to treat negative symptoms of schizophrenia have led psychiatric researchers on a search for alternatives that would both be more effective and not cause tardive dyskinesia, a motor disorder that consists of involuntary movements of the mouth, arms, and trunk of the body. Because of the many complexities in the biological treatment of individuals with schizophrenia, researchers and clinicians increasingly recognize the need to take the individual's medical and psychiatric profile into account.
- From a psychological perspective, with increasing evidence suggesting specific genetic and neurophysiological variations in the brains of people with schizophrenia, researchers are becoming increasingly interested in finding out more about the role of cognitive and social cognitive deficits in causing the disorder.
- For many years, the most common psychological interventions for people with schizophrenia were behavioral treatments, but this method is no longer practical, given that most individuals with schizophrenia receive treatment in the community. In addition, there is little data on its effectiveness, and the profession cannot justify its use. More promising is cognitive behavioral therapy including third-wave cognitive behavioral therapy, as well as family treatment based on cognitive behavioral principles. Clinicians using cognitive behavioral therapy to treat individuals with symptoms of psychosis (CBTp) do not try to change their delusions or eliminate their hallucinations, but instead try to reduce their distress and preoccupation with these symptoms.
- There have been many theories regarding schizophrenia from a sociocultural perspective. Contemporary researchers have approached the issue by trying to predict the outcome or recovery of adults hospitalized for schizophrenia. The index of expressed emotion (EE) provides a measure of the degree to which family members speak in ways that reflect criticisms, hostile feelings, and emotional overinvolvement or overconcern. Family treatment, however, is beginning to focus not on the entire family but on the communication processes with caregivers as well as ways to improve daily coping. Moving beyond the family environment, researchers have also studied broader social factors, such as social class and income, in relationship to schizophrenia. Other sociocultural risk factors for schizophrenia, or at least for symptoms of psychosis, include adversity in childhood such as parental loss or separation, abuse, and bullying.
- From a biopsychosocial perspective, treatment has moved beyond the provision of medication to greater use of evidence-based psychological interventions. Researchers appear to be gaining greater appreciation of the role of sociocultural influences. Together, these advances are increasing the chances that individuals with these disorders will receive integrated care, maximizing their chances of recovery. Clinicians also increasingly understand schizophrenia from a life-span perspective. The idea that schizophrenia is a neurodevelopmental disorder highlights this important new focus and provides a basis for interventions that take into account individual changes over time.

KEY TERMS

Active phase
Asociality
Assertive community treatment (ACT)
Avolition
Bleuler's "Four A's"
Brief psychotic disorder
Catatonia
Cognitive behavioral therapy for psychosis (CBTp)
Delusion
Delusional disorder
Developmental cascade hypothesis
Disorganized speech
Downward drift
Erotomanic type of delusional disorder
Expressed emotion (EE)
Developmental risk factor model
Extrapyramidal symptoms (EPS)
First-rank symptom (FRS)
Grandiose type of delusional disorder
Hallucination
Inappropriate affect
Jealous type of delusional disorder
Loosening of associations
Migrant
Negative symptoms
Neologisms
Neurodevelopmental hypothesis
Neuroplasticity
Paranoia
Persecutory type of delusional disorder
Positive symptoms
Restricted affect
Schizoaffective disorder
Schizophrenia
Schizophrenia spectrum
Schizophreniform disorder
Shared psychotic disorder
Social cognition
Somatic type of delusional disorder
Tardive dyskinesia
Vulnerability

CHAPTER 7

Depressive and Bipolar Disorders

OUTLINE

Learning Objectives

7.1 Explain the key features of major depressive disorder and persistent depressive disorder, including prevalence.

7.2 Compare and contrast bipolar I, bipolar II, and cyclothymic disorder.

7.3 Describe theories and treatments of depressive and bipolar disorders.

7.4 Discuss the relationships among age, gender, and suicide.

7.5 Analyze the biopsychosocial model of depressive and bipolar disorders.

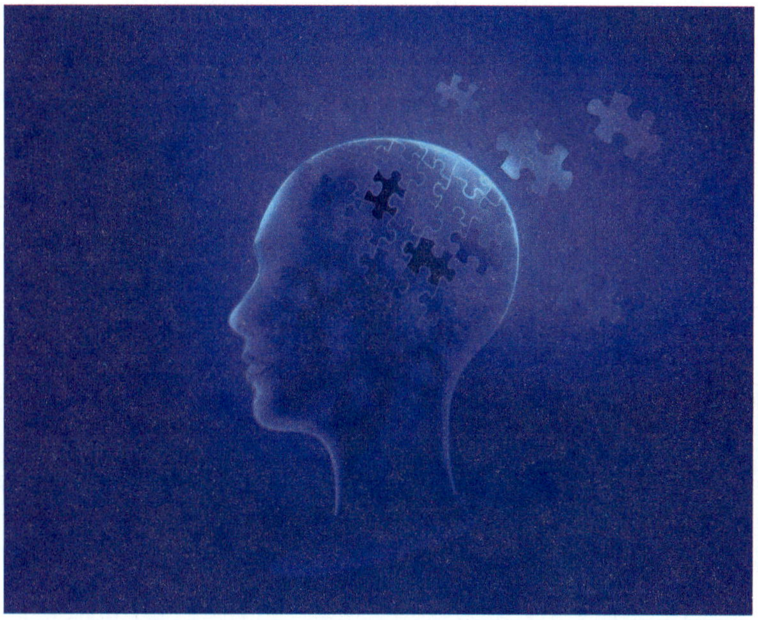

O-IAHI/Shutterstock

Case Report

Janice Butterfield

Demographic information: 47-year-old married Black heterosexual cisgender woman. Janice's pronouns are she/her/hers.

History of present illness: Janice was referred for psychotherapy after a recent hospitalization following a suicide attempt. Janice reported that the precipitant to her suicide attempt was the loss of her job in a real estate company, where she had worked for 25 years. Although her company had downsized due to the impact of the COVID-19 pandemic, she found herself feeling profoundly guilty for the negative impact her unemployment would have on her family. Janice reported she has been married for 27 years and has three daughters, one of whom lives at home. Another is in college, and her youngest will be attending college at the start of the next school year. Janice reported she had become increasingly overwhelmed by stress about her financial situation, because her family mainly relied on her income.

Along with feelings of guilt, Janice reported she had felt so depressed and down that she had spent many days in the past 2 weeks in bed and often found herself thinking of ending her life. She stopped taking the pain pills prescribed for her chronic backaches, "to save up if I needed them later." One evening when her husband was out, she attempted suicide by taking all her saved-up medications at once. Janice's husband returned to find her unresponsive and rushed her to the hospital just in time to save her life. She was hospitalized in an inpatient psychiatric unit and given medication until her suicidal thoughts and severe depression decreased enough so that the doctors deemed her no longer a threat to herself. She followed the referral given to her by the psychiatrists on the inpatient unit to attend weekly psychotherapy for follow-up. She had never been in therapy before.

During her first therapy session, Janice reported that she had thought about going to therapy many times before. She explained that her depressive episodes usually lasted about 1 month, but sometimes as long as 3 months. During these episodes, she missed a few days of work but would manage to go about her normal routine, although with much difficulty. She described how, while she was at work, she would go out to her car to cry because it was too painful to be around others. "I just didn't want anything to do with life at those points," she recalled. Her depression would eventually improve on its own, and she would lose interest in getting treatment as a result. She reported that she had occasionally thought about suicide in the past when feeling depressed, but she had never before made and carried out a plan as she had during the most recent episode. Janice cited her family as her main reason for never taking her thoughts about suicide more seriously. She also noted that her religion sees suicide as a sin.

Janice went on to explain how her depressed moods always caught her off guard, because they would occur directly after long periods when she felt happy and energetic. She stated these moods usually started after she had made a large real estate sale and felt "invincible" afterward. During these times, she described how she often needed very little sleep due to the seemingly endless amounts of energy she possessed, and she would begin to take on many new projects and clients at work—much more than would be expected of her. She also splurged on lavish clothing or jewelry, and during her last energetic period she had purchased new cars for herself and her husband. These expenditures were uncharacteristic of Janice; she described herself as usually being quite frugal.

Due to her constantly moving thoughts, Janice found it difficult to concentrate and was so distracted she was rarely able to finish anything she began to take on at work. She would feel disappointed that she had to give up some of her projects, and her joyful feelings would turn to irritability and anger. She reported that her husband usually experienced the brunt of her irritable mood, and this caused major problems in their marriage. Janice further reported that she felt like she ignored her family altogether due to her work habits when she was feeling particularly energetic. She remarked, "When I'm feeling that good, I can only think about myself and what feels good to me. I stop being a mother and a wife." Her extreme spending periods eroded her family's savings, which was especially a concern now that she had lost her job. She also felt incredibly guilty for not being able to pay for her daughters' college tuition. Janice had never talked directly with her husband or her children about her vast mood shifts. She worried that if she told her family about her personal difficulties, they would "see me as a weakling, instead of the head of the household."

Case Report *continued*

Psychiatric history: Janice had never received psychiatric treatment or therapy in the past, though she reported she had experienced mood swings since she was 19. She estimated that she had severe mood episodes (either manic or depressive) about three to four times per year. When reflecting on the severity of her mood episodes, she stated that she felt her behaviors had been more "extreme" in more recent years than when she was younger. Janice reported that she noticed the patterns in her mood swings always began with an energetic period, directly followed by a depressive episode, and then a period of several months of stability. More recently, though, she noted that the periods of stability had only been lasting 1 or 2 months, and her mood episodes had been lasting longer.

Risk level: Moderate-high, due to Janice's recent suicide attempt, stress related to loss of employment and financial difficulties, and symptoms of depression. Protective factors include social support through family, religion, and willingness to engage in mental health treatment.

Case formulation: Janice's initial diagnosis from the psychiatric unit was major depressive episode, and her current presentation also met this criteria. However, in the initial therapy session she reported also having a history of manic episodes that were followed by periods of depression, which she had not mentioned while she had been hospitalized. The symptoms of the manic episode she described caused significant financial problems for Janice, due to her excessive spending sprees. In combination with losing her job, these financial problems caused significant stress and may have contributed to the severity of her most recent depressive episode, which eventually led to a suicide attempt. Therefore, her diagnosis is bipolar I disorder, most recent episode depressed.

Treatment plan: It is recommended that Janice continue to attend weekly psychotherapy. In therapy, it will be necessary to make a suicide safety plan, given her history of suicidal ideation and recent suicide attempt. Therapy should initially focus on psychoeducation, symptom management, and mood monitoring. She will also be referred to an outpatient psychiatrist for medication reconciliation, given that psychotherapeutic medication is clinically recommended in the treatment of bipolar disorder.

Sarah Tobin, PhD

People can experience day-to-day highs and lows, but when their disturbances of mood reach a point of clinical significance, they may be considered to have a depressive or bipolar disorder. In *DSM-5-TR*, these two disorders (sometimes referred to as mood disorders) carry a set of criteria that allow clinicians to establish whether their clients show alterations in mood that significantly deviate from the individual's baseline or ordinary emotional state.

7.1 Depressive Disorders

A **depressive disorder** is characterized by periods in which, among other symptoms, an individual experiences an unusually intense sad mood, known as **dysphoria.**

depressive disorder
A disorder characterized by periods in which, among other symptoms, an individual experiences an unusually intense sad mood.

dysphoria
An unusually elevated sad mood.

Major Depressive Disorder

Major depressive disorder consists of acute but time-limited periods of depressive symptoms that are called **major depressive episodes**. You can read about these criteria from the *DSM-5-TR* in Table 1.

major depressive disorder
A disorder in which the individual experiences acute but time-limited episodes of depressive symptoms.

major depressive episode
A period in which the individual experiences intense psychological and physical symptoms accompanying feelings of overwhelming sadness (dysphoria).

Clinicians rate the severity of a depressive disorder according to the specifiers of mild, moderate, or severe. These make it possible to indicate not only how many symptoms are present above and beyond the minimum for diagnosis, but also degree of functional disability.

Considered one of the priority conditions covered by the World Health Organization (WHO), followed by low back pain and headache disorders, major depressive disorder is the third-leading cause of disability worldwide, with an estimated prevalence of 14.3 percent (James et al., 2018). Adding to the burden of disease, individuals with this disorder have an increased risk for suicide.

TABLE 1 Criteria for a Major Depressive Episode

For most of the time during a 2-week period, a person experiences at least five or more of the first nine symptoms in addition to the last two. They must experience a change from previous functioning, and at least one of the first two symptoms must be present. During this 2-week period, most of these symptoms must be present nearly every day.

1. Depressed mood most of the day
2. Markedly diminished interest or pleasure in all or most daily activities
3. Significant unintended weight loss or unusual increase or decrease in appetite
4. Insomnia or hypersomnia
5. Psychomotor agitation or retardation observable by others
6. Fatigue or loss of energy
7. Feelings of worthlessness or excessive or inappropriate guilt
8. Difficulty maintaining concentration or making decisions
9. Recurrent thoughts of death or having suicidal thoughts, plans, or attempts

In addition:

The symptoms are not attributable to a medical condition or use of a substance

The symptoms cause significant distress or impairment

In the United States, the lifetime prevalence of major depressive disorder is estimated to be 20.6 percent of the adult population with most rated as moderate or severe. Lifetime prevalence among women is 26.1 percent, and among men is 14.7 percent, Native Americans have the highest lifetime prevalence (28.2 percent), compared with Americans who are White (23.1 percent), Black (15.2 percent), Hispanic (16.2 percent), or Asian/Pacific Islander (12.2 percent) (Hasin et al., 2018).

Black-White paradox
The fact that the prevalence for depression is lower in Black adults than White adults despite the exposure of Black adults to more life stressors.

A number of factors can contribute to these demographic variations. In what is known as the **Black-White paradox** (Barnes & Bates, 2017), despite their exposure to greater stress and discrimination, Blacks are less likely to be diagnosed with major depressive disorder. Prevalence rates are lower in adults 65 and older (14.4 percent) potentially reflecting the fact that depressive symptoms may be reported as physical rather than psychological concerns in older adults (Schaakxs et al., 2017).

As shown in Figure 1 the 1-year prevalence of a major depressive episode is estimated to be 8.3 percent of all adults in the United States (National Institute of Mental Health, 2023), with

FIGURE 1 Past Year Prevalence of Major Depressive Episode Among U.S. Adults (2021)

Data Courtesy of SAMHSA

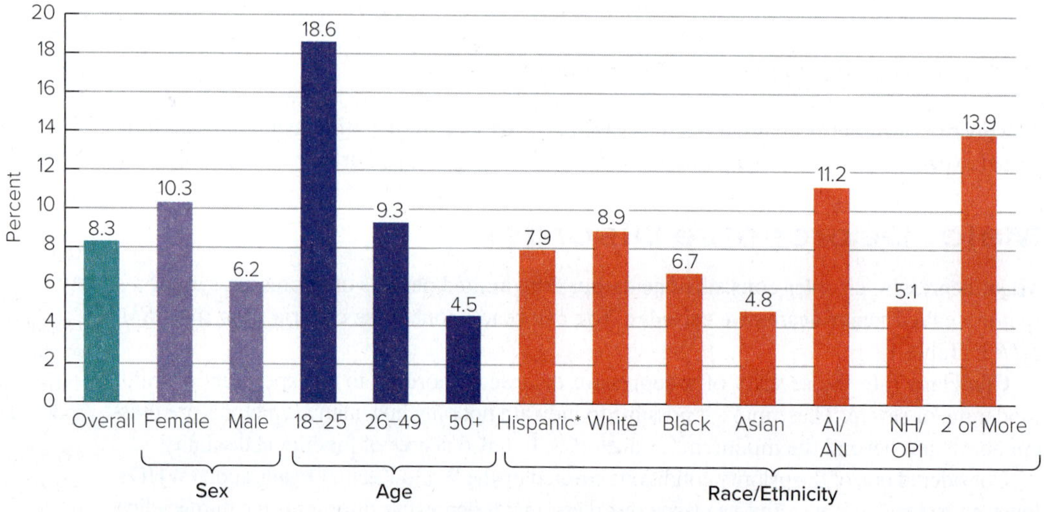

*Persons of Hispanic origin may be of any race; all other racial/ethnic groups are Non-Hispanic I AI/AN = American Indian / Alaskan Native I NH/OPI = Native Hawaiian / Other Pacific Islander.

MINI CASE

Major Depressive Disorder, Recurrent Episode

Daryll is a 37-year-old African American married gay cisgender man. His husband recently took him to a psychiatric facility for evaluation. Although Daryll has been functioning normally for the past several years, he suddenly became severely disturbed and depressed. At the time of admission, Daryll was agitated, dysphoric, and suicidal, even going as far as to purchase a gun to kill himself. He had lost his appetite and had developed insomnia during the preceding 3 weeks. As each day went by, he found himself feeling more and more exhausted, less able to think clearly or to concentrate, and uninterested in anyone or anything. He had become hypersensitive in his dealings with neighbors, co-workers, and family, insisting that others were being too critical of him. This was the second such episode in Daryll's history, the first having occurred 5 years earlier, following the loss of his job due to a massive layoff.

patterns comparable to those reported for lifetime prevalence, as is evident from this figure. The current prevalence estimates represent an increase from the 7.1 percent reported in 2021, potentially reflecting the impact of COVID-19. Yet, treatment rates have not increased commensurately, contributing to what experts believe is an ongoing mental health crisis (Goodwin et al., 2022).

Persistent Depressive Disorder

The mood disturbance occurring with major depressive disorder may take a chronic, enduring form. People with **persistent depressive disorder** have, for at least 2 years (1 year for children and adolescents), a more limited set of the symptoms that occur with major depressive disorder, including sleep and appetite disturbances, low energy or fatigue, low self-esteem, difficulty with concentration and decision making, and feelings of hopelessness. Individuals diagnosed with persistent depressive disorder alone currently do not meet the criteria for a major depressive episode, which requires that the client meet five of the criteria outlined in Table 1.

persistent depressive disorder
Chronic but less severe mood disturbance in which the individual does not experience a major depressive episode.

Prevalence data reported from the United States National Comorbidity Study Replication estimated a lifetime rate of 2.5 percent of the adult population (Kessler, Berglund, et al., 2005). The 1-year prevalence for persistent depressive disorder based on this study was estimated at 1.5 percent of the U.S. population, with almost half these cases (0.8 percent of the adult population) classified as severe (Kessler, Chiu, et al., 2005). More recently, a population study conducted in Finland reported the same lifetime prevalence of 2.5 percent, with a range for men of 1.3 to 2.5 percent and for women 2.2 to 3.8 percent (Vandeleur et al., 2017).

As in major depressive disorder, in persistent depressive disorder the symptoms take on a different form among older adults, who are more likely to report disturbances in physical than in psychological functioning (Oxman, Barrett, Sengupta, & Williams, 2000). Persistent depressive disorder is also associated with elevated risk of suicide as well as increased numbers of suicide attempts. Additionally, individuals with a lifetime history of persistent depressive disorder are at greater risk, compared to those with major depressive disorder, of higher numbers of sick days, days with activity limitations, poorer self-rated quality of life, and more symptoms reflecting physical conditions (Nübel et al., 2022).

Disruptive Mood Dysregulation Disorder

The diagnosis of **disruptive mood dysregulation disorder (DMDD)** is used for children who exhibit chronic and severe irritability and have frequent temper outbursts that occur, on average, three or more times per week over at least 1 year and in at least two settings. For a child to receive this diagnosis, these outbursts must be developmentally inappropriate,

disruptive mood dysregulation disorder (DMDD)
A depressive disorder in children who exhibit chronic and severe irritability and have frequent temper outbursts.

MINI CASE

Persistent Depressive Disorder

Kimiko is a single 34-year-old Japanese American heterosexual cisgender woman. She currently works as a community college instructor, and for the past 3 years has had persistent feelings of depressed mood, inferiority, and pessimism. She realizes that, since her graduation from college, she has never felt really happy and that, in recent years, she has struggled with thoughts of worthlessness and sad mood. Her appetite is low, and she struggles with insomnia. During waking hours, she lacks energy and finds it difficult to do her work. She often finds herself staring out the window of her office, consumed by thoughts of how inadequate she is. She fails to fulfill many of her responsibilities and has received consistently poor teacher evaluations for the past 3 years. Getting along with her colleagues has become increasingly difficult. Consequently, she spends most of her free time alone in her office.

meaning that, for example, in an older child or young teen they take the form of the behavior of a much younger child.

Between outbursts, children with this disorder remain angry or at least extremely irritable. The criteria specify that the diagnosis should not be made for the first time for children whose first episode occurs when they are younger than 6 or older than 18. However, either by directly observing the child or from the child's history, the clinician must determine that the disorder had its onset before the age of 10. In other words, a teen of 13 must be reported by parents or teachers, for example, to have been subject to angry episodes prior to turning 10 years old.

A potential criticism of this disorder is that it might be characterized as pathologizing a child's "temper tantrums," but the *DSM-5-TR* authors believed it was important to have a disorder earmarked for children and teens who in the past would have been diagnosed with bipolar disorder. Comparisons of children diagnosed with DMDD and those diagnosed with major depressive or bipolar disorder suggest that, although they share some characteristics, children with DMDD are more likely to experience problems at school, at home, and with their peers (Benarous et al., 2020). In addition to their higher levels of irritability, children with DMDD may also have reduced cognitive flexibility, reflecting potential executive control dysfunction unique to their disorder (Brænden et al., 2023).

Premenstrual Dysphoric Disorder

premenstrual dysphoric disorder (PMDD)
Changes in mood, irritability, dysphoria, and anxiety that occur during the premenstrual phase of the monthly menstrual cycle and subside after the menstrual period begins for most of the cycles of the preceding year.

People who experience depressed mood or changes in mood, irritability, dysphoria, and anxiety during the premenstrual phase that subside after the menstrual period begins for most of the cycles of the preceding year may be diagnosed with **premenstrual dysphoric disorder (PMDD)**. This disorder can carry with it the risk for increased suicidality (Yan, Ding, & Guo, 2021).

Biological factors may play a role in PMDD, with genetics influencing an individual's vulnerability to fluctuations in sex hormones affecting the brain's neurochemistry (Hantsoo & Payne, 2023). Additionally, a history of childhood maltreatment may contribute to the adult woman's development of PMDD along with personality and current life stresses (Morishita et al., 2022).

Critics argue that the PMDD diagnosis pathologizes the normal variations in mood that can occur over the course of a person's monthly menstrual cycle. However, the counterargument is that the majority of people who menstruate do not experience monthly mood alterations so severe that they would show such extreme symptoms and that biological factors appear to play a contributing role. Including PMDD as a diagnostic entity by the *DSM-5-TR* authors reflects, then, a decision in which the benefits appear to outweigh the harm (Stein, Palk, & Kendler, 2021).

7.2 Disorders Involving Alterations in Mood

Two sets of disorders are characterized by alterations in mood that go beyond everyday variations in a person's feelings of sadness or happiness. **Bipolar disorder** is diagnosed if an individual experiences an intense and disruptive period, for at least 1 week, known as a **manic episode** (see Table 2). During a manic episode, the individual may experience unusually high levels of **euphoria**, which is a feeling state that is more cheerful and elated than average, possibly even ecstatic. In a **hypomanic episode**, the individual experiences the symptoms of a manic episode for up to 4 days rather than at least 1 week.

bipolar disorder
A mood disorder involving manic episodes–intense and disruptive experiences of heightened mood, possibly alternating with major depressive episodes.

manic episode
Acute but time-limited period of intense and unusual elation.

euphoria
A feeling state that is more cheerful and elated than average, possibly even ecstatic.

hypomanic episode
A period of elated mood lasting for up to 4 days.

Bipolar Disorder

The key requirement for a diagnosis of bipolar disorder is that the individual has experienced or is having a manic episode. In contrast to what is implied by the commonly used term *manic depression*, the diagnosis does not require that the individual has ever experienced a major depressive episode.

A diagnosis of **bipolar I disorder** describes a clinical course in which the individual experiences one or more manic episodes with the possibility, although not the necessity, of experiencing one or more major depressive episodes. A diagnosis of **bipolar II disorder** means the individual has had one or more major depressive episodes and at least one hypomanic episode with symptoms not severe enough to interfere with functioning or require hospitalization. Clinicians diagnosing these disorders do so because the symptoms are not better explained by schizoaffective disorder and not superimposed on a schizophrenia spectrum or other psychotic disorder.

In rating the severity of bipolar disorders, the same ratings are used for a major depressive episode, but manic episodes are rated according to a different severity scale. As the *DSM-5-TR* authors point out, it is impossible for a manic episode to be "mild." Instead, the severity of a manic episode depends on the number of symptoms, the extent of increase in

bipolar I disorder
A clinical course in which the individual experiences one or more manic episodes with the possibility, although not the necessity, of experiencing one or more major depressive episodes.

bipolar II disorder
A clinical course in which the individual has had one or more major depressive episodes and at least one hypomanic episode.

TABLE 2 Criteria for a Manic Episode

A distinct period of atypically and persistently elevated, expansive, or irritable mood and atypically and persistently increased activity or energy must last at least 1 week and the symptoms must be present most of the day, nearly every day (or for any duration if hospitalization is necessary).

During the period of mood disturbance and increased energy or activity, three (or more) of the following symptoms are present to a significant degree (four if the mood is only irritable) and represent a noticeable change from usual behavior:

- Inflated self-esteem or grandiosity
- Decreased need for sleep (the client feels rested after, say, only 3 hours of sleep)
- More talkative mood than usual or pressure to keep talking
- Flight of ideas or subjective experience that thoughts are racing
- Distractibility (attention is too easily drawn to unimportant or irrelevant external stimuli), as reported or observed
- Increase in goal-directed activity (either socially, at work or school, or sexually) or psychomotor agitation
- Excessive engagement in activities that have high potential for painful consequences (such as unrestrained buying sprees, sexual indiscretions, or foolish business investments)

This episode must represent a clearly observable change in functioning or be severe enough to require hospitalization to prevent harm to self or others.

REAL STORIES

Carrie Fisher (1956–2016)

Carrie Fisher was an American actress, screenwriter, novelist, and lecturer who appeared in over 40 films—most notably as Princess Leia Organa in the *Star Wars* movies. She wrote four books, one of which, *Wishful Drinking* (Fisher & Ravetch, 2008) was turned into a one-woman play performed in venues across the country. In the book, she chronicles her life—from growing up in a Hollywood family, her rise to fame, her struggles with drugs and alcohol, and her battles with bipolar disorder. Fisher talks about her experiences with humor and honesty, revealing the reality of her mental illness.

Born in 1956 in Beverly Hills, California, Fisher was the daughter of actress Debbie Reynolds and singer Eddie Fisher. As the product of a Hollywood marriage, she seemed to have been destined to be a Hollywood star from the very beginning. When she was 2 years old, Fisher's father left her mother for Elizabeth Taylor, her mother's best friend. The media highly publicized this story, although in her book, Fisher states that she doesn't believe her childhood experiences had a major impact on any of the problems she encountered later in life.

Fisher first began acting at the age of 12, appearing in Las Vegas with her mother. She later dropped out of high school in order to perform with her mother on tour. In 1973, Fisher appeared with her mother in the Broadway musical *Irene*, and 2 years later, after attending drama school in London, she made her film debut in the 1975 film *Shampoo* with Warren Beatty. Two years after that, at 21, she instantly became an icon and an international celebrity for her role as Princess Leia in the *Star Wars* film series. According to Fisher, it was at this point that she began to heavily abuse cocaine and alcohol, having already experimented with marijuana at the age of 13. Looking back on her drug abuse, Fisher recalls that she used drugs as a way to self-medicate her extreme mood episodes. She first received a diagnosis of manic depression (as it was called at the time) when she was 24 years old. Although she did not pursue any treatment at that point, she began to understand what was driving much of her heavy substance use. In the book, she describes how she did not accept her diagnosis and even felt personally insulted by it. Rather than taking medication as recommended by her psychiatrist, she dropped out of treatment and impulsively moved from Los Angeles to New York, marrying singer Paul Simon shortly after.

Fisher and Simon were married from 1983 to 1984, though they dated on and off for a total of 12 years. In 1992, Fisher had a daughter, Billie, with her partner Bryan Lourd.

Despite her chronic battles with substance abuse and bipolar disorder, Fisher continued to appear in films and television shows throughout the 1980s. Her substance abuse led to a hospitalization in the mid-1980s, inspiring her first novel, *Postcards from the Edge*, a semi-autobiographical account of an actress suffering from substance abuse, published in 1987. The book became a successful movie for which she received critical acclaim.

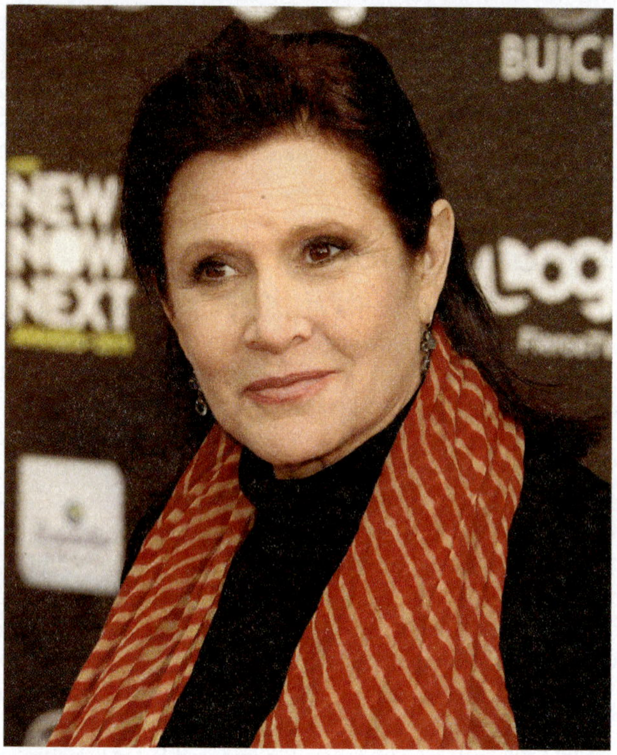

After struggling for many years with substance abuse and bipolar disorder, Carrie Fisher became an activist for the destigmatization of psychological disorders.

Jason LaVeris/FilmMagic/Getty Images

Throughout the 1990s, Fisher continued to appear in films and became well known in Hollywood for her screenwriting talents. In 1997, she suffered a psychotic break after she sought medication to treat her chronic depression. She describes that experience in *Wishful Drinking:* "Now, anyone who has stayed awake for six days knows that there's every chance that they'll wind up psychotic. Anyway, I did, and part of how that manifested was that I thought everything on television was about me. . . . I watched CNN, and at the time Versace had just been killed by that man Cunanin, and the police were frantically scouring the Eastern seaboard for him. So, I was Cunanin, Versace, and the police. Now this is exhausting programming." She was hospitalized for 6 days and then spent 6 months receiving outpatient treatment.

After having accepted her diagnosis of bipolar disorder and finally come to terms with her need for treatment, Fisher set out to educate the public about the stigmatization of mental illness. In the years leading up to her death, she was an active voice in speaking out about the need for government funding for mental health treatment and for greater public acceptance of mental illness.

In *Wishful Drinking*, Fisher describes her experiences switching between mania and depression. "I have two moods. . . . One is Roy, rollicking Roy, the wild ride of a mood. And Pam, sediment Pam, who stands on the shore and sobs . . . sometimes the tide is in, sometimes it's out." Fisher also writes of some of the various treatments for her illness that she has received, including electroconvulsive therapy (ECT).

She recalls her mix of emotions and reactions to receiving ECT, including fear, humiliation, and concern about dangerous side effects, particularly given the way the treatment had been portrayed in popular culture. However, she eventually decided that her symptoms were becoming far too severe and needed more intensive treatment.

"I'd been feeling overwhelmed and pretty defeated. I didn't necessarily feel like *dying*–but I'd been feeling a lot like not being alive. The second reason I decided to get ECT is that I was depressed. Profoundly depressed. Part of this could be attributed to my mood disorder, which was, no doubt, probably the source of the emotional intensity. That's what can take simple sadness and turn it into sadness squared." Fortunately for Fisher, ECT proved to be an effective treatment for combating her intense depressive episodes.

"At times," she writes at the end of *Wishful Drinking*, "being bipolar can be an all-consuming challenge, requiring a lot of stamina and even more courage, so if you're living with this illness and functioning at all, it's something to be proud of, not ashamed of."

Fisher passed away on December 27, 2016, at the age of 60. The cause of her death was confirmed to be cardiac arrest, though there were also traces of several drugs in her system. In *Wishful Drinking*, she writes what she hoped to be in her obituary one day: "I want it reported that I drowned in moonlight, strangled by my own bra."

activity or impairment in judgment, and degree of supervision required to prevent physical harm to the self or others.

In the United States, bipolar disorder has a lifetime prevalence rate of 1 percent and a 12-month prevalence of 0.6 percent. Globally, including the United States, these rates are 0.6 and 0.4 percent, respectively (Merikangas et al., 2011).

People with bipolar disorder are at risk of more severe chronic health problems than others their own age. They have higher rates of heart disease and diabetes (Silarova et al., 2015) and higher levels of cholesterol (Kessing, Vradi, McIntyre, & Andersen, 2015). These may be the reasons that, according to a comprehensive population study conducted in Denmark, bipolar disorder is associated with lower life expectancy across a variety of causes (Kessing et al., 2015). In addition to higher mortality due to illness, people with bipolar disorder also have elevated rates of suicide and other forms of violent death (Hayes et al., 2015) that can amount to as high as 20- to 30-times greater than in the general population, as noted in the *DSM-5-TR*.

In looking at lifetime outcomes of bipolar disorder, it is important to consider, additionally, the role of adherence to treatment, particularly among different cohorts. Individuals who are younger, those who received a recent diagnosis, and those with multiple psychiatric hospitalizations were found in one large Finnish study to be less likely to adhere to their prescribed medications. Psychoeducation along with monitoring people with bipolar disorder early in the course of treatment could potentially mitigate against the negative health outcomes associated with this disorder (Lintunen et al., 2023).

MINI CASE

Bipolar I Disorder, Current Episode Manic

Isabel is a single 38-year-old bisexual Hispanic American woman. She works as a software engineer at a large tech company, where she has worked for about 10 years. For the past week, she has shown signs of uncharacteristically outlandish behavior, beginning with thoughts of quitting her job so that she could develop her own software company out of her apartment. Isabel went without sleep for 3 days, spending most of her time at her computer developing a business model for the company. Within a few days, she took out nearly $1 million in loans, although she had few resources to finance even one of them. She visited several banks and other investors, each time making a scene with anyone who expressed skepticism about her plan. While at a bank, she became so upset when she was denied a loan that she angrily pushed over the banker's desk, and screamed at the top of her lungs that the bank was keeping her from her multimillion-dollar profit. The police were called, and Isabel was brought to an emergency room, from which she was transferred for intensive evaluation and treatment at a nearby psychiatric hospital.

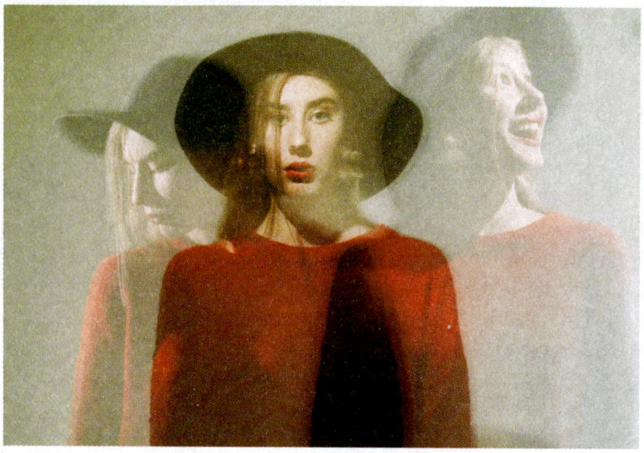

Individuals with bipolar disorder experience a range of moods, from euphoric through balanced and depressed.

Olena Holubova/Alamy Stock Photo

Clinicians diagnose people as having **bipolar disorder, rapid cycling** who have had four or more episodes within the previous year that meet the criteria for manic, hypomanic, or major depressive disorder. In some individuals, the cycling may occur within 1 week or even 1 day. Individuals who experience bipolar disorder, rapid cycling are at higher risk of suicide than others with bipolar disorder, and also of a longer duration of the disorder (Gigante et al., 2016).

Cyclothymic Disorder

Cyclothymic disorder is diagnosed when an individual experiences fluctuations between depressive and hypomanic symptoms but has never met the criteria for a hypomanic episode nor the criteria for a major depressive episode. There is an element of time involved in the diagnosis, in that clinicians must establish that the individual has experienced symptoms for at least 2 years (1 year in children), with symptoms present at least half the time, each period lasting at least 2 months.

MINI CASE

Cyclothymic Disorder

Larry is a divorced 60-year-old White heterosexual man who works as a bank cashier. For much of his adult life, co-workers, family, and friends have repeatedly told him he is very moody. He acknowledges that his mood never feels quite stable, although at times others tell him he seems more calm and pleasant than usual. Unfortunately, these intervals are quite brief, lasting for a few weeks and usually ending abruptly. Without warning, he may experience either a somewhat depressed mood or a period of elation.

During his depressive periods, Larry's confidence, energy, and motivation are very low. During his hypomanic periods, he willingly volunteers to extend his workday and to undertake unrealistic challenges at work. On weekends, he might decide to put in long shifts at a homeless shelter without getting any sleep. Larry disregards the urging of his family members to get professional help, insisting that it is his nature to be high-energy at times. He also states that he doesn't want some "shrink" to steal away the periods during which he feels on top of the world.

bipolar disorder, rapid cycling
A form of bipolar disorder involving four or more episodes within the previous year that meet the criteria for manic, hypomanic, or major depressive disorder.

cyclothymic disorder
A mood disorder with symptoms that are more chronic and less severe than those of bipolar disorder.

7.3 Theories and Treatment of Depressive and Bipolar Disorders

Biological Perspective

From the biological perspective, people diagnosed with mood disorders are understood as having symptoms caused by a combination of genetics and biochemical variations.

Biological Theories

Supporting the role of genetics in understanding the contributions to depressive disorders are moderately high heritability estimates, ranging from 33 to 54 percent. Genetic inheritance seems to have a greater effect on the development of depression in younger than in older adults (Wium-Andersen et al., 2020).

Bipolar disorder has an even stronger pattern of genetic inheritance, with an estimated heritability, based on familial inheritance studies, ranging from 60 percent to as high as 85 percent (Berrettini & Lohoff, 2017). SNP-based heritability estimates for bipolar disorder are, however, considerably lower, amounting to 25 to 45 percent, and involving as many as 30 separate genetic locations (Stahl et al., 2019). These discrepancies in heritability estimates may reflect imprecise measurement and overestimates based on the data from twins reared together (Gordovez & McMahon, 2020).

Moving from genetics to the biochemical variations, increasing evidence points to the role of altered serotonin and norepinephrine levels in causing the mood changes associated with major depressive disorder. However, not everyone with genetic predisposition shows these mood-changing alterations in neurotransmitter levels. If exposed as adults to life stressors and other environmental factors, the genetically predisposed can experience a series of changes in the neural pathways active in regulating mood. Contributing further to their chances of developing depression are variations in brain-derived neurotrophic factor (BDNF), a protein that helps keep neurons alive and able to adapt and change in response to experience (Naoi, Maruyama, & Shamoto-Nagai, 2018).

These alterations in neurotransmitters can further influence the mood of individuals with major depressive disorder by causing activation within the brain's internally based attentional circuits, the default mode network. Rather than focus their attention outward, individuals with major depressive disorder become overly preoccupied with their thoughts and feelings (Kaiser, Andrews-Hanna, Wager, & Pizzagalli, 2015). As a result, the depressed person turns those thoughts and feelings in a negative direction (Guo et al., 2015).

Brain scan and neuropsychological testing of individuals with bipolar disorder suggest that they too have difficulties in the default mode network as well as altered executive function consistent with variations in the prefrontal lobe (Abé et al., 2015). These changes may have their origins in altered genetics which, in turn, place individuals at risk when they are exposed to life stressors, particularly early in life (Pfaffenseller, Kapczinski, Gallitano, & Klamt, 2018).

Potentially reflecting a combination of genetic or other biochemical variations is an increased risk of major depression in adults who have experienced an ischemic stroke, in which blood supply is suddenly cut off from a section of the brain. The loss of function associated with a stroke and its associated disability may be a factor on its own, but there appear to be biochemical causes as well related to changes in brain neurotransmitters (Ji et al., 2023).

Antidepressant Medications

Antidepressant medication is the most common form of biologically based treatment for people with major depressive disorder. Clinicians prescribe antidepressants from four major categories: **selective serotonin reuptake inhibitors (SSRIs)**, **serotonin and norepinephrine reuptake inhibitors (SNRIs)**, tricyclic antidepressants (TCAs), and monoamine oxidase inhibitors (MAOIs).

selective serotonin reuptake inhibitor (SSRI)
Category of medications that target serotonin pathways in the brain.

serotonin and norepinephrine reuptake inhibitor (SNRI)
Category of medications that target serotonin and norepinephrine pathways in the brain.

The choice of antidepressant depends on the client's presenting symptoms, as well as the clinician's preference for a particular class of medications. Ultimately, the medications the individual receives may be selected by trial and error as the clinician attempts to identify which work best for their specific symptoms and produce the fewest, or least intrusive side effects.

SSRIs block the uptake of serotonin, making more of this crucial neurotransmitter available to act at the receptor sites of receiving neurons. SSRIs include fluoxetine (Prozac), citalopram (Celexa), escitalopram (Lexapro), paroxetine (Paxil), and sertraline (Zoloft). Balancing their positive effects on mood are their side effects. The most commonly reported are nausea, agitation, and sexual dysfunction. A newer class of antidepressants, approved for use in the United States in 2013, are serotonin modulators (such as vortioxetine).These antidepressants target the postsynaptic serotonin receptors rather than the reuptake of serotonin in the synapse.

SNRIs increase both norepinephrine and serotonin levels by blocking their reuptake. They include duloxetine (Cymbalta), venlafaxine (Effexor), and desvenlafaxine (Pristiq). These medications also carry with them a number of undesirable side effects including suicidal thoughts or attempts as well as allergic symptoms, gastrointestinal disturbances, weakness, nausea, vomiting, confusion, memory loss, irritability, and panic attacks, among others. Compared to SSRIs, the SNRIs show statistically significant effects in experimental studies, but clinically they seem to hold no advantages.

TCAs, which derive their name from the fact that they have a three-ring chemical structure, include amitriptyline (Elavil, Endep), desipramine (Norpramin), imipramine (Tofranil), and nortriptyline (Aventyl, Pamelor). These medications are particularly

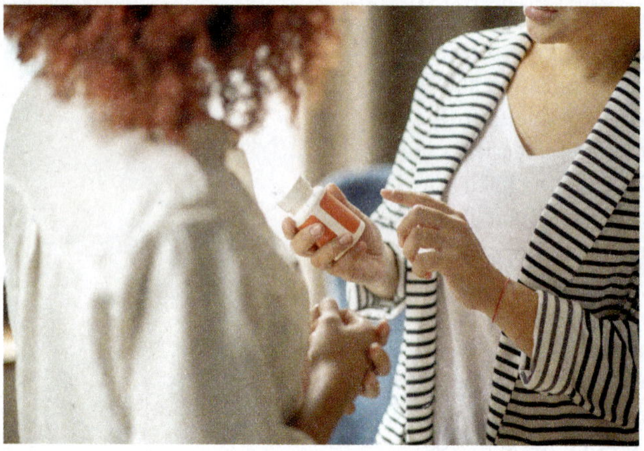

Before prescribing an antidepressant medication, a clinician must balance efficacy against side effects.
Dmytro Zinkevych/Shutterstock

effective in alleviating depression in people with disturbed appetite and sleep. Although the exact process by which TCAs work remains unclear, researchers believe that they block the premature reuptake of biogenic amines back into the presynaptic neurons, thus increasing their excitatory effects on the postsynaptic neurons.

The antidepressant effects of MAOIs, such as phenelzine (Nardil) and tranylcypromine (Parnate), prolong the life of serotonin and norepinephrine in the synapse, thereby increasing their actions in the central nervous system. MAOIs are particularly effective in treating chronic depression in people who have not responded to other medications. However, they have serious side effects that can be life-threatening when people taking them are also on allergy medications or ingest foods or beverages such as beer, cheese, and chocolate, all of which are high in a substance called tyramine. As a result, clinicians do not prescribe MAOIs as commonly as other types of antidepressant medications.

Antidepressant medications take time to work, requiring 2 to 6 weeks to take effect. Once the symptoms have subsided, the clinician will urge the client to remain on the medication for 4 or 5 additional months, and much longer for people with a history of recurrent, severe depressive episodes. It is best for the clinician and client to work together to develop therapeutic programs that include regular visits early in treatment, expanded educational efforts that focus on the medications, and continued monitoring of treatment compliance.

lithium carbonate
Naturally occurring salt used to treat bipolar disorder.

Bipolar Disorder Medications

The traditional treatment for bipolar disorder is **lithium carbonate**, referred to as lithium, a naturally occurring metallic salt found in small amounts in drinking water that, when used medically, replaces sodium in the body. Clinicians advise people who have frequent manic episodes (two or more a year) to remain on lithium continuously as a preventive measure. The drawback is that, even though lithium is a natural substance in the body, it can have undesirable side effects. These include mild central nervous system disturbances, gastrointestinal upsets, and more serious cardiac effects. As a consequence, people who experience manic episodes may be reluctant or even unwilling to take lithium continuously, which can lead them to experience relapse (Samalin & Belzeaux, 2023).

From the client's perspective, lithium can be seen to interfere with the euphoria that can accompany the beginnings of a manic episode. Consequently, people with this disorder who enjoy those pleasurable feelings may resist taking the medication. Unfortunately, by the time their euphoria escalates into a full-blown episode, it is often too late because their judgment has been clouded by their manic symptoms of grandiosity and elation. To help overcome this dilemma,

What's in the *DSM-5-TR*

Depressive and Bipolar Disorders

Modifications to the category of mood disorders in the *DSM-5* (versus the *DSM-IV-TR*) were intended to provide greater precision in the diagnosis by refining the criteria for major depressive episode, manic episode, and hypomanic episode. One of the major problems in the *DSM-IV-TR* was a failure to differentiate these episodes from a person's typical level of activity, sadness, or disturbance. In particular, the failure to distinguish bipolar disorder from attention-deficit/hyperactivity disorder might, in turn, have led to overdiagnosis of children and adolescents with bipolar disorder. Thus, the changes represent a slight but important improvement and will lead to greater specificity.

As noted in the text, a highly controversial decision in the *DSM-5* was the addition of premenstrual dysphoric disorder (PMDD), which is retained in the *DSM-5-TR*. This change was met with criticism for pathologizing normal experiences in women. Similarly, critics argue that disruptive mood dysregulation disorder pathologizes children's normal experience of temper tantrums. The rationale for proposing this new diagnosis, however, was that it would reduce the frequency of bipolar disorder misdiagnoses in children.

Finally, the *DSM-5* authors angered many critics when they decided to leave out the "bereavement exclusion" present in *DSM-IV-TR*. This change means that an individual who meets the criteria for a major depressive episode and who has lost a loved one in the past 2 months (which was the bereavement exclusion) can receive a psychiatric diagnosis. Thus, prior to the *DSM-5*, losing a loved one in the past 2 months excluded people from receiving this diagnosis. The argument in favor of making this change was that, in a vulnerable individual, bereavement could trigger a major depressive episode that would be appropriate to diagnose. The *DSM-5-TR* terminology is now "persistent grief disorder (PGD)," a diagnosis consistent with that of the *ICD-11*.

clinicians may advise their clients to participate in lithium groups, in which members who use the medication on a regular basis provide support to each other and reinforce the importance of staying on the medication.

Because of the variable nature of bipolar disorder, other medications can be beneficial in treating symptoms apart from the mania itself. For example, people in a depressive episode may need to take an antidepressant medication in addition to the lithium for the duration of the episode. However, this can be problematic for a person who is prone to developing mania, because an antidepressant might provoke hypomania or mania. Those who have psychotic symptoms may benefit from taking antipsychotic medication such as clozapine (Li, Tang, Wang, & de Leon, 2015).

People who experience rapid cycling present a challenge for clinicians because of the sudden changes that take place in their emotions and behavior. Psychopharmacologists report that rapid cyclers, especially those for whom lithium has not been sufficient, seem to respond positively to prescriptions of anticonvulsant medication, such as carbamazepine (Tegretol) or valproate (Depakote), although these alone are not as effective as lithium (Zivanovic, 2017).

Alternative Biologically Based Treatments

For some clients with mood disorders, medication is either ineffective or slow in alleviating symptoms that are severe and possibly life-threatening. Even with the best treatment, 60 percent of individuals with major depressive disorder do not achieve symptom relief after a 2-year period (Bockting et al., 2018).

Research is beginning to support the value of improving the efficacy of medications through **pharmacogenetics**, the use of genetic testing to identify who will improve with a particular medication. This method has the potential to allow clinicians to make informed decisions prior to prescribing an antidepressant, thus leading to more rapid improvement (Wang, Wang, Zhang, & An, 2023). Its value in treating depression is using an individual's own genetic profile to help determine which particular medication can provide symptom relief (Scherf-Clavel et al., 2022). Similarly, pharmacogenetic studies involving lithium not only show potential benefits but also point to the need for a better genetic understanding of bipolar disorder before the method can have more widespread utility (Vecera et al., 2021).

pharmacogenetics
The use of genetic testing to identify who will and will not improve with a particular medication.

transcranial magnetic stimulation
The use of repetitive electromagnetic pulses to stimulate nerve cells in the brain associated with mood regulation and depression.

circadian rhythms
Biological clocks that set patterns of sleepfulness and wakefulness on approximately a 24-hour basis.

Clinicians also have several somatic alternatives to medication for addressing treatment-resistant depression. One such alternative is electroconvulsive therapy (ECT) (Lisanby, 2007). Clinicians and clients are not sure exactly how ECT works, but most current hypotheses center on ECT-induced changes in neurotransmitter receptors and in the body's natural opiates which, in turn, cause structural changes in the brain (Yrondi et al., 2018).

A second option in the somatic treatment of depression is **transcranial magnetic stimulation (TMS)**, the use of repetitive electromagnetic pulses to stimulate nerve cells in the brain associated with mood regulation and depression. Administered via a "figure 8" coil to deliver pulses just below the brain's surface, TMS may also be administered inside a padded helmet to provide "deep" TMS. Shown to be effective in reducing symptoms, the effects of TMS may be attributed to changes it promotes in the prefrontal cortex (Shanok et al., 2023).

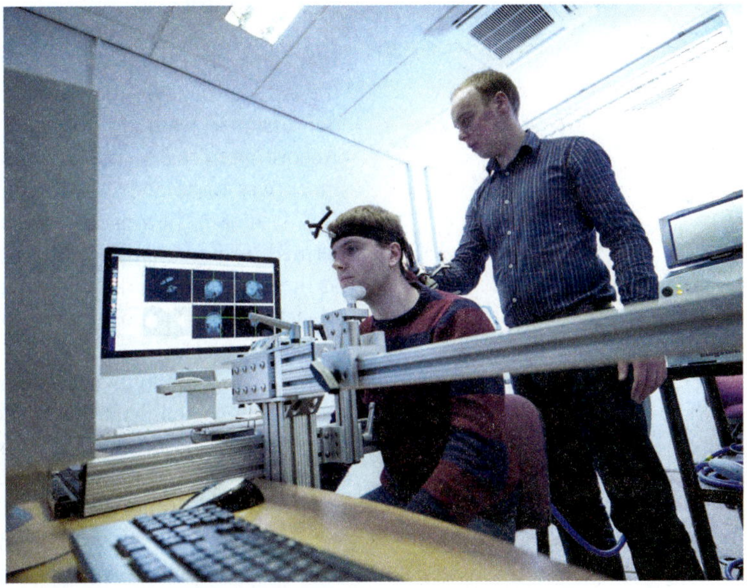

Transcranial magnetic stimulation involves administered electromagnetic pulses to an individual's brain through a coil placed on the head.
Image Source Trading Ltd/Shutterstock

Based on the hypothesis that at least some mood disorders reflect a disruption in daily biological clocks known as **circadian rhythms**, there are treatments that "reset" the individual's bodily clock. Such treatments include light therapy, in which the individual is seated in front of a bright light for a period of time, such as 30 minutes in the morning. Although rates of remission vary from 33 to 77 percent, a distinct advantage of light therapy is that its side effects are minimal and almost entirely disappear after the dosage is reduced or treatment discontinued (D'Agostino et al., 2020).

Psychological Perspective

From the psychological perspective, mood disorders reflect disturbances in the ways that individuals experience their thoughts and emotions. Relationships with others, particularly significant people in an individual's life, are also viewed as contributors to mood disorders, particularly depressive disorder.

Psychodynamic Approaches

Early psychoanalytic theories based on the psychodynamic approach proposed that people with depressive disorders had suffered a loss early in their lives that affected them at a deep, intrapsychic level (Abraham, 1911/1968). It was attachment theory, however, that focused attention on people's feelings of security or insecurity arising from the way their caregivers reared them in childhood. Bowlby (1980) proposed that people with an insecure attachment style have a greater risk for developing a depressive disorder in adulthood. Following up on Bowlby's ideas, Bemporad (1985) proposed that insecurely attached children become preoccupied with the need to be loved by others. As adults, they form relationships in which they overvalue the support of their partners. When such relationships end, they become overwhelmed with feelings of inadequacy and loss.

Psychoanalytic explanations of bipolar disorder propose that manic episodes are defensive responses through which individuals stave off feelings of inadequacy, loss, and helplessness. Clients are thought to develop feelings of grandiosity and elation or become hyperenergetic as an unconscious defense against sinking into a state of gloom and despair. Supporting the role of early childhood experiences, researchers have identified a link, through the use of immature defense mechanisms, to risk for bipolar II disorder (Wang et al., 2021).

Contemporary approaches to treatment within the psychodynamic perspective focus on helping individuals manage their symptoms rather than attempting to repair the core of the individual's disturbed attachment. These approaches consist of short (8- or 10-session), focused treatments. Although this regimen is effective, clinicians working in this perspective note that longer-term treatment may be recommended for clients with more severe symptoms (Driessen et al., 2013).

Behavioral and Cognitive Behavioral Approaches

One of the earliest behavioral formulations of theories of depression regards the symptoms of depression as resulting from lack of positive reinforcement (Lazarus, 1968; Skinner, 1953). According to this view, depressed people withdraw from life because they no longer have incentives to be active. Contemporary behaviorists base their approach on Lewinsohn's (1974) model. Lewinsohn maintained that depressed people have a low rate of what he termed "response contingent positive reinforcement behaviors," which increase in frequency as the result of performing actions that produce pleasure. According to the behaviorist point of view, the lack of positive reinforcement elicits the symptoms of low self-esteem, guilt, and pessimism.

behavioral activation
Behavioral therapy for depression in which the clinician helps the client identify activities associated with positive mood.

In the method known as **behavioral activation** for depression, based on these behaviorist principles, the clinician helps the client identify activities associated with positive mood. The client keeps a record of the frequency of engaging in these rewarding activities and sets small weekly goals that gradually increase in frequency and duration. These activities are preferably consistent with the client's core values. Some clients may prefer to explore the arts, whereas others spend time in physical activity. Behavioral activation seems particularly well suited for clients who are not "psychologically minded," for group therapy, and for settings such as hospitals, nursing homes, and substance-abuse treatment centers (Sturmey, 2009). This approach may also have potential for individuals with bipolar disorder whose daily lives are punctuated by episodes of extreme mood swings (Kim, 2020).

Clinicians are increasingly integrating behavioral with cognitive approaches that focus on the role of dysfunctional thoughts as causes of, or at least contributors to, mood disorders. People with depressive disorders, according to the cognitive behavioral perspective, think in repetitively negative ways that perpetuate their negative emotions. Beck (1967) defined these depressive thoughts as the **cognitive triad**—that is, a negative view of the self, the world, and the future.

These negative views lead depressed individuals, in turn, to experience a profound loss of self-esteem, convinced they will never have what they need to feel good about themselves. They assume they are worthless and helpless and that their efforts to improve their lives are doomed to fail. In the course of their daily experiences, the depressed, in this perspective, make faulty interpretations that keep alive the cycle of negative thoughts and emotions (Beck, Rush, Shaw, & Emery, 1979; Beck & Weishaar, 1989). Each of these faulty interpretations, or cognitive distortions, has its own unique qualities (see Table 3), but they share a failure to draw logical conclusions from the individual's experiences.

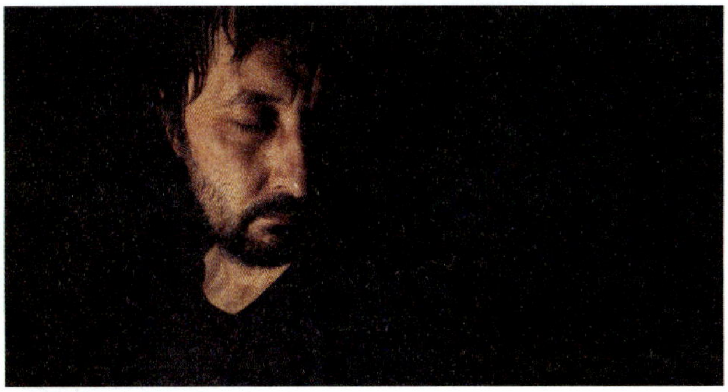

According to the cognitive perspective, people with major depressive disorder experience negative views about themselves, the world, and the future.

Igor Stevanovic/Alamy Stock Photo

cognitive triad
According to the cognitive theory of depression, the view that a depressed person's dysphoria results from a negative view of the self, the world, and the future.

Behavioral therapy with clients who have depressive disorders follows the general principles outlined in the chapter "Theoretical Perspectives" in which clinicians help their clients develop more positively reinforcing experiences. In this approach, clinicians begin with a careful assessment of the frequency, quality, and range of activities and social interactions in their client's life, focusing on sources of positive and negative reinforcement. Based on this analysis, the clinicians work with their clients to institute changes in their environments while also teaching them social skills to improve the quality and number of their positive interactions. An important focus of the work done by behaviorally oriented clinicians is to encourage clients to increase their participation in activities they find inherently rewarding. These rewarding activities, in turn, can help boost the client's mood.

Behaviorally oriented clinicians also believe that education is an essential component of therapy. They regard individuals with depressive disorders as perpetuating their negative emotions by setting unrealistic goals, which they are then unable to achieve. To counteract these, clinicians working in the behavioral perspective assign homework exercises that encourage clients to make gradual behavioral changes, which will increase the probability that they can achieve their goals and thus feel rewarded.

TABLE 3 **Examples of Cognitive Distortions**

Type of Distortion	Definition	Example
Overgeneralizing	If it's true in one case, it applies to any case that is even slightly similar.	"I failed my first English exam, so I'm probably going to fail all of them."
Using selective abstraction	Taking seriously only events that represent failures, deprivation, loss, or frustration.	"Even though I won the election for the student senate, I'm not really popular because not everyone voted for me."
Taking excessive responsibility	Feeling responsible for all bad things that happen to you or to others to whom you are close.	"It's my fault that my friend didn't get the internship—I should've warned her about how hard the interview would be."
Assuming temporal causality	Assuming that if it has been true in the past, it's always going to be true.	"My last date was a wipeout, my next date will probably hate me too."
Making excessive self-references	Feeling at the center of everyone else's attention and assuming everyone can see your flaws and errors.	"When I tripped over the branch in the sidewalk, everyone could see how clumsy I am."
Catastrophizing	Always thinking the worst and being certain that it will happen.	"Because I failed my accounting exam, I will never make it in the business world."
Engaging in dichotomous thinking	Seeing everything as either one extreme or another rather than as mixed or in between.	"I can't stand people who are liars because I can never trust them."

SOURCE: Beck, A. T., Rush, A. J., Shaw, B. F., & Emery, G. (1987). *Cognitive therapy of depression.* Guilford Press.

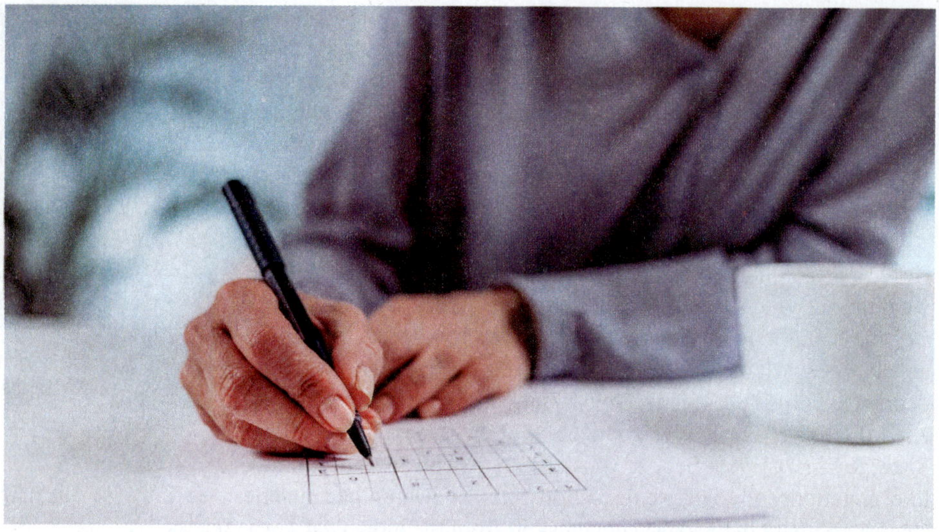

A clinician working in the behavioral perspective might take advantage of this client's enjoyment of puzzles as self-reinforcement in therapy.
Microgen/Shutterstock

Another technique used by the behavioral clinician combines behavioral contracting with self-reinforcement. For example, the clinician and client may agree that a client would benefit from the opportunity to socialize outside the home more often. Together, they would then set up a schedule of rewards in which they pair the social activity with something the client identifies as a desirable reward compatible with the goals of treatment (the clinician would not recommend that the client use the rewards of alcohol, drugs, or online gambling). Other methods the behaviorally oriented clinician would use include more extensive instruction, modeling, coaching, role playing, rehearsal, and perhaps working with the client in a real-world setting.

The focus of cognitive behavioral therapy (CBT) for major depressive disorder is on helping clients try to change their dysfunctional thought processes that in turn will improve their mood. Like behaviorally oriented therapy, CBT requires an active collaboration between the client and the clinician. In contrast to behaviorally oriented therapy, however, CBT also focuses on the client's dysfunctional thoughts and how to modify them through cognitive restructuring. Mindfulness training, as an additional component of a cognitive behavioral intervention, can help clients develop a greater sense of self-efficacy, an extra boost to its positive effects on mood (Eisendrath et al., 2015). CBT plus mindfulness can also be useful interventions for individuals from Latinx communities experiencing ongoing exposure to adversity and stress associated with immigration (Fortuna et al., 2020).

Another CBT technique known as mood monitoring can further help clients learn ways to track their mood over time and look for patterns in mood fluctuation. This is particularly helpful in the case of clients with bipolar disorder, who through the mood monitoring technique can become more aware of worsening symptoms, so they can intervene using skills or other methods to avoid a full-blown manic or depressive episode (Driessen & Hollon, 2010).

Psychoeducation is an especially important aspect of treating people with bipolar disorder to help them understand its nature, as well as the reasons medication is so important in controlling symptoms (Bond & Anderson, 2015).

interpersonal therapy (IPT) A time-limited form of psychotherapy for treating people with major depressive disorder, based on the assumption that interpersonal stress induces an episode of depression in a person who is genetically vulnerable to this disorder.

Interpersonal Approaches

Developed as a brief intervention, **interpersonal therapy (IPT)** is a focused approach intended to last between 12 and 16 weeks. In IPT, clients are helped to manage the interpersonal stress associated with their depressive episodes, which themselves are seen as a function of genetic predisposition. Administered according to a set of guidelines, interpersonal therapy provides clinicians with a clear model to follow so that treatment can proceed within the scheduled time frame. The IPT manual has the additional advantage of ensuring some consistency across therapists, making it possible to evaluate its effectiveness empirically.

Clinicians administer interpersonal therapy in three broad phases. In the first phase, the clinician assesses the magnitude and nature of the individual's depression using quantitative assessment measures and semi-structured interviews. Depending on the type of depressive symptoms the individual shows, the therapist may consider combining treatment with antidepressant medications along with psychotherapy.

In the second phase, the therapist and the client collaborate on formulating a treatment plan that focuses on the primary problem. Typically, these problems are related to grief, interpersonal disputes, role transitions, and problems in interpersonal relationships stemming from inadequate social skills.

The therapist carries out the treatment plan in the third phase, varying the methods according to the precise nature of the client's primary problem. The IPT approach encourages clinicians to combine such techniques as encouraging self-exploration, providing support, educating the client on the nature of depression, and offering feedback on the client's ineffective social skills. A primary focus of therapy is on the here and now, rather than on past childhood or developmental issues.

For clients who cannot take antidepressant medications or for whom it is impractical to use medications, IPT is an especially valuable intervention, in that nonmedical staff can administer it, or clients, with instruction, can learn it themselves (Weissman, 2007). Research continues to support its use as an alternative to CBT (Bruijniks et al., 2022).

Interpersonal and social rhythm therapy (IPSRT) (Frank, 2007) is a biopsychosocial approach to treating people with bipolar disorder that incorporates the concepts of stressful life events and disturbances in circadian rhythms (such as altered sleep/wake cycles, appetite, and energy level) into a focus on the individual's personal relationships. According to the IPSRT model, mood episodes are likely to emerge from medication nonadherence, stressful life events, and disruptions in social rhythms.

The goal of IPSRT is to increase the stability of a client's social rhythms. A meta-analysis of randomized controlled trials showed support for this method in improving life skills for people with bipolar disorder, but not for reducing symptoms, suggesting this is best thought of as an adjunct rather than first-line method of treatment (Lam & Chung, 2021).

Looking across the results of virtually all published studies on interventions for mood disorders, Hollon and Ponniah (2010) concluded that cognitive behavioral and behavioral therapy meet the criteria for evidence-based treatments, receiving strong support particularly for individuals with less severe or chronic depression. Individuals with more severe depressive or bipolar disorders also benefit from cognitive behavioral, interpersonal, and behaviorally oriented therapy above and beyond the effects of medication, and perhaps even instead of medication entirely, particularly over the long term (McHugh et al., 2013).

Sociocultural Perspective

According to the sociocultural perspective, individuals develop depressive disorders in response to external life circumstances. These circumstances can be specific events such as sexual victimization, chronic stress such as poverty and single parenting, or episodic stress such as bereavement or job loss.

minority stress model
Approach to psychological disorders that emphasizes the role of discrimination due to minority status.

Acute and chronic stressors seem to play a differential role in predisposing an individual to experiencing depressive symptoms. Exposure to an acute stress such as the death of a loved one or an automobile accident could precipitate a major depressive episode. However, exposure to chronic strains from poor working conditions, health or interpersonal problems, or financial adversity can interact with genetic predisposition and personality to lead certain individuals to experience more persistent feelings of hopelessness. Moreover, once activated, an individual's feelings of depression and hopelessness can exacerbate the effects of exposure to stressful environments, which, in turn, can further increase the individual's feelings of chronic strain through a process of stress sensitization (Monroe, Anderson, & Harkness, 2019).

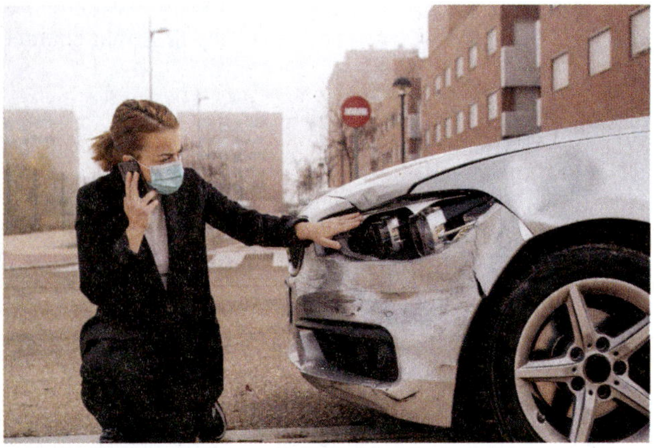

A combination of personal stressors and the large-scale stress due to the COVID-19 pandemic placed individuals at risk of developing a depressive disorder.
Addictive Creative/Shutterstock

The **minority stress model** posits that individuals in marginalized groups who are affected by societal oppression such as racism and homophobia are exposed to chronic levels of high stress due to this discrimination. Lower perceived levels of safety and belongingness can increase depression in individuals who are subject to this type of discrimination (Wilson & Liss, 2020). Oppression-based trauma differentially affecting minoritized populations due to the COVID-19 pandemic and social unrest in the spring of 2020, following high-profile murders of unarmed Black people by the police, further exacerbated these sources of stress (De Leon et al., 2023).

On the positive side, strong religious beliefs and spirituality may combine with the social support that membership in a religious community provides to lower an individual's chances of developing depression, even among those with high risk. People who identified as religious showed, in combination with other social resources, greater resilience in the face of COVID-19 (Kimhi et al., 2021). The effect of religiosity extended to adults with chronic diseases, a group who might otherwise have been particularly prone to depressive symptoms during the pandemic (Davis et al., 2021). Thus, although sociocultural factors can contribute to psychological disorders, it is possible for individuals to draw on the support provided by their community.

7.4 Suicide

suicide
A fatal self-inflicted destructive act with explicit or inferred intent to die.

suicidal ideation
Thinking about ending one's life.

suicide attempt
Undertaking nonfatal suicidal behavior.

The definition of **suicide** is "a fatal self-inflicted destructive act with explicit or inferred intent to die" (Goldsmith, Pellmar, Kleinman, & Bunney, 2002, p. 27). Suicidal behavior runs along a continuum of thinking about ending one's life, or **suicidal ideation**, to developing a plan, to undertaking nonfatal suicidal behavior or **suicide attempt**, to the actual commission of suicide. Although not a diagnosable disorder, suicidality is one potential diagnostic feature of a major depressive episode and is also associated with a number of diagnoses, as specified in the *DSM-5-TR*.

Around the world, there are approximately 800,000 suicides each year, which translates to a death rate of 10.6 per 100,000 in the populations. There are significant differences in suicide rates between high-income and low-middle-income countries. Young adults and older women in low-middle-income countries have higher rates of suicide. Middle-aged men in high-income countries, in contrast, are the segment of the population at highest risk for suicide (World Health Organization, 2021).

In the United States, suicide is the 10th leading cause of death, having claimed the lives of over 48,000 people in 2021. Firearms account for nearly half of all deaths due to suicide, particularly for men. Women in the United States are more likely to take their lives by suffocation and poisoning. As you can see from Figure 2, showing racial and ethnic variations in the United States, non-Hispanic American Indian/Alaska Natives have the highest suicide rates. Additionally, although fewer in number within the population, individuals 65 and older have the highest rates; the highest actual numbers are among those 45 to 64 years old, accounting for nearly one-third of all suicides (Centers for Disease Control and Prevention, 2023).

The biopsychosocial perspective is particularly appropriate for understanding why people commit suicide and in many ways parallels the understanding gleaned from an integrative framework for major depressive disorders. Biological theories emphasize the genetic and physiological contributions that also contribute to the causes of mood disorders. Psychological theories focus on distorted cognitive processes and extreme feelings of hopelessness that characterize suicide victims. From a sociocultural perspective, the variations

FIGURE 2 The Racial/Ethnic Groups with the Highest Rates in 2021 were Non-Hispanic American Indian and Alaska Native People and Non-Hispanic White People

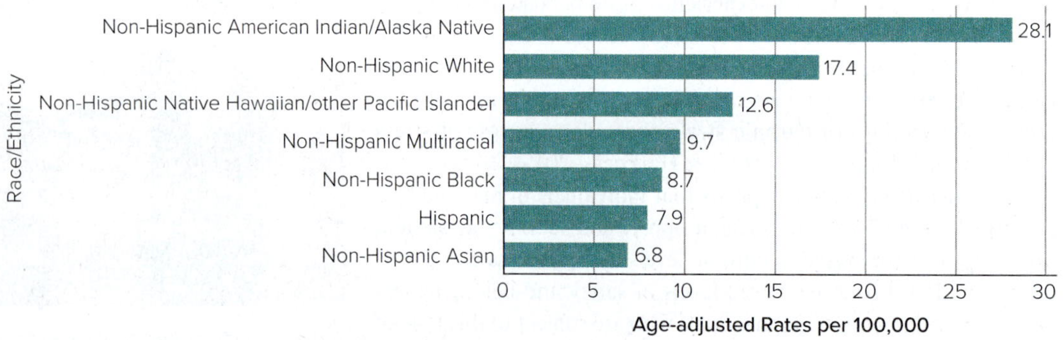

Source: Centers for Disease Control and Prevention. (2023). Facts about suicide. https://www.cdc.gov/suicide/facts/index.html

You Be the Judge

Do-Not-Resuscitate Orders for Suicidal Patients

The question of whether physicians should assist patients in ending their own lives, a process known as physician-assisted suicide, came to public attention in the 1990s when Dr. Jack Kevorkian, a Michigan physician, began providing terminally ill patients with the means to end their lives through pharmacological injections. Kevorkian's very public involvement sprang from what he saw as a righteous campaign to alleviate people's suffering and allow them to "die with dignity." He was imprisoned for 8 years following the televised assisted suicide he performed on a man with amyotrophic lateral sclerosis (ALS), a terminal nervous system disease.

Medical professionals are required to direct patients, terminally ill or not, to direct them—in an "advance directive" or "living will"—by stating whether they wish to have artificial life support should they be unable to survive on their own. The advance directive often includes a DNR or "do-not-resuscitate" order in which the patient specifies that no heroic life-support measures should be taken to prolong life with, for example, life-support machines. Medical professionals respect the conditions of the DNR when they must make life-and-death decisions. In contrast, when individuals who have psychological disorders and wish to end their lives embark upon the same plans as a medical patient with a life-threatening illness, clinicians treat them to prevent them from committing suicide. The treatment may include involuntary hospitalization.

The obligation to respect end-of-life wishes may present an ethical conflict for mental health professionals when treating suicidal individuals who complete a DNR stating that they do not wish to be given life support. The question is whether having a serious psychological disorder that is incapacitating, resistant to treatment, and debilitating is any different from having a similarly untreatable and painful medical illness.

Q: *You be the judge:* Does the individual's right to autonomy, respected with a DNR, differ in this type of case (Cook, Pan, Silverman, & Soltys, 2010)?

between and within countries suggest contributions relating to an individual's religious beliefs and values and the degree to which the individual is exposed to life stresses.

The perspective of positive psychology provides a framework for understanding why individuals who are at high risk for the reasons stated nevertheless do not commit suicide. The buffering hypothesis of suicidality (Siegmann et al., 2018) describes resilience as a separate dimension from risk. Individuals may be at risk of committing suicide, but if high on resilience, are unlikely to do so (Sher, 2019).

Personality may play a role in promoting resilience in the face of stress as a protection against suicide. In one long-term study of Mexican-origin youth, researchers found that a combination of the traits of high conscientiousness and low neuroticism predicted an ability to remain positive in the face of stress, which reduced suicide risk compared to that of youth who were lower in both personality traits (Lawson et al., 2021).

Interventions based on the resilience model would not only address the individual's specific risk factors, but also assess and then strengthen the individual's feelings of personal control and perceived abilities to handle stress. CBT is one such intervention shown to be effective on reducing suicide attempts in college campus clinics (Farabaugh et al., 2019) and members of the military with a history of suicide attempts (Rudd et al., 2015).

7.5 Depressive and Bipolar Disorders: The Biopsychosocial Perspective

The disorders you read about in this chapter span a range of phenomena, from chronic but distressing sad moods to rapidly vacillating alternations between mania and depression. Although these disorders clearly indicate disturbances in neurotransmitter functioning, they also reflect the influences of cognitive processes and sociocultural factors. Because individuals may experience the symptoms of depressive disorders for many years, clinicians are increasingly turning to nonpharmacological interventions, particularly for cases in which individuals have mild or moderate symptoms. The situation for clients with bipolar disorder is more complicated, because lifelong maintenance therapy on medication is more likely to be necessary. Nevertheless, these individuals can benefit from psychological interventions to help keep their symptoms monitored and under control.

Even individuals whose mood disorder symptoms reflect a heavy influence of biology, however, should have access to a range of therapeutic services. With the development of evidence-based approaches, which integrate interventions across the individual's multiple domains of functioning, the chances are good that people with these disorders will increasingly have the ability to obtain treatment that allows them to regulate their moods and lead more fulfilling lives.

Return to the Case: Janice Butterfield

After several weeks of therapy, Janice's depression had started to show improvement. Once her depression remitted, however, she stopped taking her medication. As she discussed in her initial therapy session, Janice found it important to appear strong to her family and associated psychological problems with weakness. Despite her concerns about admitting her psychological struggles, Janice continued to come to her weekly psychotherapy, and the sessions focused on her feelings about her diagnosis and the importance of taking her medication to prevent future mood swings, though she felt stable at the time. Reminded of examples of the past consequences of her mood swings, however, Janice was slowly able to better understand that the impact on her family would be far worse should she continue to go through mood cycles than if she worked at maintaining stability.

Dr. Tobin's Reflections: Though it is a natural reaction to feel down when faced with a challenge such as losing a job and having to find a way to support your family, Janice's response went beyond the typical depression most people feel, and she met diagnostic criteria for a major depressive episode. Janice's description of her past depressive episodes was also consistent with this diagnosis. It was also revealed that Janice experienced manic episodes in the past that had not only greatly affected her life but had put her family at great financial risk. Unfortunately, it wasn't until Janice had attempted suicide that she finally sought the help she needed. It is not unusual for individuals with bipolar disorder to be noncompliant with medication, because they go through long periods of feeling "normal" or being at their baseline. This was especially true of Janice, who had gone her entire life without seeking treatment and had difficulty understanding the need to take medication when she was not feeling depressed or manic.

Janice described experiencing a worsening of her mood episodes over time. This is typical for individuals with bipolar disorder who go without treatment for many years. Though she has been hesitant to talk about her problems with her family, it will be important to include them in her treatment because they can help Janice understand when her mood may start to shift. Individuals with bipolar disorder may struggle to be aware of these changes in mood. Over time, it will be important for Janice to continue to explore her concerns about the stigma of mental health treatment, given that this had been a major barrier to her reaching out for help in the past.

SUMMARY

- Depressive and bipolar disorders reflect a disturbance in a person's emotional state or mood. People can experience this disturbance in the form of extreme depression, excessive elation, or a combination of these emotional states. An episode is a time-limited period during which specific intense symptoms of a disorder are evident.
- Major depressive disorder is characterized by acute but time-limited episodes of depressive symptoms, such as feelings of extreme dejection, a loss of interest in previously pleasurable aspects of life, bodily symptoms, and disturbances in eating and sleeping behavior. Individuals with major depressive disorder also have cognitive symptoms, such as a negative self-view, feelings of guilt, inability to concentrate, and indecisiveness. Depressive episodes can be melancholic or seasonal. Persistent depressive disorder consists of depression that is not as deep or intense as that experienced in major depressive disorder but has a longer-lasting course. People with persistent depressive disorder have, for at least

2 years, depressive symptoms such as low energy, low self-esteem, poor concentration, decision-making difficulty, feelings of hopelessness, and disturbances of appetite and sleep. Disruptive mood dysregulation disorder, diagnosed in individuals 6 to 18 years of age, consists of chronic and severe irritability, and premenstrual dysphoric disorder occurs in women prior to their monthly menstrual periods.

- Bipolar I disorder is characterized by an intense and highly disruptive experience of extreme elation, or euphoria, called a manic episode, which manifests in heightened levels of thinking, behavior, and emotionality that cause significant impairment. Bipolar episodes in which both mania and depression are displayed can be labeled with specifiers to indicate severity. Bipolar II disorder is diagnosed when briefer, less intense, and less disruptive states called hypomanic episodes, are present. Cyclothymic disorder consists of a vacillation between dysphoria and hypomanic episodes.
- Clinicians have explained depressive and bipolar disorders in terms of biological, psychological, and sociocultural approaches. Biological theories focus on genetics and neurotransmitter hormonal functioning. Psychological theories have moved from early psychoanalytic approaches to more contemporary viewpoints that emphasize the behavioral, cognitive, and interpersonal aspects of mood disturbance. The behaviorist viewpoint assumes that depression is the result of a reduction in positive reinforcements, deficient social skills, or the disruption caused by stressful life experiences. According to the cognitive perspective, depressed people react to stressful experiences by activating a set of thoughts called the cognitive triad: negative views of the self, the world, and the future. Cognitive distortions are errors people make in the way they draw conclusions from their experiences, applying illogical rules such as arbitrary inferences and overgeneralizing. Interpersonal theory posits a model of understanding depressive and bipolar disorders that emphasizes disturbed social functioning. Sociocultural approaches emphasize the role of stress in the environment, resulting both from discrimination and from large-scale events affecting populations as a whole.
- Clinicians base depressive and bipolar disorder treatments on biological, psychological, and sociocultural perspectives. Antidepressant medication is the most common form of somatic treatment for people who are depressed, and lithium carbonate is the most widely used medication for people who have bipolar disorder. In cases of incapacitating depression and some extreme cases of acute mania, the clinician may recommend a form of somatic therapy. The psychological interventions most effective for treating people with depressive and bipolar disorders are those rooted in the behaviorist, cognitive, and cognitive behavioral approaches. Sociocultural and interpersonal interventions focus on the treatment of mood symptoms within the context of an interpersonal system, such as an intimate relationship.
- Although no formal diagnostic category specifically applies to people who commit suicide, many suicidal people have depressive or bipolar disorders, and suicidality is a risk factor in other disorders. Clinicians explain the dramatic act of suicide from biological, psychological, and sociocultural perspectives. The treatment of suicidal clients varies considerably, depending on the context, intent, and lethality. Most intervention approaches incorporate support and direct therapy, with a focus on building an individual's resilience.

KEY TERMS

Behavioral activation
Bipolar disorder
Bipolar disorder, rapid cycling
Bipolar I disorder
Bipolar II disorder
Black-White paradox
Circadian rhythms
Cognitive triad
Cyclothymic disorder
Depressive disorder
Disruptive mood dysregulation disorder (DMDD)
Dysphoria
Euphoria
Hypomanic episode
Interpersonal therapy (IPT)
Lithium carbonate
Major depressive disorder
Major depressive episode
Manic episode
Minority stress model
Persistent depressive disorder
Pharmacogenetics
Premenstrual dysphoric disorder (PMDD)
Selective serotonin reuptake inhibitor (SSRI)
Serotonin and norepinephrine reuptake inhibitor (SNRI)
Suicidal ideation
Suicide
Suicide attempt
Transcranial magnetic stimulation

CHAPTER 8

Anxiety, Obsessive-Compulsive, and Trauma- and Stressor-Related Disorders

OUTLINE

Learning Objectives

8.1 Summarize characteristics of anxiety disorders.

8.2 Describe obsessive-compulsive and related disorders.

8.3 Identify the trauma- and stress-related disorders.

8.4 Explain the biopsychosocial perspective on anxiety, obsessive-compulsive, and trauma-and stressor-related disorders.

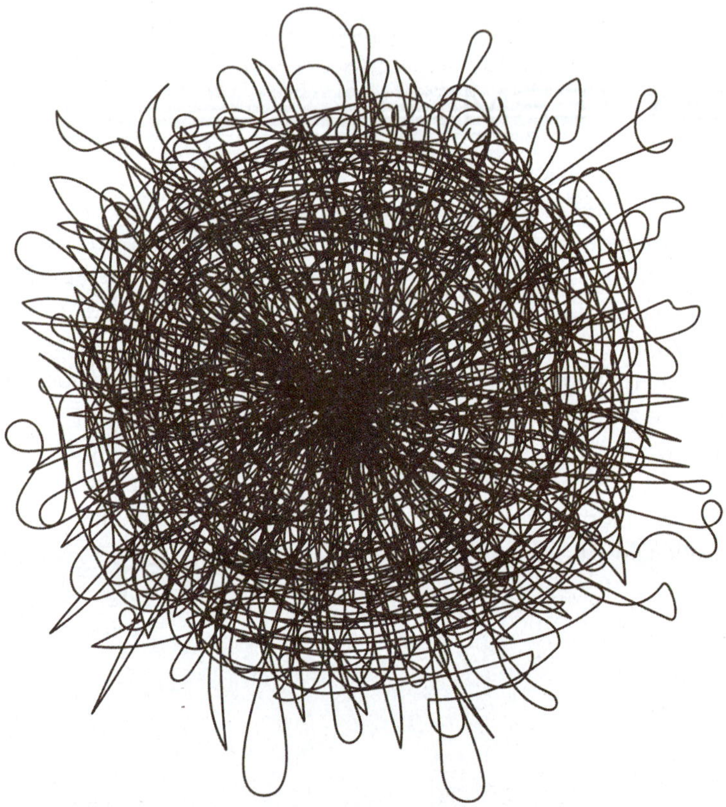

Mironov Konstantin/Shutterstock

Case Report

Barbara Wilder

Demographic information: 30-year-old White gay cisgender woman. Barbara's pronouns are she/her/hers.

History of present illness: At age 18, Barbara enlisted in the Army to help pay for college. Shortly after she graduated with a bachelor's degree in business, the United States invaded Iraq and Barbara was sent on her first tour of duty, which lasted 18 months. She returned for three more tours before she was injured so severely in a military police raid that her lower left leg required amputation and she received a medical discharge.

While Barbara was receiving medical treatment at the Veterans Affairs (VA) Medical Center, her doctors noticed that she seemed constantly "on edge." When asked to provide details about her leg injury, she would grow anxious and withdrawn. She stated that she had difficulty sleeping because of frequent nightmares. Suspecting that she could be suffering from post-traumatic stress disorder (PTSD), the VA physicians referred her to the PTSD specialty clinic. Barbara reported that she had indeed been suffering a great deal of psychological stress since returning from her final tour of duty. She described her time in Iraq as incredibly dangerous and stressful. She worked on the military police unit and was in charge of guarding prisoners of war. Her station was often attacked, and gunfire fights were a frequent occurrence. Barbara also witnessed numerous incidents in which civilians and fellow soldiers were injured and killed.

Although she was under constant threat of injury or death while in Iraq and witnessed many grotesque scenes, Barbara stated that for the first three tours she was generally able to stay focused on her work without being unduly fearful. Over time and with repeated long tours of duty, however, she found it increasingly difficult not to be affected by the events around her. At the start of what was to be her last tour of duty, Barbara recalled that she felt as if she were starting to "mentally break down." When she was injured in the raid, she was certain she had been killed and remained in a state of shock for nearly 12 hours. Once she regained consciousness, Barbara recalled, she "just lost it" and began screaming at the medical staff around her. She now remembers very little of that day, but she recalls the feeling of total fear that overcame her and that remains with her to the present time.

In addition to the emotional difficulties she faced when she came home from the war, Barbara also was required to readjust to life in her community and to no longer living the life of a soldier. This adjustment was difficult not only because she had been away from her friends and family for so long, but also because she felt overwhelming distress associated with combat memories. Nevertheless, Barbara was recovering well from her injury—undergoing physical therapy at the VA and getting used to life without her leg. However, there was no denying that she was a different person than she had been before her time as a soldier, due to both her injury and the horrifying experiences she had survived during her time in Iraq.

Barbara originally planned to return to school to receive a degree in business administration after she completed her military service. However, since returning to the United States 6 months ago, she has given up on this plan. She rarely leaves the house where she resides with her parents. For the first 2 months after her return stateside, she drank alcohol excessively on a daily basis. She eventually noticed that drinking only seemed to make her anxiety worse, and so she stopped altogether. Though she stated she never talks about her experiences in Iraq, at least once every day Barbara is haunted by disturbing, vivid flashbacks to violent images she witnessed while in the war. These visions also come to her in nightmares. She remarked that she must have replayed the image of seeing her leg blown up thousands of times in her mind. She reported feeling as if she were in a state of constant anxiety and that she was particularly sensitive to loud, unexpected noises. As a result, Barbara reported she was often irritable and jumpy around other people, growing angry quite easily. She expressed fears that she would never be able to make anything of her life, and that she barely felt motivated to make strides toward independence. Once social and outgoing, she no longer has any desire to see her friends or date, and mostly ignores her parents. She described being emotionally "numb" and very detached from her feelings—a great departure from her usual temperament.

Psychiatric history: Barbara reported that she had always been "somewhat anxious," but that she never experienced this anxiety as an interference with her daily functioning. She described herself before her military

Case Report *continued*

enlistment as a normal, outgoing person who was mostly content with her life. She reported no history of mental illness in her immediate family.

Symptoms: Barbara reported that since her return from Iraq, she has frequently experienced a number of distressing symptoms that have significantly interfered with her life. These include difficulty sleeping, nightmares, flashbacks, restlessness, feelings of detachment from others, diminished interest, emotional "numbness," avoidance of talking about the trauma, hypervigilance, increased anger, and irritability for the past 6 months.

Case formulation: Barbara's symptoms over the past 6 months meet the required *DSM-5-TR* criteria for post-traumatic stress disorder: intrusive recollection, avoidance/numbing, hyperarousal, duration (at least 1 month), and interference with functioning. During her three tours of duty in Iraq, she was repeatedly exposed to dangerous or life-threatening situations and witnessed many gruesome events as a soldier. Though she was initially able to cope with these experiences, over time her resolve was shaken and she began to respond to her surroundings with fear and horror, especially pertaining to the incident in which she lost part of her left leg. Despite drinking heavily for a period of weeks, she has been abstinent for several months and did not meet enough criteria for a *DSM-5-TR* diagnosis of alcohol use disorder.

Risk level: Low. Barbara denies suicidal ideation and has no history of suicide attempts.

Treatment plan: After the psychological assessment determined that Barbara was suffering from PTSD, she was referred for weekly individual psychotherapy as well as a weekly PTSD therapy group at the VA. Psychotherapy for PTSD often consists of some exposure to the trauma via talking and/or writing about it in detail. Some treatments include reflecting on the ways in which trauma has affected the individual's general beliefs about trust and safety. The purpose of group therapy is to provide social support for those suffering from the disorder and to work on coping skills training. Group therapy can sometimes be utilized in place of individual therapy.

Sarah Tobin, PhD

8.1 Anxiety Disorders

anxiety disorders
Disorders characterized by excessive fear and anxiety and related disturbances in behavior.

anxiety
A future-oriented and global response, involving both cognitive and emotional components, in which an individual is inordinately apprehensive, tense, and uneasy about the prospect of something terrible happening.

fear
The emotional response to real or perceived imminent threat.

The central feature of **anxiety disorders** is the experience of a chronic and intense feeling of **anxiety** in which people feel a sense of dread about what might happen to them in the future, and engage in significant amounts of worry. The intense and often unshakable worry and dread experienced by people with anxiety disorders causes them to have great difficulty functioning on a day-to-day basis. This feeling goes beyond the typical worries people have from time to time about performing their everyday activities at work or home, or in their interactions with other people.

People with anxiety disorders also experience **fear**, which is the emotional response to real or perceived imminent threat. Again, like the experience of anxiety, the sense of fear that people with these disorders experience goes beyond ordinary or even rational concern over the possible dangers of the situations in which they find themselves.

Avoidance is another important component of the lives of people with anxiety disorders, who go to great lengths to avoid situations that provoke the emotional responses of anxiety and fear. When they are unable to avoid such situations, they will have difficulty performing jobs, enjoying leisure pursuits, or engaging in social activities with friends and families. Avoidance in this sense can be either behavioral, for instance avoiding specific situations or objects that provoke anxiety, or psychological, such as avoidance of painful memories or feelings.

Across all categories, anxiety disorders have a lifetime prevalence rate in the United States of 28.8 percent and an overall 12-month prevalence of 12.7 percent (Kessler et al., 2012). Of all 12-month prevalence cases, nearly 23 percent are classified as severe. The percent of people reporting lifetime prevalence across all anxiety disorders peaks between the ages of 30 and 44, with a sharp dropoff to 15.3 percent among people 60 years and older

(Kessler, Chiu, et al., 2005). The annual prevalence drops from the high at ages 30–44 to 9 percent at ages 60 and older (Figure 1). The average age of onset across all anxiety disorders is 21.3 years of age, with ranges from 15 years and younger to up to 39 years, depending on the nature of the disorder (de Lijster et al., 2017).

The COVID-19 pandemic is largely acknowledged as having produced negative mental health consequences, particularly involving anxiety. A meta-analysis of over two million people from around the world suggests that anxiety as a symptom became extremely widespread, affecting 35.1 percent of the population. Among cases identified as meeting the criteria for an anxiety disorder, as many as 25 percent were rated as mild to moderate, and 10 percent as severe (Delpino et al., 2023).

Unfortunately, for the as many as 20 percent of clients seen by their primary care health providers who meet the criteria for an anxiety disorder, less than half (44.5 percent) receive a correct diagnosis. In part, the reasons for the failure to diagnose these individuals in primary care settings is due to the presence of physical symptoms (such as chest discomfort or heart palpitations) that can mask the anxiety disorder, and these clients will not receive appropriate treatment (Shuzany & Simon, 2022).

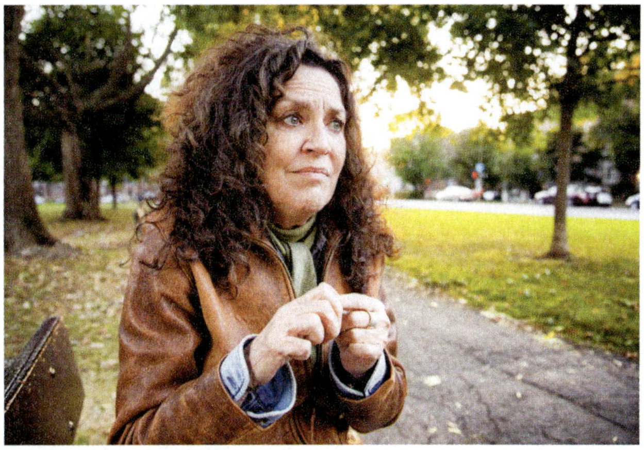

People with anxiety disorders become unable to function due to strong feelings of dread and fear.

NicolasMcComber/E+/Getty Images

Separation Anxiety Disorder

Individuals with **separation anxiety disorder** have intense and inappropriate anxiety about leaving home or being left by their attachment figures, the people close to them in their lives. Children with this disorder may cling so closely to a parent they will not let the parent out of their sight. Adults who meet the criteria for this disorder have intense anxiety about being separated from the person to whom they are most emotionally attached, usually their romantic partner.

separation anxiety disorder
A childhood disorder characterized by intense and inappropriate anxiety, lasting at least 4 weeks, concerning separation from home or caregivers.

Prior to the *DSM-5*, the condition of separation anxiety disorder was considered specific to children. However, recognizing that there are a significant number of adult-onset cases, *DSM-5* lifted the disorder's age restriction to make the diagnosis applicable to adults as well as children, and this remains true in the *DSM-5-TR*. Although the key features of the disorder can vary according to the individual's age, always included is the criterion that the individual becomes excessively distressed when separated from the home or the attachment figure or even at the thought of such separation occurring.

Part of the anxiety people with the disorder experience is worry about harm befalling their attachment figure, such as them being kidnapped, a fear that can become extreme and irrational. This worry leads them to try to avoid spending any time apart or away from home, interfering with their ability to work or go to school. They need to sleep near their attachment figures and may have nightmares about separation. The prospect of separation may lead them to develop physical complaints such as headaches, stomachaches, or even nausea and vomiting. They may carry with them possessions of their attachment figures in an effort to maintain emotional closeness (Niemyjska & Parzuchowski, 2020).

Worldwide, epidemiologists estimate that 5.3 percent of individuals experience separation anxiety disorder at some point in life, with 43.1 percent of those developing the symptoms in adulthood. Regardless of when the symptoms first become evident, people with this disorder were more likely to have suffered adversities during their childhood or traumatic events at some point in their lives. Women are more likely than men to

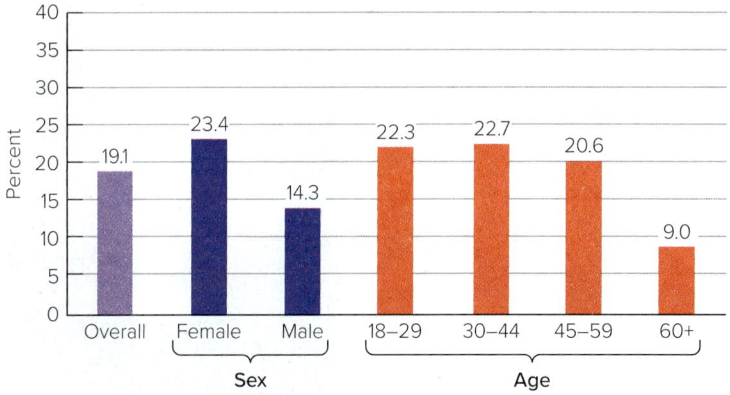

FIGURE 1 Past-Year Prevalence of Any Anxiety Disorder among U.S. Adults (2001–2003)

SOURCE: U.S. Department of Health and Human Services. Any Anxiety Disorder. https://www.nimh.nih.gov/health/statistics/any-anxiety-disorder.shtml

experience separation anxiety disorder. People who develop this disorder are at greater risk of subsequently developing other anxiety disorders and depressive disorder ("internalizing" disorders) as well as ADHD and conduct disorder (Silove et al., 2015).

Theories and Treatment of Separation Anxiety Disorder

Although twin studies supported the role of genetic contributions to this disorder, a novel children-of-twins study conducted by Swedish researchers suggested that anxiety is passed down from parents to children through environmental, rather than genetic, mechanisms. In other words, children with anxious parents learn to develop anxiety through modeling the behavior of their parents (Eley et al., 2015).

Sociocultural factors also play a role in predisposing certain individuals to developing separation anxiety disorder. The symptoms of the disorder seem to be more severe in countries that promote an individualistic, independent culture than in those with a more collectivist set of cultural norms (Eley et al., 2015). Remaining with attachment figures may seem more acceptable in collectivist cultures, so the behavior of individuals with separation anxiety disorder may not appear so out of the ordinary.

Research on separation anxiety disorder in adults suggests that exposure to trauma can play a significant role throughout the life span. Among nearly 39,000 adults studied in 18 countries within the World Health Organization, both childhood adversity and lifetime trauma were shown to increase an individual's likelihood of developing the disorder (Silove et al., 2015).

Investigations of the effectiveness of therapy for separation anxiety disorder in children suggest that cognitive behavioral therapy (CBT), including internet-based CBT, can have beneficial effects on symptom reduction in children as young as 7 years old. Although children receiving this type of treatment respond best when their parents have higher quality relationships, they can still show improvement in anxiety symptoms with a 10-week course of treatment that persists for at least 1 year following treatment completion. Moreover, compliance tends to be high in internet-based therapy, which also makes possible higher rates of participation of the child's parents (Spence, Prosser, March, & Donovan, 2020).

Selective Mutism

selective mutism
A disorder originating in childhood in which the individual consciously refuses to talk.

Refusing to talk in specific situations is the core feature of **selective mutism**. Children with this disorder are capable of using normal language, but they become almost completely silent under certain circumstances, most commonly the classroom. This is a relatively rare

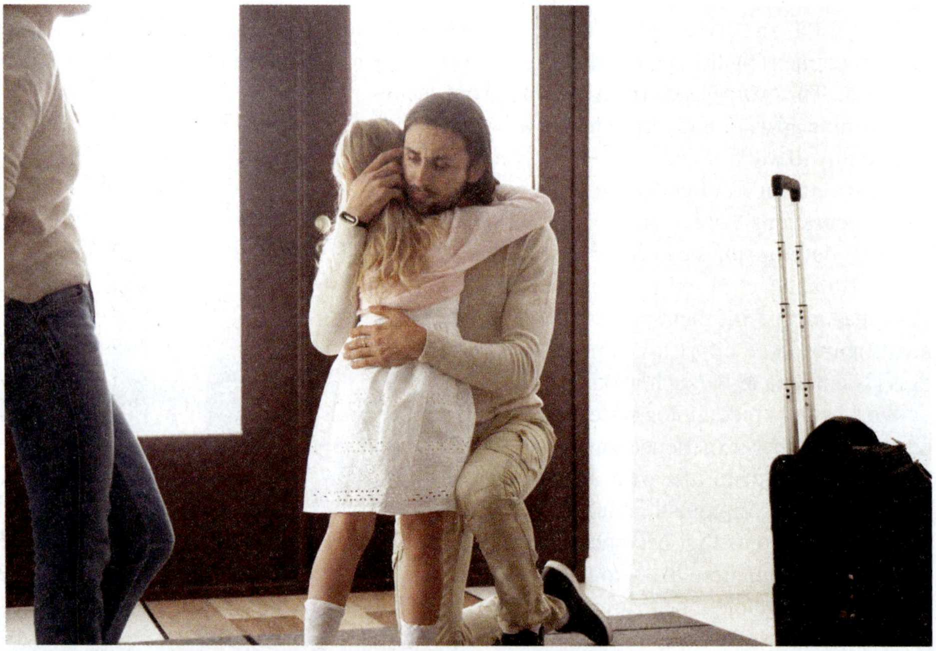

Children with separation anxiety disorder experience extreme distress when they are apart from their primary caregivers.
Aleksandr Davydov/Alamy Stock Photo

disorder, with estimates of its prevalence ranging from a low of 0.2 percent to a high of 2 percent and beginning between the ages of 3 and 6 years; frequency is equal among boys and girls (Kearney & Vecchio, 2007). Here is evidence to suggest a connection between selective mutism and autism spectrum disorder (Muris & Ollendick, 2021).

From a treatment standpoint, nonpharmacological interventions appear to be more acceptable to families of children with selective mutism. Efficacy data on these interventions, which include behavior therapy and cognitive behavioral therapy, have shown support, but a recent meta-analysis found that there are gaps in the literature. There are few randomized controlled trials, outcome measures show large variations, and the methods of delivery varied considerably such as whether the intervention was delivered at home, in the school, or both. Those remaining studies considered to have used acceptable methods show support for a combination of family systems and behavioral or cognitive behavioral interventions (Hipolito et al., 2023).

Specific Phobias

You can perhaps attest to the fact that it is common to have some fear of or at least a desire to avoid such things as spiders or situations with enclosed spaces or heights. In a **specific phobia**, however, the fear or anxiety is so intense that it becomes incapacitating. As is true for other anxiety disorders, there is a strong avoidance component to specific phobia. People with specific phobia go to great lengths to avoid the feared object or situation. If they can't get away, they endure the situation but only with marked anxiety and discomfort. Unlike an aversion or dislike for a given object, a specific phobia induces significant distress. Moreover, diagnosis requires that the phobia is not a fleeting condition but must be present for at least 6 months.

specific phobia
An irrational and unabating fear of a particular object, activity, or situation.

Although the possible varieties of specific phobias may seem endless, they fall into four major categories: insects and animals, the natural environment (storms or fires), blood-injection-injury (seeing blood, having an invasive medical procedure), and engaging in activities in particular situations (riding an escalator, flying). A fifth category includes a variety of miscellaneous stimuli or situations such as fear of vomiting.

Overall, the lifetime prevalence for specific phobia in the United States is 18.4 percent and 12-month prevalence is 12.1 (Kessler et al., 2012). The highest lifetime prevalence rates are for fear of natural situations, particularly heights, and are estimated to be between 3.1 and 5.3 percent. Animal phobia ranges in prevalence from 3.3 to 7 percent. That these are the two most common forms of specific phobia is indicated by the fact that among people with any form of specific phobia, 50 percent have a fear of animals or a fear of heights (LeBeau et al., 2010). A comparison of lifetime prevalence rates among 22 countries shows similar rates of 12.5 percent in the United States, Colombia, and Brazil, with the lowest rates in China (2.6 percent). Animal phobias are the most prevalent overall (3.8 percent), followed by fear of medical procedures (3.0 percent), then still water and weather events (2.3 percent). Worldwide, specific phobias were less prevalent in adults 60 and older than in younger people, and in men than in women (Wardenaar et al., 2017).

Theories and Treatment of Specific Phobias

Within the biological perspective, researchers believe the anxiety associated with specific phobias may relate to brain variations, potentially specific to a given phobia. For example, individuals with acrophobia (fear of heights) show altered functioning in the prefrontal (responsible for planning) and vision-related areas of the cortex (Hang et al., 2022). The amygdala, which moderates the fear response, also seems to play a role in specific phobias, particularly those acquired through learning in which people associate a given stimulus with the emotion of fear (Garcia, 2017).

Treatment of specific phobias following from the biological perspective focuses on symptom management through administration of benzodiazepines, but only if a client does not respond to other nonpharmacological treatments (Kimmel, Roy-Byrne, & Cowley, 2015). Unlike other forms of anxiety disorder, specific phobias are more circumscribed in nature and the situations are generally more easily avoided. Thus, clinicians would prescribe medications only when the specific phobia interferes with the individual's ability to carry out ordinary activities to such a degree that they cannot function on a daily basis or when psychological interventions fail to produce improvement.

The behavioral approach to specific phobias emphasizes the conditioning that occurs when the individual learns to associate unpleasant physical sensations with a certain kind of stimulus or situation. Behaviorists assume there may be some adaptive value to having such reactions, because the situations may truly be ones we should fear, such as poisonous snakes. The symptoms become maladaptive, according to this view, as individuals begin to generalize an appropriate fear reaction to all stimuli in that category, including harmless ones.

There are developmental aspects to specific phobias. Very young children tend to fear objects or situations they can see; as they get older, feared objects become more abstract in nature (such as "the bogeyman") (Davis & Ollendick, 2011). Further, older children may view the objects and situations they fear as more catastrophic than younger children with the same phobias do (Ollendick et al., 2017). Specific phobias in childhood may change, but it is also possible that they are predictive of generalized anxiety or panic disorder (Warner et al., 2023). At the other end of the age spectrum, older adults with specific phobias may not report symptoms but instead misattribute their anxiety to a physical condition (Coelho et al., 2010). It is also possible that, due to age-related changes in mobility, older adults develop a "fear of falling" that could reach the proportions of a specific phobia (Grenier et al., 2019).

According to the cognitive behavioral view, individuals with specific phobias have overactive alarm systems for danger, and they perceive things as dangerous because they misinterpret harmless stimuli. For example, the mistaken perception of an object or a situation as uncontrollable, unpredictable, dangerous, or disgusting is correlated with feelings of vulnerability. These attributions might explain the common phobia of spiders, a creature about which people have many misconceptions and apprehensions. In blood-injection-injury phobia, in contrast, disgust and fear of contamination play a prominent role (de Jong & Peters, 2007).

People with phobias also tend to overestimate the likelihood of a dangerous outcome after becoming exposed to the feared stimulus (de Jong & Merckelbach, 2000). They may be particularly likely to show what is called a "looming cognitive style" in which they unrealistically envision the threatening stimulus to be moving closer to them in time and space in rapid and uncontrollable escalation (Yeo, Hong, & Riskind, 2020).

Behavioral approaches to specific phobias focus on changing the symptoms by changing the ways in which individuals respond to the feared stimulus. In exposure therapy, positive reinforcement is used to lead clients to substitute adaptive responses (relaxation) for maladaptive ones (fear or anxiety). The four methods of exposure therapy vary in the way this basic procedure is carried out (see Table 1). Systematic desensitization presents the client with progressively more anxiety-provoking images while the client is being trained to relax. The idea is that the client cannot feel both anxious and relaxed at the same time, and that over the course of treatment, anxiety will be completely replaced with relaxation. A key component of this method, then, is **relaxation training**, a behavioral technique used in the

relaxation training
A behavioral technique used in the treatment of anxiety disorders that involves progressive and systematic patterns of muscle tensing and relaxing.

MINI CASE

Specific Phobia, Natural Environment

Aarman is a 32-year-old South Asian heterosexual cisgender man seeking treatment for his irrational fear of thunderstorms. He has had this phobia since age 4, and throughout life he has developed various strategies for coping with his fear. Whenever possible, he avoids going outside when a storm is forecast. Not only will he stay within a building, but he will ensure that he is in a room with no windows and no electrical appliances. As his job as a lawyer has grown in responsibility, Aarman has found that he can no longer afford to take time off because of his fear, which he knows is irrational.

TABLE 1 **Methods of Exposure Used in Behavioral Therapy of Phobias**

	Graduated Exposure	Immediate Full Exposure
Imagery	Systematic desensitization	Imaginal flooding
Live	Graded *in vivo*	*In vivo* flooding

treatment of anxiety disorders that involves progressive and systematic patterns of muscle tensing and relaxing.

In the behavioral technique called **flooding**, clients are totally immersed in the feared situation, where they feel the anxiety with full force. ***In vivo* flooding** exposes the client to the actual feared situation, such as the top floor of a tall building for a client who fears heights. Another variant of flooding is **imaginal flooding**, in which the clinician exposes the client virtually to the feared situation.

In vivo flooding is perhaps the most stressful of any of the treatments described and therefore has a high dropout rate (Choy, Fyer, & Lipsitz, 2007). An alternative is the **graded** *in vivo* method in which clients initially confront situations that cause only minor anxiety and then gradually progress toward those that cause greater anxiety. Often the therapist tries to be encouraging and to model the desired nonanxious response. In treating a client who has a fear of enclosed spaces, the therapist could go with the client into smaller and smaller rooms. Seeing the therapist showing no signs of fear could lead the client to model the therapist's response. The therapist could also offer praise to further reinforce the new response the client is learning. As illustrated in Table 1, behavioral treatments vary according to the nature of the client's exposure to the phobic stimulus (live or imaginal) and the degree of intensity with which the stimulus is confronted (immediate full exposure or exposure in graduated steps).

The most recently tested variant of exposure therapy uses **virtual reality exposure therapy (VRET)**, in which clients become immersed in computer-generated environments that resemble the situations they fear. Safer than *in vivo* therapy for obvious reasons and more realistic than imaginal methods, VRET would seem to be an ideal way to provide clients with experiences that can allow them to unlearn their fears, showing success in treatment of fear of heights and fear of spiders (Morina, Ijntema, Meyerbröker, & Emmelkamp, 2015) and blood-injury phobia (Jiang, Upton, & Newby, 2020). VRET can also be used to treat individuals who prefer virtual to physical exposure to the feared stimulus, or as a bridge between virtual to in vivo exposure (Scheveneels, De Witte, & Van Daele, 2023).

Cognitive behavioral therapy for specific phobias also has strong empirical support and has demonstrated effectiveness for at least 12 months after treatment (van Dis et al., 2020). However, the length of time required (6 to 12 weeks) can prove to be a deterrent in the treatment of children. A method known as **One Session Treatment (OST)**, also dependent on principles of CBT, was therefore developed as a more cost-effective approach to treatment of specific phobias in children. Although called "one session," OST takes place over two sessions, with the first devoted to assessment and treatment planning. In the second session (lasting 3 hours), the clinician provides a series of graded exposure tasks along with the setting of homework for clients to use on their own. Its efficacy plus cost-effectiveness makes OST a desirable option from a larger mental health standpoint in treating specific phobias (Wang et al., 2022).

flooding
A behavioral technique in which the client is immersed in the sensation of anxiety by being exposed to the feared situation in its entirety.

***in vivo* flooding**
A behavioral technique in which the client is immersed in the actual feared situation.

imaginal flooding
A behavioral technique in which the client is immersed through imagination into the feared situation.

graded *in vivo*
A procedure in which clients gradually expose themselves to increasingly challenging anxiety-provoking situations.

virtual reality exposure therapy (VRET)
A method of exposure therapy that uses virtual reality, in which clients become immersed in computer-generated environments that resemble the situations they fear.

One Session Treatment (OST)
A treatment for specific phobias in which cognitive behavioral therapy is condensed into one 3-hour session involving exposure and homework.

Social Anxiety Disorder

The primary feature of **social anxiety disorder** is a fear of becoming humiliated or embarrassed in front of other people. Extending beyond the ordinary concerns people may have about looking foolish or making a mistake during a performance, this disorder makes people anxious even at the prospect of eating or drinking in front of others. Thus, the fear is not

social anxiety disorder
An anxiety disorder characterized by marked, or intense, fear or anxiety in social situations in which the individual may be scrutinized by others.

What's in the *DSM-5-TR*

Definition and Categorization of Anxiety Disorders

The *DSM-5* unveiled major changes in the definition and categorization of anxiety disorders. Agoraphobia became a separate disorder, much as it is now in the *ICD-11*. In addition, social phobia in *DSM-IV-TR* was renamed social anxiety disorder. The change reflects the fact that social anxiety disorder is not a phobia in the sense of representing fear of other people. In the *DSM-5*, "social phobia" appeared in parentheses but this term was completely removed in the *DSM-5-TR*. The *DSM-5* moved obsessive-compulsive disorder (OCD) into the same category as body dysmorphic disorder, hoarding disorder, trichotillomania (excessive hair pulling), and skin picking. Acute and post-traumatic stress disorders moved into their own category of "Trauma- and Stressor-Related Disorders." Finally, several disorders formerly in the group that originated in childhood (a designation now dropped) were moved into the anxiety disorder grouping.

of other people (i.e., it is not a phobia), but rather of what other people may think of the individual. In *DSM-IV-TR,* the disorder was referred to as social phobia; it was renamed in *DSM-5* with "social phobia" in parentheses but this term was completely eliminated in the *DSM-5-TR*.

Social anxiety disorder has a lifetime prevalence of 13 percent in the United States with a 12-month prevalence of 7.4 percent (Kessler et al., 2012). Of those who develop this disorder over a 12-month period, nearly 30 percent have cases classified as severe (Kessler, Berglund, et al., 2005).

Theories and Treatment of Social Anxiety Disorder The biological underpinnings of social anxiety disorder may, some researchers believe, be related to partly heritable mechanisms (Stein & Gelernter, 2014). The intense anxiety experienced by an individual with social anxiety disorder, from this perspective, is essentially a form of intense shyness combined with the personality trait of neuroticism. These qualities in turn either cause or are caused by alterations in areas of the brain responsible for attention. Individuals with social anxiety disorder, according to this view, become excessively self-focused and therefore exaggerate the extent to which others look critically upon them.

Of the possible medications that can be used to treat social anxiety disorder, the selective serotonin or norepinephrine reuptake inhibitors (SSRIs and SNRIs) are regarded as having the greatest effectiveness. Other medications that may work as well have considerable drawbacks. Benzodiazepines have significant potential for abuse; moreover, they may actually interfere with treatment that includes psychological methods such as exposure to feared situations. MAOIs, which can also effectively manage social anxiety symptoms, have potentially dangerous side effects (Jorstad-Stein & Heimberg, 2009).

Among psychological approaches, the cognitive behavioral perspective regards people with social anxiety disorder as unable to gain a realistic view of how others really perceive them. Further, behavioral avoidance in social anxiety disorder causes individuals to avoid or suffer through various forms of social situations, thus perpetuating the fear response by blocking individuals with the disorder from gaining experience and confidence in social settings. As in other forms of cognitive behavioral therapy, the clinician working from this perspective attempts to reframe the client's thoughts in combination with real or imagined exposure.

Related to the cognitive behavioral approach is the view of social anxiety disorder as reflecting a core fear of interacting with new people in new situations. Rather than viewing the various symptoms of the disorder as having independent origins, researchers working within this network model believe the specific fears (such as being unable to look new

MINI CASE

Social Anxiety Disorder, Performance Only Type

Theo is a 19-year-old White bisexual transgender man. He is a sophomore in college and reports that he is terrified at the prospect of speaking in class. His anxiety is so intense that he enrolls only in very large lecture classes, where he sits in the back of the room, slouching in his chair to make himself as invisible as possible. On occasion, one of his professors randomly calls on students to answer certain questions. When this occurs, Theo begins to sweat and tremble. Sometimes he rushes from the classroom and frantically runs back to his dormitory for a few hours and tries to calm himself down.

people in the eye or to take a test in front of others) may all be interrelated via a central connection to that core fear of strangers. Following this approach, therapy would attempt to treat the core set of fears, which would then have a cascade effect on the more peripheral symptoms (Heeren & McNally, 2018).

Social anxiety disorder may also become manifest in new ways, with the changes caused by COVID-19 in the use of videocalls for both professional and social interactions. Because they can see themselves on the screen during one of these calls, people with this disorder can readily become overwhelmed by the feeling that others are negatively evaluating them. One possible intervention based on the cognitive behavioral approach is to encourage clients to focus on the positive aspects of their presentation rather than seeing themselves in only a negative light (Romano, Moscovitch, Saini, & Huppert, 2020).

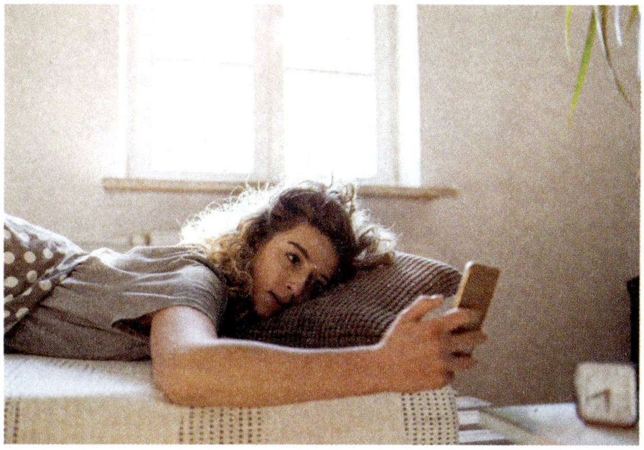

For individuals with social anxiety disorder, the use of smartphone apps that allow them to be seen by others can create increased stress.

pikselstock/Alamy Stock Photo

For clients who do not respond to psychotherapy or medication, there are promising signs about the benefits of alternate methods, including motivational interviewing, acceptance and commitment therapy, and mindfulness/meditation. Their common element, also present in CBT, is the practice of stepping back from situations to identify and challenge automatic thoughts (Kocovski et al., 2015). Mindfulness training, specifically, can also help reduce social anxiety symptoms by reducing an individual's bias toward seeing threat in social situations (Packard, Molloy, & Anderson, 2022).

Panic Disorder and Agoraphobia

In *DSM-IV-TR*, agoraphobia was not considered a diagnosis separate from panic disorder. The *DSM-5-TR*, consistent with emerging research and the *ICD*, now separates the two disorders, although the two diagnoses may both be assigned if the individual meets the criteria for both. Research findings tend to be reported in terms of the two disorders combined.

Panic Disorder

People with **panic disorder** experience periods of intense physical discomfort known as **panic attacks**. During a panic attack, the individual feels overwhelmed by highly unpleasant physical sensations that can include heart palpitations, respiratory distress (chest pain, shortness of breath, hyperventilation, feeling of choking), autonomic disturbances (sweating, nausea, stomach distress, shaking or trembling, heart palpitations), and sensory afflictions (dizziness, numbness, or tingling). They may feel that they are "going crazy" or losing control. Symptoms specific to culture, such as headache, uncontrollable screaming, or crying do not count toward the diagnosis.

panic disorder
An anxiety disorder in which an individual has panic attacks on a recurrent basis or has constant apprehension and worry about the possibility of recurring attacks.

panic attack
A period of intense fear and physical discomfort accompanied by the feeling that one is being overwhelmed and is about to lose control.

DSM-5-TR includes 13 specifiers for panic attacks that make it possible to clarify the nature of the symptoms the individual experiences, such as palpitations, sweating, trembling, chest pain, nausea, chills, fear of "going crazy," and fear of dying. Of these symptoms, palpitations and dizziness are the most commonly reported (Craske et al., 2010).

Having an occasional panic attack is not enough to justify a diagnosis of panic disorder. To meet the diagnostic criteria, the individual must experience panic attacks on a repeated basis and be accompanied by fear of having another. People with this disorder also might engage in avoidance behaviors, staying away from situations in which another panic attack might occur. The distress these individuals feel places them at elevated risk for suicide attempts and thoughts.

Agoraphobia

In **agoraphobia**, the individual feels intense fear or anxiety triggered by real or anticipated exposure to situations such as using public transportation, being in an enclosed space such as a theater or an open space such as a parking lot, and being outside the home alone. People with agoraphobia are fearful not of the situations themselves but of the possibility that they will either be unable to escape or get help, or that while there, they will fall or otherwise have embarrassing or incapacitating symptoms even though the actual

agoraphobia
Intense anxiety triggered by the real or anticipated exposure to situations in which individuals may be unable to get help should they become incapacitated.

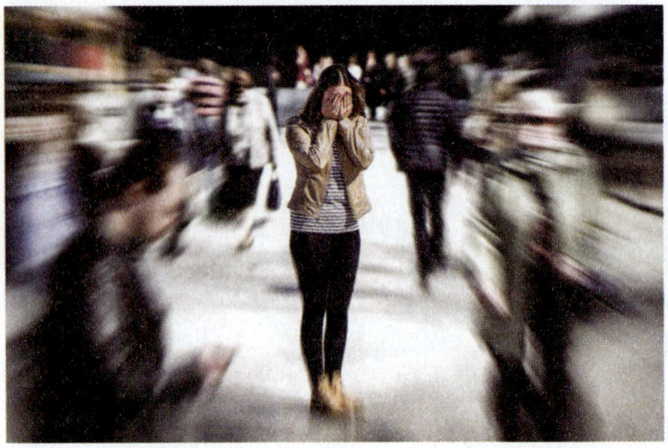

People with agoraphobia feel intense fear or anxiety when they feel they cannot escape crowded situations.

risk may be very small. If they cannot avoid the situation, they become highly anxious and fearful, and to cope, they might require the presence of a companion. As in other psychological disorders, these symptoms must persist over time (in this case, at least 6 months), cause considerable distress, and not be due to another psychological or medical disorder.

Panic attacks are somewhat common, in that they are estimated to occur in 20 percent or more of adults; panic disorder has a much lower lifetime prevalence of between 3 and 5 percent. Across a variety of studies, settings, and diagnostic criteria (from the *DSM-IV-TR*), one-quarter of those who have panic disorder with the agoraphobia syndrome would have met diagnostic criteria for agoraphobia alone (Wittchen et al., 2010). Depressive symptoms and substance use disorders may occur as a result of agoraphobia.

Theories and Treatment of Panic Disorder and Agoraphobia Researchers studying biological contributions to panic disorder focus on norepinephrine, the neurotransmitter that helps prepare the body to react to stressful situations. Higher levels of norepinephrine can make the individual more likely to experience fear, anxiety, and panic. Serotonin may also play a role in increasing a person's likelihood of developing panic disorder, as deficits in serotonin are linked to anxiety (Kalk, Nutt, & Lingford-Hughes, 2011). Heightened sensitivity in the areas of the brain involved in fear conditioning may further contribute to the panic disorder, leading individuals with this disorder to be less able to reverse the effects of conditioning through the behavioral process of extinction (Schwarzmeier et al., 2019).

anxiety sensitivity theory
The belief that panic disorder is caused in part by the tendency to interpret cognitive and somatic manifestations of stress and anxiety in a catastrophic manner.

Furthermore, according to **anxiety sensitivity theory**, people who develop panic disorder have heightened responsiveness to the presence of carbon dioxide in the blood. They are also more likely to panic due to their tendency to overestimate the seriousness of their sensations and underestimate their ability to cope with the situation (Cho, Choi, & Kim, 2021).

The most effective antianxiety medications for panic disorder and agoraphobia are benzodiazepines, which increase the availability of the inhibitory neurotransmitter GABA. However, because benzodiazepines can lead clients to become dependent on them or to abuse them, clinicians may prefer to prescribe SSRIs or SNRIs (Pollack & Simon, 2009).

Psychological perspectives consider predisposing factors involving personality and emotions as contributing to panic disorder and agoraphobia. Thus, people with panic disorder and agoraphobia may have personality traits that exacerbate their symptoms, including high levels of neuroticism and low levels of extraversion (Zugliani, Martin-Santos, Nardi, & Friere, 2017). Their tendency to ruminate, to prefer not to experience strong emotions, and to keep to themselves may serve to maintain their symptoms above and beyond whatever was their prior exposure to anxiety-provoking situations (Spinhoven, van Hemert, & Penninx, 2017).

conditioned fear reactions
Acquired associations between an internal or external cue and feelings of intense anxiety.

From a classical conditioning perspective, panic disorder results from **conditioned fear reactions** in which the individual associates bodily sensations such as difficulty breathing with memories of the last panic attack, causing a full-blown panic attack to develop.

MINI CASE

Panic Disorder and Agoraphobia

Frieda is a 31-year-old Latina heterosexual cisgender woman. She is a former delivery driver who sought treatment because of recurrent panic attacks that have led her to become fearful of driving. She has become so frightened of the prospect of having an attack on the job that she has asked for medical leave. Although initially she would leave the house when accompanied by her mother, she now is unable to go out under any circumstances, and her family is concerned that she will become a total recluse.

The cognitive behavioral model proposes that people with panic disorder, upon feeling the unpleasant sensations of the panic attack begin, believe it is unpredictable and uncontrollable and that they will not be able to stop it (White, Brown, Somers, & Barlow, 2006). CBT, accordingly, focuses on changing the ways that individuals interpret their bodily sensations during a panic attack. Effective in reducing panic disorder symptoms for as long as 31 years (Bilet, Olsen, Andersen, & Martinsen, 2020), CBT is also effective as an online treatment approach (Stech, Lim, Upton, & Newby, 2020). There may also be a role in the psychological treatment of panic disorder and agoraphobia of short-term psychodynamic therapy, with both methods shown to be efficacious in a large-scale review of randomized controlled treatments (Papola et al., 2022).

Generalized Anxiety Disorder

The key feature of **generalized anxiety disorder** is that, unlike the disorders you have learned about so far, the feelings of fear and dread that people with this disorder has no particular focus. People with generalized anxiety disorder feel anxious for much of the time, even though they may not be able to say exactly why they feel this way. In addition, they worry a great deal, apprehensively expecting the worst to happen to them. Their symptoms span a range of physical and psychological experiences including general restlessness, sleep disturbances, feelings of fatigue, irritability, muscle tension, and trouble concentrating or the mind going blank. There is no particular situation they can identify as lying at the root of their anxiety, and they find it difficult to control their worrying. Some individuals may worry about a few specific topics, based on life stressors, and others may have a more vague sense of worry and dread in general.

generalized anxiety disorder
An anxiety disorder characterized by anxiety and worry that is not associated with a particular object, situation, or event but seems to be a constant feature of a person's day-to-day existence.

Generalized anxiety disorder has a lifetime prevalence of 6.2 percent. Over a 12-month period, the prevalence is reported to be 2.9 percent; of these cases, 32 percent are classified as severe (Kessler et al., 2012). As noted in the *DSM-5-TR*, it can be very disabling, accounting for 110 million disability days per year in the entire U.S. population. It is also the most frequent psychological disorder associated with completed suicides.

There are differences between older and younger adults in the nature of generalized anxiety disorder. Older individuals worry more about their own health and family well-being, and young adults worry more about their own future and the health of other people. Older adults also show more sleep disturbances, are less likely to seek reassurance, and show higher rates and severity of depression accompanying their anxiety (Altunoz et al., 2018).

Theories and Treatment of Generalized Anxiety Disorder

Biologically based theories of generalized anxiety disorder focus on disturbances in the responses of the amygdala, the part of the brain involved in processing fear. Individuals with generalized anxiety disorder seem to be primed to anticipate negative events even when anticipating what other people may perceive as ambiguous. Researchers

MINI CASE

Generalized Anxiety Disorder

Jin is a 32-year-old Korean heterosexual cisgender woman and the single mother of two children. She is seeking professional help for her longstanding concerns about anxiety. Despite the fact that her personal and financial life are relatively stable, she worries most of the time that she will develop financial problems, that her children will become ill, and that the political situation in the country will make life for her and her children more difficult. Although she tries to dismiss these concerns as excessive, she finds it virtually impossible to control her worrying. Most of the time, she feels uncomfortable and tense, and sometimes her tension becomes so extreme that she begins to tremble and sweat. She finds it difficult to sleep at night. During the day she is restless, keyed up, and tense. She has consulted a variety of medical specialists, each of whom has been unable to diagnose a physical problem.

believe that this pre-programmed response to fear may have a genetic basis (Schienle, Hettema, Cáceda, & Nemeroff, 2011). Clinicians treating generalized anxiety disorder from the biological perspective rely on benzodiazepine medications. However, these come with risk for abuse and therefore should be administered with caution (McHugh et al., 2020).

The cognitive behavioral approach to generalized anxiety disorder builds on the assumption that the anxiety people with this disorder experience results from cognitive distortions in their interpretation of daily events, leading to excessive worrying. Clinicians using this approach attempt to break the cycle of negative thoughts and worries by helping clients learn how to recognize anxious thoughts, to seek more rational alternatives to worrying, and to take action to test these alternatives. Once the cycle of worry has been broken, the individual can develop a sense of control over the worrying behavior and become better able to manage and reduce anxious thoughts when they threaten to become overwhelming.

Another compounding factor in generalized anxiety disorder from the cognitive behavioral perspective is the individual's inability to tolerate uncertainty or ambiguity. People with this disorder seek to reduce uncertainty by trying to know exactly what will happen when, without taking into account the fact that it is not always possible to know the outcome of every situation. Cognitive behavioral therapy can be of benefit in helping individuals with the disorder come to accept such ambiguities (Bomyea et al., 2015). Behavioral therapy, as an alternative, includes uncertainty awareness training, in which clients learn to recognize when they are letting their worries about ambiguous situations lead them to catastrophize that the worst is about to happen to them (Hebert & Dugas, 2019).

Researchers are continuing to explore variations in the basic cognitive behavioral approach to give individuals a broader set of options. Acceptance and commitment therapy (ACT) is thought to have similar mechanisms to CBT and is gaining evidence as a standalone treatment for various anxiety disorders (Arch et al., 2012). Digitally based CBT provided through smartphone apps is also proving to have benefits and has the advantage of being deliverable on a more widespread basis than individually based CBT (Carl et al., 2020). However, clinicians should consider factors that can affect the outcome of combined ACT-CBT; older adults appear to benefit less from the combination than from CBT alone (Witlox et al., 2022).

8.2 Obsessive-Compulsive and Related Disorders

An **obsession** is a recurrent and persistent thought, urge, or image that the individual experiences as intrusive and unwanted. Individuals try to ignore or suppress the obsession or to neutralize it by engaging in some other thought or action. The thought or action the person uses to try to neutralize the obsession is known as a **compulsion**, a repetitive behavior or mental act the person feels driven to carry out according to rigid rules. Compulsions need not, however, be paired with obsessions.

In **obsessive-compulsive disorder (OCD)**, individuals experience either obsessions or compulsions to such an extent that they find it difficult to conduct their daily activities. As part of the disorder, they may experience significant distress or impairment in their ability to work and have a satisfying family or social life.

Rated as one of the top 10 debilitating disorders by the World Health Organization (Veale & Roberts, 2014), OCD has a lifetime prevalence in the United States estimated at 1.6 percent. The 12-month prevalence is slightly lower, 1 percent; of these cases, about half are classified as severe (Kessler, Berglund, et al., 2005). The 12-month prevalence of subthreshold OCD (cases not meeting all diagnostic criteria) is estimated at 4.5 percent, and for OCD symptoms at 8.3 percent (Adam, Meinlschmidt, Gloster, & Lieb, 2012). Individuals with OCD have a 14 percent risk of suicide attempts and 44 percent risk of suicidal thoughts according to the latest *DSM-5-TR* information.

The most common compulsions experienced by people with OCD are repeated behaviors such as washing and cleaning, counting items, putting items in order, checking, or requesting assurance. These compulsions may also take the form of mental rituals, such as

obsession
An unwanted thought, word, phrase, or image that persistently and repeatedly comes into a person's mind and causes distress.

compulsion
A repetitive and seemingly purposeful behavior performed in response to uncontrollable urges or according to a ritualistic or stereotyped set of rules.

obsessive-compulsive disorder (OCD)
A disorder characterized by recurrent obsessions or compulsions that are inordinately time consuming or that cause significant distress or impairment.

counting up to a certain number every time the individual has an unwanted thought. Some individuals with OCD experience tics, which are uncontrollable motor movements such as twitches, vocalizations, and facial grimaces.

Table 2 lists items from the Yale–Brown Obsessive-Compulsive Symptom Checklist, an instrument commonly used for assessing individuals with OCD. You can read through these items to get a sense of the types of thoughts and behaviors experienced by people with this disorder. Central dimensions that appear to run through these individual scales include incompleteness, or the feeling that something is not "just right," and the experience of disturbing or alarming thoughts (Cervin et al., 2021).

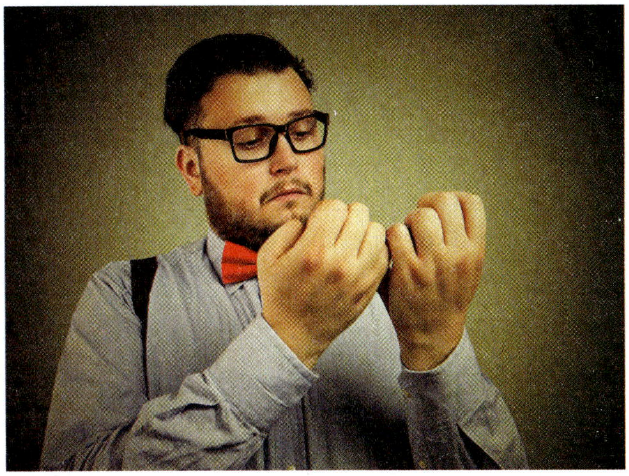

In one form of obsessive-compulsive disorder, individuals become preoccupied with dirt and must constantly engage in cleansing rituals.

Ivan Chiosea/Alamy Stock Photo

Theories and Treatment of Obsessive-Compulsive Disorder

Given the prominent role in OCD of motor movements such as cleaning and ordering, the biological basis for the disorder is thought to originate in variations in the basal ganglia, the subcortical areas of the brain active in motor control. Further contributing to the motor symptoms is failure of the prefrontal cortex to inhibit unwanted thoughts, images, or urges. Brain scan evidence supports these explanations, showing disrupted pathways in the brain's motor control centers involving the basal ganglia and frontal lobes (Liu et al., 2020).

Pharmacological treatments for OCD include SSRIs such as fluvoxamine or sertraline (Goodman, Storch, & Sheth, 2021). In extreme cases in which no other treatments provide symptom relief, people with OCD may be treated with psychosurgery. Deep-brain stimulation to areas active in motor control can help relieve symptoms by reducing the activity of the prefrontal cortex, which in turn may help reduce the frequency of obsessive-compulsive thoughts (Roth et al., 2020).

The cognitive behavioral perspective on OCD proposes that maladaptive thought patterns contribute to the development and maintenance of OCD symptoms. Individuals with OCD may be primed to overreact to anxiety-producing events in their environment. These experiences become transformed to disturbing images, which the individuals then try to suppress or counteract by engaging in compulsive rituals. CBT may be combined with exposure therapy. Given the disorder's effects on daily life, individuals with OCD can also benefit from family and couple therapy integrated into CBT (Stewart, Sumantry, & Malivoire, 2020).

Complicating their symptoms are beliefs about the danger and meaning of their thoughts, or their "metacognitions," which lead people with OCD to worry, ruminate, and feel they must monitor their every thought (Solem et al., 2009). People with OCD may also be high

MINI CASE

Obsessive-Compulsive Disorder, with Poor Insight

Cesar is a 16-year-old Latino cisgender male adolescent. He was referred for treatment by one of his teachers, who became disturbed by Cesar's irrational concern about the danger posed by an electrical outlet at the front of the classroom. Cesar pleaded daily with the teacher to have the outlet disconnected to prevent someone from accidentally getting electrocuted while walking by it. The teacher told Cesar his concerns were unfounded, but he remained so distressed that he felt driven, when entering and leaving the classroom, to shine a flashlight into the outlet to make sure a loose wire was not exposed. During class time, he could think of nothing else but the outlet.

TABLE 2 **Sample Items from the Yale–Brown Obsessive-Compulsive Symptom Checklist**

Scale	Sample Items
Aggressive obsessions	Fear of harming oneself Fear of blurting out obscenities Fear of being responsible for something else terrible happening (e.g., fire, burglary)
Contamination obsessions	Concerns or disgust with bodily waste or secretions (e.g., urine, feces, saliva) Bothered by sticky substances or residues
Sexual obsessions	Forbidden or perverse sexual thoughts, images, or impulses Sexual behavior toward others (aggressive)
Hoarding/saving obsessions	Worrying about throwing away seemingly unimportant things that might be needed in the future
Religious obsessions	Concerned with sacrilege and blasphemy Excess concern with right/wrong, morality
Obsession with need for symmetry or exactness	Accompanied by magical thinking (e.g., concerned that another will have an accident unless things are in the right place)
Miscellaneous obsessions	Fear of saying certain things Lucky/unlucky numbers Colors with special significance Superstitious fears
Somatic obsessions	Concern with illness or disease Excessive concern with body part or aspect of appearance (e.g., dysmorphophobia)
Cleaning/washing compulsions	Excessive or ritualized hand-washing Excessive or ritualized showering, bathing, toothbrushing, grooming, or toilet routine
Checking compulsions	Checking locks, stove, appliances, and so on Checking that nothing terrible did not/will not harm self Checking that did not make mistake completing a task
Repeating rituals	Rereading or rewriting Need to repeat routine activities (e.g., in/out door, up/down from chair)
Counting compulsions	Constantly counting objects for no actual reason
Ordering/arranging compulsions	Straightening out objects in ones living space and becoming upset if this order is disturbed
Hoarding/collecting compulsions	Picking up items that have no apparent usefulness
Miscellaneous compulsions	Excessive list making Need to tell, ask, or confess Need to touch, tap, or rub Rituals involving blinking or staring

SOURCE: Adapted from Goodman, W. K., Price, L. H., Rasmussen, S. A., Mazure, C., Delgado, P., Heninger, G. R., & Charney, D. S. (1989). The Yale-Brown Obsessive-Compulsive Scale II validity. *Archives of General Psychiatry, 46*, 1012–1016.

in the personality trait of perfectionism, a component of neuroticism, that can be thought of as a cognitive vulnerability unique to this disorder (Naragon-Gainey & Watson, 2018).

Cognitive behavioral therapy is currently regarded as the most effective treatment for OCD (Mc Donald et al., 2023). In addition to reducing target symptoms, cognitive behavioral therapy has beneficial effects on the individual's everyday quality of life (Carpenter et al., 2018). Exposure and response prevention are also considered first-line treatments; these expose clients to anxiety-inducing stimuli while preventing them from engaging in overt or covert rituals (Rector, Richter, Katz, & Leybman, 2019). Internet-based, self-guided CBT is also proving effective, allowing individuals with this disorder to overcome the treatment barriers posed by barriers such as shame, guilt, and fear of stigmatization (Schröder et al., 2020).

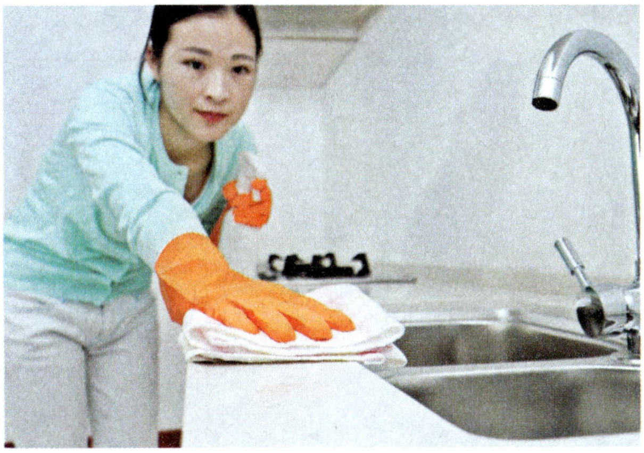

Some people with obsessive-compulsive disorder worry incessantly about germs and dirt and feel irresistible urges to clean and sanitize.

baona/iStock/Getty Images

Body Dysmorphic Disorder

People with **body dysmorphic disorder (BDD)** are preoccupied with the idea that a part of their body is ugly or defective. Their preoccupation goes far beyond the ordinary dissatisfaction many people feel about the size and shape of their body or appearance of a particular body part. People with BDD may check themselves constantly, groom themselves to an excessive degree, or constantly seek reassurance from others about how they look.

body dysmorphic disorder (BDD)
A disorder in which individuals are preoccupied with the idea that a part of their body is ugly or defective.

Repetitive behaviors, such as checking the mirror or seeking reassurance, are included as criteria for BDD, criteria not present prior to the *DSM-5*'s reclassification of BDD (Schieber, Kollei, de Zwaan, & Martin, 2015). Table 3 illustrates these types of repetitive behaviors seen in people with BDD, which include items from the Body Dysmorphic Disorder version of the Yale-Brown Obsessive-Compulsive Disorder Scale (BDD-YBOCS) (Phillips, Menard,

You Be the Judge

Psychosurgery

As you read in the chapter "Theoretical Perspectives," psychosurgery is increasingly being used to give clinicians a tool for controlling the symptoms of obsessive-compulsive disorder. However, to what extent is surgical intervention justifiable to control the occurrence of psychological symptoms? This surgery is not reversible.

The debate over psychosurgery goes back to the mid-twentieth century when physician Walter Freeman traveled around the United States, performing approximately 18,000 psychosurgeries in which he severed psychiatric patients' frontal lobes from the rest of their brains to control their unmanageable behaviors. Will future generations look upon psychosurgery and similar interventions as excessively punitive and even barbaric? On the other hand, with symptoms that are so severe and disabling, is any method that can control them valid even if imperfect?

Gillet (2011) raised these issues regarding the use of current forms of psychosurgery. By altering the individual's brain through such radical techniques, psychiatrists are tampering with a complex system of interactions that make up the individual's personality. Just because they "work" and no other methods are currently available, does this justify making permanent changes to the individual's brain? The victims of the leukotomies performed by Freeman "improved," in that their behavior became more docile, but they were forever changed.

Q: *You be the judge:* Is it appropriate to transform the person using permanent methods whose basis for effectiveness cannot be scientifically established? As Gillet (2011) concludes, "burn, heat, poke, freeze, shock, cut, stimulate or otherwise shake (but not stir) the brain and you will affect the psyche" (p. 43).

TABLE 3 Body Dysmorphic Disorder Modification of the Yale–Brown Obsessive-Compulsive Scale (BDD-YBOCS)

This modification of the Yale–Brown Obsessive-Compulsive Scale uses the following criteria to determine the severity of the client's symptoms regarding the presumed body defect or defects:

1. Time occupied by thoughts about body defect
2. Interference due to thoughts about body defect
3. Distress associated with thoughts about body defect
4. Resistance against thoughts about body defect
5. Degree of control over thoughts about body defect
6. Time spent in activities related to body defect such as mirror checking, grooming, excessive exercise, camouflaging, picking at skin, asking others about defect
7. Interference due to activities related to body defect
8. Distress associated with activities related to body defect
9. Resistance against compulsions
10. Degree of control over compulsive behavior
11. Insight into the nature of excessive concern over defect
12. Avoidance of activities due to concern over defect

SOURCE: Phillips, K. A., et al. (1997). Body dysmorphic disorder modification of the Y-Bocs (Bdd-Ybocs). http://www.veale.co.uk/wp-content/uploads/2010/11/BDD-YBOCS-Adult.pdf

Fay, & Pagano, 2005), a measure found to satisfy psychometric criteria of validity and reliability (Patel et al., 2023).

As many as 87 percent of women are dissatisfied with some aspect of their body's appearance (Mond et al., 2013). Overall, however, at any one point in time, the prevalence of BDD is a much lower 1.9 percent across groups of different ages. Estimates place the prevalence at as high as 13 percent of patients seen in general cosmetic surgery practices (Veale, Gledhill, Christodoulou, & Hodsoll, 2016).

BDD is frequently accompanied by major depressive disorder, social anxiety disorder, obsessive-compulsive disorder, and eating disorders. The distress clients experience clearly can become intense. People with BDD have higher risk of suicidal thoughts and suicide attempts, particularly if they also have other major psychological disorders (Angelakis, Gooding, & Panagioti, 2016).

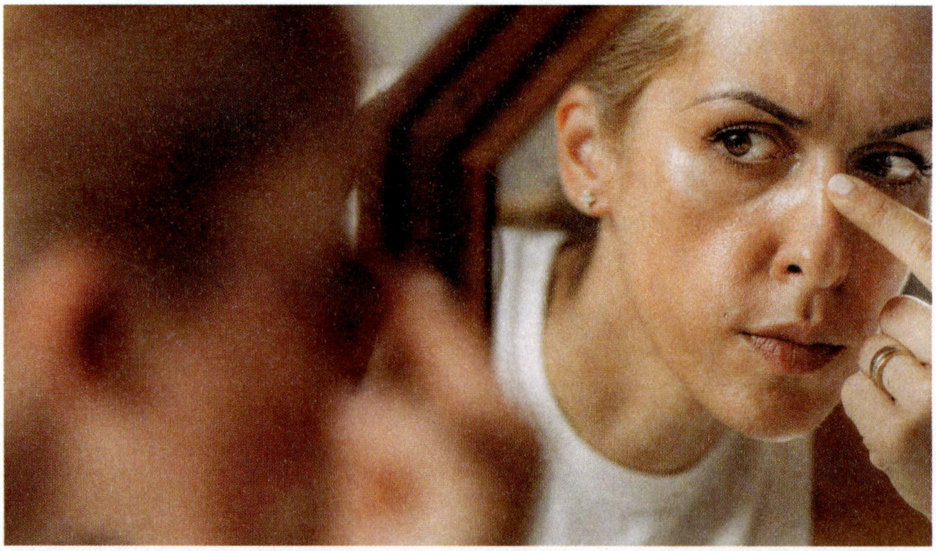

Caption: Individuals with body dysmorphic disorder become preoccupied with what they believe is their flawed appearance.

MICROGEN IMAGES/SCIENCE PHOTO LIBRARY/Alamy Stock Photo

MINI CASE

Body Dysmorphic Disorder, with Poor Insight

Lydia is a 63-year-old White lesbian cisgender woman whose local surgeon referred her to an outpatient mental health clinic. For the past 8 years, Lydia has visited plastic surgeons across the country to find one who will perform surgery to reduce the size of her hands, which she perceives as "too fat." Until she has this surgery, she will not leave her house without wearing gloves. The plastic surgeon concurs with Lydia's family members and friends that Lydia's perception of her hands is distorted and that plastic surgery would be inappropriate and irresponsible.

BDD has cross-cultural aspects. In Japan, the belief that physical appearance is offensive to others is called *shubo-kyufo*, a subtype of *taijin kyofusho* or "fear of interpersonal relations." The syndrome *koro* or *suoyang* ("disappearance of the penis" in Chinese) includes other BDD symptoms as well (Fang & Hofmann, 2010).

Treatment of BDD from a biological perspective includes medications, particularly SSRIs, that can reduce the associated symptoms of depression and anxiety as well as the more obsessive symptoms of distress, bodily preoccupations, and compulsions. Once on SSRIs, people with BDD can experience improved quality of life and overall functioning and perhaps gain insight into their disorder (Bjornsson, Didie, & Phillips, 2010).

Psychological and sociocultural perspectives focus on experiential and cultural contributions to BDD. For example, individuals may develop unusual sensitivity about their appearance as the result of teasing by peers during a time when their identities were in a critical period of formation. Once they start to believe that their bodily appearance is defective or deviates from the ideal to which they aspire, they become preoccupied with this belief, setting off a series of dysfunctional thoughts and repetitive behaviors. Their selective attention to this presumably unattractive body part is accompanied by the belief that no one could possibly like them, which in turn can lead them to avoid social situations and engage in rituals such as looking in the mirror and frequently studying this imagined defect. Adding to their distress can be the use of social networking sites that focus primarily on bodily appearance (Ryding & Kuss, 2020).

Clinicians treating clients with BDD from a cognitive behavioral perspective focus on helping them to understand that appearance is only one aspect of their total identity, while challenging them to question their assumptions that their appearance is, in fact, defective. The clinician may also help these individuals realize that other people looking at them may not even be thinking about their appearance at all, or if so, not critically (Fang & Wilhelm, 2015).

Acceptance-based approaches, such as acceptance and commitment therapy (ACT), provide a specific route to addressing feelings of shame, thought to be an important component of body dysmorphic disorder. In ACT, clients learn to weaken the influence of self-critical thoughts that can contribute to shame. Compassion-focused therapy (CFT) adds the element of self-compassion, helping clients become able to cultivate feelings of warmth and a sense of kindness toward themselves (Linde et al., 2023). The ability to be mindful about self-critical thoughts and feelings, and then cultivate self-compassion can thus help reduce feelings of shame especially with regard to body image.

From a sociocultural perspective, factors such as feelings of lack of acceptance by members of marginalized groups may serve as risk factors for BDD. Examining the role of specific stressors in a sample of gay men, researchers identified the risk factors of fear of rejection, sexual orientation concealment, internalized homophobia, and discrimination/prejudice, finding rates of BDD symptoms at nearly 50 percent (Oshana, Klimek, & Blashill, 2020).

Hoarding Disorder

In **hoarding disorder**, people have persistent difficulties discarding or parting with their possessions, even those that are not of much value. These difficulties include any form of discarding, including putting items into the garbage. People with hoarding disorder believe

hoarding disorder
A disorder in which people have persistent difficulties discarding things, even if they have little value.

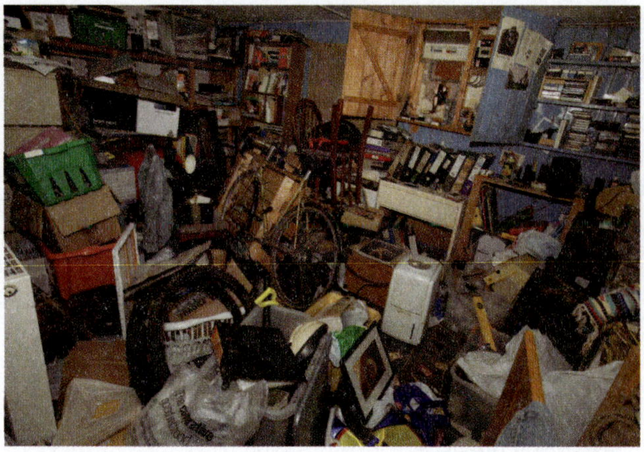

In extreme cases of hoarding disorder, individuals can accumulate literally mountains of clutter filled with items that no longer are of any use.

Simon Cook/Alamy Stock Photo

these items have utility or aesthetic or sentimental value, but in reality they often consist of items with no actual worth such as old newspapers, bags, or leftover food.

When faced with the prospect of discarding the items, these individuals become distressed, while their homes can become unlivable due to the clutter that accumulates over the years. The rooms fill up with a mixture of objects that actually are of value and items that ordinarily would be thrown away, such as old magazines. Unlike ordinary collectors, who organize their items in a systematic way, people with hoarding disorder accumulate items without any form of organization.

Because the disorder became a diagnosis on its own in *DSM-5*, the only prevalence data available are the estimates the authors cite, from 2 to 6 percent of adults. Prior work suggests that a substantial percentage of adults with hoarding disorder also have comorbid depressive symptoms (Hall, Tolin, Frost, & Steketee, 2013). Older adults who develop hoarding disorder are likely to become physically and cognitively impaired, experiencing significant effects on their daily functioning (Ayers, Najmi, Mayes, & Dozier, 2015). Hoarding also appears cross-culturally, but clinicians need to take into account the extent to which a culture values thrift and storing of possessions, according to the *DSM-5-TR*.

A biopsychosocial approach appears to be most effective in treating hoarding disorder. Biological treatments have traditionally included SSRIs, but these have mixed effectiveness. There may be a neurocognitive component that warrants treatments through addressing cognitive function. Hoarding disorder is also becoming understood from a developmental perspective as reflecting adverse life experiences in childhood, and in later adulthood from stressful life events (Chia et al., 2021).

Taking all possible contributions into account, CBT is considered the gold standard of treatment (Lin et al., 2023). Home visits in which the therapist uses cognitive behavioral methods can show beneficial effects in as short as a 12-week treatment period (Rowa et al., 2020). Compassion-focused therapy can also be used effectively through its facilitation of the de-shaming of individuals with hoarding disorder. Such an approach can also prove of use for clients who do not respond to CBT (Chou et al., 2020).

One important caution in the treatment of hoarding disorder involves what are called "involuntary clean-outs." If you have ever watched an episode of one several popular television series on hoarders, this method may seem like a viable approach. However, researchers warn that not only is this an ineffective approach, but it is also one that can be highly traumatic for the client. To reduce the harm when the individual's living situation has become unsafe, community workers can engage the individual in reducing clutter through active decision-making (Kysow, Bratiotis, Lauster, & Woody, 2020).

Trichotillomania (Hair-Pulling Disorder)

trichotillomania (hair-pulling disorder)
An impulse-control disorder involving the compulsive, persistent urge to pull out one's own hair.

A diagnosis of **trichotillomania (hair-pulling disorder)** is given to individuals who pull out their hair in response to an increasing sense of tension or urge. After they pull their hair, they feel temporary relief, pleasure, or gratification. People with trichotillomania are upset by their uncontrollable behavior and may find that their social, occupational, or other areas of functioning are impaired because of the disorder. They feel unable to stop the behavior, even when it results in irreversibly bald patches and lost eyebrows, eyelashes, and bodily hair including pubic hair.

The hair pulling may be automatic, in which the individual is unaware of the behavior, or focused in which they do so intentionally as a way to reduce the hair-pulling urge. Individuals who fall into the automatic category experience pronounced stress and anxiety.

The Trichotillomania Symptoms Questionnaire (see Table 4) provides you with an idea of the behaviors associated with this disorder (Shusterman, Feld, Baer, & Keuthen, 2009).

Focused hair pullers are more likely to pull from their eyelashes. Certain environmental triggers may precipitate the hair pulling, with common settings including the bathroom, bedroom, work, school classrooms, and while engaged in such activities as driving, reading, watching television, and studying. Tweezers are the most common forms of hair pulling, and a high percentage do so in front of a mirror. Surveys on trichotillomania interestingly reveal that online responders are more likely to endorse hair pulling from their pubic areas, as well as cheek, chin, nose, pets, and other people. Perhaps surprisingly, older individuals are more likely to pull from their scalp (Barber et al., 2023).

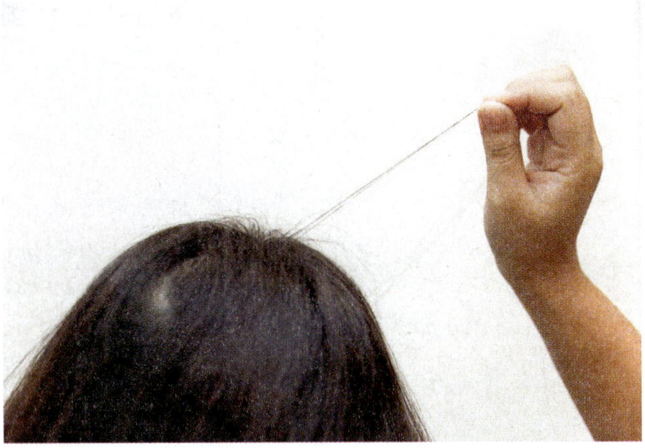
People with trichotillomania engage in frequent hair pulling, often without awareness or feeling they can control the behavior.
Quality Stock/Alamy Stock Photo

People with this disorder experience significant impairment in areas of life ranging from sexual intimacy to social activities, medical examinations, and haircuts. They can also develop skin infections, scalp pain or bleeding, and carpal tunnel syndrome. Psychologically, they may experience low self-esteem, shame and embarrassment, depressed mood, irritability, and argumentativeness. Those who also eat the hair they pull can develop hairballs, which settle in their gastrointestinal tract and cause abdominal pain, nausea and vomiting, weakness, and weight loss.

Diagnosable trichotillomania is relatively rare, with an estimated 1.7 percent of adults and occurs equally in men and women, although it develops later in men (age 19 years) than women (age 15 years). Those with this disorder are also likely to have comorbidities with a range of disorders including anxiety, depression, OCD, PTSD, ADHD (Grant, Dougherty, & Chamberlain, 2020), and hazardous alcohol use (Grant, Collins, Chesivoir, & Chamberlain, 2023). Additionally, trichotillomania is associated with significantly reduced quality of life across a number of important domains including health, relationships, home, goals and values, and self-esteem (Valle & Grant, 2022).

Genetics seems to play an important role in trichotillomania, with an estimate of 80 percent heritability of the disorder (Novak, Keuthen, Stewart, & Pauls, 2009). Researchers have also identified variations in *SAPAP3*, a gene related to glutamate, which in turn is implicated in obsessive-compulsive disorder (Zuchner et al., 2009). The neurotransmitters serotonin, dopamine, and glutamate are, in turn, thought to play a role in the development of trichotillomania (Duke et al., 2009). Brain imaging studies of individuals with trichotillomania suggest the presence of variations in white matter in the regions active in cognitive and emotional processing along with deficits in cortical control over the motor movements involved in hair pulling (Uhlmann et al., 2020).

The behavioral treatment of habit reversal training (HRT) is regarded as the most effective approach to treating trichotillomania. HRT appears to have its greatest efficacy when combined with another method known as "decoupling." In this method, the hair pulling is performed in proximity to the area where the client carries it out but is instructed to move quickly in another direction to deviate from the original target. Decoupling can also be conducted using imagery rather than at the site of the hair pulling (Moritz et al., 2023).

MINI CASE

Trichotillomania (Hair-Pulling Disorder)

Audra is a 15-year-old White cisgender adolescent female. For most of her childhood and adolescence, she lived a fairly isolated existence with no close friends. Although she never discussed her unhappiness with anyone, she often felt depressed and hopeless. As a young child, Audra lay in bed on many nights secretly tugging at her hair. Over time, this behavior increased to the point at which she plucked the hair, strand by strand, from her scalp. Typically, she pulled out a hair, examined it, bit it, and either threw it away or swallowed it. Because her hair was thick and curly, her hair loss was not initially evident, and Audra kept her hair carefully combed to conceal the bald spots. One of her teachers noticed that she was pulling her hair in class, however, and in looking more closely, she saw the bald patches on Audra's head. She referred Audra to the school psychologist, who called Audra's mother and recommended professional help.

TABLE 4 Trichotillomania Symptoms Questionnaire

1. Do you currently pull your hair out?
2. At any point in your life, including now, have you had periods of uncontrollable hair pulling?
3. Do you (or did you in the past) experience urges to pull your hair out?
4. Do you (or did you in the past) try to resist pulling your hair out?
5. Do you (or did you in the past) feel relief when pulling your hair out?
6. Do you (or did you in the past) wish that the urge to pull your hair out would go away?
7. Have you been diagnosed with trichotillomania by a professional?
8. Do you, or did you in the past, feel shame, secrecy, or distress about your hair pulling?

SOURCE: Shusterman et al., (2009). Affective regulation in trichotillomania: Evidence from a large-scale internet survey. *Behaviour Research and Therapy*. Volume 47, Issue 8, August 2009, Pages 637–644.

There are two common core elements in HRT as a treatment of trichotillomania (McGuire et al., 2020). Awareness training helps the client learn to identify the situations in which the hair pulling occurs, such as when stressed at work. The second element is competing response training, in which the individual learns a new response to compete with the habit of hair pulling, such as fist clenching. The key feature is that the new response is incompatible with the undesirable habit.

When it was first developed several decades ago, HRT was given for only one session. Since that time, clinicians have extended the length of treatment and added several cognitive components, including self-monitoring and cognitive restructuring. For example, clients may learn to challenge their cognitive distortions such as their perfectionistic beliefs. Dialectical behavior therapy (DBT) may add to these methods a combination of mindfulness training, in which clients learn to identify the cues that trigger their hair pulling, and imagery training, in which they visualize themselves in a tranquil state (Snorrason, Berlin, & Lee, 2015).

Combining acceptance and commitment therapy (ACT) with HRT is also shown to produce relief from hair-pulling symptoms. Cognitive behavioral therapy can help in treating children and adolescents with trichotillomania, with very little alteration from the basic protocol used for adults. An advantage of ACT for this disorder is that it can be administered along with cognitive behavioral treatment in a group format, with results as effective as those obtained with individual therapy (Haaland et al., 2017).

Although trichotillomania can be a highly disabling condition, there is promise in the range of therapies based on behavior therapy, cognitive behavioral therapy, and the newer approaches that help individuals identify and cope with the feelings associated with the behavior.

Excoriation (Skin-Picking) Disorder

excoriation (skin-picking) disorder
Recurrent picking at one's own skin.

Individuals are regarded as having **excoriation (skin-picking) disorder** if they repeatedly pick at their own skin. The skin picking may be of healthy skin, skin with mild irregularities (such as moles), pimples, calluses, or scabs from previous picking. People with this disorder pick at these bodily areas either with their own fingernails or with instruments such as tweezers. When they are not picking their skin, they think about picking it and try to resist their urges to do so. The skin picking must lead to lesions to be diagnosable. They may attempt to cover lesions due to skin picking with clothing or bandages, and they feel ashamed of and embarrassed about their behavior.

Because this is a new diagnosis, epidemiological data are limited, but *DSM-5-TR* estimates the lifetime prevalence at 3 percent based on online survey data. Although researchers believe skin picking is valid as a distinct diagnosis from trichotillomania (Lochner, Grant, Odlaug, & Stein, 2012), the two disorders share causes and effective treatment approaches (Snorrason, Belleau, & Woods, 2012). Additionally, personality factors may play a role in both disorders, including such traits as perfectionism and impulsiveness, as well as inattention and hyperactivity (Grant et al., 2021).

There are two types of excoriation disorder, resting along a continuum of severity (Grant et al., 2020). In the first, people pick their skin as a result of strong and frequent emotional urges over which they have little control. The second subtype has less severe symptoms, and people with it experience little distress associated with skin picking.

Treatment options for individuals with excoriation disorder are similar to those recommended for people with trichotillomania. Behavioral approaches include HRT, both alone and combined with ACT (Lochner, Roos, & Stein, 2017). Unfortunately, people with excoriation disorder may fail to benefit from the help that treatment could provide from psychotherapy due to feelings of shame about their disorder (Gallinat et al., 2019).

8.3 Trauma- and Stressor-Related Disorders

Individuals who are exposed to trauma or a stressful event may be at risk for developing a psychological disorder as shown in Figure 2 (Nakama et al., 2023). The category of trauma- and stressor-related disorders has as a diagnostic criterion the condition of an actual event that acts as a precipitant. *DSM-5* included disorders in this group that were originally in their own category within the anxiety disorders and also placed into this category a set of disorders in childhood that can be traced to exposure to stress or trauma. *DSM-5-TR* maintains this classification.

Reactive Attachment Disorder and Disinhibited Social Engagement Disorder

Reactive attachment disorder (RAD) is a diagnosis given to children involving a consistent pattern of inhibited, emotionally withdrawn behavior toward adult caregivers along with minimal responsiveness to others and limited positive affect. According to the *DSM-5-TR*, children with this disorder appear to have lost the ability to turn to attachment figures for comfort, support, protection, and nurturance.

The diagnosis of **disinhibited social engagement disorder** describes an opposite situation in which a child with a history of trauma engages in culturally inappropriate, overly familiar behavior with people who are relative strangers.

These disorders are placed among the trauma- and stressor-related disorders because they are found in children who have experienced an abuse pattern of social neglect, repeated changes of primary caregivers, or rearing in institutions with high child-to-caregiver ratios. Consequently, such children are significantly impaired in their ability to interact with other children and adults.

reactive attachment disorder (RAD)
A diagnosis given to children involving a consistent pattern of inhibited, emotionally withdrawn behavior toward adult caregivers along with minimal responsiveness to others and limited positive affect.

disinhibited social engagement disorder
Diagnosis given to children who engage in culturally inappropriate, overly familiar behavior with people who are relative strangers.

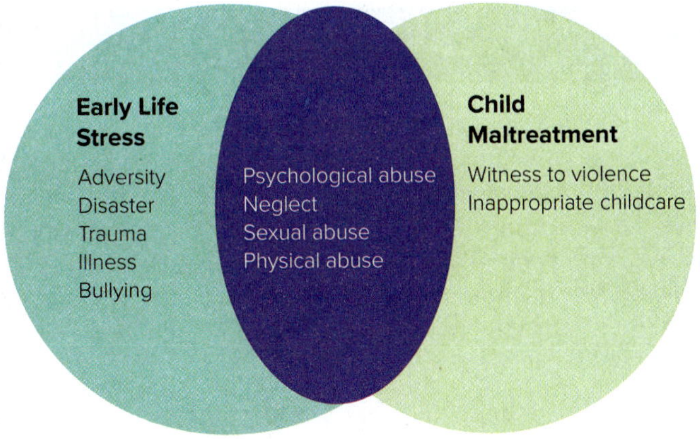

FIGURE 2 Early childhood stress, maltreatment, and abuse can increase the risk of an individual's developing a trauma- and stress-related disorder.

SOURCE: Nakama, N., Usui, N., Doi, M., & Shimada, S. (2023). Early life stress impairs brain and mental development during childhood increasing the risk of developing psychiatric disorders. *Progress in Neuro-Psychopharmacology & Biological Psychiatry*, 126, 1-8. https://doi.org/10.1016/j.pnpbp.2023.110783

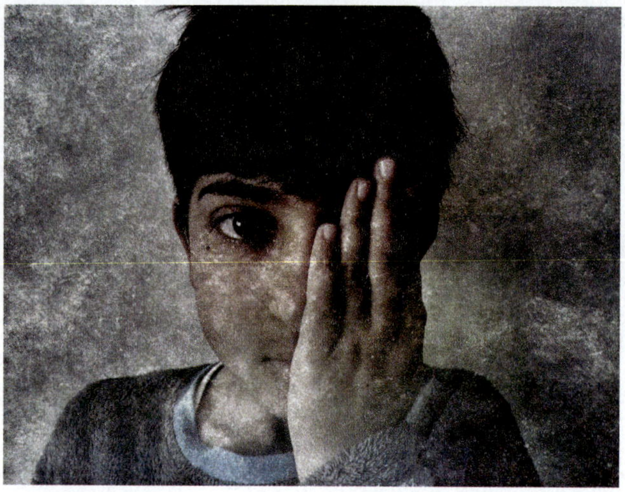

Children who are maltreated may experience lasting effects including disorders of attachment.

itanistock / Stockimo/Alamy Stock Photo

Children with reactive attachment disorder have also received poorer caregiving and are more likely to have insecure attachment styles as they grow older (Gleason et al., 2011). These effects can persist for years, lingering until at least the age of 12 (Humphreys, Nelson, Fox, & Zeanah, 2017) and placing the individual at risk for the development of other forms of psychopathology including alcohol and drug misuse (Seim et al., 2020). Additionally, their early exposure to maltreatment in the form of oppression and abuse can have lasting impact on brain development, as shown in studies on animal models. Some of these effects have also been observed in human studies including diminished volume of the frontal cortex and hippocampus, leading to long-term deficits in cognition and social skills (Nakama, Usui, Doi, & Shimada, 2023).

There are underlying similarities in the origins of the two disorders. Nevertheless, research supports the distinction between them and hence their conceptualization by *DSM-5-TR* as separate dimensions of psychopathology in childhood (Lehmann et al., 2015).

trauma
Response experienced by an individual to an event that is harmful or life threatening that can have lasting adverse effects on the individual's functioning and mental health.

acute stress disorder
An anxiety disorder that develops after a traumatic event, and lasts for up to 1 month with symptoms such as depersonalization, numbing, dissociative amnesia, intense anxiety, hypervigilance, and impairment of everyday functioning.

post-traumatic stress disorder (PTSD)
A disorder in which an individual exposed to a traumatic event continues to experience a range of distressing symptoms for more than a month that include reexperiencing the traumatic event, avoidance of reminders of the trauma, numbing of general responsiveness, and increased arousal.

Acute Stress Disorder and Post-Traumatic Stress Disorder

Trauma is a psychological response to an event that is harmful or life threatening, and can have lasting adverse effects on the individual's functioning and mental health. When people are exposed to the threat of death, or to actual or threatened serious injury, or sexual violation, they risk developing **acute stress disorder**. Being exposed to the death of others, or to any of these events, real or threatened, to others can also lead to the development of this disorder. For example, first responders to the scene of an accident or police officers who are regularly exposed to the details of child abuse cases may also experience this disorder.

The symptoms of acute stress disorder fall into four categories: intrusion of distressing reminders of the event, dissociative symptoms such as feeling numb or detached from others, avoidance of situations that might serve as reminders of the event, and hyperarousal including sleep disturbances or irritability. The symptoms may persist for a few days to a month after the traumatic event.

The events that can cause acute stress disorder may lead to the longer-lasting disorder known as **post-traumatic stress disorder (PTSD)**. If the individual experiences acute stress disorder symptoms for more than a month, the clinician assigns the PTSD diagnosis. The intrusions, dissociation, and avoidance seen in acute stress disorder are also present in PTSD. Symptoms also include loss of memory of the event, excessive self-blame, distancing from others, and inability to experience positive emotions.

The diagnosis of PTSD has a long history. In World Wars I and II, the condition was referred to with such terms as *shell shock*, *traumatic neurosis*, *combat stress*, and *combat*

MINI CASE

Acute Stress Disorder

Brendan is a 40-year-old White heterosexual cisgender man. He had no prior history of mental health concerns until 2 weeks ago when he survived a wildfire that destroyed his apartment and many buildings in his neighborhood. Since the fire Brendan has been tormented by graphic images of waking to see his room filled with smoke. Although he was treated and released within several hours from the emergency room, he described himself as feeling in a daze, emotionally unresponsive to the concerns of his friends and family, and seemingly numb. He continued to experience these symptoms for several weeks, after which they gradually subsided.

fatigue. Survivors of European concentration camps in the 1930s and 1940s also were reported to suffer long-term psychological effects, including chronic depression, anxiety, and difficulties in interpersonal relationships due to guilt over having survived when so many others were killed.

The lifetime prevalence of PTSD is 6.8 percent, with a yearly prevalence of 3.5 percent. Of those who develop PTSD within a given year, 37 percent experience severe symptoms (Kessler, Berglund, et al., 2005). Among U.S. Army soldiers returning from Afghanistan, 6.2 percent met the PTSD diagnostic criteria, and more than double that rate, 12.9 percent, was seen among soldiers returning from Iraq (Hoge et al., 2004). It is estimated that nearly 17 percent of Iraq War veterans meet the screening criteria for this disorder (Hoge et al., 2007).

Women exposed to trauma during their military service are more likely to develop PTSD after the trauma of sexual assault. Women exposed to combat-related trauma and sexual assault show a cumulatively higher risk of developing both PTSD and substance use disorders (Yalch, Hebenstreit, & Maguen, 2018). Among veterans who are men, being LGBTQ+ is another risk factor for PTSD. During their service these individuals had a higher risk of exposure to sexual trauma than other veterans, and correspondingly higher rates of PTSD (Shipherd et al., 2021).

The symptoms of PTSD and related disorders, such as depression, can persist for many years. For example, survivors of the North Sea oil rig disaster in 1980 continued to experience symptoms of PTSD along with anxiety disorders (not including PTSD), depressive disorders, and substance use disorders that were significantly higher than those of a matched comparison group (Boe, Holgersen, & Holen, 2011). Furthermore, individuals who were previously exposed to trauma are more likely to experience thoughts of suicide after exposure to a second traumatic event such as a natural disaster (Brown et al., 2018).

The COVID-19 pandemic has the potential to create large-scale, lasting traumatic reactions, particularly among front-line health care workers treating seriously ill patients under highly stressful conditions. Among medics working in Wuhan, China, in December 2019, as many as 32 percent showed PTSD symptoms when surveyed in early April 2020 (Li et al., 2020). In the United States, combat veterans with PTSD can be considered at heightened risk as well for COVID-19–related PTSD (Haderlein et al., 2020). Older adults with chronic PTSD may also be at heightened risk for exacerbation of their symptoms due to the stressors and social isolation associated with the pandemic (Rutherford et al., 2020).

Exposure to natural disasters in childhood and adolescence can become a risk factor for PTSD for as long as 2 years following such events. One meta-analysis found that between the years of 1981 and 2019, young people who were victims of floods and earthquakes in events around the world, particularly girls, were as high as 20 percent in follow-ups conducted for up to 2 years after the traumatic event (Rezayat et al., 2020).

complex post-traumatic stress disorder
Diagnosis in *ICD-11* used to apply to individuals who suffer prolonged exposure to severe stressors or multiple and repeated adverse events from which they cannot escape.

Recognizing that some individuals with PTSD experience symptoms due to prolonged exposure to severe stressors, the *ICD-11* adds the diagnosis known as **complex post-traumatic stress disorder**. People with complex PTSD develop the disorder as the result of exposure to such multiple and repeated stressors as torture, slavery, genocide campaigns, prolonged domestic violence, or repeated childhood sexual or physical abuse. Children who are victims of human trafficking, for example, may show complex PTSD symptoms as well as somatic symptoms such as headaches, backaches, and digestive disturbances (Ottisova, Smith, & Oram, 2018).

PTSD may also be experienced by individuals in other contexts who are exposed to some type of traumatic experience. One study of chronic substance users in rural counties in northern New England found that 84 percent reported experiencing probable symptoms of PTSD after witnessing an overdose (Nolte et al., 2023). Chronic food insecurity may also become a stressor that can precipitate PTSD, with an estimated prevalence in one low socioeconomic status, Latino/Hispanic sample amounting to, among the nearly half experiencing a trauma-related experience, 17.4 percent (Marshall et al., 2023).

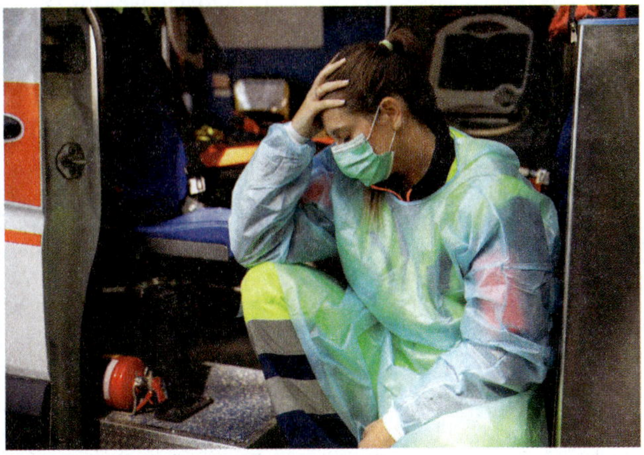

First responders, as shown in this photo of a health care worker during the COVID-19 pandemic, can themselves experience signs of stress disorder.

loreanto/Shutterstock

Individuals in various professions that place them in potentially traumatic situations can also be at risk for PTSD. In a study of Belgian police officers, 93 percent described one episode involving a shooting incident or being the victim of physical violence as traumatic, and as many as 5.9 percent reported symptoms classified as PTSD or complex PTSD (Rentmeesters & Hermans, 2023). Canadian lawyers, in another study, also appeared to be at risk for PTSD, reporting an 8-month cumulative prevalence of 17.5 percent; the risk was associated with longer time spent in the profession (Leonard, Vasiliadis, Leclerc, & Brunet, 2023).

Theories and Treatment of Post-Traumatic Stress Disorder A traumatic experience is an external event that impinges on the individual and hence does not have biological "causality." However, researchers propose that traumatic experiences have their impact in part because they lead to changes in the brain that make certain regions primed or hypersensitive to possible danger in the future. Individuals with PTSD experience alterations in the hippocampus, the structure in the brain responsible for consolidating short-term memory. As a result, these individuals become unable to distinguish relatively harmless situations (such as fireworks) from the ones in which real trauma occurred (such as combat). They continue to re-experience the event with heightened arousal and therefore avoid situations that resemble those in which they were traumatized (Lambert & McLaughlin, 2019).

SSRI antidepressants (paroxetine and sertraline) are the only FDA-approved medications for people with PTSD. However, the response rates of patients with PTSD to these medications are rarely more than 60 percent, and fewer than 20 to 30 percent achieve full remission of their symptoms. The time since the trauma occurred appears to play a role in treatment response, with better outcomes occurring in individuals whose trauma was further in the past (Nøhr et al., 2021) More recently, ketamine is proving to have a favorable effect on PTSD symptoms with as high as an 80 percent positive response rate for individuals who do not respond to traditional medications (Jumaili et al., 2022).

From a psychological perspective, research suggests that people with PTSD have a biased information-processing style that, due to the trauma they experienced, causes their attention to be highly attuned toward potentially threatening cues. Therefore, they are more likely to feel that they are in danger, and also are more likely to avoid situations they perceive as potentially threatening (Huppert, Foa, McNally, & Cahill, 2009). Personality and coping style also predict responses to trauma, including high levels of neuroticism and extreme sensitivity to internal cues of anxiety (Naragon-Gainey & Watson, 2018).

Barbara, whose case opened the chapter, seems to have been an exception in this regard; she did not appear to be high on neuroticism, attuned to negative cues, or a victim of childhood abuse. Her prolonged exposure to severe combat along with the loss of her leg seemed to account for her development of the disorder.

Generally considered the most effective psychological treatment for PTSD, cognitive behavioral therapy combines some type of exposure (*in vivo* or imaginal) with relaxation

MINI CASE

Post-Traumatic Stress Disorder

Steve is a single 35-year-old biracial heterosexual cisgender man. For the past 10 years, he has suffered from flashbacks in which he relives the horrors of his 9-month-long deployment as a marine in Afghanistan. These flashbacks occur unexpectedly in the middle of the day, and Steve is thrown back into the emotional reality of his war experiences. These flashbacks, and the nightmares from which he often suffers, have become a constant source of torment. Steve has found that alcohol provides the only escape from these visions and from the distress he feels. Often, he ruminates about how he should have done more to prevent the deaths of his fellow soldiers, and he feels that his friends should have survived rather than him.

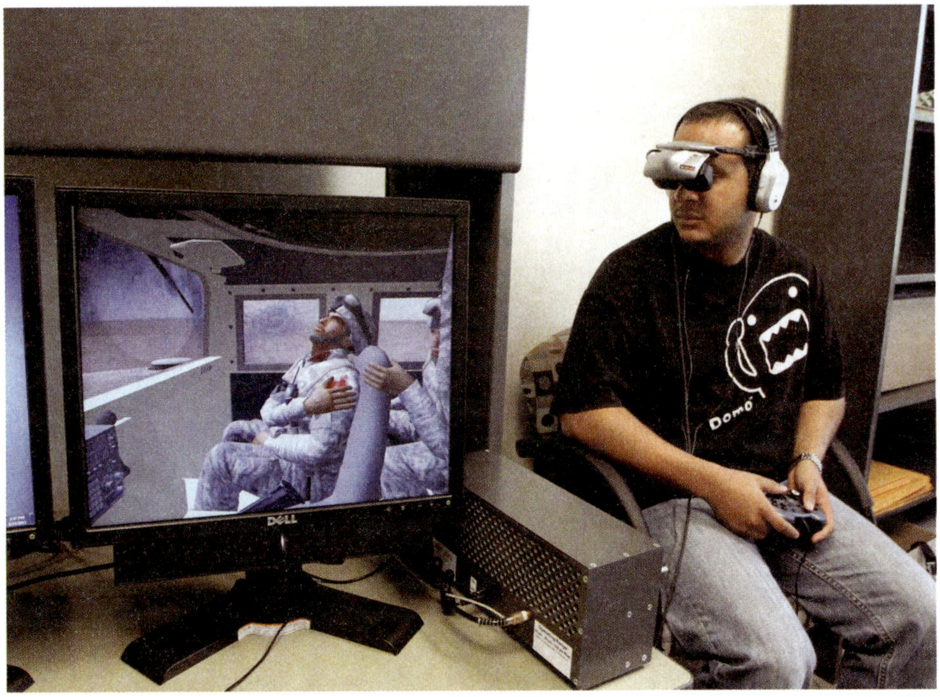

A military veteran suffering from PTSD uses virtual reality technology to expose himself to anxiety-provoking imagery as part of his treatment at a VA hospital.

George Skene/Orlando Sentinel/Tribune News Service/Getty Images

and cognitive restructuring. CBT can also be adapted to the specific cultural context of the client. Exposure-based treatments such as Cognitive Processing Therapy and Prolonged Exposure are thought to be highly effective forms of CBT-based treatment for PTSD, and are commonly used in the treatment of veterans in the VA Hospital System. Another widely utilized exposure-based treatment, which is also used within the VA System, is Eye Movement Desensitization and Reprocessing (EMDR). In this treatment, clinicians guide clients to talk through traumatic memories while focusing their eye movements on specific targets, which allows the brain to process traumatic memories in new ways, thus reducing suffering associated with the memories. Holistic approaches also show good treatment outcomes–for example, psychoeducation, meditation, and stretching exercises were found to be useful adaptations in treating Afghan refugees seen in a German clinic (Kananian, Soltani, Hinton, & Stangier, 2020). Veterans living in rural or underserved areas can also benefit from brief PTSD interventions, such as short-term prolonged exposure, through primary care outpatient clinics in the VA, where they can receive treatment outside of specialty mental health clinics (Rauch et el., 2023).

Specific trauma-focused psychotherapy that focuses on memory of the traumatic event or its meaning is also recommended for adults with PTSD, and it has the advantage of being an effective online approach (Ehlers et al., 2023). Trauma-focused psychotherapy can also be adapted for use with adolescents and children as young as preschool age (McGuire, Steele, & Singh, 2021). Mindfulness-based, internet-delivered psychotherapy can also be effective with young adults, in part through having favorable effects on sense of sense and qualities of relationships (Dumarkaite et al., 2021).

Couples therapy is another method that can prove beneficial in reducing symptoms as well as reducing distress both in the individual and in the individual's partner (Morland et al., 2022). Such an approach can help lower reintegration stress in both partners, improving their communication and expression of intimacy and reducing the number of disagreements about parenting. Adding to CBT, mindfulness-based approaches can also be useful with couples in which one partner is a veteran (Davis et al., 2021).

Because trauma is so often a component of other disorders, including substance use disorders, the U.S. government's Substance Abuse and Mental Health Services Administration (SAMHSA) has compiled a treatment manual for clinicians working in behavioral health (SAMHSA, 2014). This manual is based on the principles of **trauma-informed care**, a model

trauma-informed care
An approach to treatment that acknowledges the role that trauma can have on the mental health of individuals.

REAL STORIES

Lady Gaga (born Stefani Germanotta, 1986-Present)

As Lady Gaga rose to worldwide fame at the age of 21, the world knew her as a talented young singer-songwriter with a daring or edgy sense of style. By the time she entered the worldwide pop music stage, she was an experienced performer who had gotten her start as a teenager in New York City, where she attended New York University's Tisch School of The Arts. She dropped out, though, so she could pursue her own creative endeavors, and was briefly signed to Def Jam records in 2005. After being released by the label, she continued to perfect her music and fashion through club performances and work with rock bands. In 2007, she was signed to Interscope records and then released two major hits that propelled her to international fame, "Just Dance" and "Poker Face" (Biography, 2021). Since then, she has released six studio albums, starred in major film and television roles, and received critical praise and awards including an Academy Award and multiple Grammys.

It wasn't until years after her success had been cemented that Lady Gaga revealed that while she was rising to major success and acclaim, she was also struggling with mental illness and chronic pain.

In 2016, in an appearance on a segment of the *Today Show* in which she visited a shelter for homeless LGBTQ+ youth, Lady Gaga revealed to the world that she suffered from PTSD related to being raped at 19. In the interview, she expressed that she hadn't been able to talk about the rape until 2014, and that she had been in treatment.

In a 2020 interview with Oprah Winfrey, Lady Gaga reflected on coping with the aftermath of her experience of rape: "I all of a sudden became a star and was traveling the world going from hotel room to garage to limo to stage, and I never dealt with it, and then all of a sudden I started to experience this incredible intense pain throughout my entire body that mimicked the illness I felt after I was raped." In the interview she also connected developing PTSD and pain with the fact that she did not process or cope with the assault at the time it happened (Lady Gaga, 2020).

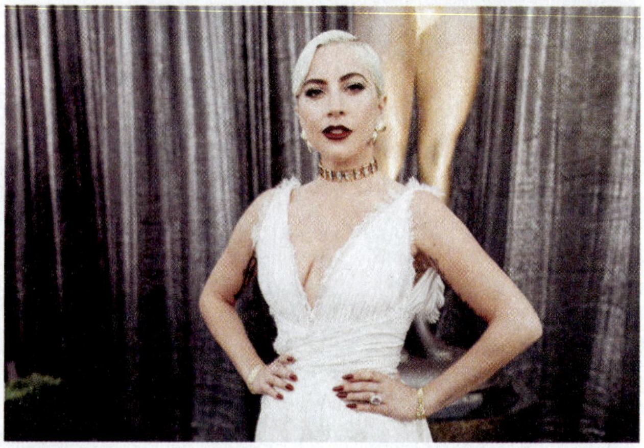

Lady Gaga in 2009 attending the Monster Cable Party at the Tube Club, Berlin, Germany.

Emma McIntyre/Staff/Getty Images

Even before she revealed her diagnosis and mental health struggles, Lady Gaga was advocating for those experiencing mental health issues, particularly young people. In 2012, she co-founded the Born This Way Foundation with her mother, Cynthia Germanotta. The Foundation seeks to raise awareness of mental health issues among youth and provides resources and global campaigns aimed at reducing stigma around these problems.

On the Foundation's website, Lady Gaga posted a letter to her fans in 2016 in which she described her experiences with mental health treatment. She vividly recounts issues such as dissociations, depression, and somatization of her anxiety. In her words: "It's like the panic accelerator in my mind gets stuck and I am paralyzed with fear" (Lady Gaga, 2016).

In many of the lyrics in her music, Lady Gaga is candid about symptoms she has experienced during her mental health struggles. For example her 2020 song "911" vividly describes taking antipsychotic medications: "Turning up emotional faders/Keep repeating self-hating phrases/I have heard enough of these voices/Almost like I have no choice" (Barbour, 2020). The video for the song "911" uses visual metaphors to highlight these experiences as well. In an Instagram post about the video, Lady Gaga explained, "Something that was once my real life everyday is now a film, a true story that is now the past and not the present. It's the poetry of pain" (Lady Gaga, 2020).

In addition to advocating for mental health awareness, Lady Gaga has also been a fierce advocate for LGBTQ+ rights and became an important voice for President Biden's 2020 campaign. "The highest honor of [her] lifetime," as she has referred to it, came on January 20, 2021 when she sang the Star-Spangled Banner at President Biden's inauguration (Nelson, 2021).

Lady Gaga's talent and bravery have inspired her fans worldwide, and her willingness to be vulnerable and frank about her mental health has helped fight stigma and provide hope for those who struggle. In opening up about her disorder and sharing her experiences, she has also helped destigmatize PTSD related to sexual assault, and she has been candid that PTSD should not be seen as a diagnosis that affects only military veterans.

"I have wrestled for some time about when, how and if I should reveal my diagnosis of Post-Traumatic Stress Disorder (PTSD). After five years of searching for the answers to my chronic pain and the change I have felt in my brain, I am finally well enough to tell you. There is a lot of shame attached to mental illness, but it's important that you know that there is hope and a chance for recovery" (Lady Gaga, 2016).

that promotes trauma awareness and understanding to professionals treating individuals with a history of trauma. The idea of resilience is central to this philosophy of treatment, helping individuals foster their own inner strengths as they develop a greater sense of competence. Furthermore, according to the principles of trauma-informed care, clinicians must avoid retraumatizing clients who already have histories of trauma.

An alternative view to PTSD comes from the field of positive psychology, which proposes that people can grow through the experience of trauma, a phenomenon known as **post-traumatic growth**. According to this approach, trauma can allow clients to cope by developing positive interpretations of their experiences (Achterhof et al., 2018). Social support and positive religious coping may form important components of this recovery process (Yazici, Ozdemir, & Koca, 2020).

post-traumatic growth
The personal growth that can occur following exposure to a traumatic experience.

Given the number of types of treatment and their various approaches to promoting change, often with methods that focus on past trauma, the question for the clinician becomes one of choosing the best approach. It does appear that PTSD psychotherapy does follow a "dose-response" principle, in that greater improvement is associated with a longer time in treatment, at least up to the point of a particular therapy's protocol. Therefore, clinicians must adapt their treatment according to which will allow their clients to receive "good enough" care prior to reaching the point of dropping out. One study of veterans comparing trauma-focused vs. present-centered therapy (focusing on symptom reduction) showed that although both methods were effective compared to controls, dropout rates early in treatment were higher for exposure-based therapy (Thompson-Hollands et al., 2023).

8.4 Anxiety, Obsessive-Compulsive, and Trauma- and Stressor-Related Disorders: The Biopsychosocial Perspective

The disorders you learned about in this chapter were originally classified in a single category prior to the *DSM-5*, reflecting the symptom of anxiety. However, in the *DSM-5-TR*, they fall into three sets of diagnostic categories: anxiety, obsessive-compulsive and related disorders, and trauma- and stressor-related disorders. For each set of diagnoses, the biopsychosocial perspective provides an important framework both for understanding and treatment.

In the case of anxiety disorders, biological factors can increase an individual's propensity to developing specific types of fears. However, even in the biological perspective, researchers and clinicians recognize the importance of combining treatments that include changes in the ways that their clients interpret fearful situations.

Obsessive-compulsive and related disorders also may have a strong biological component, and again, treatment may focus on changes in neurotransmitter levels that may contribute to an individual's symptoms. Psychosocial and sociocultural factors, though, clearly play a role as well. Treatments that attempt to alter an individual's cognitions while also recognizing such contributing factors as, for example, age and living situations, can be effective as stand-alone interventions without requiring medication.

Trauma- and stressor-related disorders are heavily rooted in experiential learning, in which individuals develop symptoms prompted by exposure to fear-producing events or events that cause physical harm. Sociocultural factors are therefore particularly important to consider when clinicians diagnose these disorders but, as with the other disorders covered in this chapter, can become a major focus of therapy.

Though differing in origin and symptoms, the disorders covered in this chapter therefore benefit from a true biopsychosocial approach, in which all contributions are used in the planning and delivery of treatment.

Return to the Case: Barbara Wilder

Barbara's therapist decided not to use pharmacological interventions but instead to begin treatment with cognitive processing therapy, a cognitive behavioral therapy specifically aimed at reducing symptoms of PTSD. In therapy, Barbara learned to challenge the thoughts that she was still in danger much of the time. Through the use of imaginal flooding, she became accustomed to discussing her experiences in Iraq without provoking fear or anxiety by relearning to associate her memories of the war with relaxation.

In addition to individual therapy, Barbara's therapist suggested that she participate in group therapy. In these sessions, Barbara met with seven other Iraq War veterans for 90 minutes a week for 10 weeks. She was able to talk about her traumatic memories as well as provide support to other veterans as they discussed their experiences. By interacting with veterans she could relate to, she relearned how to interact with others socially, which decreased her feelings of irritability and anger around other people in her life.

Within 1 month of beginning her treatment at the VA, Barbara began to experience some relief from her PTSD symptoms, though she continued to have occasional nightmares. Using the coping skills she learned in therapy, Barbara was able to recover from the flashbacks and began to participate in life once again. She made a full physical recovery after receiving a prosthetic leg. Within 2 months, her emotional numbing, irritability, and anxious symptoms completely subsided. Barbara often remarked to her therapist that she felt that she was "herself" again. Several months later, she took a part-time job in an electronics store and enrolled in a part-time MBA program at a nearby community college. She moved into her own apartment a few towns away from her parents' home and began to reconnect with old friends who still lived close by. Barbara continues to come to the VA for individual therapy every week, and though the events she experienced in Iraq still haunt her, she has learned to live with the memories and has begun to adjust to civilian life.

Dr. Tobin's Reflections: It was clear upon her initial presentation that Barbara was presenting with classic symptoms of PTSD. Fortunately she was able to utilize the resources available for her to get help and provide relief from her suffering. Early intervention for those with PTSD is critical in preventing the prolonging of symptoms throughout the life span, and Barbara was able to put her life back together as a result of addressing her PTSD through treatment early on. For many veterans of wars fought in earlier eras (such as Vietnam), the needed resources were not available when they returned home from war. These veterans currently make up a large population of the Veterans Affairs system, though the rates of PTSD continue to increase for soldiers fighting in the wars in Iraq and Afghanistan.

SUMMARY

- Anxiety disorders are characterized by the experience of physiological arousal, apprehension or feelings of dread, hypervigilance, avoidance, and sometimes a specific fear or phobia.
- Separation anxiety disorder is characterized by intense and inappropriate anxiety about being separated from home or caregivers. Many infants go through a developmental phase in which they become anxious and agitated when they are separated from their caregivers. In separation anxiety disorder, these emotions continue far longer than is age appropriate. Even the prospect of separation causes extreme anxiety. Although there appears to be a strong genetic component to separation anxiety disorder, environmental factors also contribute. Cognitive behavioral techniques may be most effective. Another disorder appearing in childhood and thought to center on anxiety is selective mutism, in which a child refuses to speak in specific situations, such as the classroom. Behaviorist methods using shaping and exposure seem particularly well suited to treating children with selective mutism.
- Specific phobias are irrational fears of particular objects or situations. Cognitive behaviorists assert that previous learning experiences and a cycle of negative, maladaptive thoughts cause specific phobias. Treatments recommended by the behavioral and cognitive behavioral approaches include flooding, systematic desensitization, imagery, *in vivo* exposure, and virtual reality exposure therapy (VRET) as well as procedures aimed at changing the individual's maladaptive thoughts, such as cognitive restructuring and thought stopping. Treatment based on the biological perspective involves medication.
- Social anxiety disorder is a fear of being observed by others while acting in a way that will be humiliating or embarrassing. Cognitive behavioral approaches to social anxiety disorder regard the disorder as due to an unrealistic fear of criticism, which causes people with the disorder to lose the ability to concentrate on their performance, instead shifting their attention to how anxious they feel, which then causes them to make mistakes and, therefore, to become more fearful.

Behavioral methods that provide *in vivo* exposure, along with cognitive restructuring and social skills training, seem to be the most effective in helping people with social anxiety disorder. Medication is the treatment recommended within the biological perspective for severe cases of this disorder.

- Panic disorder is characterized by frequent and recurrent panic attacks—intense sensations of fear and physical discomfort. Agoraphobia presents with intense anxiety around the thought or experience of being in a public place, particularly with a fear of being unable to escape. Biological and cognitive behavioral perspectives are particularly useful for understanding and treating this disorder. Treatment based on the cognitive behavioral perspective involves methods such as relaxation training and cognitive restructuring. Medications can also help alleviate symptoms, with the most commonly prescribed being antianxiety and antidepressant medications.
- People who are diagnosed as having generalized anxiety disorder have a number of unrealistic worries that spread to various spheres of life. The cognitive behavioral approach to generalized anxiety disorder emphasizes the unrealistic nature of these worries and regards the disorder as a vicious cycle that feeds on itself. Cognitive behavioral treatment approaches recommend breaking the negative cycle of worry by teaching individuals techniques that allow them to feel they control the worrying. Biological treatment emphasizes the use of medication.
- In obsessive-compulsive disorder, individuals develop obsessions, or thoughts they cannot rid themselves of, and compulsions, which are irresistible, repetitive behaviors. A cognitive behavioral understanding of obsessive-compulsive disorder regards the symptoms as the product of a learned association between anxiety and the thoughts or acts, which can temporarily produce relief from anxiety. A growing body of evidence supports a biological explanation of the disorder, with the most current research suggesting that it is associated with an excess of serotonin. Cognitive behavioral methods involving exposure and thought stopping are considered highly effective. Body dysmorphic disorder involves preoccupation with the idea that a part of the body is ugly or defective. Other disorders related to OCD include hoarding disorder, trichotillomania, and excoriation disorder.
- Individuals who are exposed to trauma or stressors may develop one of a set of disorders. This set of disorders include, as a diagnostic criterion, the condition that there is an actual event that precipitates the symptoms. Children with reactive attachment disorder have severe disturbances in the way they relate to others and are emotionally withdrawn and inhibited. In contrast, children with disinhibited social engagement disorder engage in culturally inappropriate, overly familiar behavior with people who are relative strangers. Both of these disorders are found in children who have experienced social neglect through repeated changes of primary caregivers or being reared in institutions with high child-to-caregiver ratios. Research indicates that children with these disorders continue to have problems even if their circumstances improve.
- In post-traumatic stress disorder, the individual is unable to recover from the anxiety associated with a traumatic life event, such as tragedy, an accident, participation in combat or work as a front-line professional during a disaster or pandemic. The aftereffects of the traumatic event include flashbacks, nightmares, and intrusive thoughts that alternate with the individual's attempts to deny that the event ever took place. Some people experience a briefer but troubling response to a traumatic event; this condition, called acute stress disorder, lasts from 2 days to 4 weeks and involves the kinds of symptoms that people with PTSD experience over a much longer period of time. Cognitive behavioral approaches are considered highly effective treatment, although SSRIs may also be recommended. Additional approaches include mindfulness-based CBT, trauma-informed psychotherapy, couples-based CBT, and culturally adapted CBT. From a positive psychology perspective, post-traumatic growth can also occur, particularly if individuals are able to access social support.

KEY TERMS

Acute stress disorder
Agoraphobia
Anxiety
Anxiety disorders
Anxiety sensitivity theory
Body dysmorphic disorder (BDD)
Complex post-traumatic stress disorder
Compulsion
Conditioned fear reactions
Disinhibited social engagement disorder
Excoriation (skin-picking) disorder
Fear
Flooding
Generalized anxiety disorder
Graded *in vivo*
Hoarding disorder
Imaginal flooding
In vivo flooding
Obsession
Obsessive-compulsive disorder (OCD)
One Session Treatment (OST)
Panic attack
Panic disorder
Post-traumatic growth
Post-traumatic stress disorder (PTSD)
Reactive attachment disorder (RAD)
Relaxation training
Selective mutism
Separation anxiety disorder
Social anxiety disorder
Specific phobia
Trauma
Trauma-informed care
Trichotillomania (hair-pulling disorder)
Virtual reality exposure therapy (VRET)

CHAPTER 9

Dissociative and Somatic Symptom Disorders

OUTLINE

Learning Objectives

9.1 Specify the symptoms of dissociative disorders.

9.2 Identify symptoms and treatments of somatic symptom disorders.

9.3 Recognize psychological factors affecting other medical conditions.

9.4 Explain the biopsychosocial perspective for dissociative and somatic symptom disorders.

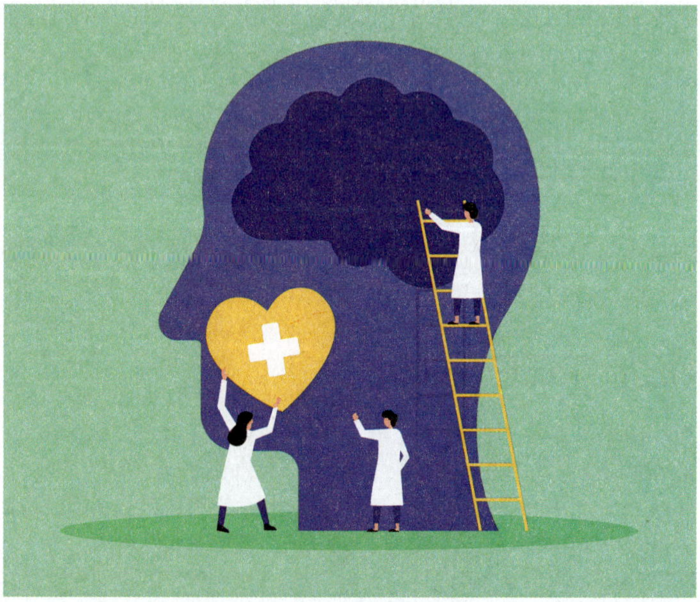

mnaufal design/Shutterstock

Case Report

Rose Marston

Demographic information: 37-year-old White transgender woman who identifies as pansexual. Rose's pronouns are she/her/hers.

History of present illness: Rose was referred for a psychological evaluation by her physician, Dr. Stewart, who became concerned that Rose may have been experiencing symptoms of a psychological disorder. For the past year, Rose had made weekly appointments with Dr. Stewart as well as other health practitioners due to her concern that she was suffering from a severe physical condition. Dr. Stewart diagnosed Rose with early-onset lactose intolerance. However, this did not seem to correspond with the intense and frequent stomach pains Rose complained of, which persisted even after she cut dairy out of her diet.

During the psychological evaluation, Rose reported she was dissatisfied with Dr. Stewart's conclusions, and she consulted with alternative health care practitioners such as homeopathic physicians and even a Reiki master. She admitted she had been hoping that one of the practitioners would discover she had a diagnosable medical condition, and many had even suggested she receive a psychological evaluation, which she refused. She finally agreed to Dr. Stewart's recommendation and scheduled an appointment at an outpatient mental health clinic for an evaluation, after much persistence from him.

Rose reported she had recently lost her job after calling in sick nearly every day over the past 3 months. She stated she felt it was more important to spend her time consulting health care practitioners, and she also preferred not to leave her house for fear of exacerbating her symptoms. She stated she was distressed about the amount of time she had spent worrying about her stomach pain, but she also was overwhelmed by feelings of guilt if she did not direct her activities toward trying to identify the cause of her physical symptoms. Rose said her symptoms originated as mild stomach irritation, and that over the past year they had escalated to the point where her stomach was causing her constant and severe pain. She reported having tried a multitude of remedies, all unsuccessful.

During the evaluation, Rose stated that she felt "devastated" about how her worry over her physical symptoms had interfered with her life but believed she had to focus on finding a diagnosis. Her boyfriend of 2 years had recently ended their relationship, and she admitted she had distanced herself from him since her concerns about her physical symptoms began. She found, in addition, that her concern about these symptoms overshadowed any thoughts about the relationship.

The clinician conducting the evaluation asked Rose to describe any recent major stressors in her life, and she reported she had lost her favorite uncle to cancer in the previous year. When describing this loss, Rose immediately became tearful and admitted she felt she had never mourned her uncle and instead pushed away her feelings about his death most of the time.

Following the evaluation, the clinician contacted Dr. Stewart to consult about her case, which Rose had consented to by signing a release of information. Dr. Stewart told the clinician he believed Rose's physical symptoms seemed to be indicative of late-onset lactose intolerance, but that she had refused to accept this diagnosis. Her symptoms may have worsened as a result of her failure to get the proper treatment. Dr. Stewart also remarked that Rose seemed to have been acting very differently since the death of her uncle.

Psychiatric history: Rose had previously seen a psychiatrist for depression in her late 20s. Her depressive symptoms began after she graduated from college and varied in severity until she endured an episode so intense she contemplated suicide. She had received a course of antidepressants that had been effective. Rose reported that she also experienced significant improvement in her symptoms of depression and overall mental health following her gender transition, which she completed at age 32. At the time of the evaluation, Rose had not been on any psychiatric medications for approximately 5 years because she felt the previous course had been effective enough for her to discontinue, and her mental health felt stable in general since transitioning.

Case formulation: Rose meets criteria for somatic symptom disorder, moderate to severe, with predominant pain. This diagnosis is based on her heightened anxiety, which is excessive, in response to her physical symptoms, to the point where her life has been significantly disrupted (loss of her job and her romantic relationship). Her concerns about her symptoms are both persistent (lasting

Case Report *continued*

longer than 6 months) and disproportionate to their actual severity. She has devoted an objectively excessive amount of time and energy to her physical symptoms and has refused to accept a relatively mild diagnosis of lactose intolerance. The onset of Rose's symptoms may originate from distress caused by the death of her uncle, due to her report that she engaged in avoidance of processing her reaction.

Risk level: Low risk. Rose denies current suicidal ideation, and she has no history of suicide attempts.

Treatment plan: Following the evaluation and consultation with Dr. Stewart, the clinician referred Rose to a therapist specializing in cognitive behavioral treatment for somatic disorders. In this evidence-based approach, Rose's therapist should focus on evaluating her excessive concerns about her physical condition with cognitive restructuring, and behavioral strategies to increase her engagement with recommendations from Dr. Stewart to improve her physical symptoms.

Sarah Tobin, PhD

9.1 Dissociative Disorders

The human mind seems almost endlessly capable of dissociating or separating attentional focus. You can think intensively about a problem while jogging, perhaps not even realizing that you ran a mile without being aware of your surroundings. In dissociative disorders, this separation of a person's mental functions occurs to a far more extreme degree than what many people experience in daily life.

Dissociative disorders raise intriguing questions about the ways in which people's sense of self evolves over time, and the way memory and sense of reality can become fragmented and distinct within the same individual. In contrast, somatic symptom disorders, discussed later in this chapter, raise equally fascinating questions about mind-body relationships.

Major Forms of Dissociative Disorders

dissociative identity disorder (DID)
A dissociative disorder in which an individual develops more than one self or personality.

You generally take for granted the idea that each individual has one personality and one sense of identity. However, in **dissociative identity disorder (DID)**, separate personalities and identities can develop within the same individual. A common trigger for these different identities to develop is trauma experienced early in life, when an individual may purposefully dissociate from physical, emotional, or sexual trauma, but then over time continue to rely on these separate identities to cope with ongoing abuse or trauma. These identities then continue to develop even past the end of the period of trauma, and into adulthood. The separate personalities seem to have their own unique characteristic ways of perceiving, thinking, and relating to others. By definition, people with DID have at least two distinct identities and, when inhabiting the identity of one, are not aware that they also inhabit the other. Their experiences therefore lack continuity. They have large gaps in important memories about themselves and their lives, often memories of a traumatic nature such as being victimized or abused. As reported in the *DSM-5-TR*, over 70 percent of individuals with DID have attempted suicide or engaged in other self-harm and high-risk behaviors.

dissociative amnesia
An inability to remember important personal details and experiences; usually associated with traumatic or very stressful events.

fugue
An episode of amnesia involving inability to recall some or all of one's past and the loss of identity, with either bewildered wandering or travel that seems focused on a particular purpose.

People with **dissociative amnesia** are unable to remember information about an event or set of events in their lives. This type of memory loss is different from the everyday slips that cause people to misplace objects or forget people's names. People with dissociative amnesia forget a specific event in their lives, most likely one of a traumatic or stressful nature. Their amnesia may even invoke a **fugue** state, an episode of amnesia that leaves them unable to recall some or all of their past and identity, along with either bewildered wandering or travel that seems focused on a particular purpose. These individuals may become suicidal when the amnesia decreases.

MINI CASE

Dissociative Identity Disorder

Maya is a 26-year-old Latina heterosexual cisgender woman. She is single, lives with two roommates, and works as a clerk at a department store. She rarely leaves her apartment except to go to work and to see her family who live close by. Her coworkers described her as being rather quiet and shy, even around customers. When she was 18, she started an intimate relationship with a middle-aged man who was physically and emotionally abusive toward her. The relationship lasted for about 2 years before she left him. Although others often remind her of this troubled relationship, Maya claims to remember very little about that time and has no recollection of the physical abuse she endured. Currently, she says she is totally uninterested in pursuing any romantic relationships. Those to whom Maya is closest know different versions of her personality or "alters" that go by different names and behave in ways that are totally incongruous with Maya's original personality. Whereas Maya is quiet and reserved, her main alter "Rita" is flamboyant, outgoing, and hypersexual. A second alter, "Joe," occasionally emerges from Maya's apartment dressed in men's clothing and speaking in deep tones. Maya's alters are oblivious to the details of her life.

Your ordinary perception of who you are includes knowing that you live within your own body. **Depersonalization** is the condition in which people feel their identities have become detached from their bodies. They may have experiences of unreality, of being an outside observer, and of emotional or physical numbing. **Derealization** is a condition in which people feel a sense of unreality or detachment from their surroundings. **Depersonalization/derealization disorder** is a condition in which people have the experience of depersonalization, derealization, or both.

depersonalization
Condition in which people feel detached from their own body.

derealization
Condition in which people feel a sense of unreality or detachment from their surroundings.

depersonalization/derealization disorder
A dissociative disorder in which the individual experiences recurrent and persistent episodes of depersonalization, derealization, or both.

Theories and Treatment of Dissociative Disorders

In normal development, people integrate the perceptions and memories they have of themselves and their experiences. You can remember many of the events from your past, which give you a sense of continuity over time. In a dissociative disorder, often due to experiencing trauma or chronic abuse early in life, the individual loses this continuity, trying to block out or separate from conscious awareness events that caused extreme psychological, if not physical, pain. There may be a physical correspondence to these traumatic memories, as indicated by evidence of reductions in the size of portions of the brain involved in memory among individuals with dissociative amnesia (Dimitrova et al., 2023).

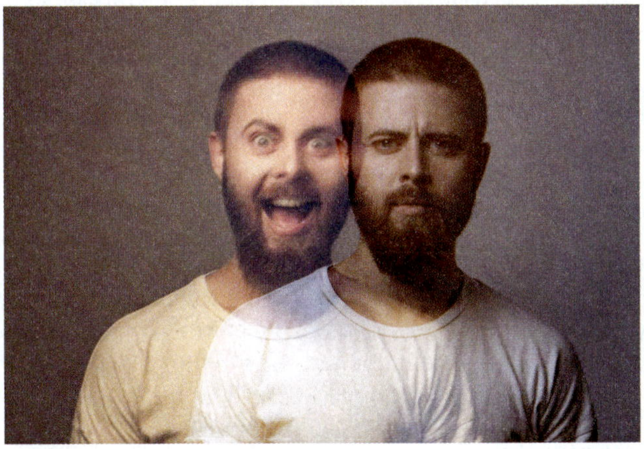

Individuals with dissociative identity disorder have learned to cope with extremely stressful life circumstances by creating "alter" personalities that unconsciously control their thinking and behavior when they are experiencing stress.

Khosrow Rajab Kordi/Alamy Stock Photo

REAL STORIES

Adam Duritz (1964–Present)

"It all fell apart within a span of 5 minutes, with one phone call and one text message. Of course there was the long downward slope leading to that moment, but I see that now only in retrospect" (Duritz, 2008).

Adam Duritz, an American singer from the rock band Counting Crows, has spoken openly about his struggles with dissociative disorder and depersonalization. He first shared his experiences with the world through an autobiographical essay published in *Men's Health* magazine in 2008. In the passage above, he is referencing a moment in which he recognized that his sense of disconnection from other people and the world around him went beyond just the physical distance that came with fame and years of success, but indicated a very real concern about his mental health.

Duritz was born in Baltimore, and moved around with his family throughout childhood, after his father was enlisted in the military during the Vietnam War. He spent no more than 2 years in any location around the United States, until he was in high school, when the family settled in California (Harkness, 2023).

In San Francisco in 1991, Duritz co-founded the Counting Crows as the main songwriter and lead singer. After signing their first record deal, the band shot to early success, and Duritz, by all accounts became a national celebrity whose life was closely followed by the media. Since debuting their first album *August and Everything After* in 1993, the band has sold over 20 million records, had multiple chart-topping songs, and was nominated for two Grammy awards, and an Academy Award for best original song from the animated film "Shrek 2." The band is still active, with their most recent record coming out in 2021 followed by a world tour (Harkness, 2023).

In Duritz's 2008 essay, he described in detail the evening when he first realized that he was struggling with unusual feelings of disconnection from the world around him, and needed to seek help. He was in Australia on tour, when he had gotten a call that his grandmother had passed away, and at the same time received a message from his girlfriend at the time that she wanted to end their relationship. His first response was to stay with his band on the tour despite his family's pleas that he travel to Baltimore for his grandmother's funeral, but due in part to symptoms of depersonalization, he was unable to acknowledge the reality of what this meant and chose not to go, instead traveling with his band to their next tour stop. It wasn't until he had a sleepless night where he felt wracked with guilt and anxiety about how much he had missed out on in his family's life, the reality of the situation hit him, and he immediately flew back home. After arriving in Baltimore, it was then that he "decided that I had completely lost touch with reality—and that I needed help" (Duritz, 2008).

Looking back at that time, he later acknowledged that because of his symptoms of depersonalization, he often felt completely disconnected from his family and romantic partners "because nothing seems real, it's hard to connect with the world or the people in it because they're not there. You're not there. That's why I rarely saw my family back then: It's hard to care when everything feels as if it's taking place in your imagination. And if you're distant with people, especially women you're romantically involved with, they eventually leave" (Duritz, 2008). At the time though, it seemed that his extremely busy life with his band provided enough reason to stay out on the road and live far away from his family, and also made relationships difficult to sustain.

After that episode in 2004, Duritz finally sought treatment, a difficult journey of finding relief from symptoms which lasted about 2 years until he found an effective medication regimen. During that time he was less active in his career, struggled with memory loss, gained a significant amount of weight, and found his mental health fluctuating due to the side effects of medications. He was eventually able to record with his band and perform a few shows during this period, but it was a torturous time for Duritz. In a 2014 interview, he recounted, "I really hoped it would go away, or that I would find the right medication so it didn't affect me anymore, or that I would just go to therapy and could think my way around it. But none of that has happened" (Clinch & Levitan, 2014). In addition to finding an effective medication regimen, Duritz also found that exercising and keeping healthy routines like staying sober (he had previously struggled with alcohol and drug abuse), and continuing to make music and tour consistently, helped to manage his symptoms and keep him stable. Throughout the most difficult years of his struggle with dissociative disorder and finding effective treatment, he and his band released a double album in 2008, which chronicled the challenges of that time, as well as the slow recovery that began after he sought help (Harkness, 2023). Since then, Duritz has continued to write, record, and tour with the Counting Crows, though he has had ups and downs with his mental health and has periods where he has had to work hard to stay consistent in his musical career.

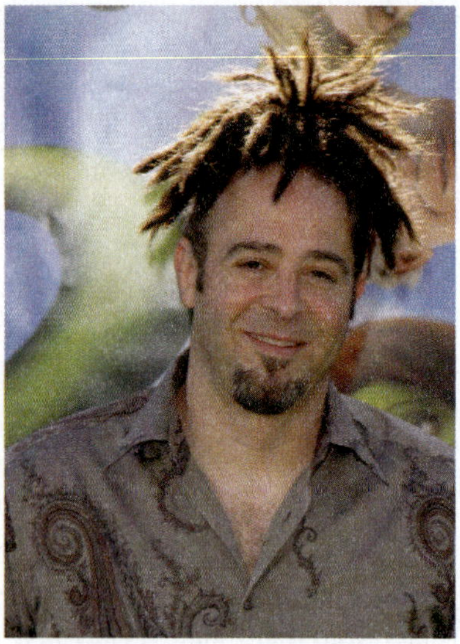

Adam Duritz, lead singer of Counting Crows at the "Shrek 2" Premiere, May 2004.

PictureLux/The Hollywood Archive/Alamy Stock Photo

Duritz often speaks to the impact of his dissociative disorder on his songwriting. "It's important to every single song I've ever written. It's the reason for all of them. I just didn't talk about it for a long time. I didn't know specifically what it was for a long time, but the feeling was always there, since I was in my early 20s" (Furness, 2015). He has also described a sense of peace with writing music, because it continually challenges him and keeps him moving forward by providing structure and purpose (Hilleary, 2021).

In Duritz's words, "I have a bottom I've reached that I don't want to reach again. Nothing is preventing me from going back down there except myself...The decision to change in and of itself means nothing. It's the work that follows that means everything" (Duritz, 2008).

MINI CASE

Dissociative Amnesia with Dissociative Fugue

Troy is a 39-year-old biracial heterosexual cisgender man. He entered the mental health crisis center in a daze, tears streaming down his face, and wearing only a T-shirt despite the frigid temperatures outside. "I have no idea where I live or who I am! Will somebody please help me?" The crisis team asked Troy to search his pockets for an ID or other identifying information, but the only thing he had on him was a picture of a young girl. Troy appeared exhausted and was taken to a bed, where he promptly fell asleep. The crisis team called the local police to find out whether there was a report of a missing child. As it turned out, the little girl in the photograph was Troy's daughter. She had been hit by a car in a shopping center parking lot. Although she had suffered a broken leg, the child was resting comfortably in a hospital pediatrics ward. Her father, however, had disappeared. Troy had apparently been wandering around the hospital for several hours, leaving his wallet and cell phone with the hospital social worker in the emergency room. When he awoke, he was able to recall who he was and the circumstances of the accident, but he remembered nothing of what had happened since.

In true cases of a dissociative disorder, when the symptoms do not appear feigned, the current consensus is that the dissociation is a response to early emotional or physical trauma (Reinders & Veltman, 2020). DID specifically appears to be related to an earlier exposure to trauma, occurring at as young as infancy and ranging up to age 6 (Raison & Andrea, 2023).

Assuming that people with dissociative disorders are reacting to trauma by developing dissociative symptoms, the treatment goal becomes primarily one of integrating the

You Be the Judge

Dissociative Identity Disorder

The possibility that an individual may not be responsible for actions committed while multiple personalities are in control of the person's behavior leads to fascinating legal questions. Theoretically, of course, it's possible for one alter to commit a crime while the other alters, or even the host, remains unaware. Obviously, however, convicting one alter means the host (along with all the other alters) is also put in prison. At another level, however, this question relates to the legal definition of insanity. Is a person with dissociative identity disorder able to control his or her own mind if part of the mind has split off and is acting independently?

There are three possible approaches to defending a client who legitimately has this diagnosis. In the "alter-in-control" approach, the defendant claims that an alter personality was in control at the time of the offense. In the "each-alter" approach, the prosecution must decide whether each personality met the insanity standard. In the "host-alter" approach, the issue is whether the host personality meets the insanity standard.

Dissociative identity disorder has rarely been successful as a legal defense after a public outcry following the ruling in 1974 that serial rapist Billy Milligan was insane due to lack of an integrated personality (*State v. Milligan,* 1978). Since that time, cases have had a variety of outcomes, ranging from the judgment that multiple personalities do not preclude criminal responsibility (*State v. Darnall,* 1980) to the ruling that alter personalities are not an excuse for inability to distinguish right from wrong (*State v. Jones,* 1998). The courts threw out two more recent cases in Washington State (*State v. Greene,* 1998) and West Virginia (*State v. Lockhart,* 2000) on the grounds that scientific evidence and/or adequate reliability standards do not exist in the diagnosis of the disorder (Farrell, 2010). The key issue for forensic psychologists and psychiatrists is identifying the difference between malingering and the actual disorder (Farrell, 2011).

In aiding accurate diagnosis, clinicians can use structured clinical interviews (see Table 1), which the profession has rigorously standardized. Such an instrument includes

TABLE 1 **Items from the SCID-D-R**

Scale	Items
Amnesia	Have you ever felt as if there were large gaps in your memory?
Depersonalization	Have you ever felt that you were watching yourself from a point outside of your body, as if you were seeing yourself from a distance (or watching a movie of yourself)? Have you ever felt as if a part of your body or your whole being was foreign to you? Have you ever felt as if you were two different people, one going through the motions of life and the other part observing quietly?
Derealization	Have you ever felt as if familiar surroundings or people you knew seemed unfamiliar or unreal? Have you ever felt puzzled as to what is real and what's unreal in your surroundings? Have you ever felt as if your surroundings or other people were fading away?
Identity confusion	Have you ever felt as if there was a struggle going on inside of you? Have you ever felt confused as to who you are?
Identity alteration	Have you ever acted as if you were a completely different person? Have you ever been told by others that you seem like a different person? Have you ever found things in your possession (for instance, shoes) that belong to you, but you could not remember how you got them?

SOURCE: Steinberg, M. (1994). *Structured clinical interview for DSM-IV dissociative disorders—Revised (SCID-D-R)*. American Psychiatric Association.

a careful structuring, presentation, and scoring of questions. The professionals who developed and conducted research on this instrument emphasize that only experienced clinicians and evaluators who understand dissociative diagnosis and treatment issues must administer and score it.

The *DSM-5-TR* considers the diagnosis of dissociative identity disorder to be valid. The precedents created by rulings that the diagnosis is not admissible due to failure to meet scientific standards may in time be overturned. Nevertheless, the diagnosis is challenging at best and potentially easy to feign, particularly if a clinician inadvertently plants the idea of using it as a defense.

Q: *You be the judge:* Should dissociative identity disorder be considered admissible in criminal cases? Why or why not?

disparate parts of self, memory, and time within the person's consciousness. Treatment guidelines for dissociative identity disorder emphasize best practices such as establishing and maintaining a strong therapeutic alliance, not playing favorites with any of the alters, and, from a positive psychology perspective, helping clients see themselves and their worlds in a more favorable manner by restoring their shattered assumptions (Ducharme, 2017).

As a specific technique, cognitive behavioral therapy is well suited to helping clients with dissociative identity disorder develop a coherent sense of themselves and their experiences.

MINI CASE

Depersonalization/Derealization Disorder

Robert is a 49-year-old Black heterosexual cisgender man. He entered the psychiatrist's office in a state of extreme agitation, almost panic. He described the terrifying nature of his "nervous attacks," which began several years ago but had now reached catastrophic proportions. During these "attacks," Robert feels as though he is floating in the air, above his body, watching everything he does but feeling totally disconnected from his actions. He reports that he feels as if his body is a machine controlled by outside forces: "I look at my hands and feet and wonder what makes them move." However, Robert's thoughts are not delusions. He is aware that his altered perceptions are not normal. The only relief he experiences from his symptoms comes when he strikes himself with a heavy object until the pain finally penetrates his consciousness. His fear of seriously harming himself adds to his main worry that he is losing his mind.

The Unified Protocol for the Transdiagnostic Treatment of Emotional Disorders in treatment of DID includes 18 to 22 sessions focused on helping clients recognize and accept their emotions and learn to incorporate their perceptions of having multiple personalities into a single sense of self. As part of this treatment, clinicians take the client through a series of graded exposures in response to fear-evoking memories and triggers. At each stage of these fear hierarchies, clients learn to accept emotions that earlier were either avoided or went out of control. At the end, clients internalize an "inner therapist" so they can continue to invoke these methods after treatment has ended. By confronting and then changing their cognitions, then, clients can gain a sense of control that will allow them to incorporate those memories into their sense of self (Mohajerin, Lynn, Bakhtiyari, & Dolatshah, 2019).

9.2 Somatic Symptom and Related Disorders

In the group of disorders in which **somatic symptoms** are prominent, people experience physical problems and/or concerns about medical symptoms. The term *somatic* comes from the Greek word *soma*, meaning "body." Somatic symptom disorders are psychological in nature, because although people with these disorders may or may not have a diagnosed medical condition, they seek treatment for their physical symptoms and associated distressing behaviors, thoughts, and feelings.

somatic symptoms
Symptoms involving physical problems and/or concerns about medical symptoms.

Somatic Symptom Disorder

People with **somatic symptom disorder** have physical symptoms that may or may not be accounted for by a medical condition; they also have maladaptive thoughts, feelings, and behaviors. People with this disorder think to a disproportionate degree about the seriousness of their symptoms, feel extremely anxious about them, and spend a great deal of time and energy on the symptoms or their concerns about their health. Although it may appear that people with this diagnosis are intentionally manufacturing symptoms, they actually are not consciously attuned to the ways in which they express these psychological problems physically.

somatic symptom disorder
A disorder involving physical symptoms that may or may not be accounted for by a medical condition and accompanied by maladaptive thoughts, feelings, and behaviors.

Due in part to its comorbidity with depressive disorders, somatic symptom disorder presents an individual at higher risk of suicidal thoughts and suicide attempts. The severity of their symptoms alone nevertheless, as pointed out in *DSM-5-TR*, may also lead to an increased risk of suicidality.

Although somatic symptom disorder may develop in an individual at any time, the COVID-19 pandemic may have presented a unique set of risk factors. Even after the acute infection subsides, individuals may develop somatic symptom disorder regarding what they

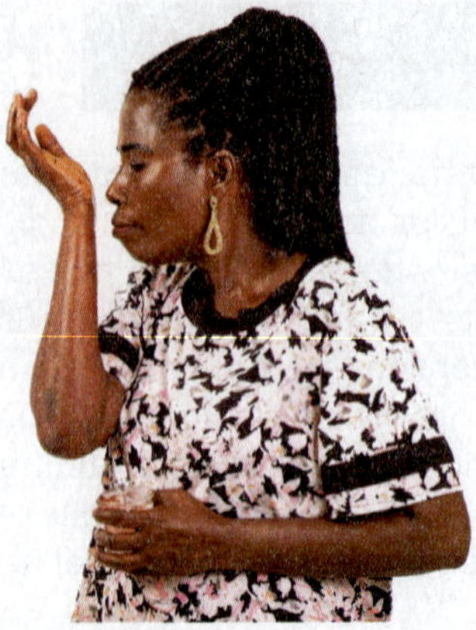

Individuals who were infected during the COVID-19 pandemic may be at risk for somatic symptom disorder, believing that they continue to have physical symptoms, such as this woman who believes she has lost her sense of smell.

vystekimages/Alamy Stock Photo

believe are persistent symptoms, especially given the prevalence of "long COVID." In one investigation carried out in France between the first two waves of the pandemic (early and late 2020), over half continued to experience at least one physical symptom, and 10 percent met the diagnostic criteria for somatic symptom disorder. Those with somatic symptom disorder were more likely to be older women, infected during the second wave, and having probable PTSD (Horn et al., 2023).

The French study illustrates the difficulty that clinicians have in discerning somatic symptoms that do and do not have a physical cause, particularly when the very symptoms are ones that are associated with a known disease entity.

Illness Anxiety Disorder

illness anxiety disorder
A somatic symptom disorder characterized by the misinterpretation of normal bodily functions as signs of serious illness.

In contrast to somatic symptom disorder, in which individuals report symptoms that have no physical basis, people with **illness anxiety disorder** fear or mistakenly believe that normal bodily reactions represent the symptoms of a serious illness. In other words, they do not experience actual "symptoms." Their anxiety leads them to easily become alarmed about their health and go out to seek unnecessary medical tests and procedures. Even though they have no "symptoms," they fear that they are at risk for a serious illness.

As was true for somatic symptom disorder, the COVID-19 pandemic had the potential to heighten people's illness anxiety and, similarly, making it difficult for clinicians to separate the disorder from more or less ordinary concern about becoming infected. However, "COVID anxiety" is not a universal experience. One British study reported a 22 percent rate of extreme fear of COVID, with 34 percent consuming COVID-related media stories many times per day. There were significant consequences for people with extreme COVID anxiety, including not leaving the home at all, engaging in excessive handwashing and disinfecting, and even washing their clothes every time they did have to leave the house. Over half reported experiencing severe social and occupational dysfunction, with rates higher among individuals from an ethnic group at increased risk for COVID-19 (King et al., 2023).

The identification of this particular variant of illness anxiety disorder suggests that its symptoms may respond to external factors related to social and historical context. Although too soon for COVID anxiety to become a part of the diagnostic system, it does appear from research conducted thus far that, should it linger beyond the ending of the pandemic, there will be a need to ensure that the "disorder" remains separated from what might be adaptive illness-prevention behaviors.

MINI CASE

Somatic Symptom Disorder, with Predominant Pain

Helen, a 34-year-old White bisexual cisgender woman, is seeking treatment because her physician said there was nothing more he could do for her. When asked about her physical problems, Helen recited a litany of complaints, including frequent episodes when she could not remember what had happened to her and other times when her vision was so blurred that she could not read the words on a printed page. Helen enjoys cooking and doing things around the house, but she becomes easily fatigued and short of breath for no apparent reason. She often is unable to eat the elaborate meals she prepares, because she becomes nauseated and is prone to vomit any food with even a touch of spice. According to Helen's husband, she has lost all interest in sexual intimacy, and they have intercourse only about once every few months, usually at his insistence. Helen complains of painful cramps during her menstrual periods and at other times says she feels that her "insides are on fire." Because of additional pain in her back, legs, and chest, Helen wants to stay in bed for much of the day. She lives in a large, old Victorian house, from which she ventures only infrequently "because I need to be able to lie down when my legs ache."

MINI CASE

Illness Anxiety Disorder, Care-Seeking Type

Hannah is a 48-year-old Japanese American heterosexual cisgender woman. She is a mother of two children, both of whom have recently moved away from home. Within the past year, her menstrual periods have become much heavier and more irregular. Seeking an explanation, Hannah began to spend days reading everything she could find on uterine cancer. Although medical books specified menstrual disturbance as a common feature of menopause, one newspaper article mentioned the possibility of uterine cancer. Hannah immediately made an appointment with her gynecologist, who tested her and concluded that her symptoms were almost certainly due to menopause. Convinced that her physician was trying to protect her from knowing "the awful truth," Hannah visited one gynecologist after another in search of someone who would properly diagnose what she was certain was a fatal illness. She decided to give up her job as a restaurant hostess. First, she was concerned that long hours of standing at the cash register would aggravate her medical condition. Second, she felt she could not be tied down by a job that was interfering with her medical appointments.

A further consideration in the diagnosis of illness anxiety disorder is the possibility that it is conceptually difficult to distinguish from somatic symptom disorder. Instead, researchers suggest that the concept of "pathological health anxiety" could justifiably be applied to both somatic symptom and illness anxiety disorder with both potentially related to an anxiety or obsessive-compulsive spectrum disorder (Axelsson & Hedman-Lagerlöf, 2022).

Yet another factor to consider is the role of a diagnosed health condition in contributing to symptoms of depression and anxiety. In what is referred to as "diabetes distress," individuals who are diagnosed with Type 2 (adult-onset) diabetes can become despondent as they face the challenge of adopting changes in lifestyle associated with the need to reduce their blood glucose levels. Estimates place the 10 percent with diagnosable depression and up to 22 percent with depressive symptoms, suggesting that the direction between illness and psychological factors can operate in both directions. Furthermore, individuals who experience diabetes distress can give up on making those necessary lifestyle adaptations, only decreasing the likelihood that they will be able to manage their diabetes within acceptable limits (Schmitt et al., 2021).

Functional Neurological Symptom Disorder (Conversion Disorder)

Individuals with **functional neurological symptom disorder (conversion disorder)** experience an actual change in a bodily function which cannot be linked to an underlying medical condition. The kinds of changes these individuals experience can range from being unable to move normally such as becoming paralyzed, unable to walk, to losing the ability to speak, and developing vision or hearing loss.

functional neurological disorder (conversion disorder)
A somatic symptom disorder involving the translation of unacceptable drives or troubling conflicts into physical symptoms.

Reflecting prior theory on this disorder, the term *conversion* that you see in parentheses in the name of the disorder reflects its historical origins that can be traced back to Freud, who named it after seeing a number of his patients showing symptoms that he believed reflected unconscious conflict (i.e., "conversion" of the psychological to the physical). The current term *functional neurological* refers to the fact that the individual's symptoms are experienced as neurological or sensory impairments that affect their ability to carry out certain behaviors.

Unfortunately, for individuals with this disorder, it may be difficult to get the type of psychological intervention that could benefit them if they seek treatment only from a medical professional. Diagnoses of functional neurological disorder are made as

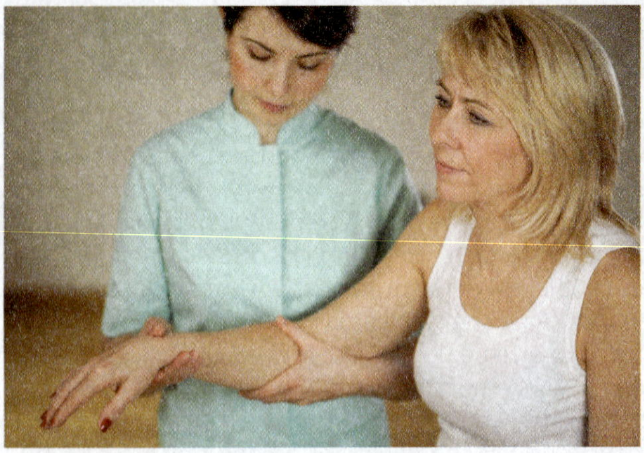

Medical personnel may fail to refer individuals with functional neurological disorders for appropriate treatment due to biases against the legitimacy of the diagnosis.

Ground Picture/Shutterstock

"exclusionary," rather than from the perspective of the diagnostic criteria for the disorder (Forejtová et al., 2023). Biases against the legitimacy of the disorder may further result in a lower likelihood of the individual being referred to the type of therapy that could alleviate their symptoms (Begley et al., 2023). The *ICD-11* classifies functional neurological disorder together with dissociative disorders with the new diagnosis of *dissociative neurological symptom disorder*. For the first time, this places what was considered a "psychological" disorder into the same area within the *ICD-11* as neurological disorders. As a result, individuals with these disabling symptoms may receive treatment to restore the functions that they have lost.

Conditions Related to Somatic Symptom Disorders

As you have just learned, psychological factors can manifest as physical symptoms, or anxiety over real or imagined physical symptoms can become the source of a psychological disorder. Although there may be no physiological basis for the disorders, the symptoms feel very real to those who are experiencing them. In contrast, **malingering** consists of deliberately feigning the symptoms of physical illness or psychological disorder for an ulterior motive such as receiving disability or insurance benefits.

In the *DSM-5-TR*, malingering is included as a condition that might be a focus of clinical attention, rather than as a diagnosis. The situations in which it might present include forensic evaluations and occupational or military settings in which the possibility that clients are feigning symptoms must be ruled out. Although malingering might serve an adaptive function, it is also likely that some of these situations can produce **primary gain**–namely the direct benefits of occupying the sick role. Structured malingering assessments can improve the evaluation of suspected malingerers and protect the practitioners who are faced with making the determination (Weiss & Van Dell, 2017).

In **factitious disorder imposed on self**, people show a pattern of falsifying symptoms that are either physical, psychological, or a combination of the two. The individual falsifies these symptoms not to achieve economic or material gain but for the purpose of adopting the sick role, known as **secondary gain**, which is the sympathy and attention they receive from other people when they are ill. In extreme cases, known informally as

malingering
The fabrication of physical or psychological symptoms for some ulterior motive.

primary gain
The relief from anxiety or responsibility due to the development of physical or psychological symptoms.

factitious disorder imposed on self
A disorder in which people fake symptoms or disorders not for the purpose of any particular gain but because of an inner need to maintain a sick role.

secondary gain
The sympathy and attention that a sick person receives from other people.

MINI CASE

Functional Neurological Disorder, with Sensory Loss

Brayden is a 24-year-old White queer non-binary person. They are pursuing a PhD in engineering and constantly feel stressed by their rigorous academic workload. They have always thought of themselves as a person to whom weird things happen and have commonly made more of situations than was warranted. Driving on a snowy night, Brayden accidentally hit an older adult man who was walking on the side of the road, causing the man a near-fatal injury. In the months that followed, Brayden became caught up in lengthy legal proceedings, which distracted them from their work and caused them tremendous emotional stress. On awakening one Monday morning, Brayden found themself staggering around, unable to see anything other than the shadows of objects in the room. At first they thought they were just having a hard time waking up. As the morning progressed, however, Brayden realized they were losing their vision. They waited 2 days before going to the emergency clinic on campus. When they did go, they were oddly unconcerned about what seemed like such a serious physical condition.

instances of Munchausen's syndrome, the individual's entire existence becomes consumed with the pursuit of medical care. A related disorder is **factitious disorder imposed on another** or Munchausen's syndrome by proxy. The individual with this disorder feigns the symptoms of another person, potentially motivated by the need for attention or to be seen as a martyr or good parent. However, this is a disorder that instead is better viewed as a form of maltreatment given that the target of this behavior is usually a child. In the United States, such behavior is considered a form of medical child abuse (Bursch, Emerson, & Sanders, 2021).

factitious disorder imposed on another
A condition in which a person induces physical symptoms in another person who is under that person's care.

Theories and Treatment of Somatic Symptom and Related Disorders

Some of the most famous cases studied by Freud included what now would be considered a somatic symptom disorder or functional neurological disorder. Freud's writing included the listing of the many inexplicable symptoms of his patients along with the development of his methods of treatment that included hypnosis, free association, and dream analysis. With the assumption that the symptoms were the expression of unconscious conflict, Freud and his fellow psychoanalysts used terms such as "hysteria" (meaning, literally, "wandering uterus") as explanations for what they saw as repressed sexual desires that became manifest in bodily or neurological symptoms whose source could not be traced to any physical dysfunction.

Although present-day psychoanalysts no longer believe in the "wandering uterus" theory, they maintain that unconscious conflicts are important contributors and regard the aim of treatment to be one of identifying and bringing these conflicts into conscious awareness, allowing the client to gain the insight and self-awareness that will make it possible to express emotion directly, rather than through physical manifestation. Psychodynamically based clinicians also seek to identify and treat these disorders from a trauma informed perspective, using methods based in part on the Core Conflictual Relationship Theme method (Van Nieuwenhove et al., 2020).

From the cognitive behavioral perspective, the dissociative, somatic symptom, and related disorders are viewed in terms of the maladaptive thoughts that become linked to the client's physical symptoms. The underlying model is based on the premise that people with these disorders are subject to cognitive distortions that lead them to misinterpret normal bodily sensations through a "perception filter" mechanism. Once they start to exaggerate the importance of their symptoms, they become even more sensitized to internal bodily cues, which in turn leads them to conclude that they are truly ill (Schulz et al., 2020).

In applying cognitive behavioral therapy to clients with somatic symptom and related disorders, clinicians help their clients gain a more realistic appraisal of their body's reactions. One advantage of this approach is that it can be delivered by nurse practitioners working in primary care settings (Sitnikova et al., 2019). Importantly, to be successful, though, a client's treatment preferably begins at an early stage of the disorder (Berezowski et al., 2022).

Hypnotherapy and medication are two additional approaches that clinicians use specifically for treating functional neurological disorder. In hypnotherapy, the therapist instructs the hypnotized client to move the paralyzed limb. The therapist then makes the posthypnotic suggestion to enable the client to sustain the movement after the therapist brings the client out of the hypnotic trance. Clinicians who are unable to see their clients on a face-to-face basis

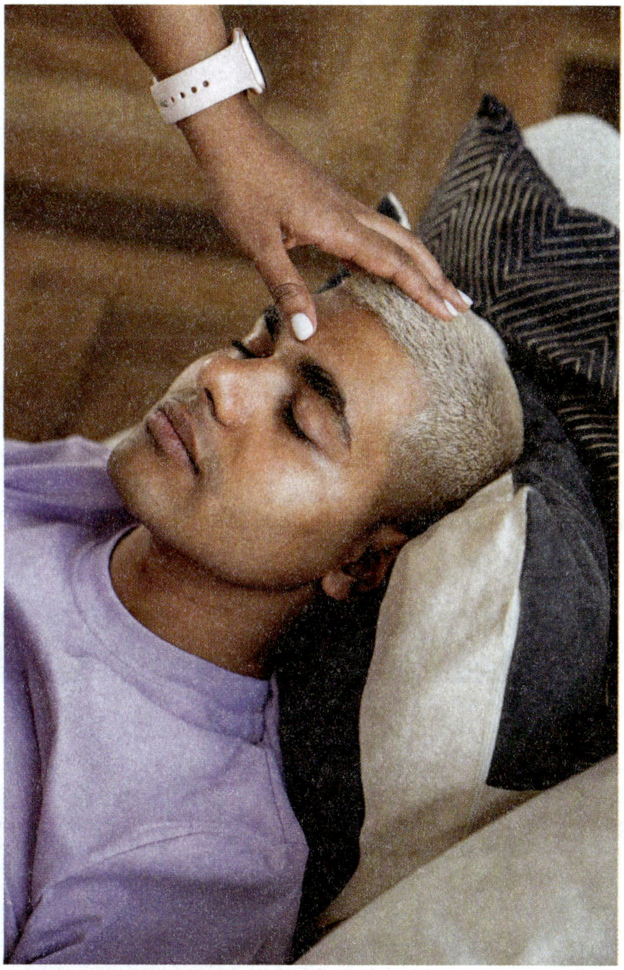

In hypnotherapy, individuals with functional neurological disorder may be encouraged to recount memories that are too troubling to consciously recall.

Westend61 GmbH/Alamy Stock Photo

What's in the *DSM-5-TR*

Somatic Symptom and Related Disorders

The *DSM-5* brought a number of significant changes to the entire category of what we now call somatic symptom disorders. The authors of the *DSM-5* acknowledged that the terminology for what were called somatoform disorders in *DSM-IV-TR* was potentially confusing. They also recognize that somatic symptom disorders, psychological factors affecting other medical conditions, and factitious disorders all include the presence of physical symptoms and/or concern about medical illness. Furthermore, they recognize that the mind and body interact, so clinicians cannot separate physical symptoms from their psychological basis, nor vice versa. Further complicating the prior system, according to the *DSM-5* authors, was the fact that it is never entirely possible to determine that a psychological symptom has no physical basis.

The term *illness anxiety disorder* replaced *hypochondriasis*. Clinicians will give those individuals who have no physical symptoms but are highly anxious this diagnosis, specifying whether it includes care-seeking.

In the *DSM-5-TR*, functional neurological disorder retains "conversion disorder" in parentheses following the diagnosis, indicating that the individual shows atypical nervous system functioning. However, to receive the diagnosis, the person must have symptoms that cannot be explained by a nervous system disease. Individuals will need to have a full neurological examination before health care professionals conclude that their symptoms have no neurological basis.

Other than improving the terminology, the *DSM-5-TR* authors hope their revisions will lead to improved data collection on this group of disorders. Inconsistencies in the diagnostic criteria, combined with the main theoretical focus shifting from the psychodynamic to the cognitive behavioral, have produced a situation in which there are not yet solid epidemiological data on a group of disorders whose prevalence we can now more accurately estimate.

can also deliver hypnotherapy effectively through telepsychology (Hasan, Pearson, Morris, & Whorwell, 2019). For those clients who are treated by practitioners working from an integrated neurological-psychological approach, physical therapy can also be included as a way to restore lost functioning (Maggio et al., 2020).

Cognitive behavioral therapy for individuals with illness anxiety disorder focuses on their high levels of **health anxiety**, or undue concern about physical symptoms and illness. In therapy, individuals learn to restructure their maladaptive beliefs about their physical symptoms and gain more realistic interpretations of their body's reactions. Countering COVID-19-related illness anxiety, Internet-based cognitive behavioral therapy focusing specifically on symptoms developed after the pandemic, can also be effective (Sharrock et al., 2021). In severe cases, where clients either do not want to enter or stay in individual therapy, group therapy using principles of ACT may provide an effective alternative (Eilenberg et al., 2016).

health anxiety
Undue concern about physical symptoms and illness.

psychological factors affecting other medical conditions
Disorder in which clients have a medical disease or symptom that appears to be exacerbated by psychological or behavioral factors.

9.3 Psychological Factors Affecting Other Medical Conditions

So far you have learned about disorders in which individuals are experiencing physical symptoms that do not correspond to any known physiological cause. The diagnostic category called **psychological factors affecting other medical conditions** includes conditions in which a client's physical functioning is adversely affected by one or more psychological states. These can include depression, anxiety, stress, denial of a diagnosis, or engaging in poor or even dangerous health-related behaviors.

MINI CASE

Psychological Factors Affecting Other Medical Conditions

Rohan is a 41-year-old South Asian heterosexual cisgender man. He currently works as a manager of a large discount chain store, a position he worked his way up over the past few years. Despite his success, Rohan struggles with an agitated depression, which causes him to feel impatient and irritable most of the time. He recognizes that his emotional problems relate to long-standing issues with his parents, and he resents the fact that he chronically suffers from an inner tension that has always been part of his personality. The youngest in a family of four children, Rohan perceived that throughout his childhood he had to do "twice as much" as his siblings to gain his parents' attention and affection. Now, as an adult, he is caught up in a drive toward success that literally makes him physically sick. He has intense headaches and stomachaches on most days, yet he is reluctant to seek medical help because he doesn't want to take time away from work.

TABLE 2 **Psychological Factors Affecting Other Medical Conditions**

Medical Condition	Possible Psychological Factor
Hypertension (high blood pressure)	Chronic occupational stress increasing the risk of high blood pressure
Asthma	Anxiety exacerbating the individual's respiratory symptoms
Cancer	Denying the need for surgical interventions
Diabetes	Being unwilling to alter lifestyle to monitor glucose levels or reduce intake
Chronic tension headache	Continuing family-related stresses that contribute to worsening of symptoms
Cardiovascular disease	Refusing to visit a cardiac specialist for evaluation despite chest discomfort

Table 2 outlines several examples of medical conditions that can be affected by psychological factors. Specifying the interaction of psychological factors with medical conditions provides health professionals with a clearer understanding of how the two interact. Once this interaction has been identified, the clinician can address the issues and work to help the client's medical condition improve.

Relevant Concepts for Understanding Psychological Factors Affecting Other Medical Conditions

Psychological disorders, stress, emotional states, personality traits, and poor coping skills are factors that can affect an individual's physical health and well-being. This category of disorders acknowledges the complex interactions through which psychological and physical conditions can affect each other.

Stress and Coping

Within psychology, the term **stress** refers to the unpleasant emotional reaction experienced when a person perceives an event to be threatening. This emotional reaction may include heightened physiological arousal, reflecting increased reactivity of the sympathetic nervous system. A **stressful life event** is a stressor that disrupts the individual's life. A person's efforts to reduce stress is called **coping**. It is when coping is unsuccessful, and the stress does not subside, that the individual may seek clinical attention for medical or psychological problems that have developed as a consequence of the constant physiological arousal caused by the experience of chronic negative emotions.

stress
The unpleasant emotional reaction that a person has when an event is perceived as threatening.

stressful life event
An event that disrupts the individual's life.

coping
The process through which people reduce stress.

What types of events qualify as stressors? The most common way to describe stressors is through stressful life event rating scales, which are intended to quantify the degree to which individuals were exposed to experiences that could threaten their health. One of the best known of these is the Social Readjustment Rating Scale (SRRS) (Holmes & Rahe, 1967), which assesses life stress in terms of life change units (LCUs). In developing the LCU index, researchers calculated how strongly each type of event was associated with physical illness. The rationale behind this measure is that the more an event causes you to adjust your life circumstances, the more deleterious it is to your health.

Life events scales have merit because they are relatively easy to complete and present a set of objective criteria that clinicians can use to assess an individual's potential for experiencing stress. Some of these include major life events such as loss of a partner or close family member, or being laid off from a job. Others are smaller, seemingly less significant, but still can represent sources of stress. From a cognitive perspective, the key factor is how much life adjustment is required by the event. However, smaller stressful events can also create coping challenges. You and your best friend may each experience the same potentially stressful event, such as being late for an advising appointment, but you may be far more perturbed by this situation than your friend. Your day will thus be far less pleasant than your friend's, and if you are constantly running late for important meetings, class, or work, you might be at risk for a stress-related illness.

The cognitive model of stress places greater emphasis on the way you interpret events than on whether you experienced a given event. Like the cognitive approach in general, the cognitive model of stress proposes that the appraisal of an event as stressful determines whether it will have a negative impact on your emotional state. Not only do people differ in the way they interpret events, the circumstances surrounding the event also affect them. If your friend's professor doesn't take class attendance but yours does, this would help explain why you feel more stressed about being late than your friend.

As this example shows, stress is in the mind of the beholder. Even a relatively minor event can lead you to experience stress if you interpret it negatively. The cognitive model assumes, furthermore, that these "little" events can have a big impact, especially when they build up in a short period of time. Events called **hassles** can have significant effects on health when there are enough of them and you interpret them negatively. If you are not only late but get into an argument with your friend, stub your toe, spill your coffee, and miss your bus home, you will have as many potentially stress-causing events in one afternoon as someone experiencing a "bigger" life event such as being laid off from work.

hassles
Relatively minor events that can cause stress.

On the positive side, you can balance your hassles with what researchers call **uplifts**, which are events on a small scale that boost your feelings of well-being. Perhaps you're browsing through a social media feed and someone has sent you a friendly message. The smile this greeting brings to your face can help make up for some of the stress of the hassles you just experienced. Uplifts are especially important within the positive psychology movement, which views them as contributing to people's feelings of day-to-day happiness.

uplifts
Events that boost your feelings of well-being.

It's wonderful when life sends a few uplifts your way, but when it doesn't, you need to find other ways to reduce stress through coping if you are to maintain your mental health. Two basic ways of coping are **problem-focused coping** and **emotion-focused coping** (Lazarus & Folkman, 1984). In problem-focused coping, you attempt to reduce stress by acting to change whatever it is that makes the situation stressful. If you're constantly late for work because the bus is overcrowded and tends to arrive 5 or 10 minutes after it's supposed to, then you can cope by getting an earlier bus, even if it means you have to wake up 10 minutes ahead of schedule. In contrast, in emotion-focused coping, you don't change the situation but instead change the way you feel about it. Rather than think about a stressful experience, you just put it out of your mind.

problem-focused coping
Coping in which the individual takes action to reduce stress by changing whatever it is about the situation that makes it stressful.

emotion-focused coping
A type of coping in which a person does not change anything about the situation itself but instead tries to improve feelings about the situation.

A third way of coping does not neatly fit into the problem- vs. emotion-focused distinction. In **social support**, individuals seek connections with others in order to reduce stress. Those they seek help from may provide practical suggestions or actual assistance in addressing the situation (problem-focused) while also allowing individuals to relieve stress by feeling that they are understood (emotion-focused). Talking to your friends about the challenges you have in balancing your many demands at school, or problems in your relationships, can give you both a mood boost and a way to potentially fix those problems.

social support
A method of coping in which individuals seek connections with others in order to reduce stress

Which is the best coping method to use? The answer is, it depends. People cope with some situations more effectively through problem-focused coping. In changeable situations, you are most likely better off if you use problem-focused coping. If you're stressed because your grades are in a slump, rather than not think about the problem, you would be well advised to try to change the situation by studying harder. If you're stressed because you lost your Internet connection while taking a mandatory online exam, there is nothing you can do to change the situation (though later you can try asking your professor to let you make it up). If you're not sure what to do or just want to see what your friends have to say, then social support would be an excellent way to alleviate stress.

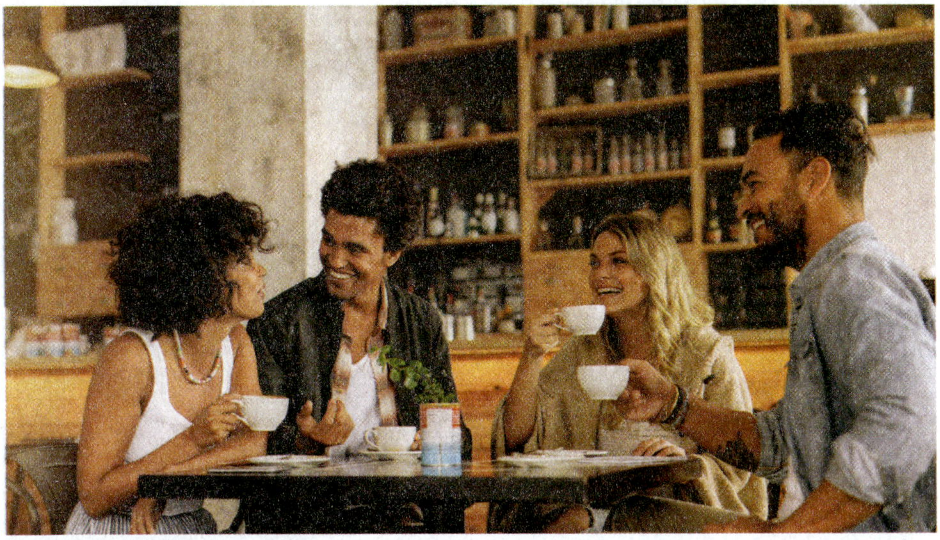

Having people to share your experiences with can be an important way to cope with stress.
Jacob Lund/Alamy Stock Photo

Personality also plays a role in affecting how much stress individuals experience as a result of exposure to potential stressors. In general, people with high levels of optimism are more resilient to stress. As you can probably recall from your own experience, the first year of college is associated with a great deal of stress, both academically and socially. Using measures of optimism and exposure to stressors, researchers found that both independently predicted the levels of subjective well-being undergraduates reported during their transition to the new academic environment (Yovita & Asih, 2018).

A combination of optimism and what's called a "proactive" personality may also help reduce the stress associated with the COVID-19 pandemic. People with this personality type look for new opportunities, show initiative, and persevere in the face of obstacles. In a study of Chinese health care workers at the height of the pandemic, those with this proactive orientation had higher levels of performance in their jobs than their counterparts whose personalities did not provide them with the same degree of resilience (Yi-Feng Chen et al., 2021).

Conversely, personality traits may operate in the opposite direction, particularly when combined with coping methods that do not serve the function of reducing stress. In a study of older adults with lymphoma (cancer of the lymphatic system), researchers in the Netherlands reported that individuals high in neuroticism were higher on levels of distress, particularly if they also used maladaptive emotion-focused coping methods of feeling helpless and hopeless, becoming anxiously preoccupied, or avoiding the reality of their condition (Arts et al., 2021).

Not only can personality influence the way in which individuals cope with stress, but stress exposure can initiate a set of reactions within the body that lowers its resistance to disease. The large-scale study conducted in the United Kingdom known as "Whitehall II" demonstrated that workers exposed to such chronic stressors as lack of control over work schedules, heavy psychological workloads, and insufficient social support can contribute to such negative outcomes as higher rates of depression as well as increased risk of cardiovascular disease (Piantella et al., 2021).

Sociocultural factors also play a role in causing and aggravating an individual's level of stress. One of these sociocultural factors is that of minority status stress. In one study of Hispanic female-identified college students, minority status stress was compared to typical college stress as predictors of intention to remain in college and grade point average. Both forms of stress independently predicted depressive symptoms which, in turn, predicted whether students saw themselves as remaining in college. Among the sources of college minority status stress were a negative university social climate such as racist practices and policies, discrimination based on race, pressures from within one's own race about how to act, and lack of academic confidence (Arbona, Fan, & Olvera, 2018).

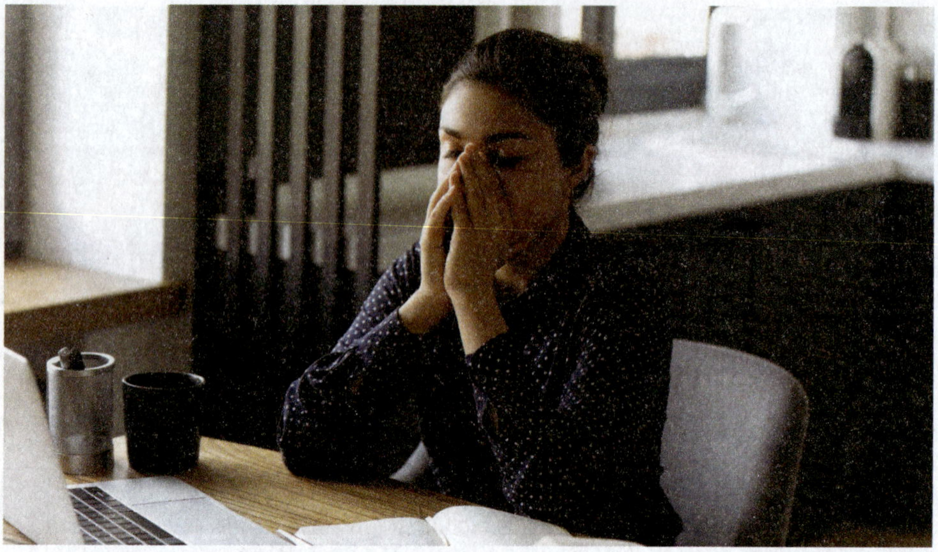

Heavy psychological workloads, in addition to other occupational stress factors, can have a significant impact on both physical and mental health.
fizkes/Shutterstock

Emotional Expression

Coping with stress by controlling your negative emotions is one way to reduce your levels of perceived stress. However, there are times when expressing your emotions, even if they are negative, can improve your physical and mental well-being. In one classic study, researchers instructed a group of first-year college students to write about the experience of coming to college, a highly stressful one, as previously noted. A control group wrote about superficial topics. Those who wrote about coming to college reported being more homesick than the control subjects. Even though they experienced more negative emotions, however, they made fewer visits to physicians and, by the end of the year, were doing as well as or better than the control subjects in terms of grade point average and the experience of positive moods. The researchers concluded that confronting feelings and thoughts about a stressful experience can have long-lasting positive effects, even though the initial impact of such a confrontation may be disruptive (Pennebaker, Colder, & Sharp, 1990).

Pennebaker and his colleagues have expanded their findings to a variety of populations. In a meta-analysis of 146 randomized studies, disclosure had a positive and significant effect on people with a wide range of emotional concerns (Frattaroli, 2006). Researchers have even identified positive mental health effects of writing on social media sites, including blogging (Ko & Kuo, 2009).

As a strategy for reducing stress, emotional expression can also have benefits for individuals coping with one of life's most significant life events, the loss of a spouse. In a study of Dutch adults, primarily widows, emotional expression along with other adaptive coping strategies, was associated with lower bereavement-related depression. Additionally, however, the use of mindfulness further contributed to fewer depressive symptoms across a 6-month period (Eisma, Janshen, Huber, & Schroevers, 2023).

Keep in mind, however, that although the person expressing these feelings may feel better, the person who listens to the retelling of a sad or difficult story may suffer negative emotional consequences (Kellas, Horstman, Willer, & Carr, 2015). This is one of the reasons individuals who work in the helping professions may experience burnout, otherwise known as "compassion fatigue" (West, 2015). Contributing to compassion fatigue may be the individual's tendency to ruminate, which can particularly trouble those who are also high in empathy (Liu et al., 2021).

As discussed in Chapter 8, first responders can be at risk for developing PTSD after exposure to a natural disaster. In an in-depth interview study of first responders, researchers identified a number of factors that participants believed could help to mitigate against stress. These included the response preparedness of their organization for handling disasters, the opportunity to debrief with their colleagues after the disaster along with general peer support, recognition of their efforts, and access to workplace resources such as gyms and meditation rooms (Alavi, Kia-Keating, & Nerenberg, 2023).

Personality

One of the most thoroughly researched connections between personality and health is the **type A behavior pattern**, a set of behaviors that purportedly include being hard-driving, competitive, impatient, cynical, suspicious of and hostile toward others, and easily irritated. As popular as the idea has become, even entrenched into everyday language, a retraction initiated by Kings College London (2019) of all published articles pertaining to this quality requires that the entire concept be rethought (e.g., Eysenck, 2021).

type A behavior pattern
Set of behaviors that purportedly include being hard-driving, competitive, impatient, cynical, suspicious of and hostile toward others, and easily irritated.

The problems in the original research documenting this personality-health link provide a valuable lesson in the importance of transparency by researchers as well as the need for replication. The investigation that prompted the retractions noted a number of serious problems, ranging from ethical violations to actual data fabrication. In the aftermath of the retraction, personality researchers now take a far more conservative approach when demonstrating any health effects of personality and related behavior that may contribute to a particular physical disease.

Does the retraction of the Type A body of research mean that personality plays no role in predisposing individuals to chronic physical disease, including those that involve the cardiovascular system? Continuing investigations into linkages between Five Factor Model traits and health suggest that such linkages do exist, but not in the simple manner originally proposed within the context of Type A research. Instead, it appears more likely that personality traits can predict certain health-related behaviors that would, in turn, either improve or worsen an individual's chance of developing a chronic disease. Across 15 international samples, a team of psychologists and public health researchers found a small, but significant contribution of conscientiousness to such behaviors as likelihood of visits to dentists and general practitioners. Those lower in conscientiousness and agreeableness but higher in neuroticism were more likely to be admitted to hospitals. The authors warn, however, that the effects were small in magnitude, suggesting that personality alone cannot explain people's risks of developing disease (Willroth et al., 2023).

type D personality
A personality type seen in those who experience emotions that include anxiety, irritation, and depressed mood.

behavioral medicine
An interdisciplinary approach to medical conditions affected by psychological factors that is rooted in learning theory.

There does, however, continue to be evidence to support the so-called **type D personality**. The "D" in type D stands for "distressed." Type D personalities experience emotions that include anxiety, irritation, and depressed mood, but they have difficulty expressing these emotions. Their higher rates of heart disease appear to be related both to the presence of these negative emotions and to their tendency to inhibit rather than express them (Lin et al., 2018).

Applications to Behavioral Medicine

Because psychological factors that contribute to a medical condition have such a wide range, clinicians must conduct a careful assessment of the way each particular client's health is affected by their behavior. The field of **behavioral medicine** refers to an interdisciplinary approach to medical conditions affected by psychological factors that is rooted in learning theory. In addition, clinicians working in behavioral medicine often team up with psychologists and other mental health professionals to help clients learn and maintain behaviors that will maximize their physical functioning. By improving patients' compliance with medical treatment, clinicians can help them achieve better health and avoid further complications (Wilson, 2015).

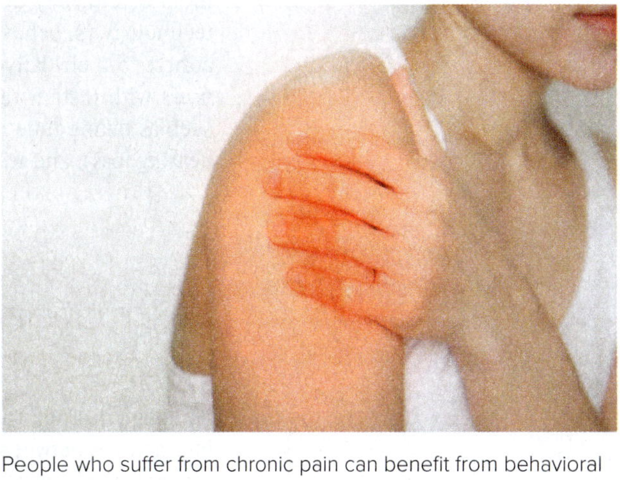

People who suffer from chronic pain can benefit from behavioral medicine approaches, including the use of cognitive behavioral therapy.
ANN PATCHANAN/Shutterstock

Psychoeducation is an important component of behavioral medicine. Clients need to understand how their behavior influences the development or worsening of the symptoms of chronic illness.

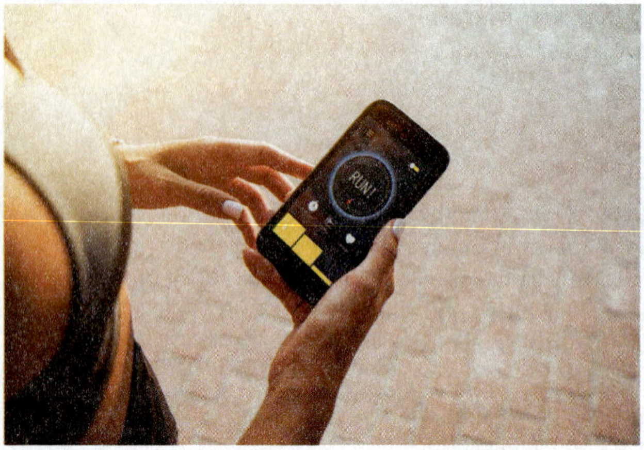

Smartphone applications can provide individuals with useful prompts to monitor their daily levels of physical activity, among other health-related behaviors.

Westend61 GmbH/Alamy Stock Photo

Then the clinician can work with them to develop specific ways to improve their health habits. For example, a balanced diet and exercise are key to preventing and reducing the serious complications of cardiovascular disease. Time spent outdoors, even if not in active exercise, can also reduce stress levels (Beyer, Szabo, Hoormann, & Stolley, 2018). The clinician can teach clients ways to build these new health habits into their daily regimens. Other applications include coaching people with sleep disorders to improve their bedtime habits with such methods as avoiding daytime naps, exercising late in the day, and staying off electronic devices prior to going to bed.

Learning to manage chronic pain is another application of behavioral medicine. Cognitive behavioral therapy, along with other pain management techniques, was found in one large-scale review of research to produce beneficial effects both on chronic neck pain as well as anxiety and depression. Additionally, patients became less likely to catastrophize about the cause and nature of their pain (Ploutarchou et al., 2023).

Treatments can also include involvement of family members, particularly those who serve in a caregiving role to a long-term partner, child, or friend. Not only are these individuals vital for maintaining the health of those they care for with respect to a particular physical condition, but the quality of their relationship can also influence the ability of a medical patient to recover from or cope with a serious illness. As an example, researchers studying recovery from a post-cardiac event found that both patients and their spouses who were satisfied with their relationship reported a higher quality of life (Bouchard et al., 2023).

Behavioral medicine is also moving increasingly toward interventions the profession once considered alternative, including mindfulness training, relaxation, and meditation. In these approaches, clinicians teach clients to monitor their internal bodily states (such as heart rate and breathing), as well as their perceptions, affective states, thoughts, and imagery, without judging. By observing their bodily reactions in this objective fashion, clients gain a more differentiated understanding of which aspects of their experiences illness affects and which it does not. Mindfulness training has the added advantage of being translatable into online technology when combined with an intervention focused on the individual's medical condition, including strategies to maintain a healthy weight (Carpenter et al., 2019).

Wearable technologies, such as smartwatches and smartphones, could become important tools in behavioral medicine as these provide user-friendly and widely accessible ways to monitor a variety of health indicators. In a comparison of self-prompts through wearable technology vs. behavioral feedback, researchers found that participants were more likely to adhere to their daily physical activity goals (Conroy et al., 2023). In addition to providing users with instant readings, these applications can also promote other healthy behaviors such as taking time to engage in mindfulness activities, keep noise levels down (to prevent hearing loss), and wind down before bedtime.

9.4 Dissociative and Somatic Symptom Disorders: The Biopsychosocial Perspective

Although distinct, the disorders you've learned about in this chapter all reveal the complex interactions between mind and body and call for distinctions between "real" and "fake" psychological symptoms. They also all raise questions about the nature of the self. Mind-body interactions also play a role in the way in which stress relates to medical illnesses and physical symptoms.

Biology clearly plays a role in making some individuals more vulnerable to psychological disorders, and particularly these disorders. A person may have a known or undiagnosed physical condition that certain stressors particularly affect, which then triggers the symptoms for a somatic symptom or related disorder. However, whatever the role of biology, cognitive behavioral explanations provide useful approaches for treatment. Even people whose medical condition is clearly documented, as in chronic pain disorder, can benefit from learning how to reframe their thoughts about their disorder, if not also their actual health-related behaviors.

It is quite likely that the mind–body connections underlying these disorders will come under even closer scrutiny as work on *DSM-5-TR* evolves. The historical connections between these and the so-called "neurotic" disorders that seemed to affect many of Freud's patients will fade. Nevertheless, dissociative and somatic symptom disorders will undoubtedly maintain their fascination, if not their names.

Return to the Case: Rose Marston

Rose underwent 16 weekly individual therapy sessions, focusing on specific CBT techniques such as psychoeducation, cognitive restructuring techniques, exposure and response prevention, perceptual retraining exercises, and self-monitoring techniques in which she recorded the number of minutes spent thinking about her symptoms every day. These exercises focused on teaching Rose to look at her body in a more holistic, objective way and take the focus away from her stomach. During each session, Rose and her therapist discussed what happened during the previous week, reviewed "homework," and set an agenda for the session. Using this highly structured approach, Rose began to feel relief from her symptoms after the first few weeks of treatment. In addition, she began to treat her lactose intolerance through a combination of diet control and over-the-counter medication. By the end of the 16 weeks, Rose's pain was gone, and she had reconciled with her boyfriend, recognizing the strain put on their relationship by her constant concerns over her stomach pain. Her depression had also lifted, and she and her clinician agreed that taking an antidepressant would not be necessary. Rose continued to visit her clinician once per month for check-in visits to review her progress and assess for recurrence of symptoms.

Dr. Tobin's reflections: Rose's apparent sensitivity to her rather mild physical symptoms likely contributed to her previous depression. Though that had been temporarily treated with antidepressants, it was clear that her concerns continued until the concomitant stressors of breaking up with her boyfriend and losing her job led to an exacerbation of symptoms. It was helpful in Rose's case that she was highly motivated for treatment, which contributed to her positive outcome. Although individuals with somatic symptom disorder may be uncomfortable disclosing the extent of their symptoms and thoughts about them, Rose's motivation allowed her to reveal her thoughts and beliefs about her stomach discomfort. This information allowed her clinician to successfully tailor treatment to her specific concerns. Although Rose will require constant monitoring of her lactose intake, fortunately she will be able to keep her physical symptoms under control, which will ameliorate the source of her psychological preoccupation and distress.

SUMMARY

- This chapter covered three sets of conditions: dissociative disorders, somatic symptom disorders, and psychological factors affecting other medical conditions. Each of these conditions involves interactions between physical functioning and psychological symptoms or behaviors.
- Dissociative disorders occur when the human mind seems capable of dissociating, or separating, mental functions. Major forms of dissociative disorders include dissociative identity disorder (DID), dissociative amnesia, depersonalization, derealization, and depersonalization/derealization disorder. These disorders appear in many cases to have a connection to traumatic life experiences.
- Somatic symptom and related disorders are a group of conditions in which an individual's major symptoms involve what the individual experiences as physical problems and/or concerns about medical illness. Illness anxiety disorder involves mistaken fears about normal bodily reactions. The COVID-19 pandemic may have heightened people's illness anxiety due to the realistic nature of the threat presented by the risk of infection.

- The essential feature of functional neurological symptom disorder (conversion disorder) as defined in the *DSM-5-TR* is that the individual experiences a change in a bodily function not due to an underlying medical condition. A renaming from *DSM-5*, the term *conversion* now appears in parentheses, as a reference to what prior theories refer to as presumed transformation of psychological conflict to physical symptoms.
- Conditions related to somatic symptom disorders include malingering, the deliberate feigning of symptoms of physical illness or psychological disorder for an ulterior motive such as receiving disability or insurance benefits; and factitious disorder, where people show a pattern of falsifying symptoms that are either physical, psychological, or a combination of the two, in some cases involving a second person as the target of falsification.
- The diagnostic category called psychological factors affecting other medical conditions includes conditions in which a client's physical illness is adversely affected by one or more psychological states such as depression, stress, denial of a diagnosis, or engaging in poor or even dangerous health-related behaviors.
- Psychological disorders, stress, emotional states, personality traits, and poor coping skills can affect an individual's medical conditions. This category of disorders acknowledges the complex interactions through which psychological and physical conditions can affect each other.
- Coping can help regulate the emotion of anxiety and hence reduce stress. However, there are times when expressing emotions can improve both physical and mental well-being. Actively confronting the emotions that arise from an upsetting or traumatic event can have long-term health benefits.
- Because psychological factors that contribute to a medical condition have such a wide range, clinicians must conduct a careful assessment of how each particular client's health is affected by behavior. The field of behavioral medicine applies the growing body of scientific evidence regarding mind–body relationships to helping improve people's physical health by addressing its relationships to the psychological factors of stress, emotions, behavior patterns, and personality.
- Biology clearly plays a role in making some individuals more vulnerable to psychological disorders, and particularly so in these disorders. A person may have a known or undiagnosed physical condition that may be affected by certain stressful life events, which then trigger the symptoms for a somatic symptom disorder. However, whatever the role of biology, cognitive behavioral explanations provide useful approaches for treatment.

KEY TERMS

Behavioral medicine
Coping
Depersonalization
Depersonalization/derealization disorder
Derealization
Dissociative amnesia
Dissociative identity disorder (DID)
Emotion-focused coping
Factitious disorder imposed on another
Factitious disorder imposed on self
Fugue
Functional neurological disorder (conversion disorder)
Hassle
Health anxiety
Illness anxiety disorder
Malingering
Primary gain
Problem-focused coping
Psychological factors affecting other medical conditions
Secondary gain
Social support
Somatic symptom disorder
Somatic symptoms
Stress
Stressful life event
Type A behavior pattern
Type D personality
Uplifts

Feeding and Eating Disorders; Elimination Disorders; Sleep-Wake Disorders; and Disruptive, Impulse-Control, and Conduct Disorders

CHAPTER 10

OUTLINE

Learning Objectives

10.1 Identify characteristics, theories, and treatments of eating disorders.

10.2 Discuss symptoms and theories of elimination disorders.

10.3 Recognize indicators of sleep-wake disorders.

10.4 Differentiate among disruptive, impulse-control, and conduct disorders.

10.5 Analyze the biopsychosocial model for eating, elimination, sleep-wake, and impulse-control disorders.

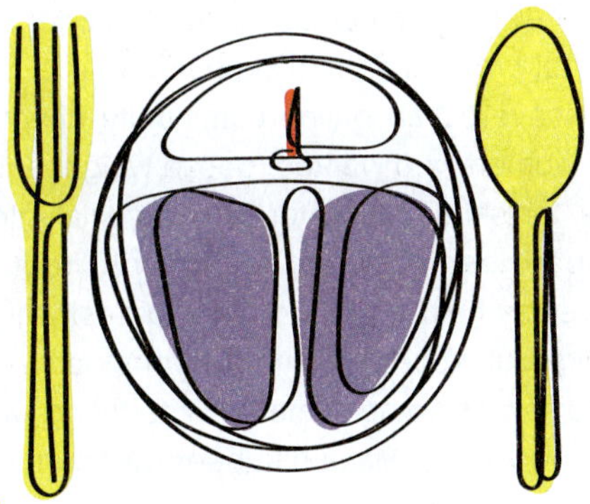

M7Studio/Shutterstock

Case Report

Maria Nomirez

Demographic information: 25-year-old Puerto Rican Latina heterosexual cisgender woman. Maria's pronouns are she/her/hers.

History of present illness: Maria self-referred to a community mental health center due to concerns about feeling depressed. During the initial intake evaluation, Maria stated that she had been feeling down and depressed for several months, and since her depression had not improved on its own, she had decided to seek treatment. She stated this was not an easy decision for her, because she usually was able to handle difficult emotions on her own. Maria also reported that those close to her were worried about her health and had been urging her for some time to seek treatment, although she couldn't understand why they were concerned.

The clinician noted that Maria appeared severely underweight and frail. Maria said she was feeling depressed, mainly because, as she described it, "I feel like a huge monster all the time." She estimated that these feelings originated while she was pregnant with her daughter, now 2 years old. She stopped working after giving birth in order to focus on raising her daughter, while her husband worked full time. Maria said she had had a difficult time returning to her normal weight after giving birth, and that she believed she still appeared pregnant: "All I can see in the mirror is my stomach and how enormous it makes me look all over." She reported that she did not know her current weight and was afraid to weigh herself for fear that she was continuing to gain weight. She exclaimed, "I feel so ashamed that I am so bigstill. I feel like I'll never look normal again."

Maria reported that she followed a diet consisting of about 300 to 400 calories per day, and that she had been "working her way down" in terms of daily caloric consumption ever since her concerns about her weight began. At that time, Maria had searched online for diet tips and discovered an online community devoted to supporting women who wanted to lose weight and stay thin. These "pro-ana" (slang for pro-anorexia) sites, as she described them, offered her support from other users, as well as helpful tips not only for restricting her caloric intake but also for hiding it from others, whose concern she saw as bothersome and interfering with her goals of losing weight. Maria had been visiting the sites daily for about 6 months. Her husband discovered them on their computer and, recognizing the danger they posed, pleaded with Maria to stop visiting them. She said she didn't understand why, because maintaining a low body weight was so important to her and the thought of gaining weight caused her intense feelings of anxiety.

Although she said she rarely felt interested in sex and had not menstruated for about 4 months, Maria explained that she and her husband had been trying to conceive another child for about 6 months. The clinician asked about any other physiological changes she might have noticed. Maria said she felt tired much of the time, but beyond that, she denied any difficulties. "I usually just think about my daughter and about staying thin. There isn't really time to worry about much else." She said further that while out in public, she often compared her body to those of others. This had become a source of overwhelming anxiety, so she typically preferred to stay home to avoid feeling "judged for being fat."

According to Maria, her family had been "constantly bothering" her about her weight. "They just don't understand how I feel. They try to force me to eat and it just makes me feel so uncomfortable and depressed. It feels like they are mocking me because they know how disgusting I am, so I usually just avoid spending time with them now." Her parents had moved from Puerto Rico to the mainland United States when Maria was an infant, and since then several other relatives had moved close by. Although Maria described the family as close-knit, she explained that it was difficult for her older relatives to understand the differences between Puerto Rican and mainland U.S. culture, which she felt exerted pressure to be thin and attractive. "It's just not that way where they are from, and so they don't know what it's like for me."

Psychiatric history: Maria reported that as a teenager she occasionally had episodes of bingeing and purging by vomiting, although she found the effects of the purging aversive. She explained that she has been concerned about her body weight "for as long as I can remember," and that she generally tries to maintain a low body weight. However, her restrictive eating behaviors became more severe following the birth of her daughter. She denied a family history of eating disorders.

Case Report *continued*

Case formulation: Maria meets diagnostic criteria for anorexia nervosa, binge-eating/purging type. Criterion A states the individual must maintain a body weight significantly lower than what is expected for age and height. With permission, the clinician obtained Maria's weight from her most recent physician visit and found that it was less than 85 percent of her expected weight—significantly lower than the minimal expectation for a woman her age. Maria also meets Criterion B because she has been intensely fearful of gaining weight, even though she is of lower-than-average body weight. She meets Criterion C because she fails to recognize the seriousness of her low body weight.

Although Maria reported often feeling depressed, the clinician determined that it appears that her symptoms of depression are directly related to her heightened concern about her weight. Therefore, the clinician will not give her an additional diagnosis of depression. It is clear that Maria's concern about her weight has alienated her from those to whom she is closest, namely her husband and her immediate family.

Risk level: Low risk. Maria denies current suicidal ideation and has no history of suicide attempts.

Treatment plan: Maria was resistant to the clinician's advice that she should receive treatment for her anorexia. With her permission, the clinician reached out to Maria's husband and family, who agreed that treatment was crucial for her. After discussing the matter with her husband, Maria agreed to present for an initial consultation at a day treatment program that specializes in eating disorders. After the evaluation there, Maria decided that pursuing treatment would be the best decision for her family and would help reduce her feelings of depression. She agreed to sign a contract to participate in the treatment program for at least 2 months.

Sarah Tobin, PhD

The disorders we cover in this chapter include eating disorders, elimination disorders, and a range of disorders in which individuals exhibit a lack of control over their impulses. Eating disorders are characterized by difficulties individuals have regarding food and control over their eating, dieting, or elimination of food. Elimination disorders specifically affect primarily children or adolescents who are having difficulty controlling the biological functions of urination and defecation, generally due to psychological disturbances. People with sleep-wake disorders lack control over biological processes that often have a relationship to psychological functions. Finally, the impulse-control disorders reflect disturbances in the individual's ability to regulate one or more of a range of behaviors related to particular desires, interests, and the expression of emotions.

10.1 Eating Disorders

People who have **eating disorders** experience persistent disturbances of eating or eating-related behavior that change the way they eat or digest their food. These disorders go beyond dieting or occasional overeating, significantly impairing the individual's physical and psychosocial functioning.

eating disorders
Diagnosis for people who experience persistent disturbances of eating or eating-related behavior that result in the person's altering the consumption or absorption of food.

Globally, the prevalence of eating disorders by early adulthood is estimated to be 6 to 18 percent of self-identified women and 0.6 to 2 percent among self-identified men. Lifetime prevalence, correspondingly, is 0.8 to 6.3 percent of women and 0.1 to 0.3 percent of men. For anorexia nervosa, lifetime prevalence is 0.8 to 6.3 percent of women and 0.1 to 0.3 percent of men. For bulimia nervosa, lifetime prevalence globally is 0.8 to 2.6 percent of women and 0.1 to 0.2 percent of men. Binge eating disorder ranges from 0.6 to 6.1 percent of women and 0.3 to 0.7 percent of men (Silén & Keski-Rahkonen, 2022).

Eating disorders are associated with disorders related to abuse of substances, particularly tobacco, caffeine, and alcohol (Bahji et al., 2019). Ethnic differences in rates of eating disorder appear to be minimal (Cheng et al., 2019), but symptoms may vary, with women of color more likely to engage in purging but less likely to have concerns about their shape (Perez et al., 2021).

Compared to rates among cisgender heterosexual adults, the prevalence rates of eating disorders and disordered eating behaviors are nearly two times higher in non-heterosexual individuals and those with expansive gender identities. Based on the reporting of health care professionals, 10.5 percent of transgender men and 8.1 percent of transgender women are estimated to have an eating disorder, with lifetime prevalence rates for anorexia nervosa estimated to equal slightly over 4 percent and for bulimia nervosa to be 3 percent (Nagata, Ganson, & Austin, 2020). Contributing to these higher prevalence rates is the experience of discrimination against individuals with expansive gender and sexualities, particularly those diagnosed with anorexia nervosa (Kamody, Grilo, & Udo, 2020).

orthorexia nervosa
An unhealthy obsession with staying away from low-quality ingredients or food that may not be properly prepared.

Perhaps ironically, people can also develop a preoccupation with healthy eating that takes on dangerous proportions. Although it is not a diagnosis in *DSM-5-TR,* researchers are drawing attention to the pattern of behaviors referred to as **orthorexia nervosa**, an unhealthy obsession with staying away from low-quality ingredients or food that may not be properly prepared. Unlike people with the eating disorders now included as psychological disorders, people with orthorexia nervosa are not preoccupied with their weight (Hay, 2021). It is important to distinguish the obsession to avoid low-quality or poorly prepared food from a "healthy" type of orthorexia which is an interest in or fixation on healthy eating that does not lead to significant distress or impairment (Cosh, Olson, & Tully, 2023). In fact, a certain degree of concern over healthy eating becomes adaptive if it is limited to things like being concerned about food additives or avoiding tainted foods that have been recalled. However, those who are diagnosed with orthorexia are rigidly adherent to their beliefs about food and food quality and may use online or other resources to fuel their preoccupation.

Characteristics of Anorexia Nervosa (AN)

anorexia nervosa (AN)
An eating disorder characterized by severely restricted eating, an intense fear of gaining weight, and distorted body perception.

Clinicians diagnose individuals as having **anorexia nervosa (AN)** when they show three basic types of symptoms: severely restricted eating, which often leads to an unhealthily low body weight; intense and unrealistic fear of getting fat or gaining weight; and disturbed self-perception of body shape or weight. In other words, people with AN restrict their food intake, become preoccupied with gaining weight, and feel they are already overweight even though they may be seriously underweight.

At the heart of the experience of AN is a core disturbance in the individual's body image. As illustrated in Figure 1, theories of body image propose that it is made up of three interacting components. The cognitive-affective component of body image includes self-evaluation of the person's own appearance (satisfied or dissatisfied) and the importance of weight and shape for the individual's self-esteem. The perceptual component of body image includes the way individuals mentally represent their bodies. Individuals with anorexia nervosa typically overestimate their own body size. The behavioral component includes body checking, such as frequent weighing or measuring of body parts, and avoidance, which is the wearing of baggy clothing or avoiding social situations that expose the individual's body to viewing by others (Cash & Smolak, 2011).

FIGURE 1 Components of Body Image

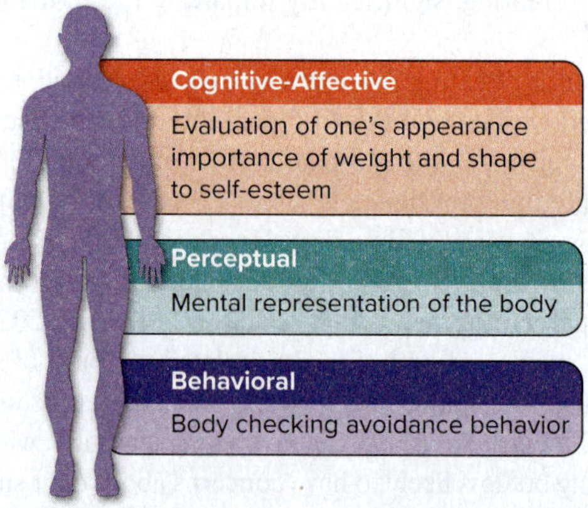

In addition to having the psychological consequences of AN, people who meet the criteria for the diagnosis develop a series of serious health changes that can, in the extreme, become life threatening. Constant undereating causes cardiac and respiratory problems, thinning bones, changes in gastrointestinal functioning, and loss of energy. Most individuals with AN become thin and gaunt, but there is also an atypical form of AN in which people with higher weight also develop body image disturbance that leads them to engage in unhealthy eating behaviors (Johnson-Munguia et al., 2023). People with AN can also suffer hair loss, and their nails become weak and brittle. Changes in their hormones caused by constant food deprivation can also lead them to become infertile as well as creating disturbances in their sexual functioning (Gonidakis, Kravvariti, & Varsou, 2015). Other risks include higher rates of obesity prior to adolescence associated with self-reports of more frequent attempts at weight loss in girls as young as 8 years old (Harnois-Leblanc et al., 2021).

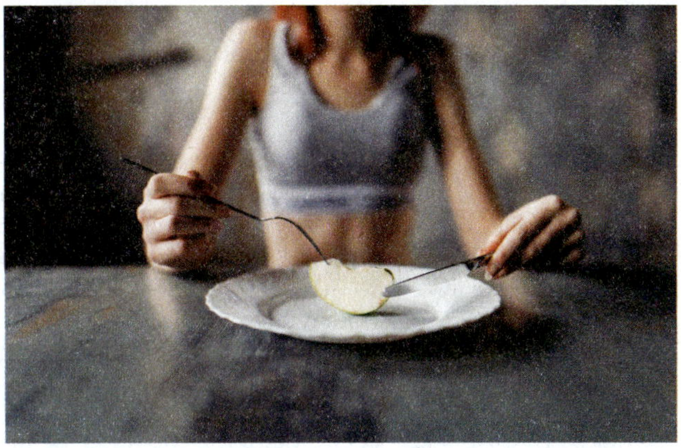

Individuals with anorexia nervosa engage in severe eating restrictions due to disturbances in their bodily self-image.

Sergiy Tryapitsyn/Alamy Stock Photo

The higher risk of mortality in people with AN has been firmly established including a risk for suicide that *DSM-5-TR* estimates as an 18-fold rate. The longer individuals have the disorder, the greater their risk (Franko et al., 2013). Although the majority of deaths from AN occur in young adults, a Norwegian study found that 43 percent of AN-related deaths occurred in women age 65 and older (Reas et al., 2005). A meta-analysis conducted on 52 separate studies revealed a prevalence of non-suicidal self-injury of 40 percent, with 51 percent experiencing suicidal ideation, and 22 percent having made a suicide attempt, with considerable overlap among all three sets of behaviors (Amiri & Khan, 2023).

Characteristics of Bulimia Nervosa (BN)

People with the eating disorder **bulimia nervosa (BN)** engage in episodes of **binge eating**, during which they rapidly eat an inordinately excessive amount of food, perhaps amounting to several thousand calories in a sitting. During these episodes, they experience a lack of control, which makes them feel they cannot stop eating or regulate how much they eat. Following the binge, they then engage in **purging**, a behavior that they use to rid themselves of their excess caloric consumption by forcing themselves to vomit, taking laxatives or diuretics, and fasting or exercising excessively. It should be noted that for an individual to receive a bulimia nervosa diagnosis, these episodes must not occur exclusively during episodes of anorexia nervosa.

bulimia nervosa (BN)
An eating disorder involving alternation between the extremes of eating large amounts of food in a short time, and then compensating for the added calories either by vomiting or other extreme actions to avoid gaining weight.

binge eating
The ingestion of large amounts of food during a short period of time, even after reaching a point of feeling full, and a lack of control over what or how much is eaten.

purging
Eliminating food through unnatural methods, such as vomiting or the excessive use of laxatives.

MINI CASE

Anorexia Nervosa (AN) Restricting Type

Blake is an 18-year-old White bisexual cisgender man in his first year of college. Growing up, Blake was usually low-average in weight, but in his first few months of college, he began to lose significant amounts of weight. His parents first noticed that he looked underweight when he came home for Thanksgiving break, but when they asked him about it, he denied that he had been trying to lose weight intentionally. He told his parents that he sometimes forgot to eat meals in the dining common because he was so busy with school, but he assured them he would try to eat regular meals more often. It turned out that Blake was indeed obsessed with dieting and exercise and had been keeping very careful food diaries and exercising daily since high school, but he did not tell anyone. Since coming to college, he felt he was able to restrict his eating more without his parents noticing. By the end of his first year, he had gone down from 130 to 95 lbs, though he assured his family that he felt "fine."

REAL STORIES

Lily Collins, 1989-Present

In a 2017 book of autobiographical essays about her life, *Unfiltered: No Shame, No Regrets, Just Me* (Collins, 2017), British-American actress Lily Collins describes in vivid detail her long struggle with eating disorders from around the age of 16. The collection of essays also details her struggles with abusive relationships, her perspective on her rise to success as an actress, and the relationship dynamics with her parents. Since the book was published, Collins' film career continued to grow, and in 2020 she starred in Netflix's comedy series "Emily in Paris," perhaps the role she is known best for.

Collins was born in the United Kingdom, and at age 5 she moved to Los Angeles after her parents separated. She grew up in L.A. living with her mother and maintained a distant relationship with her father, Phil Collins, one of the most successful musical artists of the 1980s and 1990s. In her book, Collins reflects on her relationship with food during her childhood, noting that she loved food and never thought twice about what she ate. She describes the many happy memories and associations with food she had growing up, connecting the memories to holidays, family, and places—especially England where she would often visit as a child. She also recalls how no one judged or criticized her body, but it was her own perception that shifted as she reached adolescence and experienced major life changes.

At the age of 16 Collins' relationship with food and her body started to shift drastically. At this point in her life, Collins was struggling with major new stressors, including her father separating from her stepmother, and attending a prestigious high school while starting her career in modeling and film work. In her book, she recalls viewing her body with a newer, more critical perspective, due in part to working in the entertainment industry, and she gradually and secretly started to restrict her food intake and exercise excessively.

Collins developed highly specific rules and restrictions around what types of food she allowed herself to eat, and obsessed over the calorie count of foods she did eat. She learned to withstand the effects of caloric restriction, by becoming dependent on gum and coffee for energy. And she started to drop significant amounts of weight. Recalls Collins, "As I did get thinner, more people started to notice. I was flattered by the stares and comments. I thought I looked amazing, and if anyone said anything negative, I assumed they were envious. I assumed everyone just wanted to be skinny like me. Losing weight and attaining my version of perfection became my focus. It was then that I really started my battle with anorexia."

Collins also started cycles of bingeing and purging, which she attributes to her severe food restrictions. "I'd go to the supermarket late at night and load up on every type of junk food possible and return home to my bedroom and just eat and eat . . . and then go into my bathroom and throw it all up . . . It was a 'successful' session if I could purge it all."

Collins eventually started to abuse diet pills and laxatives, which caused significant reductions in her energy and led to headaches and increased heart rate. At the time, she convinced herself these were "helping" her in losing weight. As a result of the weight loss, she developed common but devastating effects of eating disorders—she stopped getting her period, had brittle and weak nails and hair, and esophageal pain and discomfort. And her weight fluctuated despite the caloric restrictions.

Throughout the most intense years of her eating disorder, Collins kept her struggles a secret from everyone in her life. In part, Collins now reflects that she was in denial but also feared giving up a sense of "perfection" around controlling her food and her body, and for many years had no desire to stop. Prior to her eating disorder, she was very close with her mother, but the disorder took a toll due to her secrecy and fear of losing control. "I know it must have been extremely confusing to see her little girl, who had always been confident and secure, suddenly be plagued with self-doubt."

Eventually, in her early 20s, Collins confessed to her mother and friends that she had been living with her eating disorder for years. Through the encouragement of her social supports, she found a therapist and started taking steps toward recovery.

Around the age of 24, Collins started to heal enough to the point where she was able to re-establish a new relationship with food, and she became passionate about cooking and baking. She was delighted to find that she was quite talented at this pursuit, and became empowered through that to enjoy a more balanced lifestyle. A few years later, Collins starred in a movie *To the Bone*, about a young woman who was struggling with an eating disorder. The role required her to lose a significant amount of weight under the supervision of a nutritionist. Though she was hesitant at first, she ended up feeling healthier and stronger for it, for sharing and portraying her truth on screen. Following that film, Collins had to put weight back on for another role, and rather than falling back into her eating disorder, she found herself being able to connect with food in a healthy and balanced way, especially now that she had worked hard to re-establish her association with food.

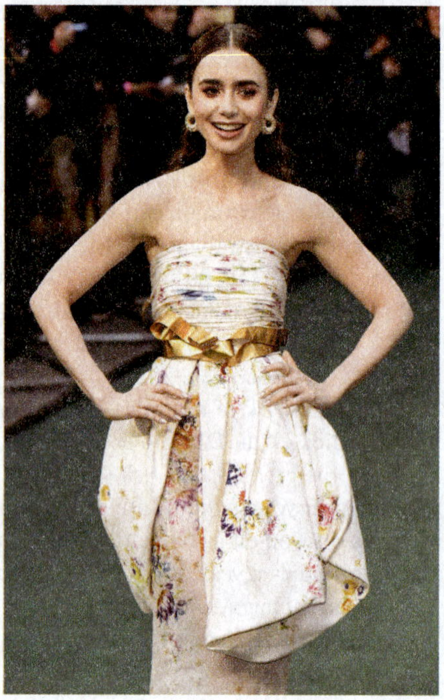

Lily Collins poses for photographers upon arrival at the 'Tolkien' premiere in London, April 29, 2019.
Featureflash Photo Agency/Shutterstock

Through her recovery process, Collins transformed from living her life in secrecy to openness and honesty with the world about her struggles, part of which involved the writing of her book of essays. In the book, she acknowledges that she still has to work at recovery through the darkest days of her disorder are behind her; "I've found comfort in knowing that treatment is forever. I don't have a time limit or deadline before I have to figure it all out. There is no end point, only progress."

MINI CASE

Bulimia Nervosa (BN)

Elena is a 26-year-old White Russian American heterosexual cisgender woman. She has struggled with her weight and body image since her early teenage years, when she was a competitive ballroom dancer. Her parents were very watchful of her eating habits during her adolescence and kept her on a very strict diet. Over time, Elena started sneaking junk food to her room late at night and then forcing herself to vomit. Since then, she has started to binge and purge nearly daily, which has led to a number of physical problems over the years, though her weight has remained about the same.

Like those who have AN, people with BN develop a number of medical problems. The most serious occur when they engage in purging by taking large doses of ipecac syrup, which can be toxic. The frequent vomiting also can lead to dental decay because the regurgitated material is highly acidic as it passes through the mouth. The laxatives, diuretics, and diet pills that people with BN use can also have toxic effects. Other health problems result from their giving themselves frequent enemas, regurgitating and then rechewing their food, and spending too much time in saunas. Constant dehydration places the individual with BN in potential risk of permanent gastrointestinal damage, fluid retention in the hands and feet, and heart muscle destruction or heart valve collapse.

Binge Eating Disorder (BED)

Binge eating disorder (BED), a new diagnosis introduced in the *DSM-5*, covers individuals who lack control over their eating and engage in binges at least twice a week for 6 months. For binge eating disorder to be diagnosed, the binges must occur with the intake of large amounts of food, go past the point of feeling full or hungry, occur while the person is alone, and be followed by self-disgust or guilt. Because the binge eating does not occur in association with compensatory behaviors, it is possible for individuals with this disorder to gain a significant amount of weight.

binge eating disorder (BED)
An eating disorder in which individuals lack control over their eating and engage in binges for at least twice a week for 6 months.

Individuals may transition between BN and AN, or they may transition to a disordered eating pattern involving purging. In one large national study of girls aged 9 to 15, as many as one-quarter transitioned between diagnoses, as well as crossing over between monthly and weekly frequency of symptoms (Glazer et al., 2019).

Although eating disorders may be associated with early life, episodes of binge eating may first emerge in the years of later adulthood. Associated with these episodes may be excessive self-blame regarding eating, feelings of loss of control, and fixation on feeling satiated. Although these themes are similar to those in younger individuals with binge eating disorder, older women's eating disturbances may more specifically take the form of internalized ageism, or beliefs in stereotypical attitudes regarding older adults (Kilpela et al., 2023).

Theories and Treatment of Eating Disorders

Eating disorders reflect a complex set of interactions among an individual's experiences with eating, body image, and exposure to sociocultural influences. The attitudes people develop throughout life toward food, eating, and body size can all play a role in influencing the risk of developing an eating disorder. Indeed, disordered eating patterns in college tend to improve over time but do not disappear completely.

Researchers working within the biological perspective focus on altered brain activity in individuals with eating disorders. In one innovative study, women with AN and women who had recovered from AN were compared on their fMRI responses to food-related cues with healthy controls after a night of fasting. Even those who were no longer symptomatic still showed lowered activation in the food reward centers and higher activation of inhibitory

What's in the *DSM-5-TR*

Reclassifying Eating, Elimination, Sleep-Wake, and Disruptive, Impulse-Control, and Conduct Disorders

Updates from *DSM-IV-TR* to *DSM-5* reflected a number of changes across categories of the disorders that fall into the scope of this chapter. In addition, diagnoses were added and removed to be consistent with emerging research on these important psychological disorders. The *DSM-5-TR* retained these major changes in classification, adding further risk factors and specifiers where necessary. It's important to understand the logic behind these changes because they do reflect a significant change in emphasis for disorders formerly regarded as restricted to childhood.

Regarding eating disorders, the most significant change was to move all the eating disorders into a new category called "Feeding and Eating Disorders" that also includes feeding disorders of childhood. Another major change from the *DSM-IV-TR* was to eliminate the two subtypes of bulimia nervosa (with and without purging).

The new category called "Binge Eating Disorder" was added to eating disorders when the *DSM-5* was written, based on a comprehensive literature review (Wonderlich et al., 2009) that showed there was sufficient validity to the diagnosis to justify its inclusion. This also reduced the number of diagnoses given for eating disorder "not otherwise specified."

The feeding disorders pica and rumination disorder were moved in the *DSM-5* revision (and retained in the *DSM-5-TR*) from the section of disorders of childhood into the same category as eating disorders. Elimination disorders became its own chapter.

Similarly, in the area of disruptive, impulse-control, and conduct disorders, the *DSM-5* authors took these out of the section on childhood and moved them into one chapter that also includes similar disorders of adulthood.

Sleep-wake disorders became reclassified in the *DSM-5* because the *DSM-IV-TR classification system* was no longer consistent with the diagnostic approach used by sleep specialists. This represents an improvement because it allows for clearer communication across health professionals in both diagnosis and treatment.

control areas of the brain, suggesting that the disorder creates lingering effects in the ways that individuals process food-related cues (Sanders et al., 2015). Further research supports the effect of AN in altered brain activity in areas responsible for processing emotions, body-related stimuli, and self-perception (Esposito, Cieri, di Giannantonio, & Tartaro, 2018).

Despite evidence of potential biological contributions, psychological perspectives are now considered the treatment of choice for eating disorders.

In cognitive behavioral therapy, clinicians first attempt to change selective biases in people with eating disorders that lead them to focus on the parts of their bodies they dislike. Second, by using exposure therapy in which clients view their own bodies ("mirror confrontation"), clinicians attempt to reduce the negative emotions they ordinarily experience. Behavioral interventions focus on reducing the frequency of body checking. Third, clinicians can address size overestimation by helping clients view their bodies while encouraging them to verbalize only positive statements about their body's appearance (Tanck et al., 2022).

CBT-based smartphone applications lend themselves to the treatment of eating disorders, particularly among high school and college-aged individuals. For the intervention provided in one exploration of this method's efficacy, women with disordered body image and eating disorder symptoms received positive body image messages that helped them learn to minimize the importance of their appearance, challenge their negative internal image, and accept imperfections in their body images in a game-like fashion (Cerea et al., 2021).

ACT, mindfulness, and other third-wave therapies continue to be explored as treatments for eating disorders. For example, yoga is safe and an acceptable option for some individuals, as shown in a large-scale meta-analysis, but it requires further, diagnostic-specific testing (Trethewey et al., 2023). In addition, interpersonal therapy is an empirically supported method that could be used as an alternative to cognitive behavioral therapy for individuals with binge eating disorder (Linardon et al., 2017).

Even as psychological perspectives emphasize body image distortions as being at the root of eating disorders, researchers working within this tradition also note the importance of sociocultural factors (Mumen & Smolak, 2019). These include normative expectations for an attractive appearance, particularly for women. For example, women athletes are considered at high risk for developing eating disorders due to concerns of appearing athletic in addition to the perceived pressures from coaches, and teammates, as well as friends, parents, and the media. These concerns may remain with them even years after their competitive days have ended, with as many as half continuing to show disordered eating patterns 6 years after leaving college sports (Thompson et al., 2020).

Occupation-specific social pressures may also affect adults with no prior history of eating disorders. For example, a study of on-camera journalists in the United States revealed higher rates of disordered eating, including unhealthy weight control behaviors such as fasting and excessive laxative use, compared to the habits of journalists who worked behind the scenes (Tran et al., 2020).

Sociocultural influences on eating disorders may also reflect larger-scale events that affect the population as a whole. During the COVID-19 pandemic, anecdotal reports continued to surface through the media of people gaining weight due to excessive economic stresses, boredom, and loneliness associated with the lockdowns. The term "COVID-19" became associated with the weight gain that people reported experiencing, and indeed, public health statistics reinforced the reality of this impact of the pandemic, particularly among individuals who reported feeling depressed or anxious (Khubchandani et al., 2022). A large-scale analysis of global reports conducted during the pandemic further showed that both binge eating and anorexia nervosa symptoms increased significantly (Güzel, Mutlu, & Molendijk, 2023).

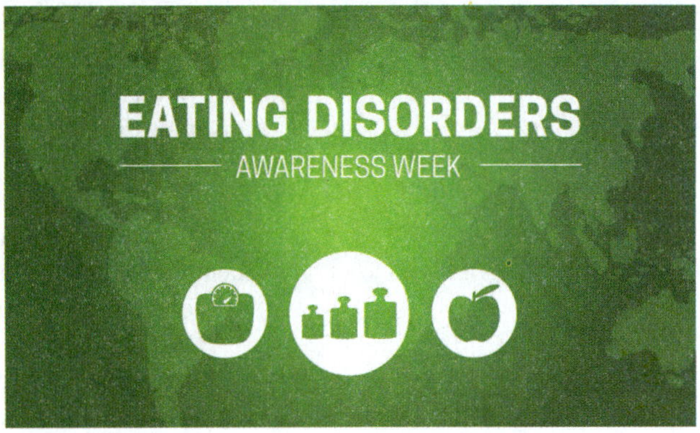

Interventions based on raising social awareness about eating disorders can benefit those who may otherwise not seek treatment on their own.

Angela Cini/Alamy Stock Photo

Early experiences in which parents or other caregivers restrict children's access to food are also understood as a potential contributor to the individual's development of an eating disorder. Restricted access may also be a function of a family's income, but it can occur in families with ample financial resources as well who themselves have complicated feelings about eating and body image. Parents may also neglect to feed their children as part of a larger constellation of adverse experiences, including emotional and physical neglect and abuse, sexual abuse, and exposure to intimate partner violence. However, even after these forms of abuse are accounted for, children from families in which parents restrict their eating have higher rates of eating disorders than families in which parents provide children with adequate nutrition (Coffino, Grilo, & Udo, 2020).

Biology may also interact with maltreatment during childhood, supporting the concept of a **maltreated ecophenotype** as an explanation of the development of eating disorders. According to this approach, early experiences of maltreatment create greater sensitivity to stressful situations in adults with eating disorders, as indicated by higher levels of cortisol, anxiety, and hunger (Monteleone et al., 2020). Individuals with eating disorders who experience childhood maltreatment may be particularly at risk for suicidal attempts (Forrest, Grilo, & Udo, 2020). These factors appear to operate similarly for individuals assigned as male and female at birth, as shown in a population-based study carried out in Denmark evaluating genetic vs. early life exposure risk on the development of anorexia nervosa (Chatwin et al., 2023).

maltreated ecophenotype
Genetic susceptibility to eating disorders that is strongly influenced by exposure to childhood maltreatment.

avoidant/restrictive food intake disorder
A disorder in which individuals avoid or restrict food eating to the point that they experience significant threats to their physical health.

Treatment based on the sociocultural perspective typically includes a family component for clients with eating disorders who are still in their teens and who have had symptoms for only a brief time (Ciao, Accurso, Fitzsimmons-Craft, & Le Grange, 2015). Family-based therapies appear to be particularly effective in reducing depressive symptoms among adolescents with bulimia nervosa (Valenzuela, Lock, Le Grange, & Bohon, 2018).

Avoidant/Restrictive Food Intake Disorder

In **avoidant/restrictive food intake disorder**, individuals show an apparent lack of interest in eating or food to the point that they experience significant threats to their physical health. They may avoid food based on its sensory characteristics such as color, smell, texture, temperature, or taste. People may also develop this disorder as the result of a conditioned negative response to having an aversive experience while eating, such as choking on a piece of food that becomes stuck in their throat. However, their restrictive food intake is not associated with feelings of disgust toward food (Breiner et al., 2023).

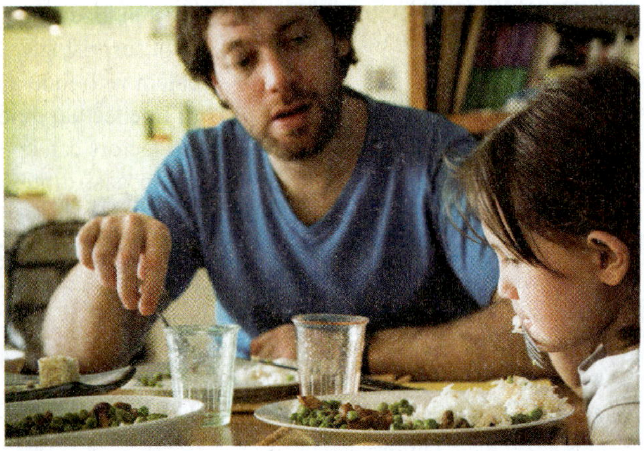

A child's chronic resistance to eating may be a sign of avoidant/restrictive food disorder.

PhotoAlto/Alamy Stock Photo

Moved in the *DSM-5* from where it was classified in *DSM-IV-TR* as a feeding disorder of infancy or early childhood and regarded as an extreme version of "picky eating" (Menzel, 2018), this diagnosis now applies to individuals of any age who do not have another eating disorder or concurrent medical condition, or whose eating patterns follow culturally prescribed eating restrictions. Their disorder causes these individuals to lose a significant amount of weight or, for children, to fail to achieve expected weight gain. By restricting their food intake, individuals with this disorder lack sufficient nutrients, they may become dependent on feeding through a stomach tube or oral nutritional supplements. All of these avoidant food behaviors interfere significantly with their psychosocial functioning.

The relative recency of the reclassification of avoidant/restrictive food disorder in addition to variations among samples in screening instruments and characteristics such as age and geographic location means that prevalence data are currently not reliable. Additionally, individuals seeking help for this disorder may have symptoms of other psychological disorders as well. Complicating the epidemiological picture further, those seeking treatment may turn to medical rather than psychological healthcare professionals (Archibald & Bryant-Waugh, 2023).

Eating Disorders Associated with Childhood

Two eating-related disorders, pica and rumination disorder, are included in *DSM-5-TR* as specific to childhood, given their likely emergence during the early years of life.

pica
A condition in which a person eats inedible substances, such as dirt or feces; commonly associated with intellectual developmental disabilities.

Individuals with **pica** eat inedible substances, such as paint, glass, string, hair, animal droppings, and paper. The term actually is derived from the Latin for "magpie," a bird known to be willing to eat almost anything. However, as used in psychological disorders, pica represents a highly serious disorder because even one incident can cause significant medical consequences due to lead poisoning or injury to the gastrointestinal tract. Although associated with childhood, pica is actually the most serious cause of self-injury to occur in people with intellectual developmental disabilities. However, it may also occur in adults, as illustrated in a case study of a well-educated woman who developed pica for foam rubber objects as well as burnt match heads ("cautopyreiophagia") (Van Wert et al., 2021).

Clinicians treating pica must reduce the individual's injurious behaviors, a method known as response interruption and redirection. This can be combined with differential reinforcement of alternative behavior can serve as a way of strengthening the individual's likelihood of eating edible items rather than those that can cause potential harm (Ruckle, Bednar, Suen, & Falligant, 2023).

rumination disorder
An eating disorder in which the infant or child regurgitates food after it has been swallowed and then either spits it out or reswallows it.

In **rumination disorder**, the child regurgitates and rechews swallowed food. Researchers investigating rumination disorder (when it was included, with feeding disorder, as a disorder of childhood) identified five common disturbances in these children: (1) delayed or absent development of feeding and eating skills; (2) difficulty managing or tolerating food or drink; (3) reluctance to eat food based on taste, texture, and other sensory factors; (4) lack of appetite or interest in food; and (5) the use of feeding behaviors to comfort, self-soothe, or self-stimulate.

Not surprisingly, 25 to 45 percent of developmentally typical children have some type of problem with food and feeding, but estimates rise to as high as 80 percent among children with intellectual developmental disorder. Complicating the clinical picture is the fact that many factors can contribute to eating problems in children, ranging from a choking experience to gastrointestinal injuries (Bryant-Waugh, Markham, Kreipe, & Walsh, 2010). However, the percent of children who meet the diagnosis for a feeding-related disorder remains relatively small (Eddy et al., 2015).

elimination disorders
Disorders characterized by age-inappropriate incontinence, beginning in childhood.

enuresis
An elimination disorder in which the child is incontinent of urine and urinates in clothes or in bed after the age when the child is expected to be continent.

10.2 Elimination Disorders

Elimination disorders are characterized by age-inappropriate incontinence and are generally diagnosed in childhood. Individuals with **enuresis** wet the bed or urinate in their clothing after they have reached the age of 5 years, at which point it is expected that they should be completely toilet trained. Children with this diagnosis must show symptoms of enuresis for three consecutive months.

One of the most frequent diagnoses for children, with 40 percent of 3-year-old children wetting the bed, declining to 22 percent by age 5, with rates estimated at three times higher for boys than girls (Thurber, 2017). There are subtypes of enuresis based on the time of day the child inappropriately passes urine (daytime only, night only, or both).

In **encopresis**, a child who is at least 4 years old repeatedly has bowel movements in clothes or other inappropriate places. The subtypes of encopresis distinguish between children who have constipation and then become incontinent due to overflow of feces, and those who do not have constipation and overflow. These distinctions are important because they can differentiate which children do and do not have a medical condition that underlies their symptoms (von Gontard, 2011). Estimates place the prevalence of encopresis at 1.5 to 7.5 percent of children ages 6 to 12 (Ritterbrand et al., 2013).

encopresis
An elimination disorder in which the child is incontinent of feces and has bowel movements either in clothes or in another inappropriate place.

Evidence-based treatment for childhood elimination disorders focuses on biobehavioral methods to establish continence (Shepard, Poler, & Grabman, 2017). Enuresis can be treated through use of a "urine alarm," a device attached to a child's underwear or pajamas that emits an auditory and/or tactile sensation in response to moisture. The child then develops a conditioned avoidance response that can trigger muscular contractions in the external sphincter of the bladder prior to the leakage of urine. Encopresis treatments supported by empirical studies include enhanced toilet training and biofeedback. In enhanced toilet training, the child is rewarded for continence, given training about appropriate defecation dynamics, and taught breathing techniques and muscle training exercises to gain control over the anal sphincters.

If children have the retentive form of encopresis, they can benefit from behavioral training that rewards them for increasing their intake of fiber and fluid and ensures that they include time on the toilet as part of their daily schedules (Kuhl et al., 2010). Enhanced toilet training, a method that combines behavioral training (such as a "star chart") with relaxation and breathing training (to address constipation) has gained support as an evidence-based treatment (Shepard, Poler, & Grabman, 2017). Another more psychologically oriented approach focuses on unresolved anger that a child may be expressing in response to family issues. Such issues can include conflict between the parents, the arrival of a newborn sibling, or the behavior of an older sibling who torments the child. Treatment that addresses these family system issues can help to reduce the child's symptoms (Reid & Bahar, 2006).

10.3 Sleep-Wake Disorders

Included as a category of disorders pertaining to altered sleep and wakefulness patterns, the *DSM-5-TR* is intended to serve clinicians not necessarily trained in sleep disorders to facilitate differential diagnosis and clarify when referral to a sleep specialist would be warranted.

DSM-5-TR organizes the sleep-wake disorders into sets based on predominant symptoms, as you can see in Table 1. To be diagnosable, symptoms must be present for a significant period of time, occur relatively frequently, and cause the individual to experience distress. Many of these diagnoses now use **polysomnography**, which is a sleep study that records brain waves, blood oxygen levels, heart rate, breathing, eye movements, and leg movements.

polysomnography
A sleep study that records brain waves, blood oxygen levels, heart rate, breathing, eye movements, and leg movements.

Sleep disorders affect a large number of individuals, including perhaps as many as 30 percent of adults in the general population in the case of insomnia alone (Cole, 2011). There was a significant spike in prevalence associated with COVID-19 lockdowns. Researchers in France reported that 74 percent of participants in a representative sample stated they had trouble sleeping during the 2020 lockdown, compared with 49 percent in the previous year when there was no lockdown. The use of sleeping pills also jumped, from 16 percent of participants prior to the lockdown to 41 percent during. Sleep-related difficulties were more likely to be reported by younger adults than those 35 and older. The stress of living in lockdown in addition to spending 24 hours in the home appeared to exacerbate symptoms (Beck et al., 2021).

Treatments for sleep-wake disorders vary considerably depending on the nature of the disorder. Cognitive behavioral therapy is regarded as highly efficacious for insomnia and,

TABLE 1 **Sleep-Wake Disorders**

Disorder (or Category)	Specific Disorders Within Category	Predominant Symptoms
Insomnia disorder		Difficulty initiating or maintaining sleep, along with early morning awakening.
Narcolepsy		Recurrent periods of an irrepressible need to sleep, lapsing into sleep, or napping within the same day. Diagnosis also requires either episodes of jaw-opening or losing facial muscle tone while laughing or showing atypical cerebral spinal fluid (CSF) or sleep disturbances on polysomnography.
Hypersomnolence disorder		Recurrent periods of sleep or lapses into sleep during the day, prolonged main sleep episodes, or difficulty being fully awake after abruptly awakening.
Breathing sleep-related disorders	Obstructive sleep apnea separate specific disorder	Frequent episodes of apnea and hypopnea while sleeping as indicated on polysomnography along with either snoring, snorting/gasping, or breathing pauses during sleep and daytime sleepiness, fatigue, or unrefreshing sleep.
	Central sleep apnea	Frequent episodes of apnea while asleep.
	Sleep-related hypoventilation	Episodes of decreased breathing (ventilation) while asleep.
Circadian rhythm sleep-wake disorders		Persistent patterns of sleep disruption due primarily to altered circadian rhythm or misalignment between the individual's internal circadian rhythm and the sleep-wake schedule required by the person's environment, or work or social schedule. Includes delayed sleep phase type (delay in timing of major sleep period), advanced sleep phase type (sleep-wake cycles that are several hours earlier than conventional), irregular sleep-wake type, non-24-hour sleep-wake type, and shift work type.
Parasomnias	Non-rapid eye movement sleep arousal disorder	Recurrent episodes of incomplete awakening from sleep accompanied by either sleepwalking or sleepwalking not associated with rapid eye movements (REMs).
	Nightmare disorder	Repeated occurrences of extended, dysphoric, and well-remembered dreams that typically involve threats to one's life.
	Rapid eye movement sleep behavior disorder	Frequent episodes of arousal during sleep associated with speaking and/or motor behaviors occurring during REM sleep.
	Restless legs syndrome (RLS)	An urge to move the legs along with uncomfortable and unpleasant sensations in the legs, urges that begin or worsen during periods of rest or inactivity that are partially or totally relieved by movement, and are worse or only occur in the evening or night.

MINI CASE

Obstructive Sleep Apnea Hypopnea

Samuel is a 68-year-old Black heterosexual cisgender man. He is seeking marriage counseling because his wife has decided she no longer wants to put up with his snoring and is insisting they sleep in separate bedrooms. In addition, he wakes feeling unrefreshed and constantly feels fatigued during the day. The counselor sends Samuel to a sleep specialist who conducts a polysomnogram, showing that Samuel goes into periods of not breathing on average every 4 minutes. Samuel is now being evaluated for treatment by the sleep specialist, who is exploring options, including a CPAP machine or implantable device, to allow Samuel and his wife to resume their previous sleeping patterns in the same bed.

along with relaxation and sleep hygiene training, for improving sleep in college student populations (Friedrich & Schlarb, 2018).

The availability of wearable technology that records length of time asleep, time awake, and even sleep stages is making it increasingly possible for individuals to gain an understanding of their own sleep patterns. As a result, more individuals may seek sleep therapy than was true in the past, when the only signal people received of a possible sleep disorder was feeling tired or experiencing frequent or unusually early awakening. Relatively new as a method of treatment for insomnia, wearable technology may also provide an effective adjunct to traditional behavioral methods (Aji et al., 2022).

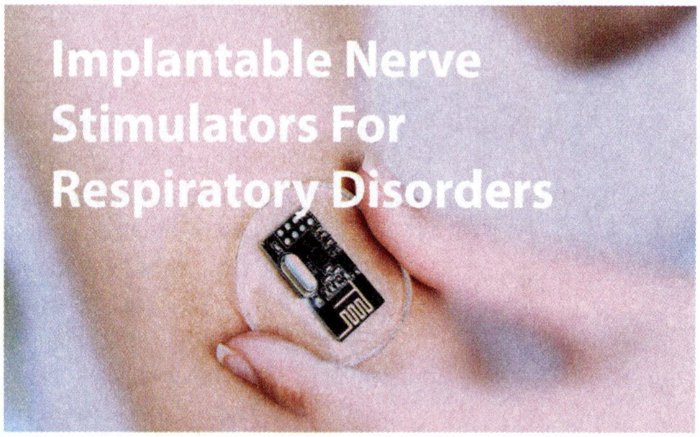

Implantable devices are now available that can help individuals control sleep apnea without a machine as intrusive as a CPAP.
Wladimir Bulgar/Alamy Stock Photo

New technologies are also helping to advance how clients can manage their own treatment in the home. Continuous positive airway pressure (CPAP) machines are mechanical devices used for treating sleep apnea. They are becoming increasingly practical and affordable (Sutherland & Cistulli, 2015). Even newer technologies allow individuals to control sleep apnea via an implantable pulse generator that stimulates the nerve that moves the tongue to produce noise (the hypoglossal nerve). This device, which improves airflow, is programmed and managed by a physician, but is operated by the individual via a remote device for use at home. One advantage over traditional CPAP machines is that the device is less intrusive and therefore promotes a high degree of compliance (Soose et al., 2022).

10.4 Disruptive, Impulse-Control, and Conduct Disorders

People with one of the disruptive, impulse-control, or conduct disorders show extreme lack of control over their behavior known as **disinhibition**. They are unable to restrain themselves from expressing what are often high levels of negative emotions. Although people with a variety of other disorders also experience difficulties in self-regulating their behavior, these particular disorders bring the individuals who have them into significant conflict with social norms or authority figures.

disinhibition
An extreme lack of inhibition or control over behavior.

Oppositional Defiant Disorder

Most children go through periods of negativism and mild defiance, particularly in adolescence, and most parents complain of occasional hostility or argumentativeness in their children. But what if such behaviors are present most of the time and are not just a phase?

Children and adolescents with **oppositional defiant disorder** display angry or irritable mood, argumentative or defiant behavior, and vindictiveness that results in significant

oppositional defiant disorder
A disorder characterized by angry or irritable mood, argumentative or defiant behavior, and vindictiveness that results in significant family or school problems.

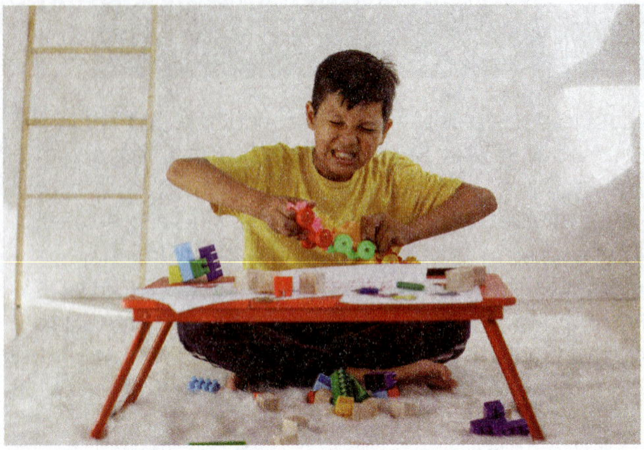

Children may show symptoms of intermittent explosive disorder in the form of what seem to be temper tantrums.

Gatot Adri/Shutterstock

family or school problems. Youths with this disorder repeatedly lose their temper, argue, refuse to do what they are told, and deliberately annoy other people. They are touchy, resentful, belligerent, spiteful, and self-righteous. Rather than seeing themselves as the cause of their problems, they blame other people or insist they are victims of circumstances. To the extent that their behavior interferes with their school performance and friendships, they risk jeopardizing their relationships with teachers and peers. These losses can, in turn, lead them to feel inadequate and depressed and perhaps cause them to act out even more.

Oppositional defiant disorder is the most common psychological disorder of childhood, with a worldwide prevalence rate of 4.9 percent in children between 1 and 7 years of age (Vasileva et al., 2020). Subthreshold rates range as high as 19 to 24 percent in children followed through the ages of 3 to 9 years old (Osa et al., 2019). *DSM-5-TR* notes that the culture-related issues are important for avoiding misdiagnosis; additionally, despite adverse circumstances, rates are lower in first-generation immigrants and refugees.

If their behavior is left unaddressed, children with oppositional defiant disorder may progress in adolescence to poorer adjustment at home and school, delinquent behavior, conduct disorder, and ultimately continued difficulties into adulthood. However, the majority of children develop sufficient emotion regulation skills so that they become protected from these maladaptive consequences (Nabokht et al., 2023).

The goal of treatment for oppositional defiant disorder is to help the child learn to exhibit appropriate behaviors, such as cooperation and self-control, and to unlearn problem behaviors, such as aggression, stealing, and lying. Therapy focuses on reinforcement, behavioral contracting, modeling, and relaxation training and may take place in the context of peer therapy groups and parent training. There are a number of effective, evidence-based approaches that use a variety of these methods, many in conjunction with parent collaboration (Kaur, Floyd, & Balta, 2022).

Intermittent Explosive Disorder

intermittent explosive disorder
An impulse-control disorder involving an inability to hold back urges to express strong angry feelings and associated violent behaviors.

People with **intermittent explosive disorder** are unable to hold back their urges to express strong angry feelings and associated violent behaviors. Their outbursts, which are unpremeditated and unprovoked, are either verbal (temper tantrums, tirades, arguments) or physical and can become assaultive or destructive in ways that are out of proportion to any stress or provocation. To be diagnosable in the *DSM-5-TR*, these outbursts must occur on at least three occasions in a 12-month period.

Estimates place the prevalence of this disorder at 2 to 5 percent of the population (Coccaro & McCloskey, 2019). People with this disorder are more vulnerable to a number of threats to their physical health, including coronary heart disease, hypertension, stroke,

MINI CASE

Intermittent Explosive Disorder

Ed is a 28-year-old White heterosexual cisgender man who works as a high school teacher. He often has unprovoked, violent outbursts of aggressive and assaultive behavior, during which he throws whatever objects he can get his hands on and yells profanities. He soon calms down, though, and feels intense regret for whatever damage he has caused, explaining that he didn't know what came over him. In the most recent episode, Ed threw a coffee pot at another teacher in the faculty lounge, inflicting serious injury. After the ambulance took the injured man to the hospital, Ed's principal called the police. Ed was taken into custody and immediately suspended from his job.

diabetes, arthritis, back/neck pain, ulcer, headaches, and other chronic pain (McCloskey et al., 2010). Epidemiological studies report high rates of comorbidity with anxiety, mood, other impulse control, and substance use disorders (Pereira et al., 2020).

Intermittent explosive disorder appears to have a strong epigenetic basis, as indicated by evidence of DNA methylation in individuals with this disorder (Montalvo-Ortiz et al., 2018). However, adverse childhood experiences can further place an individual at higher risk for the disorder, with estimates as high as a 36 percent prevalence among individuals growing up under these conditions (Turner et al., 2021).

There is also a strong cognitive component to the development of intermittent explosive disorder. People with this disorder have a set of negative beliefs that other people wish to harm them, beliefs they may have acquired as a result of being exposed to highly adverse home environments. In addition, they may have learned through modeling at home that aggression is the way to cope with conflict or frustration. Men and women are not affected equally by exposure to family violence, which is a stronger predictor of a diagnosis of intermittent explosive disorder in women compared to men (Krick et al., 2022).

Both supportive and cognitive behavioral therapy appear to provide a reduction in symptoms of this disorder. However, the evidence favors cognitive behavioral in terms of decreasing aggressive behavior in general as well as relational aggression. In one 12-session approach, known as Cognitive, Relaxation, and Coping Skills Training for intermittent explosive disorder, clinicians begin with a set of relaxation training sessions, then move on to challenging anger distortions, and then ending with imaginal exposure to anger-provoking situations (McCloskey et al., 2022).

Conduct Disorder

Individuals are diagnosed with **conduct disorder** on the basis of a history of violating the rights of others and society's norms or laws. Their delinquent behaviors include directing aggression toward people and animals such as bullying and engaging in acts of animal cruelty, destroying property, stealing, lying, and committing serious violations of rules such as being truant from school or running away from home. The *DSM-5-TR* also includes specifiers to distinguish childhood or adolescent onset (before or after 10 years of age); the presence or absence of remorse, guilt, and empathy; and the severity of the behavior, ranging from lying and truancy to physical cruelty, use of a weapon, and stealing in the presence of the victim.

conduct disorder
An impulse-control disorder that involves repeated violations of the rights of others and society's norms and laws.

Children with conduct disorder may or may not develop into adults who engage in antisocial behavior. The form of antisocial behavior that disappears after adolescence has a rate of 4.6 percent for women and 5.1 percent for men. In what is called the life course persistent pattern, the prevalence rates are far lower, amounting to 0.5 percent for women and 1.9 percent for men. These individuals, in addition to continuing to have symptoms well into adulthood, also have higher risk of developing substance use problems (Moore, Silberg, Roberson-Nay, & Mezuk, 2017).

There is increasing recognition that children raised in harsh environments that expose them to trauma, abuse, and neglect are particularly at risk for developing conduct disorder (Wang & Kenny, 2014); consequently, the *DSM-5-TR* recommends that clinicians take the individual's context into account. Sexual trauma also seems to be a precipitating factor for females, who are more likely than males to report a history of abuse in childhood (Maniglio, 2014). Additionally, Swedish researchers have identified previously unrecognized physiological risk factors for conduct disorders in children who have gastrointestinal disturbances including celiac disease, constipation, diarrhea, and lactose intolerance, along with other neurodevelopmental disorders (Kerekes et al., 2020).

Not addressed in the *DSM-5-TR*, but relevant to both conduct and oppositional defiant disorder are the personality traits referred to as "callous/unemotional." As you will learn in Chapter 14, one key component of antisocial personality disorder is the quality of psychopathy, a trait that leads individuals to disregard completely the feelings of others and to lack empathy or remorse for those they have hurt. Interventions for children with these disruptive behaviors distinguish those individuals who primarily engage in disruptive behaviors

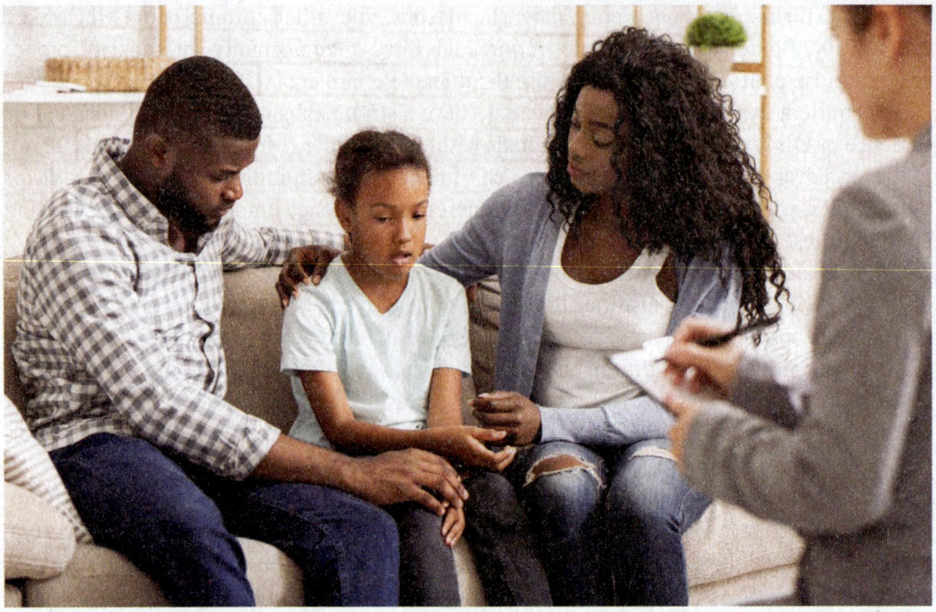

Incorporating parents into therapy for children with disruptive behavior disorders such as conduct disorder can prove beneficial, even in those children who may otherwise seem resistant to treatment.

Prostock-studio/Shutterstock

from children who show early signs of developing these precursors to psychopathy. One meta-analysis of intervention studies showed beneficial effects on therapy on both groups of children, although those with the personality traits plus a history of disruptive behavior proved to show less symptom reduction. The methods employed in these studies included a range of approaches, but those involving parents in treatment appeared to have the greatest effectiveness. These findings are encouraging given that the prevailing wisdom had been to regard children with callous/unemotional traits as untreatable (Perlstein, Fair, Hong, & Waller, 2023).

Impulse-Control Disorders

impulse-control disorder
Psychological disorder in which people repeatedly engage in behaviors that are potentially harmful, feeling unable to stop themselves and experiencing a sense of desperation if their attempts to carry out the behaviors are thwarted.

pyromania
An impulse-control disorder involving the persistent and compelling urge to start fires.

People receive a diagnosis of an **impulse-control disorder** if they engage in repetitive, behaviors that they feel are beyond their control and which often produce harm. A key feature of these disorders is that before they act on their impulses, these individuals experience so much tension and anxiety that they achieve relief only by following through on their impulses. That sense of pleasure or gratification can, however, turn into regret that they engaged in the behavior.

Pyromania

People with **pyromania** deliberately set fires, feeling tension and arousal before they commit the act. They are fascinated with and curious about fire and its situational contexts, and they derive pleasure, gratification, or relief when setting or witnessing fires or participating in their aftermath. For an individual to be diagnosed with pyromania, the firesetting must not be done for monetary reasons, and the individual must not have other medical or psychiatric conditions. Those who commit arson, by contrast, seek financial gain, and the arsonist does not experience the relief shown by people with pyromania. Individuals may also engage in firesetting for no apparent reason and without experiencing the tension and arousal shown by people with pyromania. It is therefore important to distinguish among these three types of firesetting (Palermo, 2015).

Pyromania is a rare disorder, even among arsonists, but its overall prevalence is not known. Among a sample of 90 repeat offenders, Finnish researchers found that only 3 met the criteria for pyromania (Lindberg, Holi, Tani, & Virkkunen, 2005). Slightly higher percentages were reported in one study of hospitalized psychiatric patients, in which 3.4 percent had current symptoms and 5.9 percent had lifetime symptoms consistent with a diagnosis of pyromania (Grant, Levine, Kim, & Potenza, 2005).

Pyromania appears to be a chronic condition if the individual does not receive treatment. Some individuals with pyromania may discontinue firesetting and instead switch to another addictive or impulsive behavior such as kleptomania or gambling disorder. An intensive study of 21 participants with a lifetime history of pyromania described the most likely triggers for their behavior as stress, boredom, feelings of inadequacy, and interpersonal conflict (Grant & Kim, 2007).

From a legal and forensic perspective, given its low prevalence in the population, it is challenging for clinicians to assist the courts in providing recommendations and particularly to collaborate with fire investigators and law enforcement. In this work, it can be helpful to establish an individual's previous history of firesetting which can serve as a prediction of future risk (Burton, McNiel, & Binder, 2012).

Treatment for pyromania that follows the cognitive behavioral model seems to show the most promise (Grant & Odlaug, 2010). The techniques include imaginal exposure and response prevention, cognitive restructuring of response to urges, and relaxation training.

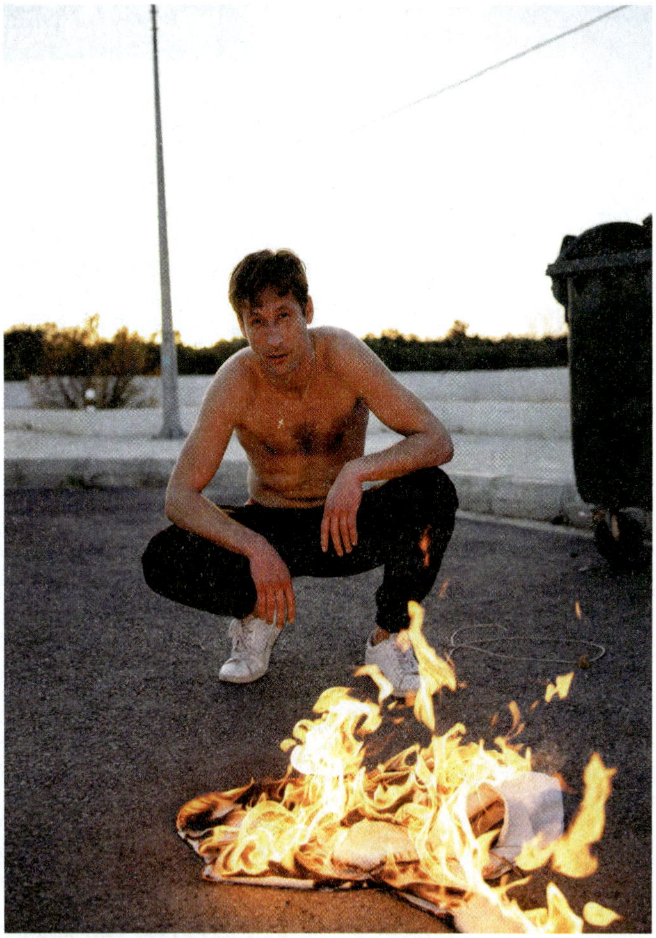

People with pyromania not only are fascinated by fire, but engage in firesetting in response to uncontrollable impulses.

BLACKDAY/Shutterstock

Kleptomania

People with the impulse-control disorder **kleptomania** are driven by a persistent urge to steal. Unlike shoplifters or thieves, they are not motivated by monetary gain but instead seek excitement from the act of stealing. Like people with other impulse-control disorders, they would prefer not to be driven to this behavior, and they feel their urge is unpleasant, unwanted, intrusive, and senseless. They steal in response to an urge or state of craving, and they experience gratification afterward. Because their focus is not on the items but on the act of stealing, individuals with kleptomania may give or throw away the stolen goods.

kleptomania
An impulse-control disorder that involves the persistent urge to steal.

As is true for firesetting, there are distinct subgroups of individuals who engage in shoplifting. Impulsive and addictive-compulsive are just two types (making up 29 percent), with the rest including individuals who are economically disadvantaged, depressed, "hobbyists," and those who have a lifetime history of trauma and loss. Although repeated shoplifters may not fit the diagnosis of kleptomania, they may still suffer negative effects due to their "reidentity stamping" as thieves. This alteration in their self-image may create a set of negative psychological outcomes (Nadeau, Rochlen, & Tyminski, 2019).

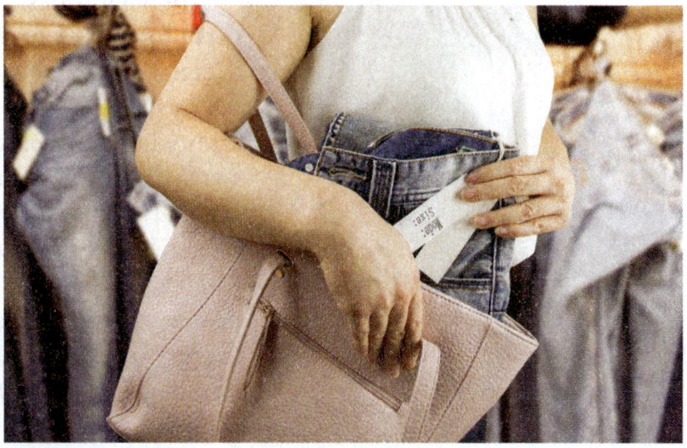

It is important to distinguish kleptomania from ordinary shoplifting, as people with kleptomania act out of an inability to control their instincts to steal.

cunaplus/Shutterstock

To make a diagnosis of kleptomania, clinicians must be unable to better account for the individual's stealing with another diagnosis of antisocial personality disorder, conduct disorder, or bipolar disorder (in a manic episode). There is overlap among the symptoms of kleptomania and mood, anxiety, and other impulse-control disorders, making it particularly important that clinicians engage in a thorough process of differential diagnosis (Grant, 2006).

You Be the Judge

Legal Implications of Impulse-Control Disorders

By definition, impulse-control disorders arise from irresistible urges. Individuals with disorders such as kleptomania and pyromania engage in the illegal acts of stealing and firesetting, respectively. Those with intermittent explosive disorder may also commit illegal acts during one of their violent outbursts. When people with these disorders encounter the justice system, then, the question arises whether we should regard them as having a disorder or as practicing a form of illegal and deviant behavior similar to psychopathy.

People with kleptomania commit acts of stealing in response to a failure to resist impulses. The stealing may give them momentary relief from their anxiety-driven urge, but ultimately it leads only to significant distress and dysfunction in their everyday lives. A key difference between kleptomania and antisocial personality disorder is that people with kleptomania feel intense regret; moreover, they do not steal for any particular monetary reason (Aboujaoude, Gamel, & Koran, 2004). Similarly, individuals with pyromania, by definition, do not seek monetary reward from their actions. Those with intermittent explosive disorder do not seek to commit violent acts but are responding to irresistible urges. People with gambling disorder steal or cheat not for the sake of material gain, but in order to support their gambling habit.

According to one view, impulse-control disorders are not "volitional" disorders, which excuse an individual from moral and legal responsibility for his or her actions. A cognitive impairment that prevents knowing or remembering the negative consequences of the person's previous addictive behaviors causes the volitional disorder. Once the behavior begins, it increases the extent of the impairment (Campbell, 2003).

The terminology the mental health profession uses to describe kleptomania and pyromania implies, however, that individuals with these disorders are somehow attracted to the opportunities to steal and start fires. In the case of pyromania, fire fighters, insurance investigators, law enforcement professionals, and even mental health professionals may fail to appreciate fully the diagnostic criteria for the disorder. One erroneous but popular belief is that serial arsonists are pyromaniacs. In fact, clinicians diagnose pyromania in a very small percent of chronic firesetters.

Q: *You be the judge:* To what extent should a defendant's diagnosis of an impulse-control disorder be a factor in a criminal trial?

Although it has received relatively little attention in research on psychological disorders (Torales, González, Castaldelli-Maia, & Ventriglio, 2020), kleptomania has a number of significant effects on the individual's life, not the least of which is the fear of or reality of arrest. In one study of 101 adults (73 percent self-identified as female), 69 percent were arrested and 21 percent were incarcerated. Over half were arrested on two or more occasions. Their symptoms started when they were 19 years old on average, and they shoplifted at least twice a week. The majority stole items of clothing, household goods, and groceries. To a lesser extent, they also stole from their friends, relatives, and places of employment. This study replicated those of smaller-scale investigations in reporting that people with kleptomania are likely to have high lifetime prevalence rates of co-occurring depressive disorders (43 percent), anxiety disorders (25 percent), other impulse-control disorders (42 percent), and drug abuse or dependence (18 percent). Suicide attempts are common among people with kleptomania (Grant, Odlaug, Davis, & Kim, 2009). These individuals may also have eating disorders and a related set of symptoms involving compulsive buying (Kim et al., 2018).

Studies of the neurobiology of kleptomania suggest that, like substance use disorders, this diagnosis is associated with altered dopamine, serotonin, and opioid receptor functions as well as changes in brain structures similar to those in people with cocaine dependence

MINI CASE

Kleptomania

Gloria is a 45-year-old White gay cisgender woman. She works as an executive for a finance company. For the past few years, she has been under considerable stress and has worked long hours as the result of reorganizations in her company. As a teenager, Gloria occasionally took small, inexpensive items, such as hair barrettes and nail polish, from the drugstore, even though she could afford to pay for them. Lately, she has started shoplifting again. This time, her behavior has an intensity she cannot control. During her lunch hour, she often visits one of the large department stores near her office building, walks around until she finds something that catches her eye, and then slips it into her purse or pocket. Although Gloria has sworn to herself that she will never steal again, every few days she finds the tension so great that she cannot stay out of the stores.

(Grant, Odlaug, & Kim, 2010). Neuroimaging also suggests that people with kleptomania respond differently than individuals who do not have the disorder to images of store shelves compared to images depicting outdoor scenery (Asaoko et al., 2023).

Individuals with kleptomania may struggle with their symptoms for years before seeking treatment (Grant et al., 2015), perhaps because they fear prosecution or because they are ashamed of their illegal yet uncontrollable actions. Cognitive behavioral treatments also are effective, particularly exposure and response prevention (Olbrich, Jahn, & Stengler, 2019). Group treatment involving both cognitive behavioral and mindfulness components also can be effective in reducing symptoms while also improving the individual's quality of life (Asami et al., 2022).

10.5 Eating, Elimination, Sleep-Wake, and Impulse-Control Disorders: The Biopsychosocial Perspective

The disorders you learned about in this chapter represent a wide range of symptoms with a combination of biological causes, emotional difficulties, and sociocultural influences. A biopsychosocial approach therefore seems appropriate in understanding each. Moreover, these disorders have a developmental course. Eating and oppositional/conduct disorders appear to originate early in life. Over the course of adulthood, individuals may develop impulse-control disorders, and late in life, physiological changes may predispose older adults to sleep-wake disorders.

In the case of each category of disorder, clients can benefit from a multifaceted approach in which clinicians take into account these developmental and biopsychosocial influences. Some disorders, such as those in the sleep-wake category, may best be diagnosed through physiological tests such as polysomnography, even though treatment may focus on behavioral control of sleep. Individuals with symptoms of eating disorders should also be evaluated medically, but effective treatment requires a multipronged and team approach among mental health and medical professionals. The psychological and sociocultural components of impulse-control disorders tend to be more prominent in both diagnosis and treatment, although there may be biological contributions to each of these as well.

This wide range of disorders provides an excellent illustration of the need for an integrative approach that takes a life-span view in understanding and treating psychological disorders. As research in these areas progresses, it is likely that individuals affected by these disorders will benefit increasingly from interventions that take advantage of this multifaceted view.

Return to the Case: Maria Nomirez

Maria maintained her attendance at the day treatment program, which consisted of twice-weekly individual psychotherapy and several group therapy sessions every week. She saw a nutritionist who helped teach her the dangers of restricting her diet, and as a condition of the treatment she maintained a diet of at least 1,500 calories per day. At first she struggled with the change in her diet, which caused her much anxiety about becoming overweight. Her work in therapy and group therapy was aimed at maintaining a healthy body image and decreasing her unrealistic beliefs about being overweight.

As the weeks progressed, Maria continued to gain weight and her distorted body image began to ameliorate. Her husband and family, once a source of tension and anxiety, became an important factor in her recovery from anorexia through their strong support and encouragement. Although Maria continued to be concerned about becoming overweight, she learned the importance of nutrition and took on a more realistic view of her body. Maria's depression remitted after the first few weeks of treatment, and she decided to stay in the program for a total of 3 months. After leaving the day treatment program, Maria continued to see her therapist on a weekly basis.

Dr. Tobin's reflections: It is rare for an individual like Maria to present for treatment due to actual concern about weight loss, given the typically distorted view these individuals have that they are overweight even when by objective standards they are severely underweight. Indeed, Maria ignored her family's encouragement to obtain treatment. Had she been under the age of 18, it would have been appropriate for her family to bring her in for treatment. In this case, however, Maria's experience of depression motivated her to seek treatment. Some symptoms of depression are typical for individuals suffering from an eating disorder, and her symptoms did not warrant an independent diagnosis of depression. Although Maria had experienced some eating-disordered behaviors as a teenager, she was able to maintain a normal weight throughout much of her young adulthood. This fluctuating pattern is quite typical in the case of eating disorders. By her report, she continued to maintain a negative body image, although this did not manifest in any symptoms until she became pregnant with her daughter and faced the reality of actual weight gain. This served as a stressor that triggered a pattern of restrictive dieting that led to extreme weight loss.

Finally, the cultural aspect of this case is important to consider. Maria's family came from a culture with different ideals around body shape and size . The gap between her experiences growing up in the mainland United States, where there is pressure for women to maintain a low body weight, and her family's Puerto Rican culture was a great source of tension for her. Her family was unable to relate to her struggles with weight and body image, which served to increase her feelings of isolation. Emphasis on physical appearance is more prominent in more economically developed countries such as the United States, which leads to higher rates of eating disorders in these countries.

SUMMARY

- The eating disorder of anorexia nervosa (AN) is diagnosed when individuals show symptoms of food refusal, refuse to or are unable to maintain normal weight, have an intense fear of gaining weight or becoming fat, and have a distorted perception of the weight or shape of their body. In the eating disorder bulimia nervosa (BN), people alternate between eating large amounts of food in a short time (binge eating) and vomiting or performing other extreme actions (purging). In binge eating disorder (BED), individuals lack control over their eating.
- Theories of eating disorders based on the biological perspective emphasize altered serotonin functioning, and treatment based on this perspective relies on medications that target this system. Psychological approaches, which now are the basis for treatments of choice, focus on distortions in body image. From the sociocultural perspective, disordered eating is understood as a function of early family experiences, particularly adverse childhood environments. Biology and sociocultural influences combine in what is described as an ecophenotype. Treatment based on sociocultural approaches uses family therapy, and more generally includes prevention through promoting public awareness.
- Avoidant/restrictive food intake disorder may develop at any age but is most likely to emerge in childhood. Pica and rumination disorders are forms of eating-related disorders associated with childhood.
- Elimination disorders are most common in children younger than age 15, but they can be diagnosed in individuals of any age. Enuresis involves incontinence of urine, and encopresis involves incontinence of feces. Biobehavioral methods appear to be most effective in treatment, as well as therapy that incorporates parent involvement.

- Sleep-wake disorders include insomnia, narcolepsy, hypersomnolence, breathing sleep-related disorders, circadian rhythm sleep-wake disorders, and parasomnias. Each of these disorders is characterized by a severe disturbance in sleeping patterns. Insomnia can be identified by an inability to fall asleep or to remain sleeping, while narcolepsy and hypersomnolence involve sleeping too frequently and at inappropriate times. Breathing sleep-related disorders and circadian rhythm sleep-wake disorders, as well as parasomnias, can be characterized by unusual bodily movements or behaviors, which can disrupt sleep or waking cycles. Treatment for these disorders include cognitive behavioral therapy and use of either wearable technology or mechanical sleep devices for sleep apnea, with implants becoming the latest advance for those who cannot or prefer not to use mechanical devices.
- People with disruptive, impulse-control, and conduct disorders repeatedly engage in behaviors that are potentially harmful. They feel unable to stop themselves and experience a sense of desperation if their impulsive behavior is thwarted. Oppositional defiant disorder is characterized by angry or irritable mood, argumentative or defiant behavior, and vindictiveness that results in significant family or school problems. Cognitive behavioral therapy addresses situations that seem to trigger the behavior.
- The diagnosis of intermittent explosive disorder applies to individuals who feel a recurrent inability to resist assaultive or destructive acts of aggression. People with pyromania are driven by the intense desire to prepare, set, and watch fires. Their behavior needs to be differentiated from firestarting and arson, clinical distinctions that may require collaboration with law enforcement and fire officials.
- In kleptomania, individuals are driven by a persistent urge to steal, not because they wish to have the stolen objects but because they experience a thrill while engaging in the act of stealing. Treatment for this disorder involves the cognitive behavioral interventions, which may be combined with mindfulness.

KEY TERMS

Anorexia nervosa (AN)
Avoidant/restrictive food intake disorder
Binge eating
Binge eating disorder (BED)
Bulimia nervosa (BN)
Conduct disorder
Disinhibition
Eating disorders
Elimination disorders
Encopresis
Enuresis
Impulse-control disorders
Intermittent explosive disorder
Kleptomania
Maltreated ecophenotype
Oppositional defiant disorder
Orthorexia nervosa
Pica
Polysomnography
Purging
Pyromania
Rumination disorder

CHAPTER 11

Paraphilic Disorders, Sexual Dysfunctions, and Gender Dysphoria

OUTLINE

Learning Objectives

11.1 Identify the patterns of sexual behaviors that represent psychological disorders.

11.2 Compare and contrast paraphilic disorders and theories of their development.

11.3 Recognize symptoms of sexual dysfunction and understand treatment methods for these dysfunctions.

11.4 Comprehend theories and symptoms of gender dysphoria.

11.5 Explain the biopsychosocial perspective of paraphilic disorders, sexual dysfunctions, and gender dysphoria.

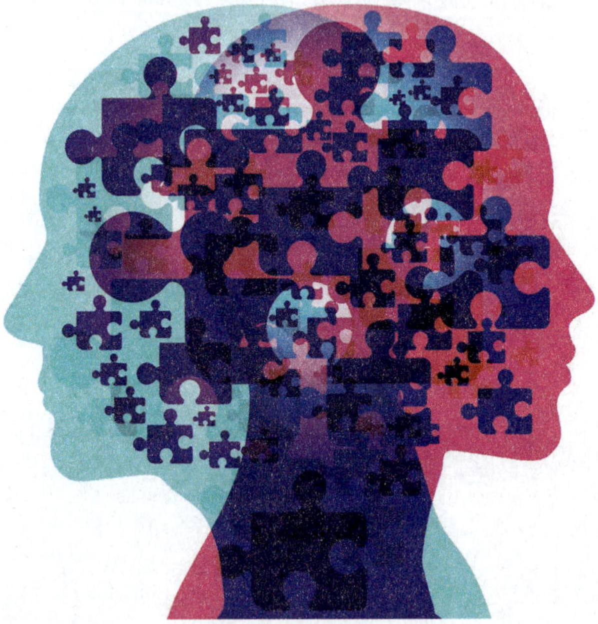

MrSquid/Shutterstock

Case Report

Shaun Boyden

Demographic information: 24-year-old White transgender man, who identifies as asexual. Shaun's pronouns are he/him/his.

History of present illness: Shaun is seeking psychotherapy for anxiety and history of gender dysphoria. At the time of intake, he reported that he was looking into options to start hormone replacement therapy (HRT) in order to start medically transitioning from female (his assigned sex at birth) to male. He was experiencing a significant increase in anxiety in the context of making that decision. Shaun added that he has limited social support in the way of people in his life who are affirming and supportive of his gender identity. He comes from a very conservative, religious upbringing, and his family has distanced themselves from him ever since he came out socially. In college, Shaun began his social transition, when he started changing his outward appearance to be more consistent with a more masculine look, stopped going by his dead name (legal name), and started using the name Shaun and he/him/his pronouns. He also started coming out to friends at that time and eventually came out to his family. Since graduating from college, Shaun has struggled to keep close friendships; a few friends stopped talking to him altogether after he came out to them as transgender. He reports that although he has always had a high baseline of anxiety in his life, he has noticed it is more challenging than ever to manage his anxious thoughts. He constantly feels tense and nervous, especially when people misgender him as female, address him by his dead name, or use she/her pronouns.

Shaun recalls that he was always a tomboy growing up, more interested in playing with boys than with girls. This was not a source of stress for him until he went through puberty and developed secondary sex characteristics, at which point he first started to feel what he now describes as gender dysphoria, or a sense that his identity did not match his biological characteristics. Shaun realized that he felt male and experienced distress around the notion that he appeared female to outside observers, and especially when he was pressured to dress in typically feminine clothing.

Given that he grew up in a small, conservative town with no visible queer or gender nonconforming people, Shaun felt ashamed and embarrassed for having these feelings, and very confused. After he started to do some research on the Internet, he realized he was not the only person who experienced these feelings, which was both relieving and terrifying to him. At one point, he ordered a breast binder online and wore it whenever he was alone in his room. At these times, he noticed his gender dysphoria decreased dramatically, and he reveled in being able to imagine himself appearing as a young man instead of a young woman. In fact, the more he did to appear male or take on male characteristics, the more he felt affirmed in his own identity.

Shaun was never interested in dating while he was a teenager and recalls that he never had any feelings of sexual attraction to other people. He learned about the term *asexual* online and joined several online support groups that connected him to others who identified similarly. He was also able to find online trans communities to connect with. The support Shaun received through his online community was a stark comparison to that in his everyday life, in which he was expected to dress in feminine attire while with his family, who disapproved of his tomboy-style clothes.

While in college, Shaun continued to struggle with gender dysphoria and found it difficult to get support from the people in his life. Over time, he started doing more research on steps to seek gender-affirming medical care, such as hormone replacement therapy (HRT) or "top" surgery (surgically removing breast tissue and creating a male-appearing chest), though he knew that his parents would never support any procedures so he would have to wait until he had his own health insurance. Shaun enjoyed having more freedom in college than he did at home, and so he felt more able to dress in stereotypically masculine attire and keep his hair short. However, much as in his hometown, there were few people on campus with whom he could relate, so he kept his thoughts about transitioning to himself.

After graduating from college, Shaun moved to a new city where he knew there was a thriving LGBTQIA+ community, in hopes of being able to get more social support and pursue a medical transition in earnest. He started to go through the relevant steps, such as legally changing his name and gender markers, and eventually he was

Case Report *continued*

able to get a job at a company where he felt he could be accepted for who he was. However, he experienced so much anxiety around meeting new people that he ended up isolated in his apartment except for going to work. Even at work he was withdrawn and kept mostly to himself.

Although there were medical providers he could consult about gender-affirming medical procedures, Shaun felt unable to make an appointment, because he thought that perhaps it was the wrong choice for him even though he knew he wanted to change his body to be more consistent with his gender identity. It was at this point that he came to psychotherapy for the first time.

Psychiatric history: Shaun has a history of mild anxiety that has never been clinically significant or impairing. He reports a history of gender dysphoria starting around the time of puberty and experiences significant distress related to it.

Case formulation: Shaun meets the relevant criteria for gender dysphoria in an adult as defined by the *DSM-5-TR,* given he has experienced dysphoria for more than 6 months and it is associated with clinically significant distress. Although he is currently experiencing some anxiety and social withdrawal, these symptoms are likely more related to his long-standing gender dysphoria and do not meet criteria for an additional diagnosis of anxiety disorder. Given that his anxiety also decreases with his dysphoria, and that he has never experienced anxiety apart from dysphoria, this further supports ruling out an additional diagnosis.

Risk level: Low risk. Shaun denies suicidal ideation and has no past history of suicide attempts.

Treatment plan: Shaun agreed to start meeting for weekly psychotherapy sessions, in order to get support for and process his feelings of gender dysphoria. Getting support in an affirmative environment such as therapy can help Shaun to think through his feelings about taking steps toward seeking gender-affirming medical procedures. Therapy can also focus on identifying ways for Shaun to start building more social support for himself in his local community and work through some of the anxiety that keeps him from connecting more with others.

Sarah Tobin, PhD

11.1 What Patterns of Sexual Behavior Represent Psychological Disorders?

When it comes to sexuality, deciding which patterns of behavior represent psychological disorders becomes a complicated process, perhaps more so than in other areas of human behavior. In any evaluation of the "normality" of a given sexual behavior, the social context takes on key importance, given that attitudes and behaviors related to sexuality vary by culture and are continually evolving over time.

Reflecting the taboo nature of sexuality for so many centuries in Western culture, there was little scientific research on sexual disorders until the mid-1900s. The three individuals credited with paving the way for contemporary research on human sexuality are Alfred Kinsey, William Masters, and Virginia Johnson. Kinsey was the first to conduct a large-scale survey of sexual behavior in the United States (Kinsey, Pomeroy, & Martin, 1948; Kinsey, Pomeroy, Martin, & Gebhard, 1953). Masters and Johnson (1966, 1970) were the first investigators to study sexual behavior in the laboratory.

The Kinsey Institute at Indiana University continues to support research on human sexuality, and the field of sexual medicine has become a specialty in its own right with journals specifically dedicated to study and treatment.

While the study of human sexuality has been established since that time, in more recent years the scope of scientific understanding about gender diversity and fluidity has significantly increased and grown highly sophisticated, enabled by multiple social and political activist movements that helped to resurrect the study of gender diversity that had been disrupted during World War II. Toward this end, researchers are now helping to provide

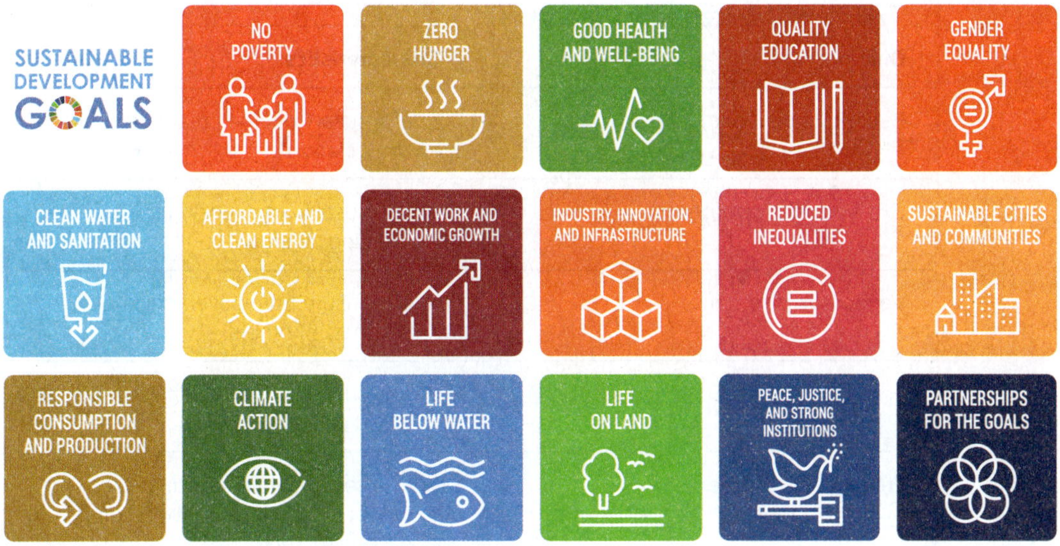

Gender equality is Sustainable Development Goal (SDG) 5 established by the United Nations in 2015. Progress toward targets is measured by indicators.

ALX1618/Shutterstock

empirical approaches that can guide clinicians and policy makers within the context of a continually shifting public landscape.

11.2 Paraphilic Disorders

As defined in the *DSM-5-TR*, paraphilic disorders cause individuals to experience impairment or distress associated with the object of their sexual attraction. **Paraphilias** are behaviors in which an individual has recurrent, intense sexually arousing fantasies, sexual urges, or behaviors related to (1) nonhuman objects, (2) children or other nonconsenting persons, or (3) the suffering or humiliation of self or partner. These disorders contrast with what might be called "unusual" or "rare" sexual interests such as attraction to dirtiness or soiled things, which do not meet the criteria for disorders because they do not cause distress or impairment even though they may involve the same or similar behavior (Schippers et al., 2021).

paraphilias
Behaviors in which an individual has recurrent, intense sexually arousing fantasies, sexual urges, or behaviors involving (1) nonhuman objects, (2) children or other nonconsenting persons, or (3) the suffering or humiliation of self or partner.

The major categories of paraphilic disorders are listed in Table 1.

The term *paraphilia* literally derives from *para* meaning "faulty" or "abnormal," and *philia* meaning "attraction." There is the danger of this term involving a value judgment, but it is important to keep in mind that clinicians will only diagnose **paraphilic disorder** when the behavior is one that causes intense distress and impairment and has lasted for at least 6 months.

paraphilic disorder
Diagnosis in which a paraphilia causes distress and impairment.

The authors of *ICD-11* take a different approach than the one used in the *DSM-5-TR*. The *ICD-11* limits paraphilic disorders to those that involve sexual arousal patterns focused on nonconsenting others or associated with substantial distress or direct risk of injury or death. These changes were intended to reflect what the authors refer to as advances in research and clinical practice, as well as major shifts in social attitudes and in relevant policies, laws, and human rights standards (Krueger et al., 2017).

Nevertheless, the fact remains that the diagnosis of a paraphilia must reflect symptoms of people who are so psychologically dependent on the particular form or target of their desire that they are otherwise unable to experience sexual arousal. Even if people with these disorders do not actually fulfill their urges or fantasies, they are obsessed with thoughts about acting upon them. Their attraction can become so strong and compelling that they lose sight of any goals other than achieving sexual fulfillment in this specific way. Making matters worse, during periods in which the individual feels especially stressed, the symptoms may become more intense.

TABLE 1 **Paraphilic Disorders**

Disorder	Characteristics
Pedophilic disorder	Sexual arousal from the presence of children or adolescents
Exhibitionistic disorder	Sexual arousal from exposing the genitals to unsuspecting strangers
Voyeuristic disorder	Sexual pleasure from observing nudity or sexual activity of others
Fetishistic disorder and partialism	Sexual arousal from an object (fetishism) or from a part of the body (partialism)
Frotteuristic disorder	Sexual urges about and sexually arousing fantasies of rubbing against or fondling a nonconsenting person
Sexual masochism and sexual sadism	Sexual arousal from being made to suffer (masochism) or from inflicting suffering on another person (sadism)
Transvestic disorder	Cross-dressing associated with intense distress or impairment

As you can see from this discussion a person's "nonnormative" sexual behavior is not pathological in and of itself. The symptoms of a paraphilia must include fantasies, urges, or behaviors that are the only way an individual can achieve "recurrent and intense sexual arousal." Neither the *DSM* nor the *ICD* regard sexual behavior that does not involve heterosexual intercourse as a criterion for a paraphilic disorder (Giami, 2015).

Note, too, that having a paraphilic disorder is not illegal, but acting on paraphilic urges may be. As a result, the person who reports having such a disorder to a mental health professional could theoretically be at risk for legal consequences such as arrest, conviction, and a court-ordered mandate to register as a sex offender. Even without these consequences the individual with a paraphilic disorder may experience other negative outcomes including feelings of shame and stigma (Grady et al., 2019). As a result, individuals with these disorders may put off or resist altogether the interventions that could benefit them.

Paraphilic disorders begin in adolescence and tend to be chronic; however, the urge to commit acts that fall into the category of a paraphilia among sex offenders appears to decline in later life (Barbaree & Blanchard, 2008). Paraphilic disorders also are more prevalent in men than women (Bártová et al., 2020). Individuals with paraphilic disorders are at risk for other psychological disorders, including anxiety disorder, depressive and bipolar disorder, sleep disorder, and psychotic disorders (Tzeng et al., 2019).

Pedophilic Disorder

pedophilic disorder
A paraphilic disorder in which an adult is sexually aroused by children or adolescents.

People diagnosed with **pedophilic disorder** are sexually aroused by children or adolescents. Clinicians use this diagnosis for adults who are at least 18 years of age and at least 5 years older than the children to whom they are attracted. The key feature of this disorder is that the individual experiences an intensity of sexual arousal when with children that may be equal to, if not greater than, that which they experience with individuals who have reached sexual maturity. This diagnosis includes people who have acted upon their urges with children as well as those whose attraction is represented by the viewing of online pornography involving children but not acting on those urges (Berlin, 2014).

MINI CASE

Pedophilic Disorder Nonexclusive Type

Kirk is a 38-year-old White heterosexual cisgender man. Shortly after getting married, Kirk began developing an inappropriately close relationship with Amy, his 8-year-old stepdaughter. It seemed to start out innocently, when he took extra time to give her bubble baths and back rubs. But after only 2 months of their living in the same house, Kirk's behavior went outside the boundary of common parental physical affection. After his wife left for work early each morning, Kirk invited Amy into his bed on the pretext that she could watch cartoons on the television in his bedroom. Kirk would begin stroking Amy's hair and gradually proceed to more sexually explicit behavior, encouraging her to touch his genitals, saying that it would be "good" for her to learn about what "daddies" are like. Confused and frightened, Amy did as she was told. Kirk reinforced compliance to his demands by threatening that, if Amy told anyone about their secret, he would deny everything and severely beat her. This continued for more than 2 years, until one day Kirk's wife returned home unexpectedly and caught him engaging in this behavior.

Given the illegality of the behavior, along with the stigmatism associated with admitting to a sexual attraction to children, it can be difficult to obtain either prevalence statistics or even specifics about the nature of the interests among people with pedophilia. One set of researchers sought to gain estimates using a crowdsourcing platform which assured anonymity. Self-selected based on recruiting criteria for people who self-identified as having pedophilic interests and/or behaviors, the results nevertheless provide useful information. Nearly one-quarter reported that they had a sexual interest in children, and of these, 32 percent either admitted to offending or showed a possible likelihood of offending. Fewer (3 percent) reported viewing online pornography (Ó Ciardha et al., 2022).

Viewing prevalence in terms of victims, the Rape Abuse and Incest National Network (RAINN) reports of sexual assault of children. Child Protective Services number over 57,000 per year, with one-third of children below the age of 12. The majority of victims (82 percent) are female, and the majority of perpetrators are men (88 percent). Over half are acquaintances, and one-third are family members (RAINN, 2021).

Exhibitionistic Disorder

People who engage in exhibitionism have fantasies, urges, and behaviors suggesting that they derive sexual arousal from exposing their genitals to an unsuspecting stranger. In **exhibitionistic disorder**, these fantasies, urges, and behaviors cause significant distress or impairment.

exhibitionistic disorder
A paraphilic disorder in which a person has intense sexual urges and arousing fantasies involving the exposure of genitals to a stranger.

Exhibitionistic disorder begins early in adulthood and persists throughout life. In one study of a small sample of male outpatients with this disorder (Grant, 2005), researchers found that almost all also had another psychiatric disorder including major depressive disorder and substance abuse. Over half experienced suicidal thoughts. This was one of the few studies in a clinical setting of people with the disorder who were not criminal offenders. In another investigation of self-identified men from a sample of police cases, approximately one-quarter also suffered from another psychological disorder (Bader, Schoeneman-Morris, Scalora, & Casady, 2008). The data from these samples are consistent with the findings from a Swedish national sample of nonclinical, noncriminal offenders, whose exhibitionism was also related to the presence of other psychological disorders (Långström & Seto, 2006).

The existence of comorbid conditions such as major depressive disorder and substance abuse, along with the reluctance of people with the disorder to come forward, present numerous challenges both for developing an understanding of the causes of the disorder and for planning its treatment (Murphy & Page, 2008). The most important step in treatment is accurately assessing both the disorder itself and these comorbid conditions (Morin & Levenson, 2008).

MINI CASE

Exhibitionistic Disorder, Sexually Aroused by Exposing Genitals to Physically Mature Individuals

Ernie is a 28-year-old Black heterosexual cisgender man. He is in jail for the fourth time in the past 2 years for public exposure. As Ernie explained to the court psychologist who interviewed him, he has "flashed" much more often than he has been apprehended. In each case, he has chosen as his victim an unsuspecting college-age woman, and he jumps out at her from behind a doorway, a tree, or a car parked at the sidewalk. He has never touched any of these girls, instead fleeing the scene after having exposed himself. On some occasions, he masturbates immediately after the exposure, fantasizing that his victim was swept off her feet by his sexual prowess and pleaded with him to make love to her. This time, his latest victim responded by calling the police to track him down. Ernie felt crushed and humiliated by an overwhelming sense of his sexual inadequacy.

Individuals who are victims of exhibitionism report a range of negative consequences including feelings of disgust and victimization. According to one large study of undergraduates at an urban university, victims are more likely to be women and, among this population, an average age of 16 years old. The participants in this study reported that the incident occurred on public transportation or in a street or public building. As reported by these students, the perpetrator was more likely to be a man who, at the time of the incident, engaged in masturbation. As upsetting as this experience was to victims, less than 10 percent reported the incident to police (Clark, Jeglic, Calkins, & Tatar, 2016).

Although exhibitionism is often examined in the context of its impact on younger women, it is possible for victims to be of any age. In an in-depth study of sexual assault against older women, researchers identified a case in which a patient in a long-term health care facility was subjected to the exhibitionism of a caregiver who removed his pants in front of her face. Instead of reporting the incident right away, she said nothing about it for a month due to her feelings of embarrassment and shame (Band-Winterstein, Goldblatt, Lev, & Harel, 2021).

Voyeuristic Disorder

voyeuristic disorder
A paraphilic disorder in which the individual has a compulsion to derive sexual gratification from observing the nudity or sexual activity of others.

People who engage in voyeurism derive sexual pleasure from observing the nudity or sexual activity of others who are unaware of being watched. Correspondingly, people with **voyeuristic disorder** are sexually aroused by observing an unsuspecting person who is naked, in the process of disrobing, or engaging in sexual activity. Voyeurism is related to exhibitionism and is the most common of the paraphilic disorders with higher prevalence in men (Castellini et al., 2018). Self-reports of voyeuristic behavior show higher rates in men compared to women (Dawson, Bannerman, & Lalumière, 2016). This difference is partly explained by higher self-reports of sex drive, the motivation to seek out sexual experiences (Levaque, Dawson, Wan, & Lalumière, 2021).

Fetishistic Disorder

fetishistic disorder
A paraphilic disorder in which the individual is preoccupied with an object and depends on this object rather than sexual intimacy with a partner for achieving sexual gratification.

partialism
A paraphilic disorder in which the person is interested solely in sexual gratification from a specific body part, such as feet.

People with **fetishistic disorder** are aroused by an object not specifically intended to be used in a sexual context. There is a wide range of objects to which people with fetishistic disorder can develop attachments. However, they do not include articles of clothing associated with dressing in clothes of another gender or objects such as vibrators that people use in tactile genital stimulation. In a related disorder, **partialism**, the individual is sexually aroused by the presence of a specific body part. Again, as with all paraphilic disorders, the attraction to objects or body parts must be recurrent, intense, and have lasted at least 6 months.

Fetishistic behavior is often conceptualized as action by a solitary individual who practices it without a partner. However, taking advantage of an online survey approach that, as noted earlier, allows for more accurate and widespread estimates of paraphilic behavior, in

MINI CASE

Fetishistic Disorder, Nonliving Objects

Johann is a 45-year-old White heterosexual cisgender man. For several years, Johann has been breaking into cars and stealing boots or shoes, and he has come close to being caught on several occasions. Johann takes great pleasure in the excitement he experiences each time he engages in the ritualistic behavior of procuring a shoe or boot and going to a secret place to fondle it and masturbate. In his home, he has a closet filled with dozens of women's shoes, and he chooses from this selection the particular shoe with which he will masturbate. Sometimes he sits in a shoe store and keeps watch for women trying on shoes. After a woman tries on and rejects a particular pair, Johann scoops the shoes from the floor and takes them to the register, explaining to the clerk that the shoes are a gift for his wife. With great eagerness and anticipation, he rushes home to engage once again in his masturbatory ritual.

one such survey, partnered fetishistic activity was rated by those reporting in this format as more sexually satisfying than solitary fetishistic activity (Rees & Garcia, 2017a). Furthermore, although having the fetishistic object may be preferred, individuals reporting this activity do not necessarily require its actual presence (Rees & Garcia, 2017b).

Also using an online survey, researchers studying internationally based social networking sites of individuals who identify as having "kinky" sexual desires found that participation in such networks provided a sense of identity. Participants regarded "kink" as a positively enjoyed personal taste, subculture, style, and way of life. For some, engagement in the fetish-oriented network framed this behavior as providing an escape from everyday life stress; others regarded their participation as an extension of their personalities (Hughes & Hammack, 2020). Again, it is worth remembering that these behaviors constitute a disorder only if they cause impairment and distress.

Frotteuristic Disorder

The term *frotteurism* derives from the French word *frotter* (meaning "to rub") and *frotteur* (the person who does the rubbing). The person with **frotteuristic disorder** has recurrent, intense sexual urges and sexually arousing fantasies of rubbing against or fondling a nonconsenting person. Among self-identified men diagnosed with paraphilic disorders, approximately 10 to 14 percent have committed acts of frotteurism (Långström, 2010).

frotteuristic disorder
A paraphilic disorder in which the individual has intense sexual urges and sexually arousing fantasies of rubbing against or fondling an unsuspecting stranger.

Cisgender men with frotteuristic disorder seek out crowded places, such as a rush-hour subway train, where they can safely rub up against their unsuspecting victims, and public transportation does seem to be a major site at which this behavior takes place. Like victims of exhibitionism, those exposed to frotteurism state that they feel violated and begin to go out of their way to avoid crowds. Also, as is true for victims of exhibitionism, most do not report the incident to police (Clark, Jeglic, Calkins, & Tatar, 2016).

MINI CASE

Frotteuristic Disorder

Bruce is a 40-year-old White heterosexual cisgender man. As a delivery messenger in a large city, he rides crowded subways throughout the day. He thrives on this opportunity to become sexually stimulated by rubbing up against unsuspecting women. Having developed some cagey techniques, Bruce is often able to take advantage of women without their realizing what he is doing. As the day proceeds, his level of sexual excitation grows, so that by the evening rush hour he targets a particularly attractive woman and only at that point allows himself to reach orgasm.

MINI CASE

Sexual Sadism and Sexual Masochism Disorders

Jalen is a 55-year-old biracial heterosexual cisgender man. For a number of years, he has insisted that his wife Camille subject him to demeaning and abusive sexual behavior. In the early years of their relationship, Jalen's requests were relatively innocent pleas that Camille pinch him and bite his chest while they were sexually intimate. Over time, however, his desire for pain increased and the nature of the pain changed. At present, the two engage in what they call "special sessions," during which Camille handcuffs Jalen to the bed and inflicts various forms of torture. Camille goes along with Jalen's requests that she surprise him with new ways of inflicting pain, and she has developed a repertoire of behaviors ranging from burning his skin with matches to cutting him with razor blades. Camille and Jalen have no interest in sexual intimacy other than that involving pain.

Sexual Masochism and Sexual Sadism Disorders

sexual masochism disorder
A paraphilic disorder marked by an attraction to achieving sexual gratification by having painful stimulation applied to one's own body.

sexual sadism disorder
A paraphilic disorder in which sexual gratification is derived from activities that harm, or from urges to harm, another person.

transvestic disorder
Diagnosis applied to individuals who dress in the clothing of the other sex and have the symptoms of a paraphilic disorder.

The term *masochism* describes the act of seeking pleasure from being in pain. People with **sexual masochism disorder** are sexually aroused by being beaten, bound, or otherwise made to suffer. Conversely, people with **sexual sadism disorder** become sexually aroused by the physical or psychological suffering of another person. *DSM-5-TR* does not classify the use of bondage, domination, and sadomasochism (BDSM) as a disorder in and of itself. Unlike "everyday sadism," which is the tendency to derive pleasure from watching or causing physical or psychological harm in others, these two disorders specifically focus on sexuality and are not particularly linked to antisocial tendencies (Sassenrath et al., 2023).

People with these disorders tend not to seek treatment because they feel no need to change, and because their behaviors often occur in the context of a consensual relationship. Even among consenting adults, acts of sexual masochism and sadism are shrouded in secrecy. Yet preference for kink and BDSM activities remains relatively common, with 46.8 percent of respondents in an online Belgian sample reporting that they had performed at least one BDSM-related activity and an additional 22 percent indicating they have or have had fantasies about it. A smaller but significant 12.5 percent of the online sample indicated performing at least one BDSM-related activity on a regular basis (Holvoet et al., 2017).

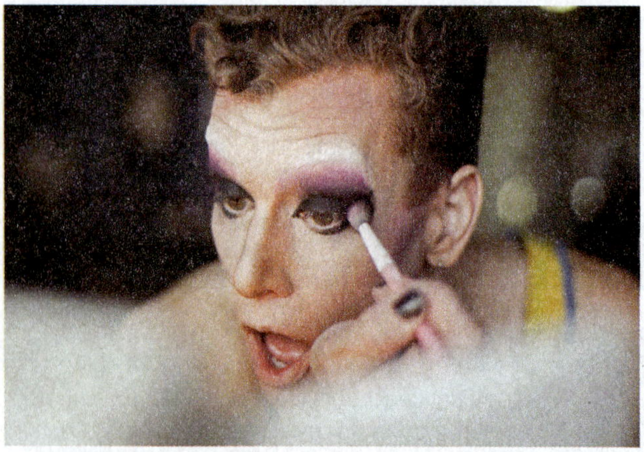

Transvestism is considered a psychological disorder only when it causes the individual to feel distress as a result of the cross-dressing behaviors. People with transvestism typically identify as cisgender.

Hex/Getty Images

Transvestic Disorder

Transvestism, also called "cross-dressing," refers to the behavior of dressing in the clothing of another gender. Cisgender men make up the large majority of individuals who show this behavior, but it is not associated with a psychological disorder. Furthermore, cisgender people who become involved in drag performance do not experience depression or gender dysphoria (Knutson & Koch, 2019).

A clinician would diagnose an individual with **transvestic disorder** only if the symptoms of a paraphilic disorder were present, namely distress or impairment associated with cross-dressing. Psychologists would not diagnose cisgender males with this disorder if they frequently cross-dress and derive sexual pleasure from this behavior (Blanchard, 2010). *DSM-IV-TR* limited this behavior to heterosexual cisgender males, but *DSM-5* opened the diagnosis to cisgender women and gay cisgender males who have this sexual interest. As previously noted, *ICD-11* eliminated the diagnosis of transvestic disorder entirely.

MINI CASE

Transvestic Disorder, with Autogynephilia

Phil is a 48-year-old White heterosexual cisgender man. In the evenings, when his wife leaves the house for her part-time job, Phil often goes to a secret hiding place in his workshop. In a locked cabinet, Phil keeps a small wardrobe of women's underwear, stockings, high heels, and dresses, and makeup and a wig. Closing all the blinds in the house and shutting off his phone, Phil dresses in these clothes and fantasizes that he is being pursued by several men. After about 2 hours, he usually masturbates to the point of orgasm as he imagines that a sexual partner is pursuing him. Then he packs up the women's clothes and puts them away. Though primarily limiting his cross-dressing activity to the evenings, Phil thinks about it frequently during the day, which causes him to become sexually excited and to wish he could get away from work, go home, and put on his special clothes. Knowing that he cannot, he wears women's underwear under his work clothes, and he sneaks off to the men's room to masturbate in response to the sexual stimulation he derives from feeling the silky sensation against his body.

Theories and Treatment of Paraphilic Disorders

Although the *DSM-5-TR* differentiates the paraphilic disorders, at the subclinical level there appear to be considerable linkages among many of them, as well as a general correspondence to degree of an individual's sex drive. Defining a high sex drive as seven or more orgasms a week for a minimum of 6 months, researchers demonstrated different patterns of relationships to paraphilic behaviors and interests based on variations in sex drives among participants in an online sample. Higher sex drive was associated with a stronger association for masochism, sadism, voyeurism, biastophilia (the act of sexually assaulting an unsuspecting person), and somnophilia (engaging in sexual activity with someone who is sleeping). However, sex drive was less strongly related to the relationship between pedophilia and blastophilia (Seto et al., 2021). The existence of themes across paraphilic interests and behavior along with the influence of sex drive suggest a need to understand these disorders from a broader perspective, rather than as completely individual entities.

From a theoretical standpoint, paraphilic disorders can be viewed as the product of biopsychosocial factors, given the roles of all three perspectives in understanding their causes and treatment. The biological perspective emphasizes altered genetic, hormonal, and sensory factors in paraphilic disorders (Guay, 2009). Biologically based treatments include antiandrogens, and luteinizing hormone-release hormone (LHRH), which acts as a suppressor in the production of testosterone. Medications that stimulate LHRH receive support as effective treatments in reducing paraphilic symptoms in men. However, they carry the drawback that by reducing testosterone below the level achieved even by castration, they also decrease conventional nonparaphilic sexual activity and desire. Medications that target LHRH also result in a number of side effects such as loss of bone mineral content, cardiovascular disease, fatigue, sleep disorders, and hot flashes and therefore are not recommended for lifelong treatment (Turner & Briken, 2018). An anti-cancer drug, degarelix, is another potential biological treatment for pedophilia that operates on hormonal activity (Landgren et al., 2020). However, its significant side effects must be balanced against its benefits, particularly because the drug does not change the extent to which individuals believe they are high risk to children (ElSayed & Gupta, 2020).

The World Federation of Societies of Biological Psychiatry (Thibaut et al., 2020), though supporting the use of such medications, nevertheless recommends that clinicians use the least intrusive methods possible and incorporate sex-drive lowering hormones only if the client is willing to take this form of treatment. Additionally, the "off-label" use of SSRI's may have benefit by working on the dopamine and serotonin systems, thought to contribute to the development of a paraphilia.

From the psychological perspective, CBT is the recommended treatment for paraphilias, with an emphasis on changing the behaviors themselves (Assumpção et al., 2014). CBT has the advantage of being translatable, with success, to online delivery (Hallberg et al., 2020). At increasing levels of severity, defined according to whether treatment is effective or not, clinicians add hormonal treatment starting with antiandrogens, progressing to progesterone, and finally neurohormones that act on the areas in the pituitary gland that control the release of sex hormones. At this point in treatment, appropriate only for the most severe cases, the goal is complete suppression of sexual desire and activity (Thibaut et al., 2020).

Another focus of treatment may be clinicians themselves, who may express prejudice, pathologizing attitudes, and other approaches that clients regard negatively. In a study of individuals who practice BDSM, researchers identified the importance of creating positive therapeutic experiences by adopting a non-judgmental view, asking client-centered questions, and encouraging a collaborative exploration of issues that are relevant to the client (Lantto and Lundberg, 2022). Clinicians can also learn through specialized training. In one intervention, researchers presented therapists in training with a 10-minute video that effectively challenged typical myths about pedophilia, such as the idea that it is a choice and that people with this disorder act upon their urges (Jahnke, Philipp, & Hoyer, 2015).

Sociocultural influences are also important to consider in understanding the development of paraphilic disorders. An analysis of popular pornography sites in the United Kingdom revealed that the sexual activity described in one out of eight titles included sexual violence, despite the fact that these would be considered offendable acts. The widespread availability of such media can be regarded from the perspective of "sexual script theory," which emphasizes the ways that individuals gain their understanding of sexuality through the resources they encounter in their environments. By normalizing sexual violence, the authors argue, this creates a cultural environment that can have an impact on users, normalizing behaviors that involve potential victims, particularly women (Vera-Gray, McGlynn, Kureshi, & Butterby, 2021).

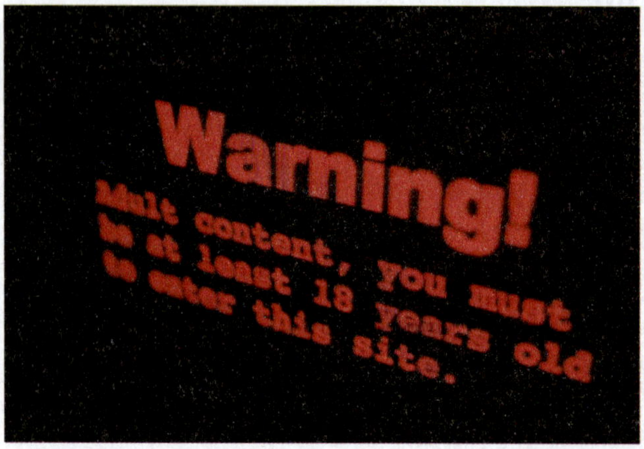

From a sociocultural perspective, sexual violence that becomes normalized in pornography is an important influence on some forms of paraphilia.
Don Farrall/Getty Images

As an example, a study conducted in Singapore analyzing Facebook comments in response to the reporting in the mainstream media of a case of sexual voyeurism against a woman showed the impact of gendered norms in response to sexual violence. Commenters both blamed the female victim and absolved the male perpetrator, supporting the view of a rape-supportive culture as shaping the perceptions of sexual violence (Tan, 2023).

You Be the Judge

Treatment for Sex Offenders

The paraphilic disorders present an ethical challenge to psychologists because of their potential link to the harming of others, particularly children and young teenagers. Treatment must balance the rights of the clients, including the right to confidentiality, informed consent, and self-determination, against the clinician's duty to prevent harm, both to others and to the client. Since treatment is often court-mandated, another question is whether it represents punishment rather than therapy.

Social workers David Prescott and Jill Levenson (2010), both of whom have an extensive background in treating sex offenders, suggest that clinicians can conduct mandated treatment in a manner consistent with the clinician's code of ethics. Mandated treatment, they argue, rather than representing punishment, is intended to assist offenders to correct the behaviors that were of harm to others and themselves. Moreover, the ethical standards that clinicians abide by regarding confidentiality are consistent with the "duty to warn" component of sex offender therapy: "Mandatory reporting trumps privilege" (Prescott & Levenson, 2010, p. 278). Second, regarding the client's right to self-determination, sex offenders are not the only individuals for whom the law mandates therapy. Child abusers and drivers arrested for operating a vehicle while intoxicated are two examples, but there are other cases in which the justice system gives family members, for example, an ultimatum to receive treatment for such behaviors as compulsive gambling.

Individuals who choose to work with sex offenders, according to Prescott and Levenson (2010), do so out of compassion and a desire to rehabilitate their clients so that they can become functioning members of society. They have found a way to empathize with clients who have committed sexually violent acts without judging the offenders and to overcome the "natural human reaction" of "disdain" (p. 282) for these individuals.

Q: *You be the judge:* Do you agree that the principles of human rights and the ethical guidelines presented by professional associations serve to protect sex offenders when they enter into therapy? Should the justice system even offer sex offender therapy, or should these individuals simply be incarcerated? On the other hand, is rehabilitation a realistic goal, as Prescott and Levenson claim, or are sex offenders beyond help?

REAL STORIES

Lamar Odom (1979–Present)

In his memoir *Darkness to Light*, renowned NBA star Lamar Odom (2019) confessed to the world, "I am a sex addict." For several years leading up until this revelation, he had been going through very public struggles with cocaine abuse, but until that point he had not been as candid about the impact of his sex addiction on his drug use.

Odom is perhaps best known for his incredibly successful NBA career, which started when he was just 19 years old. His career in the sport brought him to incredible heights and extended to other entrepreneurial ventures, including a record label and a clothing line. Odom has recalled that at the age of 7 he knew he wanted to be an NBA player. He was raised in Queens, New York, and from a very young age was struck by tragedy and loss. His beloved mother passed away suddenly from colon cancer when he was just 12 years old. Odom was then mostly raised by his grandmother and started to pursue basketball, eventually becoming the most acclaimed high school player in the country. He was eventually recruited to the University of Rhode Island, and after 1 year of playing in college, he became the fourth overall NBA draft pick and joined the Los Angeles Clippers. Odom's success in the league came early, and he was quickly recognized as a formidable player. His career highlights include winning two NBA championships with the LA Lakers, winning the NBA's prestigious Sixth Man of the Year award, and earning a bronze medal at the 2004 Olympics playing for the U.S. Men's basketball team.

While his basketball fame was on the rise, Odom confronted many personal losses and setbacks. In 2003, his grandmother passed away. Three years later to the day, his infant son died suddenly of sudden infant death syndrome (SIDS, or crib death). Odom also tragically lost several friends in the same period of time.

Odom gained worldwide fame for his whirlwind romance and marriage to Khloe Kardashian of the famous Kardashian family in 2009. In his memoir,

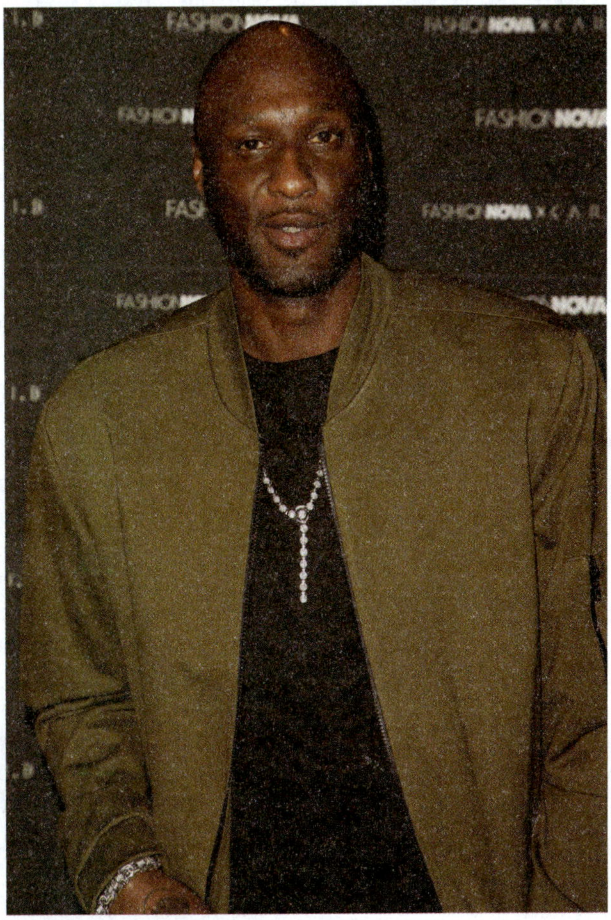

Lamar Odom at the Fashion Nova x Cardi B Collection Launch Event held at the Hollywood Palladium in May 2019.
Faye Sadou/AdMedia/ZUMA Press, Inc./Alamy Stock Photo

he recalls, "For a while, being with her was bliss and I was the happiest I've ever been ... we were one of the most famous couples in Hollywood and we made more money together than we had individually." However, after a few years of marriage, documented on television in their reality series *Khloe & Lamar* and on the successful reality show *Keeping Up with the Kardashians*, Odom's struggles with infidelity and cocaine addiction started to come to light.

His sex addiction led to lying and infidelity in his marriage, which Kardashian had discovered. Odom recalls; "I was shocked and embarrassed.... I wanted to take it back, but you can't. [I] wanted to hide it. But that sick sin was hard for me to hide ... I had a problem" (Nahas, 2019).

Odom's struggles with cocaine addiction drew public attention when he checked into rehab for drug abuse. In 2013, he was arrested for driving under the influence (DUI) and refused a chemical test, which generated widespread suspicion of struggles with drug addiction. Despite his making attempts at recovery, his multiple addictions continued to spiral and unfold as his NBA career came to its close in 2014. In October 2015, Odom's addictions to sex and drugs coalesced when he overdosed while partying in a Nevada brothel, due to a combination of cocaine, pills, and other drugs. He went into a brief coma, had kidney failure, and reportedly suffered 12 strokes, rendering him unable to walk or speak (Unity Behavioral Health, 2021).

The overdose was a wake-up call to Odom, who had been struggling with managing his drug addiction. As he said, "I wasn't in a good place mentally before [the overdose] happened.... I was basically committing suicide." After the overdose, he returned to inpatient rehab and started the recovery process, though this was not enough to save his marriage to Kardashian, and she sought a divorce in 2016. Their relationship had been very publicly on the rocks for years, with many media reports of infidelity and his struggles with cocaine addiction plaguing the marriage.

Prior to release of his 2019 memoir, Odom's sex addiction had gone unrecognized in the public specter, where most of the attention had focused on his infidelity to Kardashian. Odom himself had also downplayed these struggles (Barbour, 2019). However, it became clear to Odom (2019) after his overdose that his obsession with sex was a true addiction, and one that was intertwined with his drug addiction. In his memoir, he describes realizing that "Sex was a trigger for me to do drugs. Because you double up on [that] good feeling." Eventually, he recalls, he "ran out of porn to watch.... That's how you know when you are going a little overboard." Of his cocaine addiction, he writes, "With cocaine especially ... there's a high, and then an emotional low. You go high, and then you go low. High, low, high, low. After you do it, you feel shame. You think about all the reasons why you shouldn't have done it. Then the cycle starts again."

In his memoir, Odom (2019) admits to sleeping with more than 2,000 women during the height of his sex addiction. "There were too many strippers to count," he wrote. "It wasn't a big deal, but often I would pay them. I never thought less of them."

Since publishing his memoir, Odom has continued on his road to recovery and has been focused on the future. In the last pages of the memoir (Odom, 2019), he writes: "As for me, I'm still an addict. I still struggle. Some days I don't want to get out of bed. Some days I feel like the world and everything in it is mine. I still have my sense of humor. I can still see the bright side.... I'm hopeful. I'm determined. I am fierce. I am blessed. I am a force. I am humbled.... But mostly, I'm still figuring out who I am. I'm in a good place. I love the journey I'm on, and it's nowhere near done" (pp. 248–249).

11.3 Sexual Dysfunctions

sexual dysfunction
A marked divergence in an individual's sexual response that is accompanied by feelings of significant distress or impairment.

A **sexual dysfunction** is a marked divergence in an individual's sexual response that is accompanied by feelings of significant distress or impairment. To consider an individual as having a sexual dysfunction, clinicians must be unable to attribute this divergence to a psychological disorder, effects of a substance such as a drug of abuse or medication, or a general medical condition. The disorders themselves are categorized according to a framework that distinguishes phases of the sexual response cycle as progressing from arousal to orgasm.

The *DSM-5-TR* differentiates between sexual dysfunctions that are lifelong and those that are acquired, and it also distinguishes between those that are generalized and those that are situational. As the term implies, people with a lifelong sexual dysfunction have experienced its symptoms continually, beginning at the time at which they became sexually active. By contrast, people with acquired sexual dysfunctions were asymptomatic prior to developing the symptoms. Generalized dysfunctions affect the individual in all sexual situations. Dysfunctions that are situational occur with only certain types of sexual stimulation, situations, or partners.

Chronic health conditions along with behavioral risk factors are strongly related to the likelihood of developing sexual dysfunctions. These can include diabetes, cardiovascular disease, and genitourinary disease. Smoking and alcohol and drug use are behavioral risk factors that can contribute to sexual dysfunction (Sivaratnam et al., 2021).

The *DSM-5-TR* authors also note that cultural factors should also be considered in diagnosis. These can include expectations or prohibitions in a culture about the experience of sexual pleasure.

Not surprisingly, perhaps, reliable prevalence data on these disorders are few. Definitions of many disorders have changed periodically, leading to differing estimates (McCabe &

Connaughton, 2014), and people are reluctant to report they are experiencing symptoms. Only recently have researchers begun to arrive at measurable criteria based on the unique assessment methods these disorders require.

In a research context, the Female Sexual Function Index (FSFI) (Rosen et al., 2000) is an empirical measure used in a number of studies to investigate the prevalence of sexual dysfunctions in women and to gauge the efficacy of treatment. The FSFI is a 19-item multidimensional self-report scale that asks questions related to sexual functioning within the past month, with subscales related to specific domains of lubrication, desire, subjective arousal, orgasm, satisfaction, and pain associated with intercourse. A Spanish language translation of the FSFI is also available and shown to have similar reliability and diagnostic accuracy as the English version (Rincón-Hernández et al., 2021). Another, more behaviorally oriented approach asks individuals to record sexual events on a daily basis in the form of a self-report diary (van Nes et al., 2017).

Historically, sexual dysfunctions have been divided into categories based on an individual's assigned sex at birth (there are "male" and "female" versions of each disorder). Sexual dysfunctions are also framed in terms of heterosexual relationships and have been related to the stages leading up to and including male-female intercourse. However, researchers are beginning to examine sexual dysfunctions in same-sex relationships between men (Barbonetti et al., 2019), between women (Peixoto & Nobre, 2015), and between bisexual adults (Shepler, Smendik, Cusick, & Tucker, 2018). Research is also starting to explore sexual dysfunction in transgender individuals who have had gender-affirming medical procedures.

Given that the majority of studies on sexual dysfunctions examined heterosexual, cisgender adults, and following the American Psychological Association's (2020) guidelines for language discussing gender, the terminology you will read in this chapter will refer to *men* and *women* (and transgender men and women where specified), rather than more gender-neutral terms or the terms *male* and *female* unless the disorder is labeled in male-female terms.

Arousal Disorders

People whose sexual disorders occur during the initial phases of the sexual response cycle have low or no sexual desire or are unable to achieve physiological arousal. As a result, they may avoid having or be unable to have sexual intercourse.

Male hypoactive sexual desire disorder refers to a condition in which the individual has an atypically low level of sexual activity or may have no interest in sexual activity. In addition, a person with this disorder either has relatively few or no sexual fantasies. A person with **female sexual interest/arousal disorder** is interested in having intercourse, but their body does not physiologically respond during the arousal phase. Low sexual desire among women is reported to have a prevalence of 40 percent (Clayton & Valladares Juarez, 2017), higher in women age 65 and older (Zheng et al., 2020).

male hypoactive sexual desire disorder
A sexual dysfunction in which the individual has an atypically low level of interest in sexual activity.

female sexual interest/arousal disorder
A sexual dysfunction characterized by a persistent or recurrent inability to attain or maintain normal physiological and psychological arousal responses during sexual activity.

MINI CASE

Female Interest/Arousal Disorder, Acquired

Carol is a 33-year-old Native American heterosexual cisgender woman. With the pressures of managing a full-time advertising job and raising 3-year-old twins, Carol says that she has "no time or energy" for sexual relations with her husband, Bob. In fact, they have not been sexually intimate since the birth of their children. Initially, Bob tried to be understanding and to respect the fact that Carol was recovering from a very difficult pregnancy and delivery. As the months and years went by, however, he became increasingly impatient and critical. The more he pressured Carol for sexual closeness, the more angry and depressed she became. Carol feels that she loves Bob, but she does not think about sex and can't imagine ever being sexual again. She is saddened by the effect this change has had on her marriage but feels little motivation to try to change.

MINI CASE

Erectile Disorder, Acquired

Kai is a 34-year-old Asian American heterosexual cisgender man. He has been dating the same woman for more than a year. This is his first serious relationship, and the woman is the first person with whom he has been sexually intimate. During the past 6 months, they have frequently tried to have intercourse, but each time they have become frustrated by Kai's inability to maintain an erection for more than a few minutes. Every time this happens, Kai becomes very upset, despite his girlfriend's reassurance that things will work out better next time. His anxiety level heightens every time he thinks about the fact that he is in his mid-30s, sexually active for the first time in his life, and encountering such frustrating difficulties. He fears he is "impotent" and will never have a normal sex life.

erectile disorder
Sexual dysfunction in which a man cannot attain or maintain an erection during sexual activity that is sufficient to allow him to initiate or maintain sexual activity.

Individuals with **erectile disorder** cannot attain or maintain an erection that is sufficient to allow them to initiate or maintain sexual activity. Even if they are able to achieve an erection, they are unable to penetrate or to experience pleasure during a sexual encounter.

The prevalence of erectile disorder increases in older samples of men, from 20 percent below age 30 to over 90 percent at age 70 and older. However, increases in prevalence are also linked to medical conditions whose prevalence increases with age, most notably diabetes, prostatitis, and even periodontal (gum) disease. Cannabis use also contributes to higher rates of erectile disorder, although its relationship to age has not yet been established (Allen & Walter, 2019). As noted in the *DSM-5-TR*, cultural factors such as expectations concerning sexual performance and gender roles may contribute to variations in prevalence statistics by country.

Disorders Involving Orgasm

female orgasmic disorder
A sexual dysfunction in which a woman experiences problems having an orgasm during sexual activity.

Inability to achieve orgasm, a distressing delay in achieving orgasm, or reduced intensity of orgasm constitutes **female orgasmic disorder**. Although previous versions of the *DSM* regarded orgasm resulting from clitoral stimulation as distinct from that resulting from intercourse, the *DSM-5-TR* does not distinguish between sources of orgasm in defining the criteria for this disorder.

The factors relating to an individual's reporting of female orgasmic disorder include stress, anxiety, depression, relationship satisfaction, and age-related changes in the genital area that can lead to pain, discomfort, irritation, or bleeding (Laumann & Waite, 2008). Size and location of the clitoris also play a role (Oakley et al., 2014), as do difficulties in lubrication. In general, older women are less likely to experience orgasmic difficulties than are younger women (Rowland & Kolba, 2016).

MINI CASE

Female Orgasmic Disorder, Lifelong

Magda is a 28-year-old Latina bisexual cisgender woman. Like many of her friends, Magda often wondered as a teenager what intercourse and orgasm would feel like. When she later became sexually active in college, she realized that she was probably still missing something, since she did not feel "rockets going off" as she had imagined. In fact, she never could experience orgasm when she was engaged in any kind of sexual activity. When Magda fell in love with José, she fervently hoped that things would improve. However, even though he made her feel more sensual pleasure than anyone else, her response to him always stopped just short of climax. She approached every sexual encounter with anxiety and tended to feel depressed and inadequate afterward. To avoid making José worry, however, Magda decided it would be better to fake orgasm than to be honest with him. After 5 years together, she still has not told José that she is not experiencing orgasms, and she feels too embarrassed to seek professional help, despite her ongoing distress.

MINI CASE

Premature (Early) Ejaculation, Lifelong

Jeremy is a 45-year-old South Asian gay cisgender man. He has struggled with the problem of premature ejaculation for as long as he can remember. Since his first experience with sexual intercourse as a college student, he has been unable to control his orgasms and customarily ejaculates seconds after penetration. Because of this problem, his relationships over the years have been strained and difficult. In each instance, the person he was dating at the time became frustrated, and Jeremy felt too embarrassed to continue the relationship. For a period lasting several years, he avoided sexual relations completely, knowing that each experience of failure would leave him feeling depressed and furious.

Individuals who have a marked delay in ejaculation or who rarely if ever experience ejaculations have **delayed ejaculation**. Individuals with **premature (early) ejaculation** reach orgasm in a sexual encounter with minimal sexual stimulation before, on, or shortly after penetration and before wishing to do so (within 1 minute). Clinicians prefer to apply a psychiatric diagnosis only when the individual is distressed about the condition. The prevalence rate for premature ejaculation varies widely, from 8 to 30 percent, and seems to depend on age group and country (Lewis et al., 2010). Men who have sex exclusively with men or who have sex with both men and women, as found in a Norwegian study, have lower likelihood of premature ejaculation (Traeen, Fischer, & Grøndahl, 2022).

delayed ejaculation
A sexual dysfunction in which a man experiences problems having an orgasm during sexual activity; also known as inhibited male orgasm.

premature (early) ejaculation
A sexual dysfunction in which a man reaches orgasm well before he wishes to, perhaps even prior to penetration.

Personality traits seem to be related to premature ejaculation, including an individual's being less willing to explore novel situations and a greater tendency to avoid situations of potential risk. As a result, they are less adaptive when faced with this change in their sexuality (Gao et al., 2021).

Disorders Involving Pain

Clinicians diagnose sexual pain disorders characterized by the experience of difficulty in a sexual relationship due to painful sensations in the genitals from intercourse as **genito-pelvic pain/penetration disorder**. Genito-pelvic pain/penetration disorder can affect anyone. The individual experiences recurrent or persistent genital pain before, during, or after sexual intercourse. For women with this disorder, the pain may even be associated with a desire to avoid medical visits that include a gynecological exam (Lahaie et al., 2015).

genito-pelvic pain/penetration disorder
A sexual dysfunction affecting both males and females that involves recurrent or persistent genital pain before, during, or after sexual intercourse.

The *DSM-5-TR* notes the importance of cultural factors in influencing experience and reporting of genito-pelvic pain, including the way in which women report their symptoms. Women may feel pressured by heteronormative social narratives that emphasize the pressures to prioritize men's sexual desire and penetrative sex. Such cultural factors may also influence whether women report pain to healthcare providers and can also affect prevalence estimates.

Research on sexual dysfunction in transgender individuals who have pursued some form of gender-affirming surgery or use gender-affirming hormone therapy (HRT) is limited, though there are some studies beginning to shed light on this area. In a sample of Australian trans individuals who were assigned female at birth, 72.2% reported experiencing pelvic pain of some form following initiation of testosterone therapy (Zwickl et al., 2023). Participants in the study who had undergone a hysterectomy reported a significant reduction in pelvic pain. In an online sample of over 500 trans men and women, those who received either vaginoplasty or phalloplasty experienced greater reductions in sexual dysfunction—including arousal difficulties, sexual aversion, and low sexual desire, compared with trans individuals who received hormone therapy but not genital surgery (Kerckhof et al., 2019).

What's in the *DSM-5-TR*

The Reorganization of Sexual Disorders

The sexual disorders underwent major rethinking in the *DSM-5.* The most significant was the declaration that clinicians do not consider paraphilias disorders unless they are accompanied by distress or impairment. This change recognizes the continuum along which sexual behavior falls and removes the stigma attached to sexual behaviors that do not cause distress or impairment or harm to others.

The sexual dysfunctions also became redefined in *DSM-5.* Hypoactive sexual desire disorder is diagnosed only in people assigned male at birth; people assigned female at birth receive a diagnosis of hypoactive sexual interest/arousal. The previously separate disorders of vaginismus (inability to allow penetration) and dyspareunia (pain with intercourse) were combined into one disorder called genito-pelvic pain/penetration disorder, because they are difficult to distinguish from one another.

In other changes, the term *early* was added in parentheses after "premature" ejaculation, and male orgasmic disorder was relabeled "delayed" ejaculation. Both these changes reflect a desire, once again, to destigmatize a variant of human sexuality.

Finally, the relabeling of "gender identity disorder" in *DSM-IV-TR* to the new term *gender dysphoria,* along with other changes within this category, provides a revamped view of these disorders that not only is more consistent with the research evidence but also brings a greater understanding of people who experience the emotional distress of a mismatch between their assigned sex at birth and their own sense of gender. The *DSM-5-TR* has updated language from the *DSM-5,* and uses more inclusive language such as "experienced/expressed gender," instead of "desired gender."

Though based on empirical evidence, the *DSM-5* and *DSM-5-TR* changes in the area of sexual disorders also clarify in important ways the many varieties of normal human sexuality. As these changes take hold in the psychological and psychiatric communities, they will provide directions for successful approaches to the treatment of people whose sexuality causes them to experience distress.

Theories and Treatment of Sexual Dysfunctions

Sexual dysfunctions represent an interaction of complex physiological, psychological, and sociocultural factors, and thus the biopsychosocial perspective is well suited to understanding them. In diagnosing these disorders, it is therefore essential for the clinician to conduct a comprehensive assessment that includes a physical examination and psychological testing and including the client's partner if appropriate. In addition, the clinician must assess the individual's use of substances including not only drugs and alcohol, but also all medications, including those intended to treat psychological disorders.

Biological Perspective

As you already learned, there are higher rates of sexual disorders among people with a variety of health problems, suggesting an important role for biology. Treatments based on the biological perspectives use physical devices and pharmacological interventions that either increase an individual's level of arousal or, for men, their ability to have partnered sexual intercourse.

People are affected by hormonal changes that can influence sexuality during the **climacteric**, the gradual loss of reproductive potential that occurs in middle and later adulthood. For women, these changes occur during the years before and after menopause, when the monthly menstrual cycle ceases and estrogen production declines. For men, the corresponding changes are due to decreasing production of testosterone across middle and later adulthood.

climacteric
The gradual loss of reproductive potential that occurs in middle and later adulthood.

MINI CASE

Genito-Pelvic Pain/Penetration Disorder, Lifelong

Shirley is a 31-year-old White heterosexual cisgender woman who has been sexually active for about 10 years, with multiple male partners. Despite her ability to achieve orgasm through masturbation, she has found herself unable to tolerate penetration during intercourse. In her own mind, she feels a sense of readiness, but her vaginal muscles inevitably tighten up and her partner is unable to penetrate. It is clear to Shirley that this problem has its roots in a traumatic childhood experience when she was sexually abused by an older cousin. Although she recognizes that she should seek professional help, she is too embarrassed to do so and has convinced herself that the problem will go away if she can find the right man who will understand her problems.

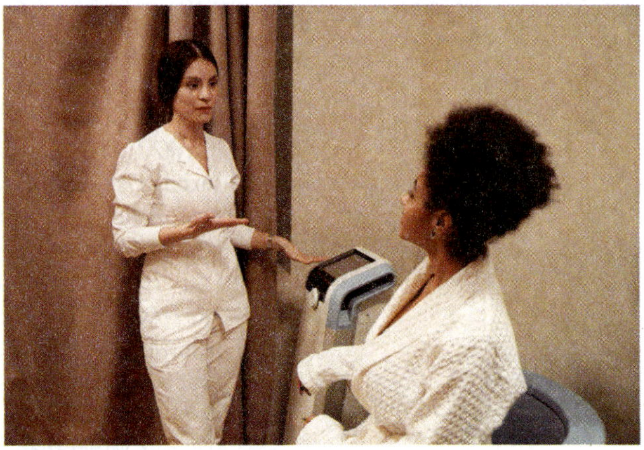

Pelvic floor therapy can be helpful for individuals who experience genito-pelvic pain/penetration disorder through using a variety of methods to promote muscular relaxation.

Svitlana Hulko/Shutterstock

The lowering of estrogen levels throughout the period of menopause can lead women to experience a number of physical symptoms that affect their sexuality, including vaginal dryness and gradual shrinking of vaginal size and muscle tone. These changes themselves do not affect their ability to achieve arousal during sexual activity, however. Cisgender females also experience a decline in free testosterone, the "male" sex hormone, but it is not clear whether this decline is related to changes in sexual desire and satisfaction.

Treatment of female sexual interest/arousal disorder that follows from the biological perspective incorporates hormonal replacement therapy (estrogen and progesterone), estrogen cream applied directly to the vagina, and testosterone therapy (Traish, Feeley, & Guay, 2009). Women with low sexual desire can also be treated with the medication flibanserin, approved by the FDA in 2015 under the trade name Addyi. Data on its efficacy suggest that flibanserin may have beneficial effects as a treatment for premenopausal women (Simon, Thorp, & Millheiser, 2019).

Medications to treat erectile disorder include the prescription drugs Viagra, Levitra, and Cialis. These are all in the category of **phosphodiesterase (PDE) inhibitors**, which work by increasing blood flow to the genital area. These medications work when accompanied by the experience of sexual excitement. PDEs, though effective, also require monitoring by a medical professional to reduce the chances of dangerous interactions with other medications an individual may be taking. Penile implants and external vacuum devices are mechanical ways that induce or make possible an erection, but they can be inconvenient to use and may require surgery.

phosphodiesterase (PDE) inhibitors
Medications for erectile disorders that increase blood flow to the genital area.

Genito-pelvic pain/penetration disorder presents a different set of treatment challenges. From a biological perspective, the physical symptoms can come from a variety of sources, including excessive tightening and tension in the muscle fibers in the pelvic area (called the "pelvic floor"). A form of physical therapy, pelvic floor therapy involves teaching the client ways to relax the pelvic floor muscles as well as manual massage by a pelvic floor specialist. More generally, persistent genital arousal disorder, which can be tied to physical pain as well as other medical contributions (such as injury or nerve damage), can be treated from a biological perspective with neuomodulators implanted under the skin, Botox (which causes the muscles to relax), and surgery (Martin-Vivar et al., 2022).

Men with erectile dysfunction can also benefit from similar forms of physical therapy as are helpful for women including pelvic floor muscle exercises, electrical stimulation, and biofeedback. Given some of the risks associated with erectile dysfunction medications, these methods provide safe and effective alternatives, as shown in a large-scale review of findings based on 912 men, ages 19 to 83 years old, across six different samples (Gbiri & Akumabor, 2023).

Psychological Perspective

People with sexual dysfunction are best understood from a psychological perspective in terms of disturbances in their thoughts about their bodies and their sexuality. These disturbances interfere with sexual functioning by shifting the individuals' attention away from the sexual situation itself and onto their own negative and distracting thoughts.

For women, preoccupation with overall body image is known to interfere with sexual functioning, perhaps interacting with attitudes toward sexuality in general (Lemer, Salafia, & Benson, 2013). A negative genital self-image specifically can also contribute to sexual dysfunction by leading them to become distracted by their thoughts about their bodies rather than focusing on their sexual sensations (Vigil, de Jong, & Poovey, 2021). For men, such cognitive disturbances can include their self-image and concern about the size of their genitals, leading them to become anxious in sexual situations (Wilcox, Redmond, & Davis, 2015).

In addition to discomfort with their bodies, individuals may hold negative "sexual self-schemas" such as feeling unloved, inadequate, and unworthy. Their self-esteem, in turn, becomes contingent on their ability to maintain a satisfactory sexual relationship (Cyranowski et al., 2020). Cultural factors about normative behaviors can contribute to these self-schemas.

It is not only the thoughts themselves that interfere with an individual's sexual functioning from a cognitive perspective, but also the tendency of individuals to engage in "meta-cognitive" thinking, meaning that they worry excessively about their thoughts. People with sexual dysfunctions who engage in this pattern of beliefs have a greater prevalence of sexual dysfunctions than individuals who do not, suggesting that their difficulty in controlling stress may contribute to their sexual difficulties (Olivari, Di Cugno, & Caselli, 2023).

Based on the view that disturbed thoughts contribute to sexual dysfunctions, therapists working within the psychological perspective rely upon principles derived from cognitive behavioral therapy. Restructuring those cognitions could therefore help alleviate sexual dysfunction symptoms. Furthermore, helping clients understand that each sexual encounter does not need to be perfect but can be "good enough" can help couples focus on sexual pleasure rather than on performance (Metz, Epstein, & McCarthy, 2018). Another approach within the cognitive behavioral perspective, one that has been found effective in increasing sexual desire and reducing distress in women with low sexual desire disorder, combines psychoeducation about female sexuality and the sexual response with mindfulness training (Gunst et al., 2019). As is true with other forms of CBT, these approaches can successfully be provided in an online format (Stephenson, Zippan, & Brotto, 2021).

For sexual pain disorders, cognitive behavioral therapists base their interventions on identifying a woman's beliefs that penetration will be painful. In one approach shown to be efficacious the clinician (a woman) supervises the client as she engages in self-performed penetration exercises. This approach helps the client to confront not only her beliefs about penetration but also the tendency to engage in catastrophic thinking about those beliefs (Ter Kuile et al., 2015).

Therapeutic efforts should not be limited on the basis of a client's age. A survey of older women (60 to 75 years of age) conducted in several European countries revealed a relatively high prevalence of between 23 and 50 percent of sexual difficulties lasting three months or longer (Graham et al., 2020). Therefore, healthcare and mental healthcare professionals should consider addressing sexual concerns expressed by individuals, regardless of their age.

11.4 Gender Dysphoria

gender dysphoria
Distress that may accompany the incongruence between a person's experienced or expressed gender and that person's birth-assigned sex.

birth-assigned sex
Term that refers to sex assigned to the individual at birth based on either genitalia and/or prenatal sex discernment.

DSM-5-TR defines **gender dysphoria** as distress due to incongruence between an individual's birth-assigned sex and their gender identity. Not everyone experiences distress as the result of this incongruence, so the term *gender dysphoria* is reserved for those who experience it and are unable to make changes so they can be affirmed in their gender identity. In other words, not all transgender or gender diverse individuals meet criteria for gender dysphoria. The criteria for the disorder, therefore, includes the feeling that **birth-assigned sex** is mismatched with gender identity, along with significant discomfort, emotional distress, and functional impairment related to a sense of inappropriateness about the person's assigned sex.

Whereas in the past the profession saw transgender people as having a "disorder," the new terminology instead focuses on the psychological distress that can emerge from not being affirmed in one's gender identity.

transgender
The identity of a person whose assigned gender does not correspond with their gender identity.

Unlike individuals with transvestic disorder, people with gender dysphoria do not derive sexual gratification from dressing in clothing of another gender cross-dressing. Further, many other identities fall in the category of **transgender**, including gender nonconforming, non-binary, and agender. These terms correspond with the notion that not all transgender people see themselves in the binary categories either man or woman, or girl or boy. Instead, they might feel they identify with several genders, or no gender at all. The term *non-binary* in particular corresponds to the notion that gender is often seen through the lens of society as a binary or either/or, when in fact gender is a social construct that exists along a spectrum of identities, behaviors, and expression.

Individuals with gender dysphoria experience depression and anxiety at higher rates than cisgender individuals. In addition, gender diverse people, and especially transgender youth, experience higher rates of suicidality, violence/victimization, and substance abuse

(Newcomb et al., 2020). Transgender women of color, in particular, are likely to be victims of violence, including murder (Ussher et al., 2020).

An important difference between the *DSM* classification of gender dysphoria and that of *ICD-11* relates to the question of whether individuals whose gender identity differs from their assigned sex require a diagnosis of dysphoria to gain access to health care. In the *ICD-11,* the former "gender identity disorder" is now reclassified as "gender incongruence," a condition related to sexual health (de Vries et al., 2021). Within the *DSM,* the diagnosis signifies a major departure from past versions, which used the term Gender Identity Disorder (consistent with past versions of the *ICD*) as a diagnosis. This was seen as highly pathologizing of gender diverse identities and was not associated with any particular health issue or psychopathology. The most recent diagnostic category focuses specifically on the psychological suffering associated with the mismatch between birth-assigned sex, and the individual's sense of their own gender. And although many social activist groups still debate the existence of gender dysphoria as a diagnosis, one of the important roles this diagnosis serves both is that it is often necessary for insurance coverage of mental health care and gender-affirming medical procedures and surgeries.

Even though transgender identity itself has been depathologized in *DSM-5-TR,* clients will nevertheless continue to face **transphobia**, the negative stereotyping and fear of transgender individuals. Transphobia can be considered a form of minority stress, leading transgender individuals to experience feelings of stigma, along with potential concealment of their transgender identities (Lindley & Galupo, 2020). From a social psychological perspective, transphobia can translate into lack of support for transgender policies and the enactment of other behaviors that continue to marginalize transgender individuals (Axt, Conway, Westgate, & Buttrick, 2021).

transphobia
The negative stereotyping and fear of transgender individuals.

Another source of discrimination that transgender people experience is lack of access to health care due to higher rates of unemployment and policies that prevent them from accessing gender-affirming care. These inequities can further contribute to anxiety, depression, and suicidality (Bretherton et al., 2020). High rates of discrimination, in turn, can also serve as precipitants to substance abuse (Connolly & Gilchrist, 2020).

Theories and Treatment of Gender Dysphoria

According to the World Professional Association for Transgender Health (WPATH), clinicians ideally provide an assessment of a client's well-being without regard to diagnostic criteria (Wylie et al., 2016). This assessment can then become the basis for determining whether a particular client is able to exercise good judgment and decision making when choosing medical treatments.

Treatment for gender dysphoria from a biological perspective focuses on **gender-affirming medical procedures**. These procedures range from hormone therapy to a variety of surgical procedures such as facial feminization surgery, chest reconstructive surgery ("top" surgery), and genital reconstructive surgery (sometimes referred to as sex reassignment surgery, or "bottom" surgery). Each of these procedures requires psychological and other evaluations to ensure that the individual does not have other psychological disorders that might affect judgment or decision making and does have documented and persistent gender dysphoria (Coleman et al., 2012). Gender affirming medical procedures have well-established positive outcomes and have shown significant long-term satisfaction and reductions in gender dysphoria for many different types of procedures (Park et al., 2022).

gender-affirming medical procedures
Biological treatments including hormone replacement therapy and surgery for people with gender dysphoria.

From a psychological perspective, clinicians who work with transgender individuals experiencing gender dysphoria can provide support through psychotherapy as well as assisting clients in the decision to seek out gender-affirming medical procedures (Dhejne, Van Vlerken, Heylens, & Arcelus, 2016). Indeed, the American Psychological Association's Guidelines for Psychological Practice with Transgender and Gender Nonconforming People (TGNP) (APA, 2015a) suggest that clients achieve the most positive outcomes when they receive social support or trans-affirmative care and are seen from an interdisciplinary perspective. Programs that train clinicians, furthermore, should prepare their trainees in psychology to work with clients who identify as TGNP.

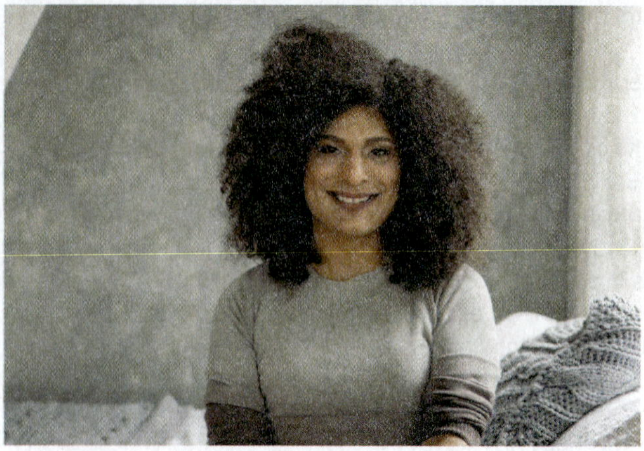

Transgender individuals with gender dysphoria can benefit from such interventions as affirmative psychotherapy.

Renata Angerami/Getty images

In **affirmative psychotherapy**, clinicians help transgender clients safely explore their gender identity, explore options for gender-affirming medical procedures, and connect with sources of social support (Austin & Craig, 2015). Clinicians can begin their treatment by using the name and pronouns used by the client, if that differs from their legal name or gender markers. Rather than assume that people's motivations, behaviors, and attitudes are based on their socially defined identities, clinicians can also recognize that these categories are conditional. For example, they can avoid using terms like *real* or *biological* gender. Clinicians should also avoid "gatekeeping," in which they exercise their power to grant or withhold access to the client's desired outcomes (Morris, Lindley, & Galupo, 2020).

Given that clinicians will continue to treat individuals with gender dysphoria, new approaches based on transgender theory are emerging that emphasize a more fluid view of gender than the binary male-female dichotomy (Nagoshi & Brzuzy, 2010), a perspective also articulated in the APA TGNP Guidelines.

affirmative psychotherapy
Approach in treating transgender clients in which clinicians help their clients safely explore their gender identity, explore options for gender-affirming medical procedures, and connect with sources of social support.

11.5 Paraphilic Disorders, Sexual Dysfunctions, and Gender Dysphoria: The Biopsychosocial Perspective

Sexual disorders constitute three discrete sets of difficulties in aspects of sexual functioning and behavior. Although many unanswered questions remain about their causes, the biopsychosocial perspective is useful in understanding how individuals acquire and maintain these diverse problems over time. Moreover, researchers and clinicians are increasingly developing models that incorporate integrated treatment. The growing research base the *DSM-5-TR* authors used reflects not only expansion of the empirical approaches to sexual disorders but also the adoption of a broader, more inclusive, and socioculturally sensitive approach to understanding and treatment.

Return to the Case: Shaun Boyden

For Shaun, being in psychotherapy was the first opportunity to talk with another person openly about his gender identity in a supportive and affirming environment. Given he had very little support in his relationships, it seems that much of Shaun's anxiety came from a sense of internalized transphobia; that is, it was difficult for him to truly accept himself, since he had not been accepted by others. The anxiety he experienced hindered him from venturing out into his community where he could find more sources of support, so in therapy he worked on setting goals for himself that included going to events and introducing himself to new people, and then building up those relationships over time. Having additional support in therapy helped him feel more affirmed in his identity, although he continued to struggle with dysphoria.

Eventually, Shaun decided he was ready to start HRT, and with the support of his therapist, he was referred to a specialist who prescribed low-dose testosterone. After starting HRT, Shaun noticed an immediate decrease in his gender dysphoria and found that taking this important step toward transitioning gave him a sense of hope. He began to feel more confident about taking additional steps, such as top surgery.

Dr. Tobin's reflections: There is never one particular path or narrative that transgender people follow in affirming their identities, so it is critical as a clinician to keep an open mind and focus on supporting transgender clients and helping them feel safe in therapy. Providing affirmative care in this way is crucial so that transgender clients can explore their feelings openly. In some cases, therapy may be one of their few sources of support. Therapists should also help connect transgender clients with resources such as medical clinics or community support services, particularly if clients have struggled to connect with these resources on their own.

Sarah Tobin, PhD

SUMMARY

- When it comes to sexual behavior, the definition of a disorder becomes even more complicated, perhaps, than in other areas of human behavior. Context is extremely important, as are customs and mores, which change over time.
- Paraphilias are behaviors in which an individual has recurrent, intense sexually arousing fantasies, sexual urges, or behaviors involving (1) nonhuman objects, (2) children or other nonconsenting persons, or (3) the suffering or humiliation of self or partner.
- When a paraphilia causes intense distress and impairment, clinicians may diagnose paraphilic disorder. Paraphilic disorders include pedophilic disorder, exhibitionistic disorder, fetishistic disorder, frotteuristic disorder, sexual masochism disorder, sexual sadism disorder, and transvestic disorder.
- From a biological perspective, paraphilic disorders involve a combination of influences including genetic, hormonal, and sensory factors in interaction with cognitive, cultural, and contextual influences. However, these changes could also be the result of early physical abuse or sexual victimization. Clinicians treating paraphilic disorders based on the biological perspective may use psychotherapeutic medications intended to alter the individual's neurotransmitter levels as well as agents that act on sexual hormones.
- From a psychological perspective, cognitive behavioral therapy is the recommended treatment for paraphilias, with an emphasis on changing the behaviors themselves.
- A sexual dysfunction is characterized by a marked divergence of an individual's response in the sexual response cycle, along with feelings of significant distress or impairment.
- Arousal disorders may be diagnosed in individuals who have low or no sexual desire, or who are unable to achieve physiological arousal during the initial phases of the sexual response cycle. As a result, they may avoid or be unable to experience orgasm. These disorders include male hypoactive sexual desire disorder, female sexual interest/arousal disorder, and erectile disorder. Inability to achieve orgasm, a distressing delay in achieving orgasm, or reduced intensity of orgasm constitutes female orgasmic disorder. Men with a marked delay in ejaculation or who rarely, if at all, experience ejaculations may have delayed ejaculation.
- Clinicians diagnose sexual pain disorders, characterized by difficulties in sexual relationships due to painful sensations in the genitals during sexual relations as genito-pelvic pain/penetration disorders.
- Treatment of sexual dysfunctions should begin with a comprehensive assessment that includes a physical exam and psychological testing, including the client's partner, if appropriate. In addition, the clinician must assess the individual's overall health and use of substances, including not only drugs and alcohol, but also all medications, including psychotherapeutic ones. Cognitive behavioral therapy is helpful for many of these disorders, as can medications or pelvic floor therapy.
- Individuals are diagnosed with gender dysphoria when they experience distress and a sense of inappropriateness about their birth-assigned sex. Both these conditions must be present for a clinician to assign the diagnosis.
- Theoretical perspectives on the experiences of transgender and gender-diverse people are undergoing radical shifts in the field of psychology. Whereas in the past the profession saw transgender people as having a "disorder," the new terminology instead focuses on the psychological distress that can emerge from not being affirmed in one's gender identity. In affirmative psychotherapy, clinicians help their clients safely explore their gender identity, consider options for gender-affirming medical procedures, and connect with sources of social support.

KEY TERMS

Affirmative psychotherapy
Birth-assigned sex
Climacteric
Delayed ejaculation
Erectile disorder
Exhibitionistic disorder
Female orgasmic disorder
Female sexual interest/arousal disorder
Fetishistic disorder
Frotteuristic disorder
Gender dysphoria
Gender-affirming medical procedures
Genito-pelvic pain/penetration disorder
Male hypoactive sexual desire disorder
Paraphilias
Paraphilic disorder
Partialism
Pedophilic disorder
Phosphodiesterase (PDE) inhibitors
Premature (early) ejaculation
Sexual dysfunction
Sexual masochism disorder
Sexual sadism disorder
Transgender
Transphobia
Transvestic disorder
Voyeuristic disorder

CHAPTER 12

Substance-Related and Addictive Disorders

OUTLINE

Learning Objectives

12.1 Explain key features of substance disorders.
12.2 Differentiate among disorders related to specific substances.
12.3 Identify symptoms of non-substance-related disorders.
12.4 Analyze the biopsychosocial perspective on the development of substance disorders.

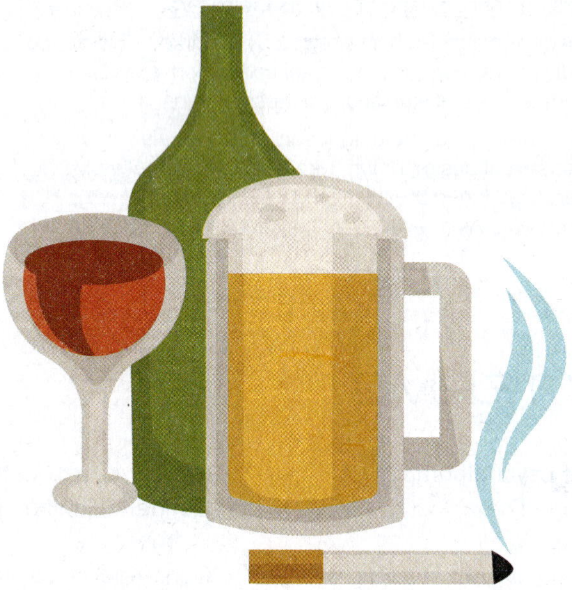

SofiaV/Shutterstock

Case Report

Carl Wadsworth

Demographic information: 32-year-old Black heterosexual cisgender man. Carl's pronouns are he/him/his.

History of present illness: Carl's sister Sharon made an appointment for Carl to see a therapist at a local outpatient therapy clinic due to concerns about his alcohol use. Sharon stated that their family was "sick of being worried" about him. She reported that Carl had been drinking more frequently and heavily over the past few years than ever before, which culminated in a recent arrest for public intoxication. Sharon explained that Carl has bipolar disorder, although he is not on medication currently, which is also very concerning to his family.

During the intake session, the therapist noticed that Carl appeared intoxicated, though he denied this when she asked whether he had been drinking recently. Consistent with clinic policy, she was forced to end the session prematurely and ensure that he received safe transportation home. When Carl presented for the next appointment intoxicated again, the therapist asked him directly whether he had been drinking prior to the session, because she was concerned that his alcohol use would interfere with therapy. Carl's reply was, "Maybe . . . just a little." The therapist asked Carl to refrain from drinking before their next appointment, to which he agreed.

When Carl showed up for the third appointment intoxicated yet again, it was clear to the therapist that treatment was necessary but could not proceed unless she was able to more directly address Carl's alcohol use with him. Carl had said he was ashamed of his alcohol use but found himself unable to cut down on his drinking, although he was slowly realizing that his years of drinking were taking a toll on him. For instance, he shared that he had been recently fired from his job after the arrest for public intoxication and was forced to live with Sharon as he could not make ends meet otherwise.

After that appointment, Carl told Sharon what had happened, and she removed all alcohol from her home and forbade Carl to go out unaccompanied. At first, Carl struggled with severe withdrawal symptoms. He then began to frequently pace around the house and was unable to sleep for 3 days due to racing thoughts and an abundance of energy. After convincing Sharon that he needed to borrow her car to go to the grocery store, Carl drove to a nearby liquor store, purchased a bottle of whiskey, and drank the entire bottle within a matter of minutes. On his way back to Sharon's home, he drove into a lamppost and was subsequently arrested for driving under the influence. He was then court-ordered to go to therapy, and his therapist allowed him to return to treatment on the condition that he attend his sessions sober.

Over the next few sessions, Carl began telling his therapist his story. He explained that he was diagnosed with bipolar disorder when he was 18 following a manic episode and treated with lithium, a medication that is often prescribed to treat the disorder. He said he preferred drinking to taking medication because he did not experience side effects, and he found weekly blood testing while on lithium "annoying." While he had not been a heavy drinker in his early adult life, his parents are both recovered alcoholics, and he worried that he might be susceptible to alcoholism.

When Carl was 28, the telecom company for which he worked downsized, and he lost his job. Carl became so depressed that he attempted suicide at his parents' home, where his mother discovered him. He was hospitalized for about 1 month and enrolled for disability status, which allowed him to receive medication and therapy. He then took up a job at a liquor store to supplement his disability, which helped him to afford his own apartment.

At the time, Carl was stable on medication and had not experienced any significant psychological impairment for several months. "I wasn't planning on drinking at work ever, but my boss sure liked to, so we started getting drunk together after closing up for the night," Carl reported. Since he found it difficult to drink heavily while on lithium, he decided to stop taking his medication so he could drink with his boss, who would taunt Carl if he declined his offer.

Since Carl was drinking mostly at night and lived by himself, no one in his family noticed he was drinking. After a few months of drinking every day at work, he started to experience withdrawal symptoms when he woke in the morning, so he began drinking immediately on awakening as well as while he was at work. He continued this routine for the next 2 years and soon was essentially unable to perform any activities outside work. His family

Case Report *continued*

grew increasingly worried, especially when he repeatedly showed up intoxicated at his parents' house. Family members urged him to try Alcoholics Anonymous (AA) and warned him of the dangers of his drinking, although Carl denied that he was having any problems. To prove this to his family, Carl would stop drinking for 1 or 2 weeks, although his desire to drink was too intense to allow him to go any longer than that. He grew increasingly depressed as he went without medication and his drinking grew more severe; however, instead of seeking treatment, Carl only drank more when he was feeling particularly depressed.

Occasionally Carl would get into an argument at work, although his boss typically did not take much notice. One day, however, Carl threatened violence against a customer, and his boss had no choice but to fire him and report him to the police, who arrested Carl for public intoxication. The police held him overnight and released him the next day when the customer chose not to press charges. Without an income, Carl was forced to move out of his apartment and move in with Sharon, who lived nearby. At that point, Sharon became more worried that Carl had spun out of control and unsure how she could help him, at which point she referred him to the therapist. Carl explained that he had been feeling hopeless about his life improving, and that he likely would not have sought help if it were not for Sharon.

Psychiatric history: Carl was diagnosed with bipolar disorder at the age of 18, following a manic episode. He managed his symptoms with medication for 10 years, at which point he lost his job and attempted suicide. Following starting his job at the liquor store, he started a pattern of daily heavy drinking. He has no prior history of treatment for substance use.

Case formulation: An important distinction to make in Carl's case is whether his alcohol use occurred secondarily as a result of his bipolar disorder, or whether it arose independently, which would qualify him for a dual diagnosis. As Carl stated regarding the episode of drinking that occurred while he lived at his sister's, he began drinking heavily while he was manic, believing he could handle a large quantity of alcohol and still drive safely. However, this was the only instance in which he reported drinking while experiencing mood symptoms.

After careful consideration of his case, it appears that Carl's initial problems with alcohol began in the absence of mood symptoms. Nor did his alcohol consumption appear to cause his mood symptoms. Because of these two distinctions, Carl qualifies for a dual diagnosis of alcohol use disorder, severe, and bipolar disorder. Further, he meets the criteria for bipolar I disorder due to the presence of manic, rather than hypomanic, episodes, which required hospitalization and severely affected his functioning.

Risk level: Low-moderate risk. Carl reported having occasional, passive suicidal ideation in the last two weeks, but he denied any intent or plan. Risk factors include a past suicide attempt 4 years ago, recent loss of employment, and symptoms of depression. Protective factors include support from his family and willingness to engage in treatment.

Treatment plan: Carl agreed to attend a local AA meeting on a daily basis in conjunction with weekly psychotherapy. He also agreed to see a psychiatrist for a medication evaluation for treatment of his bipolar disorder. It is possible that the psychiatrist will recommend medication to help with his alcohol dependence.

Sarah Tobin, PhD

substance
A chemical that alters a person's mood or behavior when it is smoked, injected, drunk, inhaled, snorted, or swallowed.

substance use disorder
A cluster of cognitive, behavioral, and physiological symptoms indicating that the individual uses a substance despite significant substance-related problems.

12.1 Key Features of Substance Disorders

A **substance** is a chemical that alters a person's mood or behavior when the person smokes, injects, drinks, inhales, snorts, or swallows it. A **substance use disorder** is a cluster of cognitive, behavioral, and physiological symptoms indicating that the individual continues using a substance even though it causes significant problems in the person's life. Clinicians diagnose substance use disorders by assessing the individual on four categories of symptoms: loss of control, social impairment, risky use, and pharmacological changes. Based on the number of symptoms the individual demonstrates, clinicians assign a severity rating from mild to severe.

Although many people refer to these disorders as representing an "addiction," the *DSM-5-TR* authors prefer the term *substance use disorder*, believing it is more precise and has fewer negative connotations. Similarly, people with these disorders are referred to not as "addicts" but as "individuals with substance use disorders." Drug addiction is not applied as a diagnostic term in the *DSM-5-TR* because of its negative connotations as well as imprecise wording. The term *addictive* appears in the chapter name as a descriptive term only.

The criteria that indicate loss of control include taking the substance in larger amounts or for a longer time than the individual originally intended. Impaired control also includes the individual's inability to cut down or regulate substance use, along with previous unsuccessful attempts to do so. The expenditure of a great deal of time to obtain the substance is a third indication of loss of control. Finally, individuals show craving, in which they have a persistent desire to take the substance, but particularly when they're in an environment where they previously used or obtained the substance.

Social impairment occurs when the substance use produces a range of significant effects in daily life. Individuals with a substance use disorder may neglect their obligations at work, which can lead to financial problems associated with loss of a job. The substance use disorders also frequently create interpersonal problems as well, due to the fact that excessive use of drugs or alcohol creates strains on relationships along with failure to carry out obligations to home and family.

Risky use associated with the substance use disorder includes behaviors that individuals engage in that are personally dangerous and put others in jeopardy, such as driving or operating machinery while intoxicated. If they are caught, or injure someone in an accident, they may be incarcerated, leading to further devastating impacts on themselves and others. Finally, an individual's health may be affected by excessive substance use. In the case of alcohol, for example, chronic diseases such as cardiovascular disease, liver disease, and diabetes may be caused by continued patterns of heavy usage. Other substances, such as cocaine, heroin, and oxycodone, may cause death due to overdose.

Substance use disorders are thus serious psychological disorders due to their potential to create harm to the self and others. Although each set of substances operates in a different fashion, misuse of any of them can become a serious threat to the quality of a person's life.

One pharmacological criteria for substance use disorders is **tolerance**, which occurs when an individual requires increasingly greater amounts of the substance in order to achieve its desired effects, or when the person feels less of an effect after using the same amount of the substance. The second pharmacological criterion is **withdrawal**, the physiological and psychological changes that occur when an individual stops taking a substance.

Substance-related disorders also include **substance-induced disorders**, which are disorders marked by development of a substance-specific syndrome due to recent ingestion of the substance itself. People receive a diagnosis of **substance intoxication** when they experience a drug's effects on their physiological functioning and show signs of significant impairment. The extent of substance intoxication depends on the specific drug, the speed with which it acts, and the duration of its effects. Efficient absorption of intravenous or smokable drugs into the

tolerance
The extent to which the individual requires larger and larger amounts of a substance in order to achieve its desired effects, or the extent to which the individual feels less of its effects after using the same amount of the substance.

withdrawal
Physiological and psychological changes that occur when an individual stops taking a substance.

substance-induced disorders
Disorders marked by development of a substance-specific syndrome due to recent ingestion of the substance itself.

substance intoxication
The temporary maladaptive experience of behavioral or psychological changes that are due to the accumulation of a substance in the body.

What's in the *DSM-5-TR*

Combining Abuse and Dependence

When the *DSM-5* was written, its authors combined abuse and dependence into the term substance use disorder, and the *DSM-5-TR* retained that combination. Individuals receive a diagnosis based on meeting only two criteria but are rated according to the degree of severity of their symptoms. Critics maintain that the revised system may diagnose substance-related disorder in too many individuals with mild symptoms who do not have an "addiction" (Martin, Steinley, Vergés, & Sher, 2011). However, the dimensional rating theoretically allows clinicians to allow for gradations from mild to severe levels of the disorder.

A second major change that took place in the *DSM-5* was the transition of caffeine withdrawal from a research-only category to a clinical diagnosis based on the argument that there is sufficient evidence from large enough populations to warrant recognition of this condition as a psychiatric diagnosis. Studies show high rates of functional impairment, as reported in the *DSM-5-TR* including severe headaches and decreased cognitive and motor performance. Since caffeine users who suffer from caffeine withdrawal may attribute their symptoms to other disorders, the presence of this diagnosis can reduce unnecessary health care utilization as well as making it possible for these individuals to receive appropriate treatment.

bloodstream can lead to a more intense kind of intoxication than occurs with drugs taken in pill form. The second category of substance-related disorders is based on the symptoms of withdrawal, whose characteristics are specific to the substance itself.

Specifiers in *DSM-5-TR* include severity ratings, remission status, and indicators of whether the individual is on maintenance therapy or using the drug in a controlled environment such as a supervised setting in substance-free jails, therapeutic communities, and locked units in hospitals.

12.2 Disorders Associated with Specific Substances

DSM-5-TR's diagnostic criteria provide a taxonomy for evaluating the scope of the problems associated with the major categories of psychoactive substances, including alcohol. Although substance use disorders and substance-related disorders share common features across a range of 11 possible substances, the specific diagnoses associated with each substance differ depending on such features as patterns of use, risks, and pharmacological effects.

Rates of Substance Use Disorders

The Substance Abuse and Mental Health Service (SAMHSA) provides data on substance use prevalence from the annual National Survey on Drug Use and Health (NSDUH). This provides a useful set of benchmarks that make it possible for epidemiologists to determine the extent to which a particular substance poses a threat to the psychological and physical health of the U.S. population.

Overall, in 2021 an estimated 61.2 million people in the United States aged 12 years and older (21.9 percent) used illicit drugs in the past year (SAMHSA, 2022). Marijuana is the most commonly used substance, with 52.5 million people 12 and older (18.7 percent) reporting use in the past year. However, not all users fit the criteria for a substance use disorder. Shown in Figure 1 are those identified in SAMHSA's 2021 report of the numbers of Americans with eight major categories of types of substance use disorder.

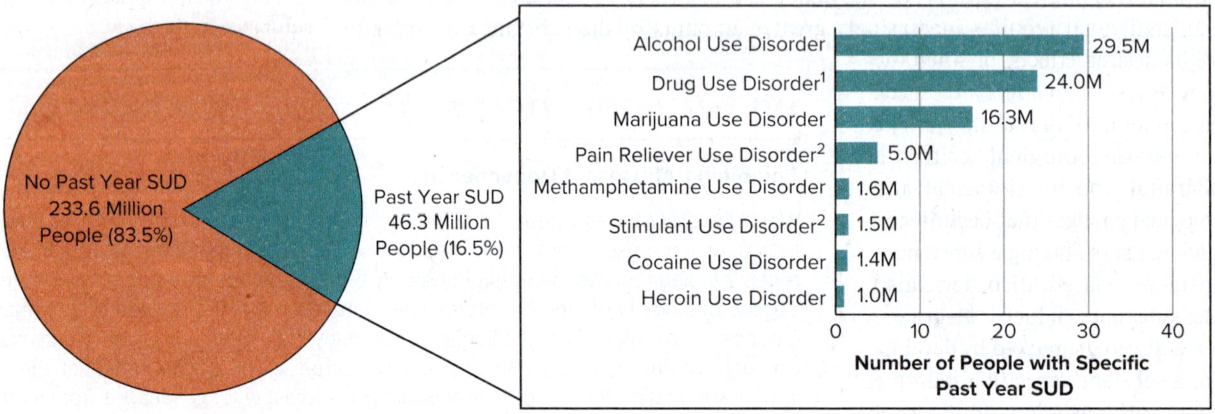

Note: The estimated numbers of people with substance use disorders are not mutually exclusive because people could have use disorders for more than one substance.

[1] Includes data from all past year users of marijuana, cocaine, heroin, hallucinogens, inhalants, methamphetamine, and prescription psychotherapeutic drugs (i.e., pain relievers, tranquilizers, stimulants, or sedatives).

[2] Includes data from all past year users of the specific prescription drug.

FIGURE 1 Rates of substance use disorder among people ages 12 or older, showing number of people with each disorder.

SOURCE: Substance Abuse and Mental Health Services Administration. (2022). *Key substance use and mental health indicators in the United States: Results from the 2021 National Survey on Drug Use and Health (HHS Publication No. PEP22-07-01-005, NSDUH Series H-57)*, Rockville, MD: Center for Behavioral Health Statistics and Quality, Substance Abuse and Mental Health Services Administration. https://www.samhsa.gov/data/report/2021-nsduh-annual-national-report

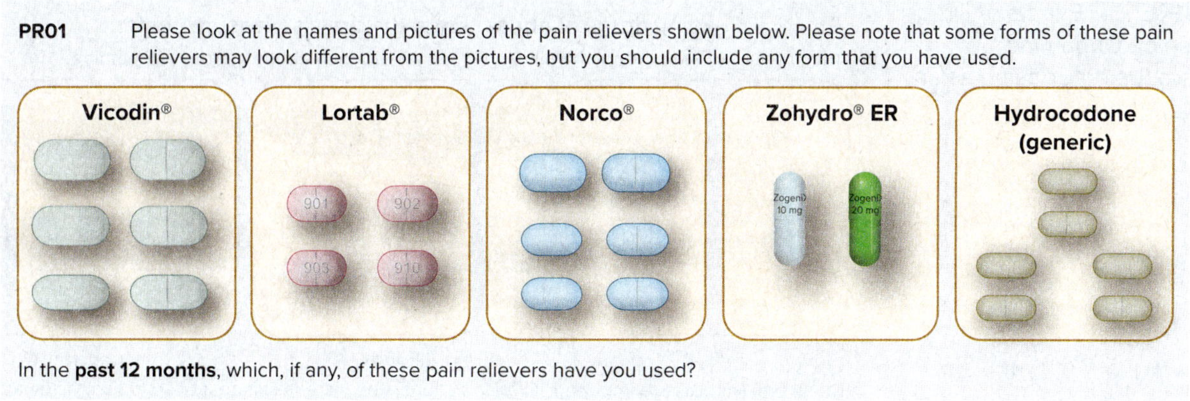

FIGURE 2 In conducting its yearly survey on drug use in the United States, SAMHSA uses images of pills that responders can choose from to help obtain accurate substance use figures.

Substance Abuse and Mental Health Services Administration. (2022). *Key substance use and mental health indicators in the United States: Results from the 2021 National Survey on Drug Use and Health (HHS Publication No. PEP22-07-01-005, NSDUH Series H-57)*, Rockville, MD: Center for Behavioral Health Statistics and Quality, Substance Abuse and Mental Health Services Administration. https://www.samhsa.gov/data/report/2021-nsduh-annual-national-report

Rates of illicit drug use by individuals 12 years of age and older vary considerably by demographic group. According to the NSDUH, the three most significant grouping characteristics are race/ethnicity, gender, and age, with variations also by geographic region. The rate of past-year illicit drug use is 36.1 percent for American Indians or Alaska Natives, followed by 34.6 percent of people who identify as multiracial, 24 percent among people who identify as Black, 22.5 percent for people who describe themselves as White, 19.4 percent of Hispanic people, and 11.1 percent for Asian American people. Males have a higher rate of drug use (14 percent) than females (9.5 percent). The rates of past year use generally decline across age groups, from the peak of 38.0 percent at ages 18 to 25 to 5.7 percent at ages 65 and older. Illicit drug use tends to be lower among college graduates, the employed, and those living in rural regions and in the Midwestern U.S. states (SAMHSA, 2022).

In reviewing these statistics, and those presented throughout this chapter, it is worth noting what they mean in terms of public trends, particularly among those who begin their patterns of drug use in their teen or even childhood years. The dangers of illicit drug use continue to receive public attention, from films and television shows depicting individuals suffering from substance use disorders. Educational programs for school-age children and adolescents continue to be implemented. Yet, these efforts only meet with measured success. In part, continued use, and particularly initiation, can be attributed to "generational forgetting," a process in which a new generation of young people adopt the drug habits that had faded since an early phase of popularity (such as LSD in the 1960s coming back in use in the 1990s). Additionally, new drugs or new modes of administering older drugs become introduced on a regular basis, including vaping, crack, crystal methamphetamine, and noninjected heroin. The known dangers of street dealers selling powerful drugs in potentially lethal forms (such as fentanyl mixed with cocaine), may also fail to act as a damper on young users, often with tragic consequences (Johnston et al., 2023).

How Drugs of Abuse Affect the Body

Most drugs of abuse directly or indirectly target the reward center of the brain by flooding its circuits with dopamine, as you can see in Figure 3. Overstimulation of the reward system produces the euphoric effects abusers seek and leads them to engage in the behavior that will allow them to repeat the experience. Drugs are more addictive than the natural "highs" produced by such activities as eating and sex because they release far more dopamine than do natural rewards, and the effects last much longer. Over time, the neurons in these

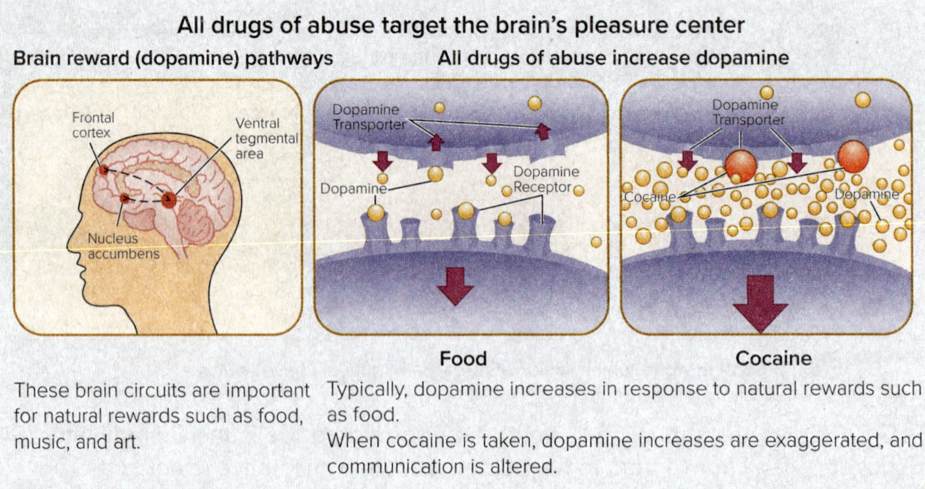

FIGURE 3 Effects of Drugs of Abuse on Dopamine Pathways (Using Cocaine as an Example)

dopamine pathways "down-regulate" in response to these surges in dopamine, meaning they produce less dopamine themselves or reduce the number of dopamine receptors. Tolerance develops when users need to take higher levels of the drugs in order to experience the effects they initially obtained.

Risk Factors for Substance Use Disorders

Individuals with other psychological disorders are more likely to abuse substances, amounting past year use percentage of 36.6 percent; marijuana use is the highest among all illicit drugs (SAMHSA, 2022). The most common conditions comorbid with substance use disorders are anxiety disorders, trauma-related disorders, mood disorders, ADHD, schizophrenia, and personality disorders. Depressive and anxiety disorders are reported in 43 percent of people in treatment for a substance use disorder involving nonmedical use of prescription painkillers. People who experience chronic pain are also at risk for a substance use disorder, as are those with cancer and heart disease (National Institute on Drug Abuse, 2020a).

There are three possible routes to the development of comorbid substance use and other psychological disorders. The first is the similarity of risk factors in substance use and other psychological disorders. Second, individuals with psychological disorders or symptoms may use drugs as a form of self-medication. Third, people who use substances may subsequently develop a psychological disorder, due either to changes in brain activity produced by the substances or to changes in lifestyle that precipitate stress, which, in turn, leads to symptoms of depression and anxiety.

Individuals who leave military service are at higher risk of substance use disorders. Among U.S. veterans, rates of admission to substance use treatment centers are reported to be as high as 10 percent, with the large majority due to heroin use. However, alcohol use disorders are the most prevalent disorders among U.S. veterans, particularly among those exposed to combat, with prevalence estimates of 65 percent among individuals seeking treatment. This rate is more than double that reported for the general population. Among veterans seeking care for the first time in the Veterans Administration system, nearly 11 percent meet the criteria for a substance use disorder. Between 37 and 50 percent of veterans of the Afghanistan and Iraq wars meet the diagnosis for a psychological disorder strongly associated with substance use disorders (National Institute of Drug Abuse, 2019).

Substance use disorders are also highly prevalent in correctional facilities. Among an international sample of more than 18,000 inmates, rates of alcohol use disorder were as high as 51 percent in men and 10 to 30 percent among women. Rates of drug use disorder averaged 30 percent in men and 51 percent in women. These high rates reflect lack of attention to treatment within the criminal justice facilities, but if treatment were instituted, there could be beneficial effects on premature mortality as well as rates of subsequent return to prison (Fazel, Yoon, & Hayes, 2017). High rates of substance use disorders among prisoners as well as sex workers and homeless individuals also place these individuals at risk of extreme health inequities, reflecting their social exclusion (Aldridge et al., 2018).

The COVID-19 pandemic presented a greater risk for individuals with substance use disorders who live within marginalized communities. In addition to the higher rates of infection within these communities, the disease itself placed a heavier burden on their psychological and social resources, further complicating their ability to avoid a relapse of their disorder. From a public health perspective, COVID-19 and addiction became dual pandemics requiring wider availability of treatment resources (Dubey et al., 2020).

Alcohol

Alcohol use is a leading risk factor for the burden of disease around the world, accounting for 2 percent of all deaths of women and 6 to 8 percent of men. The seventh leading cause of death worldwide, alcohol use is the leading risk factor for individuals 18 to 49 years old (GBD 2016 Alcohol Collaborators, 2018). Indeed, building stronger policies regarding alcohol use is one of the United Nations Sustainability Development Goals, reflecting its many social and economic impacts as well as the high percentage of global deaths attributed to alcohol consumption (Jiang, Xiang, Room, & Hao, 2016). Chronic heavy alcohol use is also associated with suicide, as reported in the *DSM-5-TR* based on international data.

Binge alcohol use is defined for women as four or more drinks on the same occasion, and for men, five or more drinks. **Heavy alcohol use** consists of four drinks for women and five for men on each of five or more days in the past month. Young adults 21 to 25 have the highest rates of binge drinking and the highest rates of heavy drinking, as shown in Figure 4. The rates of binge and heavy drinking decline sharply through age categories in adulthood; among people 65 and older, 11.4 percent engage in binge drinking and 2.8 percent in heavy drinking (SAMHSA, 2022).

binge alcohol use
Drinking four (for women) and five (for men) or more drinks on the same occasion.

heavy alcohol use
Drinking four (for women) and five (for men) drinks on each of five or more days in the past month.

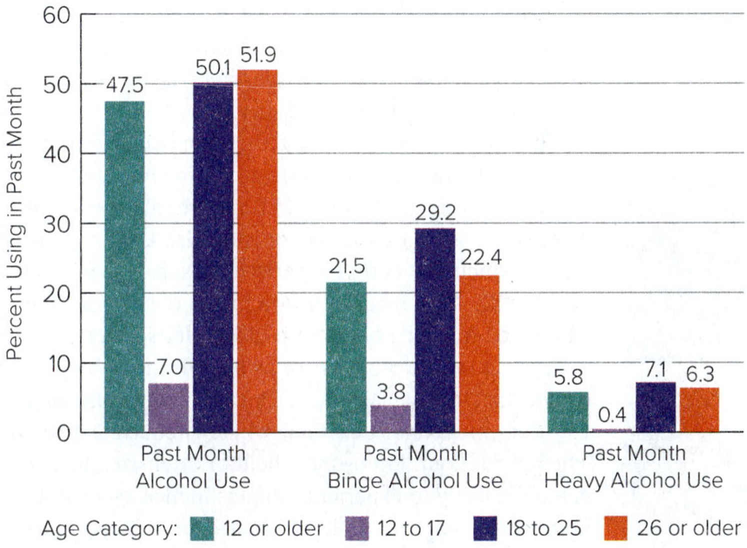

Note: Binge Alcohol Use is defined as drinking five or more drinks (for males) or four or more drinks (for females) on the same occasion on at least 1 day in the past 30 days. Heavy Alcohol Use is defined as binge drinking on the same occasion on 5 or more days in the past 30 days; all heavy alcohol users are also binge alcohol users.

FIGURE 4 Alcohol use by age group.

MINI CASE

Alcohol Use Disorder

Mala is a 55-year-old heterosexual Israeli American cisgender woman. She has been a stay-at-home parent since the birth of her and her husband's first child. Every afternoon, Mala makes herself the first in a series of daiquiris. On many evenings, she passes out on the couch by the time her husband arrives home from work. Mala lost her driver's license a year ago after being arrested three times on charges of driving while intoxicated. Although her family has urged her to obtain treatment for her disorder, she denies that she has a problem because she can "control" her drinking. The mother of three grown children, Mala began to drink around age 45, when her youngest child left for college. Before that, she kept herself extremely busy through her children's extracurricular activities. When she found herself alone every afternoon, she took solace in having an early cocktail. Over a period of several years, the daily cocktail developed into a series of five or six strong mixed drinks. Mala's oldest daughter has lately begun to insist that something be done for her mother. She does not want to see Mala develop the fatal alcohol-related illness that caused the premature death of her grandmother.

From a life-span perspective, individuals choose to engage in alcohol use by trying to cope with the challenges facing them at different periods in their lives. Alcohol use can be seen as a self-management tool in response to varying stressors. A large-scale review of previous publications showed that issues manifesting themselves in early adulthood center around the personality traits such as impulsivity, sexual behavior, and poor coping methods with stress. Throughout adulthood, psychological disorders increasingly become the focus of alcohol use as a self-management strategy. By later adulthood, individuals use alcohol as a self-management tool for coping with pain and the challenges faced by chronic health conditions (Müller et al., 2023).

From a physiological standpoint alcohol is a nervous system **depressant**, and the way it affects the individual depends on how much the drinker ingests. In small amounts, alcohol has sedating effects, and the drinker therefore feels more relaxed. With larger amounts, drinkers may begin to feel more outgoing, self-confident, and uninhibited. Beyond that point, the depressant effects become apparent, leading users to experience sleepiness, lack of physical coordination, dysphoria, and irritability. In even larger amounts, alcohol can be fatal, leading the individual's vital functions to shut down. More severe effects also occur when the individual mixes alcohol with other drugs; **potentiation** makes the effects of two drugs taken together greater than the effect of either substance alone. Combining alcohol with another depressant can have a fatal outcome, for example.

depressant
A psychoactive substance that causes the depression of central nervous system activity.

potentiation
The combination of the effects of two or more psychoactive substances such that the total effect is greater than the effect of either substance alone.

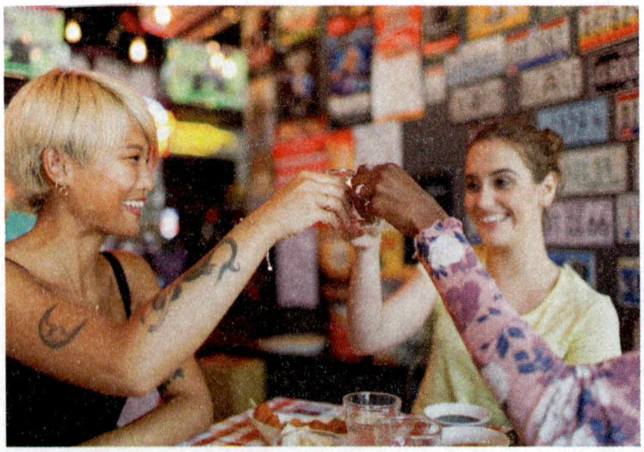

Social factors and a desire to reduce stress may contribute to the development of alcohol use disorder.

Bill Cheyrou/Alamy Stock Photo

The rate at which alcohol absorption occurs in the bloodstream depends on a number of factors, including how much a person consumes and over what time period, and whether food is present in the digestive system. Another factor is the drinker's metabolic rate (the rate at which the body converts food substances to energy). The health of the kidneys also plays a role in the rate at which alcohol is eliminated from the body, with older adults generally taking longer to eliminate waste produces of alcohol from the blood. The average person metabolizes alcohol at a rate of one-third of an ounce of 100 percent alcohol per hour, which is equivalent to an ounce of whiskey per hour. Following a bout of extensive intake of alcohol, a person is likely to experience an abstinence syndrome, or the phenomenon commonly called a "hangover." The symptoms of abstinence syndrome include a range of phenomena including nausea and vomiting, tremors, extreme thirst, headache, tiredness, irritability, depression, and dizziness. As with alcohol absorption, the extent of abstinence syndrome the person experiences reflects the amount and rate of alcohol consumption and the individual's metabolic rate.

Directly or indirectly, alcohol affects almost every organ system in the body. Long-term use can lead to permanent brain damage, with symptoms of neurocognitive disorder, blackouts, seizures, hallucinations, and damage to the peripheral parts of the nervous system. Two forms of neurocognitive disorder are associated with long-term heavy alcohol use.

Wernicke's disease is an acute and potentially reversible condition characterized by delirium, eye-movement disturbances, difficulties in movement and balance, and deterioration of the peripheral nerves to the hands and feet. It is not alcohol itself but the associated deficiency of thiamine (vitamin B_1) that causes Wernicke's disease. Long-term heavy use of alcohol damages the body's ability to metabolize nutrients, and alcohol users often have an overall pattern of poor nutrition. Adequate thiamine intake can reverse Wernicke's disease.

Wernicke's disease
A reversible form of neurocognitive disorder associated with long-term alcohol use.

Korsakoff's syndrome is a permanent form of neurocognitive disorder in which the individual develops **retrograde amnesia**, the inability to remember past events, and **anterograde amnesia**, the inability to remember new information. The chances of recovering from Korsakoff's syndrome are fewer than one in four, and about another one in four people who have this disorder require permanent institutionalization.

Korsakoff's syndrome
A permanent form of neurocognitive disorder associated with long-term alcohol use in which the individual develops retrograde and anterograde amnesia, leading to an inability to remember recent events or learn new information.

retrograde amnesia
Amnesia involving loss of memory for past events.

anterograde amnesia
Amnesia involving the inability to remember new information.

Chronic heavy alcohol consumption also causes a number of harmful changes in the rest of the body outside the nervous system, including to the liver, gastrointestinal system, bones, muscles, and immune system. When people abruptly stop ingesting alcohol after periods of chronic usage, they can experience sleep disturbances, profound anxiety, tremors, hyperactivity of the sympathetic nervous system, psychosis, seizures, or death. Additionally, older adults who use alcohol may be at greater risk for falling, placing them at risk for brain injury (Shakya et al., 2020).

Theories and Treatment of Alcohol Use Disorders

An understanding of alcohol use disorder involves considering complex biopsychosocial interactions. Treatment of this disorder also requires an integrative approach.

Measurement of the effectiveness of treatment, often used as a pre-treatment assessment, is established by administering he AUDIT, or Alcohol Use Disorders Identification Test, which is summarized in Table 1, cuts across perspectives and is used both in research and practice. It can be completed either by the clinician or the client. Ratings are made for each item on a 0 (never) to 4 (4 or more times a week) scale. A score of 8 or more is considered to represent hazardous or harmful alcohol use (National Institute on Alcohol Abuse and Alcoholism, 2007).

TABLE 1 The Alcohol Use Disorders Identification Test ("AUDIT")

1. How often do you drink alcohol?
2. How many alcoholic drinks do you typically have on a day you are drinking?
3. How often do you have six or more alcoholic drinks at one time?
4. How often have you found that you were not able to stop drinking daily once you had started?
5. How often during the past year has drinking alcohol kept you from doing something you were normally expected to do?
6. How often in the past year have you needed a first drink in the morning to get yourself going after a night of heavy drinking?
7. How often during the last year have you felt guilty or remorseful after drinking?
8. How often during the last year have you been unable to remember what happened the day before because of drinking too much alcohol?
9. Have you or someone else been hurt or harmed because of your drinking?
10. Has someone close to you or a health care professional spoken to you about your drinking or suggested that you cut down?

SOURCE: Adapted from The Alcohol Use Disorders Identification Test (AUDIT) Retrieved from https://www.drugabuse.gov/sites/default/files/files/AUDIT.pdf

Biological Perspective Twin, family, and adoption studies consistently point to the importance of genetic factors as contributors to alcohol-related disorders, with an estimated heritability of 50 to 60 percent. Pinpointing the genes responsible for alcohol-related disorders is a great challenge to researchers, however, because it is likely that multiple genes are active in their transmission (Salvatore et al., 2018). The greatest success has come from studies examining associations between genes that govern alcohol metabolism and neural transmission. Researchers are attempting to connect variations in some of these genes not only with patterns of alcohol use but also with comorbid disorders such as social anxiety disorder, personality traits, and early childhood predictors (Rambau et al., 2018). There also appears to be genetic overlap with schizophrenia, another disorder that is often comorbid with alcohol use disorder (Johnson et al., 2023).

Sociocultural influences also appear to interact with genetic vulnerability. In a large nationwide study of midlife adults, researchers found differences between twins in the level of alcohol use based on socioeconomic status. In families from lower socioeconomic levels, genetic factors seemed to play a larger role than the environment. In higher social status families, the amount of alcohol individuals use is affected by such factors as familial habits and traditions (Hamdi, Krueger, & South, 2015). Another study of children ages 9 to 11 examined genetic contributions to the anticipated effects of alcohol, the basis for **alcohol expectancy theory**, and which is considered a risk factor for alcohol use. There were no predictive effects of genetics but instead, alcohol expectancies were related to a host of sociocultural influences, including peer approval, religious beliefs, and adverse childhood experiences (Johnson et al., 2023). These studies suggest the value of examining genetic patterns of transmission within a larger social context.

alcohol expectancy theory
A perspective that emphasizes how expectations about the effects of alcohol use influence actual consumption of alcohol.

In the biological perspective, treatment of individuals with alcohol use disorders relies on prescription medications, alone or in conjunction with psychologically based therapies. Unfortunately, a large-scale research review supporting their use is limited in that they do not include females nor do they take into account race and ethnicity (Schick, Spillane, & Hostetler, 2020). Therefore, the findings on the effectiveness of various medications may be limited in terms of broader applicability beyond White males.

Turning now to the medications themselves, **naltrexone** is an opioid receptor antagonist that blocks the effects of the body's production of alcohol-induced opioids (Hillemacher et al., 2011). Individuals who take naltrexone are less likely to experience pleasurable effects of alcohol and even less likely to feel pleasure thinking about it. As a result, they will feel less of an urge to drink and will therefore be less likely to suffer a relapse of heavy drinking (Hendershot, Wardell, Samokhvalov, & Rehm, 2017).

naltrexone
An opioid receptor antagonist that blocks the effects of the body's production of alcohol-induced opioids.

Disulfiram is a medication that operates by the principles of aversion therapy. It works primarily by inhibiting the action of an enzyme that normally breaks down acetaldehyde, a toxic product of ethanol metabolism. An individual taking disulfiram who consumes alcohol within a 2-week period will experience a variety of unpleasant physical reactions, including flushing, palpitations, increased heart rate, lowered blood pressure, nausea and vomiting, sweating, and dizziness. It is possible that disulfiram's lower rates of adherence among individuals in treatment for alcohol use disorder are due to these highly noxious reactions (Walker, Korte, McRae-Clark, & Hartwell, 2019).

disulfiram
Known popularly as Antabuse, a medication used in the treatment of alcoholism that inhibits aldehyde dehydrogenase (ALDH) and causes severe physical reactions when combined with alcohol.

The third medication shown to be effective in treating alcohol use disorders is **acamprosate**, an amino acid derivative that appears to moderate glutamate receptors. Acamprosate reduces the risk of relapse by reducing the individual's urge to drink and thereby reducing the drive to use alcohol as a way of reducing anxiety and other negative psychological states.

acamprosate
An amino acid derivative that appears to moderate glutamate receptors.

With its less severe side effects, individuals using acamprosate may be more likely to remain on the medication (Donoghue et al., 2015). Acamprosate also appears to provide more benefits to people who have only recently stopped drinking and are of normal or close to normal body weight (Gueorguieva et al., 2015).

In a study of Medicaid-enrolled youth (i.e. low income), researchers found that all three biological interventions are less likely to be used, either alone or in combination with behavioral methods. Yet, these medications, in combination with behavioral treatment are recommended by SAMHSA as key to the timely treatment of individuals in this age group (Earlywine et al., 2023).

Psychological Perspective The cognitive systems that guide people's drinking behavior form the focus of psychological approaches to alcohol use disorders. According to **dual-process theory**, one cognitive system generates fast, automatic processes that trigger an impulse to drink alcohol. These automatic processes are based on learned, or conditioned positive associations with alcohol that people. The second, and slower, system consists of the controlled, laborious processing that, if used, would allow individuals to regulate and inhibit acting on those positive associations. The dual-process theory posits that the more the individual can inhibit the automatic impulse, the less likely he or she is to consume excessive amounts of alcohol. An additional influence on alcohol use, furthermore, is whether the individual has already established a behavior pattern of prior alcohol use (Hamilton, Gibbs, Keech, & Hagger, 2020). Personality may play a role in this process, because individuals who are lower in the trait of self-control are more likely to have intentions to maintain healthy behaviors, including limiting alcohol use, which they then are able to act on, making them less likely to engage in problematic drinking (Hagger et al., 2019).

dual-process theory
A theory regarding alcohol use proposing there are automatic processes that generate an impulse to drink alcohol and controlled, effortful processing that regulates these automatic impulses.

As discussed above in the context of genetic theories, alcohol expectancy theory proposes that alcohol consumption is guided by individuals' expectations about what will happen to them after they consume alcohol. Individuals develop alcohol expectancies early in life, even before they first taste alcohol. These can include the potential for alcohol to reduce tension or help them cope with social challenges, feel better or sexier, or become more mentally alert. Supporting alcohol expectancy theory, researchers established a link among college students between daily variations in expectancies regarding sociability were related to the extent to which they consumed alcohol on any given day (Stamates et al., 2023).

Cognitive factors also can influence what happens when a person consumes alcohol. According to **alcohol myopia theory**, individuals narrow their attentional focus the more alcohol they consume (Bayless & Harvey, 2017). This theory also predicts that when people drink alcohol, they also become more likely to engage in impulsive and potentially harmful behaviors, such as high-risk sexual activities. The high prevalence of binge drinking on college campuses presents a particular concern for this reason. As individuals consume greater amounts of alcohol, they are more likely to make risky choices because the immediate temptation of the moment (such as engaging in risky sex) overcomes the long-term consequences of the behavior (such as developing a sexually transmitted disease) (George, 2019).

alcohol myopia theory
Proposes that as individuals consume greater amounts of alcohol, they are more likely to make risky choices because the immediate temptation of the moment overcomes the long-term consequences of the behavior.

relapse prevention
A treatment method in which individuals are encouraged not to view lapses from abstinence as signs of certain failure.

Even individuals who engage in healthy lifestyle behaviors can be at risk for alcohol use disorders. In one large study examining alcohol use (beer) and engagement in physical activity, people who engaged in more activity were also more likely to drink beer the same day (Conroy et al., 2015). These patterns of behavior may set in as early as the first semester of college, with even those students showing increasing patterns of healthy behavior after moving away from home also increasing their alcohol consumption (Gesualdo & Pinquart, 2023). It is possible that people who believe they are engaging in healthy activity may feel they have "earned" the right to drink, negating the benefits they would otherwise gain from regular physical exercise.

There are several well-tested psychological approaches to treating alcohol use disorders. The most successful rely on cognitive behavioral interventions, motivational approaches, and expectancy manipulation. Part of effective treatment is **relapse prevention**, in which the clinician essentially builds "failure" into treatment. If the client recognizes that occasional slips from abstinence are bound to occur, then he or she will be less likely to give up on therapy altogether after suffering a temporary setback. Mindfulness training may also be added to relapse prevention to help individuals gain greater insight into the factors that trigger their relapses as well as to recognize that substance use may be a way of avoiding the present moment (Penberthy et al., 2015).

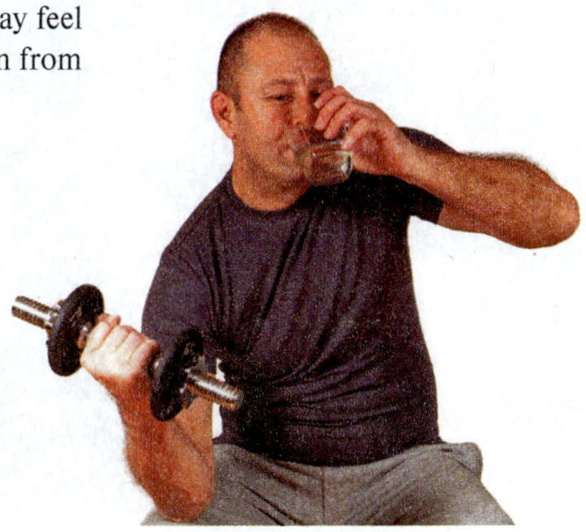

It may seem surprising, but individuals who engage in physical activity may also be at risk for alcohol misuse.
David S Swierczek/Shutterstock

Smartphone applications are also becoming available for treatment of alcohol use disorders (see Figure 5). One new approach pioneered in the United Kingdom is known as "DrinkLess" and combines a number of cognitive behavioral interventions (Garnett et al., 2021). Examples of modules available in the application include weekly drink reduction goal setting, self-monitoring and feedback, cognitive bias retraining, and identification of the emotions, situations, and events that serve as antecedents to alcohol use.

Another relatively novel approach to treatment uses physical activity as an adjunct to cognitive behavioral therapy. Its effectiveness appears to be due in part to its helping clients reduce impulsive drinking, improve emotional regulation, and reduce the craving for alcohol (Cabé, Lanièpce, & Pitel, 2021).

FIGURE 5 Sample Smartphone Application Based on DrinkLess

Drink Less. Retrived from https://apps.apple.com/gb/app/drink-less-get-help-reducing/id1020579244

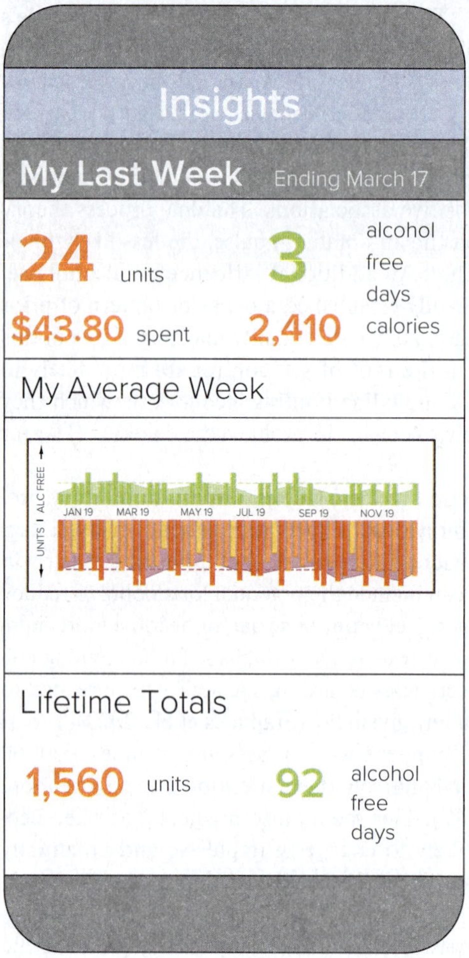

Sociocultural Perspective

Researchers and theorists working within the sociocultural perspective regard stressors in the family, community, and culture as factors that, when combined with genetic vulnerability, lead the individual to develop alcohol use disorder. As indicated earlier, socioeconomic status seems to interact with genetic vulnerability as an influence on how much alcohol individuals consume. Individuals with high socioeconomic status seem more likely to have drinking patterns influenced by familial patterns and preferences rather than by genetics.

Another approach within the sociocultural perspective takes into account the impact of socialization on patterns of alcohol use disorders while also incorporating psychological interventions. Researchers have demonstrated the benefits of cognitive behavioral therapy designed specifically for women (Epstein et al., 2018). Cognitive behavioral therapy specific for women emphasizes the themes of self-care and self-confidence as well as addressing friendships, social support, and levels of assertiveness, using female models in relevant training vignettes and worksheets.

stimulant
A psychoactive substance that has an activating effect on the central nervous system.

Acculturation is another factor evaluated by researchers working within the sociocultural perspective. Through a process of "Americanization," Hispanic and Asian Americans young adults adopt the alcohol use patterns of their age peers. Seeking to become part of American culture, individuals who become most acculturated are the ones most likely to engage in high levels of alcohol consumption, including binge drinking (Lui & Zamboanga, 2018).

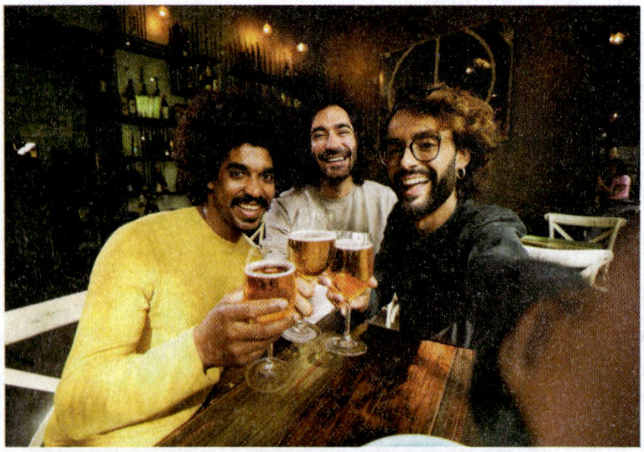

Researchers suggest that the process of "Americanization" can lead young adults from Hispanic and Asian American backgrounds to adopt alcohol use patterns of their age peers.
Gigi Delgado/Shutterstock

Treatment within the sociocultural perspective attempts to incorporate factors within the individual's social context. The Strong African American Families (SAAF) prevention program is an example of such a therapeutic model. A family-centered program for youth between the ages of 10 and 14 years of age, SAAF is a 7-week, 2-hour per week sessions in schools, community centers, and churches. Families and their children each receive separate training in such areas as racial socialization, goal-setting, setting expectations, and together attend sessions focused on family relationships, cultural pride, and values. Studies evaluating its efficacy show positive long-term effects even taking into account potential statistical bias due to self-selection on the part of program completers (Kogan, Bae, Lei, & Brody, 2019).

Other Drugs of Abuse

Stimulants The category of drugs called **stimulants** includes substances that have an activating effect on the nervous system. These differ in their chemical structure, their specific physical and psychological effects, and their potential danger to the user. In the *DSM-5-TR*, stimulants are associated with disorders related to use, intoxication, and withdrawal.

Amphetamines **Amphetamine** is a stimulant that affects both the central nervous and the autonomic nervous systems. In addition to waking or speeding up the central nervous system, it also causes elevated blood pressure and heart rate, and decreased appetite and physical activity. It may be used for medical purposes, such as to treat ADHD or as a diet pill. Even when used for medical purposes, however, amphetamine can cause dependence and have unpleasant or dangerous side effects. Increasingly large doses can make users hostile, violent, and paranoid. Users may also experience a range of physiological effects including fever, sweating, headache, blurred vision, dizziness, chest pain, nausea, vomiting, and diarrhea.

Methamphetamine is an addictive stimulant drug that is related to amphetamine but one that provokes more intense central nervous system effects. Whether taken orally, through the nose, intravenously, or by smoking, methamphetamine causes a rush or feeling of euphoria and becomes addictive very quickly. Methamphetamine overdose can cause overheating of the body and convulsions, and if not treated immediately, it can result in death. Long-term use of methamphetamine can lead users to develop mood disturbances, violent behavior, anxiety, confusion, insomnia, severe dental problems ("meth mouth"), and a heightened risk of infectious diseases including hepatitis and HIV/AIDS. The long-term effects of methamphetamines also include severe brain damage, as you can see from Figure 6.

According to (SAMHSA 2022), in 2021, 2.5 million people ages 12 and older in the United States (0.9 percent) used methamphetamines in the past year. The age group most likely to begin methamphetamine use includes people 25 and older, double that of the age groups 12 to 17 and 18 to 25. People 26 and older are also most likely to have a methamphetamine use disorder (0.7 percent or 1.5 million people).

The prescription medications Adderall and Ritalin are stimulants that teenagers can illegally obtain from friends with prescriptions or legally from a student's own healthcare professional.

Eroding the Mind
Researchers have mapped brain decay caused by methamphetamine use. The damage affected memory, emotion, and reward systems.

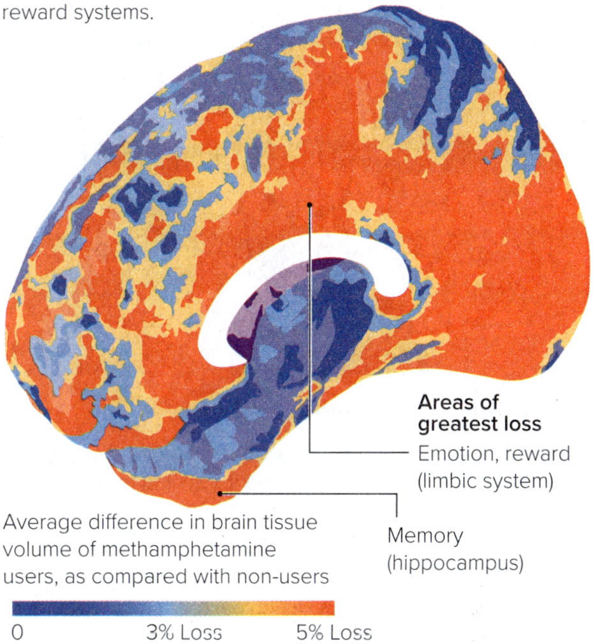

FIGURE 6 Long-Term Effects of Methamphetamine on the Brain

amphetamine
A stimulant that affects both the central nervous and the autonomic nervous systems.

methamphetamine
An addictive stimulant drug that is related to amphetamine but provokes more intense central nervous system effects.

MINI CASE

Stimulant Use Disorder, Amphetamine-Type Substance

Anya is a 23-year-old White lesbian cisgender woman. She has struggled with obesity for many years, and for the past 3 years she has tried many different strategies to lose weight. Her physician prescribed amphetamines but cautioned her about the possibility that she might become dependent on them. Anya did begin to lose weight, but she also discovered that she liked the extra energy and good feelings the diet pills caused. When she returned to her doctor after having lost the desired weight, she asked him for a refill of her prescription to help her maintain her new figure. When he refused, Anya asked among her friends until she found the name of a physician willing to accommodate her wish for ongoing refills of the prescription. Over the course of 1 year, Anya developed a number of psychological problems, including depression, paranoid thinking, and irritability. Despite the fact that she realizes something is wrong, she feels driven to continue using the drug.

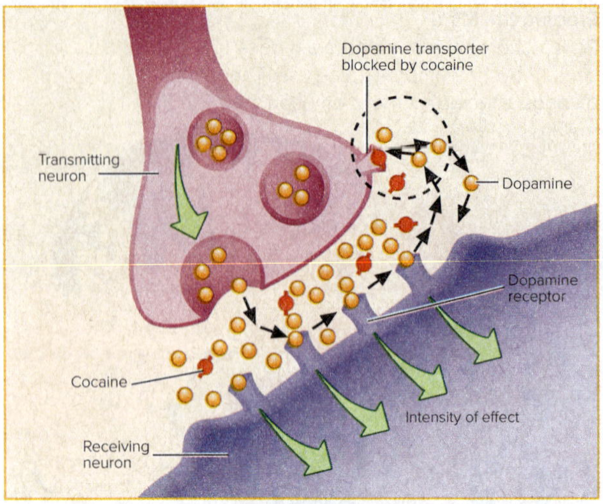

FIGURE 7 Cocaine in the Brain

In the normal communication process, dopamine is released by a neuron into the synapse, where it can bind to dopamine receptors on neighboring neurons. Dopamine is then recycled back into the transmitting neuron by a specialized protein called the dopamine transporter. If cocaine is present, it attaches to the dopamine transporter resulting in a buildup of dopamine in the synapse, which contributes to the pleasurable effects of cocaine.

In 2020, approximately 3.4 percent of high school seniors said they used Adderall, and 1.1 percent said they used Ritalin without medical supervision (Johnston et al., 2023).

Cocaine **Cocaine** is a highly addictive central nervous system stimulant that an individual snorts, injects, or smokes. Users can snort the powdered hydrochloride salt of cocaine or dissolve it in water and then inject it. Crack is the street name given to the form of cocaine that is processed to form a rock crystal that, when heated, produces vapors that the individual smokes. The effects of cocaine include feelings of euphoria, heightened mental alertness, reduced fatigue, and heightened energy. The faster the bloodstream absorbs the cocaine and delivers it to the brain, the more intense the user's high. Because this intense high is relatively short (5 to 10 minutes), the user may administer the drug again in a binge-like pattern.

Like amphetamines, cocaine increases body temperature, blood pressure, and heart rate. Cocaine's risks include heart attack, respiratory failure, stroke, seizures, abdominal pain, and nausea. In rare cases, the user can experience sudden death on the first use of cocaine or unexpectedly afterward. Other adverse effects on the body develop over time and include changes within the nose (loss of sense of smell, chronically runny nose, and nosebleeds), as well as problems with swallowing and hoarseness. Users may experience severe bowel gangrene due to a reduction of blood flow to the digestive system. Cocaine users may also have severe allergic reactions and increased risk of developing HIV/AIDS and other blood-borne diseases. When people use cocaine in binges, they may develop chronic restlessness, irritability, and anxiety. Chronic users may experience severe paranoia in which they have auditory hallucinations and lose touch with reality.

Figure 7 shows the impact of cocaine at the synapse. Like other drugs of abuse, cocaine has its effects by stimulating dopamine receptors. Researchers believe it specifically targets an area in the midbrain called the ventral tegmental area (VTA). Pathways from the VTA extend to the nucleus accumbens, a key area of the brain involved in reward. Cocaine's effects appear to be due to its blocking the removal of dopamine from the synapse, which results in an accumulation of dopamine that amplifies the signal to the receiving neurons.

cocaine
A highly addictive central nervous system stimulant that an individual snorts, injects, or smokes.

marijuana
A psychoactive substance derived from the hemp plant whose primary active ingredient is delta-9-tetrahydrocannabinol (THC).

Cannabis

Cannabis is associated with disorders related to use, intoxication, and withdrawal. **Marijuana** is a mix of flowers, stems, and leaves from the hemp plant *Cannabis sativa*, a tall, leafy, green plant that thrives in warm climates. Although the plant contains more than 400 chemical constituents, the primary active ingredient in marijuana is delta-9-tetrahydrocannabinol (THC). Hashish, containing a more concentrated form of THC, comes from the resins of the plant's flowers. Synthetic forms of THC serve some medicinal purposes, such as treating asthma and glaucoma and reducing nausea in cancer patients undergoing chemotherapy.

Most people who use marijuana smoke it as a cigarette or in a pipe. Users can also mix the drug in food or serve it as a tea. When smoked, marijuana reaches its peak blood level in about 10 minutes, but the subjective effect of intoxication does not become apparent for another 20 to 30 minutes. This effect may last 2 to 3 hours, but the metabolites of THC can remain in the body for 8 or more days.

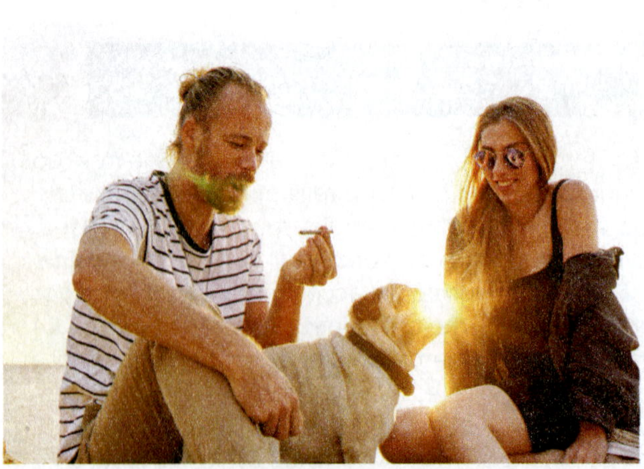

Marijuana users seek a state of euphoria and other sensory changes that they regard as pleasurable.
Aleksandra Belinskaya/Shutterstock

People use marijuana in order to alter their bodily sensations and perceptions of their environment. The effects they seek include euphoria, a heightened sense of sensuality and sexuality, and an increased awareness of internal and external stimuli. However, marijuana use also carries a number of unpleasant effects including

MINI CASE

Cannabis Use Disorder

Gary is a 22-year-old White heterosexual cisgender man. He has lived with his parents since dropping out of college midway through his first year 3 years ago. Gary was an average student in high school and, although popular, was not involved in many extracurricular activities. When he entered college, he became interested in the enticing opportunities for new experiences, and he began to smoke marijuana casually with his roommates. However, unlike his roommates, who limited their smoking to parties, Gary found that a nightly hit helped him relax. He started to rationalize that it also helped him study, because it made his thinking more creative.

As his first semester went by, Gary gradually lost interest in his studies, preferring to stay in his room and listen to music while getting high. He realized that it was easy to support his habit by selling marijuana to other people in the dorm. Although he convinced himself that he was not really a dealer, Gary became one of the primary suppliers of marijuana on campus. When he received his first-semester grades, he did not feel particularly discouraged about the fact that he had flunked out. Rather, he felt that he could benefit from having more time to himself. He moved back home and became friendly with some local teenagers who frequented a nearby park and shared drugs there. Gary's parents have all but given up on him, having become deeply discouraged by his apathy and lack of productivity. They know he is using drugs, but they feel helpless to get him to seek professional help. They have learned that it is better to avoid discussing the matter with Gary, because violent arguments always ensue.

impaired short-term memory, slowed reaction time, impaired physical coordination, altered judgment, and poor decision making. Instead of feeling euphoric and relaxed, users may experience paranoia and anxiety, particularly when they ingest high doses.

THC produces its effects by acting upon specific sites in the brain, called cannabinoid receptors. The brain regions with the highest density of cannabinoid receptors are the areas that influence pleasure but also are active in memory, thinking and concentration, perception of time, sensory responses, and ability to carry out coordinated movement. Many of marijuana's acute effects on cognitive functioning are reversible as long as the individual does not engage in chronic use.

As mentioned earlier in the chapter, marijuana is the most commonly used illicit drug in the United States. However, current prevalence statistics do not take into account the fact that recreational medical use of marijuana is now legal in 23 states, and medical use in 38 states. With these changes in legislation, the definition of an "illicit" drug will need to change in estimates of prevalence statistics.

As reported in the *DSM-5-TR*, individuals with cannabis use disorder have an intake on average 4 or more days per week, with some using throughout the day for months or years. Although researchers have attempted to determine the long-term effects of marijuana on cognitive functioning, the evidence remains equivocal, in part due to the difficulty of quantifying such factors as amount and length of exposure (Kroon, Kuhns, & Cousijn, 2021). Similarly, concerns remain about its effect on people's lives, a systematic review failed to establish a clear relationship between occupational injury and cannabis use (Biasutti, Leffers, & Callaghan, 2020). Substance use disorder, however, may present a risk in individuals who have comorbid disorders. A longitudinal investigation of Veterans established a link between those with cannabis use disorder and severity of PTSD as well as more persistent alcohol use (Livingstone et al., 2022).

Hallucinogens Included in hallucinogen-related disorders are use and intoxication, but not withdrawal. **Hallucinogens** are drugs that cause people to experience profound distortions in their perception of reality. Under the influence of hallucinogens, people see images, hear sounds, and feel sensations that they believe to be real but are not. In some cases, users experience rapid, intense mood swings. Some develop a condition called hallucinogen persisting perception disorder, in which they experience flashbacks or spontaneous

hallucinogens
Psychoactive substances that cause profound distortions in their perception of reality.

hallucinations, delusions, or disturbances in mood similar to the changes that took place while they were intoxicated with the drug. The specific effects and risks of each hallucinogen vary according to the particular substance, as you will discover.

lysergic acid diethylamide (LSD)
A form of a hallucinogenic drug that users ingest in tablets, capsules, and liquid form.

People take **lysergic acid diethylamide (LSD)** in tablets, capsules, and occasionally liquid form. Users show dramatic changes in their sensations and emotions. They may feel several emotions at once or swing rapidly from one emotion to another. With larger doses, users can experience delusions and visual hallucinations. In addition, they may feel an altered sense of time and self. They may also experience synesthesia, in which their sensory experiences blur together. For instance, they may "hear" colors and "see" sounds. These perceptual and mood alterations may be accompanied by severe, terrifying thoughts and feelings of despair, panic, and fear of losing control, going insane, or dying. Even after they stop taking LSD, users may experience flashbacks, leading them to be significantly distressed and impaired in their social and occupational functioning.

Unlike other substances, LSD does not seem to produce compulsive drug-seeking behavior, and most users choose to decrease or stop using it without withdrawal. However, it does produce tolerance, so users may need to take larger doses to achieve the effects they desire. Given the unpredictable nature of the drug's effects, such increases in doses can be dangerous. LSD can also affect other bodily functions, with effects including sweating, loss of appetite, dry mouth, sleeplessness, tremors, and increased body temperature, blood pressure, and heart rate.

peyote
A form of a hallucinogenic drug whose primary ingredient is mescaline.

Peyote is a small, spineless cactus whose principal active ingredient, mescaline, can also be produced artificially. Users chew the mescaline-containing crown of the cactus or soak it in water to produce a liquid; some prepare a tea by boiling the cactus in water to rid the drug of its bitter taste. Used as part of religious ceremonies by native peoples in northern Mexico and the southwestern United States, mescaline has long-term effects on these and recreational users that are not known. However, its effects on the body are similar to those of LSD, including increases in body temperature and heart rate, uncoordinated movements, extreme sweating, and flushing. In addition, mescaline may cause flashbacks, much like those associated with LSD.

psilocybin
A form of a hallucinogenic drug found in certain mushrooms.

Psilocybin (4-phosphoryloxy-N,N-dimethyltryptamine) and its biologically active form, psilocin (4-hydroxy-N,N-dimethyltryptamine), are substances found in certain mushrooms. Users brew the mushrooms or add them to other foods to disguise their bitter taste. The active compounds in psilocybin-containing mushrooms, like LSD, alter the individual's autonomic functions, motor reflexes, behavior, and perception. Individuals may experience hallucinations, an altered sense of time, and an inability to differentiate between fantasy and reality. Large doses may cause flashbacks, memory impairments, and greater vulnerability to psychological disorders. In addition to the risk of poisoning if the individual incorrectly identifies the mushroom, the bodily effects can include muscle weakness, loss of motor control, nausea, vomiting, and drowsiness.

phencyclidine (PCP)
A form of a hallucinogenic drug originally developed as an intravenous anesthetic.

Researchers developed **phencyclidine (PCP)** in the 1950s as an intravenous anesthetic, but it is no longer used medically because patients became agitated, delusional, and irrational while recovering from its effects. Users can easily mix the white crystalline powder with alcohol, water, or colored dye. PCP may also be available on the illegal drug market in pill, capsule, or colored powder forms that users can smoke, snort, or take orally. When individuals smoke PCP, they may apply the drug to mint, parsley, oregano, or marijuana.

PCP causes users to experience a sense of dissociation from their surroundings and their own sense of self. It has many adverse effects including symptoms that mimic schizophrenia, mood disturbance, memory loss, difficulties with speech and thinking, weight loss, and depression. Although these negative effects led to its diminished popularity as a street drug, PCP appeals to those who still use it because they feel that it makes them stronger, more powerful, and invulnerable. Despite its adverse effects, users can develop strong cravings and compulsive PCP-seeking behavior.

The physiological effects of PCP are extensive. Low to moderate doses produce increases in breathing rate, a rise in blood pressure and pulse, general numbness of the extremities, and loss of muscular coordination, as well as flushing and profuse sweating. At high doses, users experience a drop in blood pressure, pulse rate, and respiration, which may be

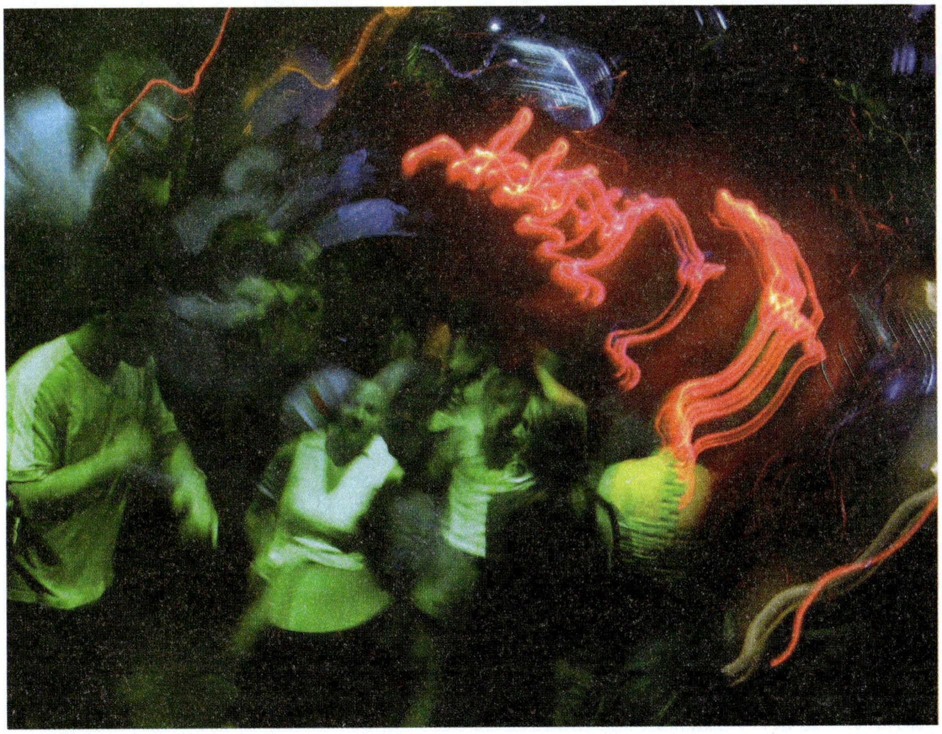

MDMA, or ecstasy, may be consumed as a way to enhance the enjoyment that users seek to experience while in large social gatherings, particularly while dancing.

Fotoman/Alamy Stock Photo

accompanied by nausea, vomiting, blurred vision, atypical eye movements, drooling, loss of balance, and dizziness. They may become violent or suicidal. In addition, at high doses users may experience seizures, coma, and death. Those who combine PCP with other central nervous system depressants (such as alcohol) may become comatose.

The chemical named **MDMA** (3,4-methylenedioxymethamphetamine) also known as **ecstasy** is a synthetic substance chemically similar to methamphetamine and mescaline. Users experience feelings of increased energy, euphoria, emotional warmth, distorted perceptions and sense of time, and unusual tactile experiences. Taken as a capsule or tablet, MDMA was once most popular among White teens and young adults at weekend-long dances known as "raves" but its use has become more widespread. Some users combine MDMA with other drugs including marijuana, cocaine, methamphetamine, ketamine, and sildenafil (Viagra), among other substances.

ecstasy (MDMA)
A hallucinogenic drug made from a synthetic substance chemically similar to methamphetamine and mescaline.

Users of MDMA may experience a range of unpleasant psychological effects, including confusion, depression, sleep problems, cravings for the drug, and severe anxiety. The drug may be neurotoxic, which means that over time users may experience greater difficulty carrying out cognitive tasks. Like stimulants, MDMA can affect the sympathetic nervous system, leading to increased heart rate and blood pressure, muscle tension, nausea, blurred vision, fainting, chills or sweating, and involuntary teeth clenching. Individuals also risk severe spikes in body temperature, which in turn can lead to liver, kidney, or cardiovascular system failure. Repeated dosages over short periods of time may also interfere with MDMA metabolism, leading to significant and harmful buildup within the body.

The main neurotransmitter involved with MDMA is serotonin. As shown in Figure 8, in which serotonin is represented by orange-colored triangles, MDMA (labeled "ecstasy") binds to the serotonin transporter responsible for removing serotonin from the synapse. As a result, MDMA extends the effects of serotonin. In addition, MDMA enters the neuron, where it stimulates excessive release of serotonin. MDMA has similar effects on norepinephrine, which leads to increases in autonomic nervous system activity. The drug also releases dopamine, but to a lesser extent.

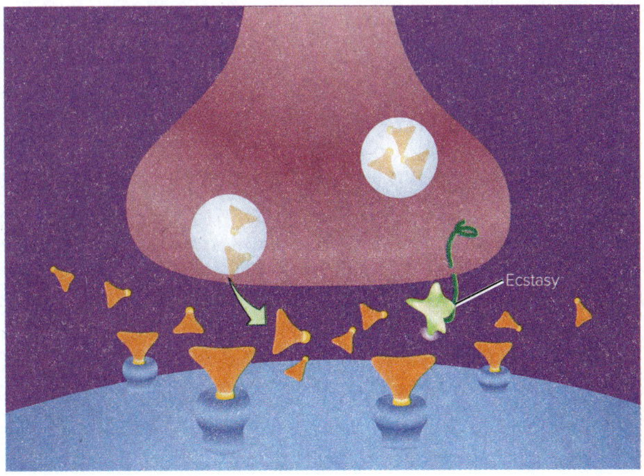

FIGURE 8 The Impact of Ecstasy (MDMA) on Serotonergic Neurons

MINI CASE

Other Hallucinogen Use Disorder

Candace is a 45-year-old White pansexual cisgender woman. An artist, she has used LSD for a number of years because she feels that doing so enhances her paintings and makes them more visually exciting. Although she claims to know how much LSD she can handle, she is occasionally caught off guard and experiences disturbing side effects. She begins sweating, has blurred vision, is uncoordinated, and shakes all over. She commonly becomes paranoid and anxious, and she may act in strange ways, such as running out of her studio and into the street, ranting incoherently. On more than one occasion, the police have picked her up and taken her to the emergency room, where doctors prescribed antipsychotic medication.

Researchers find it difficult to investigate the long-term effects of MDMA use on cognitive functioning because users typically take it with other substances. However, significant negative effects on verbal memory do occur with MDMA use alone (Thomasius et al., 2006). MDMA's effects on cognition appear to relate at least in part to the impact of the drug on the availability of an individual's cognitive resources (Roberts, Quednow, Montgomery, & Parrott, 2018). Moreover, when combined with alcohol, MDMA produces a number of long-term adverse psychological effects including paranoia, poor physical health, irritability, confusion, and moodiness.

opioid
A psychoactive substance that relieves pain.

Opioids Opioid-related disorders are connected to opioid use, intoxication, and withdrawal. An **opioid** is a substance that relieves pain. Many legally prescribed medications fall within this category, including hydrocodone (Vicodin), oxycodone (OxyContin, Percocet), morphine (Kadian, Avinza), codeine, and related drugs. Clinicians prescribe hydrocodone products most commonly for a variety of painful conditions, including dental procedures and injuries. Physicians often administer morphine before and after surgical procedures to alleviate severe pain. Codeine, on the other hand, is prescribed for mild pain. Some opioid drugs—codeine and diphenoxylate (Lomotil), for example—are used to relieve coughs and severe diarrhea, respectively.

When people take them as prescribed, these medications are effective for managing pain safely. However, because of their potential to produce euphoria as well as physical dependence, they are among the most frequently abused prescription drugs. People who abuse OxyContin may snort or inject it and suffer a serious overdose reaction as a result.

The opioids of abuse include prescription pain relievers, heroin, and synthetic opioids such as fentanyl. The "opioid crisis," the rise in the number of individuals addicted to prescription painkillers and resulting deaths, is now seen as a major public health crisis in the United States (see Figure 9).

The National Institute of Drug Abuse, based on Centers for Disease Control and Prevention data, estimates that over 80,000 deaths occurred in 2021, which was a significant

MINI CASE

Opioid Use Disorder

Jimmy is a 38-year-old biracial heterosexual cisgender man. He is experiencing homelessness and has been addicted to heroin for the past 10 years. He began to use the drug at the suggestion of a friend who told him it would help relieve the pressure Jimmy was feeling from his unhappy marriage and financial problems. In a short period of time, he became dependent on the drug and got involved in a theft ring to support his habit. Ultimately, he lost his home and moved to a shelter, where workers assigned Jimmy to a methadone treatment program.

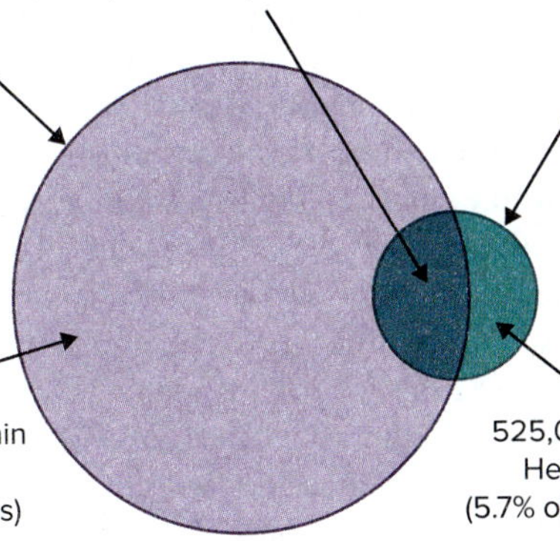

FIGURE 9 9.2 Million People Aged 12 or Older with Past Year Opioid Misuse

Source: Substance Abuse and Mental Health Services Administration. (2022). *Key substance use and mental health indicators in the United States: Results from the 2021 National Survey on Drug Use and Health (HHS Publication No. PEP22-07-01-005, NSDUH Series H-57),* Rockville, MD: Center for Behavioral Health Statistics and Quality, Substance Abuse and Mental Health Services Administration. https://www.samhsa.gov/data/report/2021-nsduh-annual-national-report

increase over the prior year (over 68,000) and almost four times as high as overdose deaths reported in 2010 (NIDA, 2023). The economic burden of prescription opioid misuse alone in the United States was estimated to be over 1 trillion dollars in 2017, with $471 million attributable to opioid use disorder. Over $92 billion was associated with lost productivity and fatal opioid overdose alone (Florence, Luo, & Rice, 2021).

Heroin is a form of opioid. It is a painkilling drug synthesized from morphine, a naturally occurring substance extracted from the seed pod of the Asian opium poppy plant. Users inject, snort, sniff, or smoke heroin. The body then converts it to morphine, which binds to

heroin
A psychoactive substance that is a form of opioid, synthesized from morphine.

You Be the Judge

Prescribing Prescription Drugs

Patients who suffer from chronic pain present a tremendous challenge to health care professionals. Long-term treatment of chronic pain through prescription medications carries the risk that patients will develop dependence. Moreover, because patients need escalating doses to achieve the same degree of relief, their pain sensitivity and levels of pain might actually increase. At the same time, patients may fear taking an opioid medication that could benefit them due to the risk of developing an addiction and thus may suffer unduly, especially if they are terminally ill. Ironically, some health care professionals as well as patients worry about the risks of addiction among patients who are in their last few months of life.

Addressing the national crisis in overuse of prescription pain medication, the National Institute of Health (2018) launched a campaign known as HEAL (Helping to End Addiction Long-Term Initiative), doubling the federal funding to accelerate scientific solutions to stemming the national epidemic.

Clearly, the development of effective, nonaddicting pain medications is a public health priority. A growing population of older adults and an increasing number of injured military service members and veterans only add to the urgency of this issue. Researchers need to explore alternate medications that can alleviate pain but have less potential for abuse. At the same time, researchers and practitioners in psychology can provide a greater understanding of effective chronic pain management, including identifying factors that predispose some patients to addiction and developing measures to prevent abuse.

Q: *You be the judge*: What is the best way to balance the patient's need for pain relief with the growing national and international crisis in abuse of prescription pain medications?

the opioid receptors throughout the brain and body, particularly those active in reward and pain perception. Opioid receptors are also located in the brain stem, which contains structures that control breathing, blood pressure, and arousal. Upon ingesting heroin, users experience a surge of euphoric feelings, along with dry mouth, warm flushing of the skin, heaviness in the arms and legs, and compromised mental functioning. Shortly afterward, they alternate between feeling wakeful and drowsy.

Heroin use is associated with a number of serious health consequences including infectious diseases (related to needle sharing), damage to the cardiovascular system, abscesses, liver and kidney disease, and fatal overdoses. As a result, people who use heroin are more susceptible to pneumonia and other pulmonary complications, as well as damage to the brain, liver, and kidneys resulting from the toxic contaminants often added to the drug.

In addition to the effects on health, heroin is highly addictive. Users can develop tolerance, and those who go through withdrawal experience severe cravings that can last for as long as a week. There are also dangers to sudden withdrawal, particularly in long-term users who are in poor health. Withdrawal symptoms can include restlessness, muscle and bone pain, insomnia, diarrhea, vomiting, cold flashes, and involuntary kicking movements.

sedative
A psychoactive substance that has a calming effect on the central nervous system.

hypnotic
A substance that induces sedation.

anxiolytic
An antianxiety medication.

Sedatives, Hypnotics, and Anxiolytics

The category of sedatives, hypnotics, and anxiolytics (antianxiety medications) includes prescription medications that act as central nervous system depressants. A **sedative** has a soothing or calming effect, a **hypnotic** induces sleep, and an **anxiolytic** is used to treat anxiety symptoms. The sedating effects of these central nervous system depressants are due to the fact that they increase the levels of the neurotransmitter GABA, which inhibits brain activity and therefore produces a calming effect. Disorders within this category include use disorder, intoxication, and withdrawal.

These medications include benzodiazepines, barbiturates, nonbenzodiazepine sleep medications such as zolpidem (Ambien), eszopiclone (Lunesta), and zaleplon (Sonata). Although safe when taken as prescribed, these medications have high potential for abuse and dependence.

In 2019, about 1.1 million people aged 12 and older in the United States used sedatives nonmedically, and 5.2 million misused tranquilizers. Individuals 60 years and older are most likely to use these medications (35.6 percent in the past year) and also have relatively high rates of misuse (1 percent within this age group) (SAMHSA, 2020). These statistics for older adults raise concern, given the potential for drug interactions with alcohol and other medications. Clinicians working with older clients therefore need to be aware of the need to regulate dosages to avoid harmful side effects (Whitbourne & Martins, 2020).

Caffeine
A stimulant found in coffee, tea, chocolate, energy drinks, diet pills, and headache remedies.

Caffeine

Caffeine is a stimulant found in coffee, tea, chocolate, energy drinks, diet pills, and headache remedies. By activating the sympathetic nervous system through increasing the production of adrenaline, caffeine increases an individual's perceived level of energy and alertness. It also increases blood pressure and may lead to increases in the body's production of cortisol, the stress hormone.

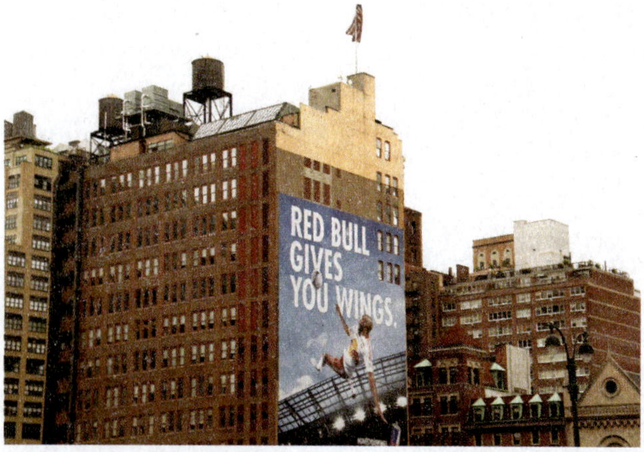

Highly caffeinated beverages are widely advertised through marketing geared toward teens and young adults.
Peter Horree/Alamy Stock Photo

Because caffeine is such a common feature of everyday life, people tend not to be aware of its dangers. When consumed in large quantities, caffeine can lead to many adverse reactions, including the development of other forms of substance dependence (Arria et al., 2017). In the United States, at least 130 energy drinks exceed the FDA-recommended limit of 0.02 percent of caffeine. The latest entries are caffeinated flavors of the liquids used in e-cigarettes, which are being marketed as energy enhancers (Lisko et al., 2017).

Disorders included in the caffeine-related category are intoxication and withdrawal, but not caffeine use disorder. Support is growing for adding caffeine use disorder as a diagnosis similar to other substance use disorders (Harstad et al., 2016) even though it might apply to only a small percentage of the population (Sweeney et al., 2020).

MINI CASE

Caffeine Intoxication

Carla is a 19-year-old White heterosexual cisgender woman. She is a sophomore in college who has felt compelled to excel at every endeavor and to become involved in as many activities as time and energy permit. As her commitments increased and her studies became more burdensome, Carla became more and more reliant on coffee, soda, and over-the-counter stimulants to reduce her need for sleep. During final examination week, Carla overdid it. For 3 days straight, she consumed approximately 10 cups of coffee a day, along with a few bottles of energy shots. In addition to her bodily symptoms of restlessness, twitching muscles, flushed face, stomach disturbance, and heart irregularities, Carla began to ramble when she spoke. Her roommate became distressed after seeing Carla's condition and insisted on taking her to the emergency room, where the intake clinician recognized her condition as caffeine intoxication.

The symptoms of caffeine withdrawal include headache, tiredness and fatigue, sleepiness and drowsiness, dysphoric mood, difficulty concentrating, depression, irritability, nausea, vomiting, muscle aches, and stiffness. Individuals who are daily consumers of caffeine are more likely to experience these withdrawal symptoms after discontinuing use. However, perhaps surprisingly, it is possible for those experiencing caffeine withdrawal to benefit from substituting decaffeinated beverages. even in people who do not believe that they will work (Mills, Lee, Boakes, & Colagiuri, 2023).

When users combine alcohol and caffeine, they may not realize how intoxicated they are and as a result may have a higher prevalence of alcohol-related consequences. In one daily-diary study of undergraduates asked to record their daily consumption of caffeine and alcohol, those who consumed caffeine in energy drinks had more alcohol-related problems (Linden-Carmichael & Lau-Barraco, 2017). Caffeine use in pre-teenage children may also present risks for alcohol use, as shown in a study of sixth graders, whose early caffeine use predicted alcohol use at 6-month follow-up (Kristjansson et al., 2022).

Tobacco **Nicotine** is the psychoactive substance found in cigarettes. The health risks of tobacco are well known; these risks are primarily associated with smoking cigarettes that, in addition to nicotine, contain tar, carbon monoxide, and other additives.

nicotine
The psychoactive substance found in cigarettes.

When nicotine enters the bloodstream, it stimulates the release of adrenaline (norepinephrine), which activates the autonomic nervous system and increases blood pressure, heart rate, and respiration. Like other psychoactive substances, nicotine increases the level of dopamine, affecting the brain's reward and pleasure centers. Substances found in tobacco smoke, such as acetaldehyde, may further enhance nicotine's effects on the central nervous system. The withdrawal symptoms associated with quitting tobacco use include irritability, difficulties with concentration, and strong cravings for nicotine.

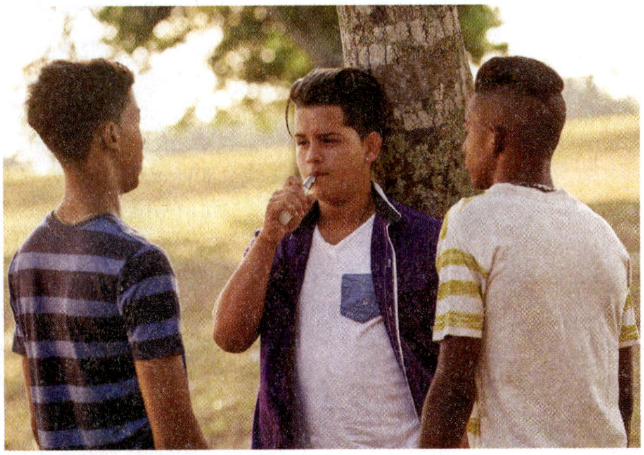

There are high rates of use of flavored e-cigarettes among underage children and teens.

Diego Cervo/Shutterstock

Increased suicide risk associated with tobacco use comes from studies in U.S. Veterans Health Administration facilities, which also controlled for other possible risk factors, as reported in the *DSM-5-TR*. Among the general population, suicide risk increases two- to three-fold.

Although cigarette smoking is significantly less widespread than in previous years, among people 12 years and older, 15.6 percent had used cigarettes in the past month, with highest rates among adults aged 26 and older (17.9 percent or 39.4 million). Among daily cigarette smokers, almost half (42 percent) smoked one or packs of cigarettes a day, rates highest for those 26 and older (SAMHSA, 2022). Young adults (18 to 25) are most likely to engage in vaping (14.1 or 4.7 million people), but underage tobacco and nicotine vaping (ages 12 to 20) rates are also high (11 percent or 4.3 million people) (SAMHSA, 2022). These numbers are of concern, because the symptoms of flavored e-cigarette use, as reported by over 2.8 million teens and young adults recruited via social media platforms, include respiratory, throat, and cardiovascular problems (Chen et al., 2020).

inhalants
A diverse group of substances that cause psychoactive effects by producing chemical vapors.

Inhalants

Inhalants are a diverse group of substances that cause psychoactive effects by producing chemical vapors. These products are not in and of themselves harmful; in fact, they are all products commonly found in the home and workplace. There are four categories of inhalants: volatile solvents (paint thinners or removers, dry-cleaning fluids, gasoline, glue, and lighter fluid), aerosols (sprays that contain propellants and solvents), gases (butane lighters and propane tanks, ether, and nitrous oxide), and nitrites (a special category of products that individuals use as sexual enhancers). Young teens (ages 12 to 15) tend to inhale glue, shoe polish, spray paint, gasoline, and lighter fluid. Older teens (ages 16 to 17) inhale nitrous oxide, and adults (ages 18 and older) are most likely to inhale nitrites. Within the category of inhalant disorders, individuals can be diagnosed as having inhalant use disorder or intoxication, but not inhalant withdrawal.

The effects of an inhalant tend to be short-lived; consequently, users try to extend their high by inhaling repeatedly over a period of several hours. Inhalants have effects similar to those of alcohol, including slurring of speech, loss of coordination, euphoria, dizziness, and, over time, loss of inhibition and control. Users may experience drowsiness and headaches, but depending on the substance, they may also feel confused and nauseated. The vapors displace the air in the lungs, causing hypoxia (oxygen deprivation), which is particularly lethal to neurons in the central nervous system. Long-term use may also cause the myelin sheath around the axon to deteriorate, leading to tremors, muscle spasms, and perhaps permanent muscle damage. The chemicals in inhalants can also cause heart failure and sudden death.

As Figure 1 shows, 2.2 million persons aged 12 and older in the United States in 2021 reported use of inhalants in the past year. Adolescents are most likely to be users of inhalants (2.4 percent or 626,000 people).

Theories and Treatment of Disorders Involving Substances other than Alcohol

Since all psychoactive substances operate on the reward and pleasure systems in the brain, similarities exist in the mechanisms through which individuals develop dependence on them. However, there are differences between alcohol and other substances in the receptor pathways for the substance, the psychosocial factors associated with dependence, and, ultimately, the best treatment methods.

Biological Perspective

Research evidence clearly supports the idea that genetics plays a role in the development of substance use disorders, including progression from age of onset to regular use, and subsequent problems associated with substance use, more so for individuals of European ancestry compared to those of African ancestry (Kranzler et al., 2023). Epigenetic studies also suggest that gene expression can be affected by specific drug-related changes (Prom-Wormley, Ebejer, Dick, & Bowers, 2017). Apart from whatever genetic contributions there may be to substance use disorders, however, treatment efforts within the biological perspective focus on medications that can reduce an individual's dependence on the substance.

Medically assisted detoxification is the first step in treatment of heroin dependence. During detoxification, individuals may receive medications to minimize withdrawal symptoms. To prevent relapse, clinicians may use one or more of three different medications. Developed more than 30 years ago, **methadone** is a synthetic opioid that blocks the effects of heroin by binding to the same receptor sites in the central nervous system. Proper use requires specialized treatment including group and/or individual counseling along with referrals for other medical, psychological, or social services. Methadone is not considered an ideal treatment because of its potential for dependence, even when combined with

methadone
A synthetic opioid that produces a safer and more controlled reaction than heroin and that is used in treating heroin addiction.

REAL STORIES

Mary J. Blige (1971–Present)

A powerhouse singer, songwriter, rapper, actor, and legend of the music industry, Mary J. Blige has survived sexual abuse, heartache, and substance addiction. Throughout much of her journey, she has used music as a way to channel her experience and connect with her audiences, and through personal strength she overcame addiction to drugs and alcohol.

Blige's career launched when she was 21 with the release of her first album, *What's the 411*. This helped lead to her early and lasting success as an R&B artist, and three decades after she set out making music, she has sold over 50 million records, with 13 albums to her name, her own record label, 9 Grammy awards, and 2 Golden Globes for both songwriting and acting, among countless other accolades. Blige's acting career took off in the 2010s with multiple roles in film and television, garnering her critical acclaim.

Blige rose from humble beginnings. Born in the Bronx, NY, she was raised in both Georgia and New York by a single mother who struggled to support Blige and her two siblings. At the age of 5, Blige was sexually assaulted by a family friend, which she kept secret for decades.

"It only happened once," she has said about the assault, "but after that there was so much else in my childhood that happened. So many dark moments–which all added up and that's what sprung on the drug addiction, trying to numb it all with the drugs. The depression. The lack of love for myself. The lack of people loving you around you. The abandonment issues. Daddy not being there all the time. Mommy not knowing how to handle it all. Although she loves you, she abandons you at some point too. I'm not saying that to be down on my mom. She was just a cursed woman as well" (Thompson, 2013).

As a teenager, Blige started drinking and using drugs to "kill the visual of what happened to me when I was five" (Lemieux, 2019). She dropped out of high school during her junior year and then started singing and recording music, eventually signing her first record deal as a solo artist in 1991.

Throughout the first half of her music career, Blige poured her life experiences, heartaches and all, into her music. Her reputation grew as an artist who was unapologetically expressive about the issues she had coped with, and she used music to continue to work through the pain in her life. As her career progressed and she grew more famous and successful, however, her addiction to cocaine and alcohol escalated.

Blige has been open in the press about what drove her substance use and addiction. In a 2019 interview, she reflected; "We numb ourselves with drugs and alcohol and people and shopping . . . to cover up what's really going on inside. . . . You're taking drugs so you can go out and feel courageous, or go out and feel beautiful or whatever. You're doing it to cover up *something*."

Throughout much of her addiction and her eventual recovery, Blige was in a highly publicized and often difficult marriage to her manager that eventually ended in 2016 after a painful divorce. She recovered from her addiction during the marriage, and at the time she credited her husband with helping her through this period. But she later revealed that she had largely overcome addiction on her own terms, without him, and had wanted to portray their relationship as perfect when instead it was crumbling behind the scenes.

This desire for privacy extended to her recovery from drugs and alcohol. Rather than go through professional treatment, Blige took her own path to recovery, using her spiritual faith as a guide. Many people actually are able to recover from substance addiction without professional intervention, though Blige's motivation went beyond her desire to use her own strength. She highly values her privacy, and in her words: "As public as I am, I'm real private. . . . I'll give you the juice and the truth, but not the stuff that's going to kill me. . . . I grew up in a neighborhood where we couldn't tell everything. It would kill us. So you 'know,' but you don't [know]. You know?" (Lemieux, 2019).

Though Blige prefers to keep many details about her personal life private, she has been vocal about her motivation for overcoming her addiction to drugs and alcohol. In many interviews, she has spoken of the impact of the deaths of other famous women in her industry, especially Whitney Houston's from overdose in 2012, on waking her up to the reality of continued addiction.

"I've seen visions of what I would look like if I kept doing drugs," she says, adding that there were also some nights when her reality may have mirrored those perhaps prophetic visualizations closely. "If I saw myself almost dying, or if I almost died, or almost O.D.'d, why would I do that again?" (Lemieux, 2019).

Blige started to work on fully facing the pain from her life and let go of substances as a way to cope. She has spoken of the importance of spirituality in her recovery: ". . . I didn't want to go to rehab. I believe that anything man himself can do for me, God can do for me in a greater way. I decided to pray and to seek God on my own. I just stayed in The Word. And it worked" (Thompson, 2013).

Now many years into her recovery, Blige continues to have a flourishing career, particularly as she picks up more acting roles in film and television. She has reflected that despite her immense success, she wants more than anything to be remembered for her strength and courage as a person. She wants the world to recognize that "I was courageous. I was a courageous woman . . . [and] I gave and gave and gave and gave and gave, when people were afraid to give. I said the things that people were afraid to say" (Lemieux, 2019).

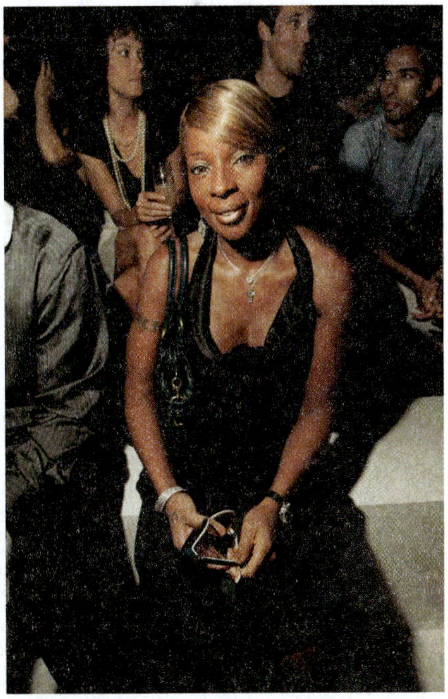

Mary J. Blige, whose film, "Mary J. Blige's My Life" chronicles her life and career.

Lars A. Niki

buprenorphine
A medication used in the treatment of heroin addiction.

psychosocial interventions. **Buprenorphine**, approved by the FDA in 2002, produces less physical dependence, a lower risk of overdose, and fewer withdrawal effects. Extended-release naltrexone is the third option for treatment of opioid use disorder. New therapies still in development include gene-targeted treatment, heroin vaccines, and agents that target cell receptors (Kuppalli et al., 2021).

Nicotine replacement therapies (NRTs), including nicotine gum and the nicotine patch, were the first FDA-approved pharmacological treatments. These deliver controlled doses of nicotine to the individual to relieve symptoms of withdrawal. Other FDA-approved products include nasal sprays, inhalers, and lozenges. Although effective when adhered to, NRTs have a low compliance rate (Mersha et al., 2021). Other biological approaches to nicotine dependence are medications that do not deliver nicotine, including bupropion (Wellbutrin), an antidepressant, and varenicline tartrate (Chantix), which targets nicotine receptors in the brain.

Psychological Perspective Whether or not individuals with dependence on substances other than alcohol receive biologically based treatment, cognitive behavioral therapy (CBT) is now widely understood to be a crucial component of successful treatment and an important counterpart to biological theories and treatments (Jain & Davis, 2021).

The principles applied in treating substance use disorders other than for alcohol through CBT are similar to those in treating alcohol dependence. Clinicians may combine CBT with motivational therapies, as well as with behavioral interventions that focus on contingency management. They can also readily adapt CBT to a range of clinical modalities, settings, and age groups.

Given the limitations of medication-only treatment, CBT also provides an effective adjunct in both inpatient and outpatient clinics. The ability to help clients develop coping skills is useful in fostering compliance with pharmacotherapies such as methadone and naltrexone as well. CBT has the additional advantage of being adaptable for computer-based interventions (Kiluk, 2019) and deliverable in culturally adapted formats (e.g., Silva et al., 2020). However, for people of color and those from collectivist cultures, there is evidence that third-wave therapies have more effectiveness, particularly when they involve use of mindfulness (Dela Cruz et al., 2023).

12.3 Non-Substance-Related Disorders

Gambling Disorder

gambling disorder
A non-substance-related disorder involving the persistent urge to gamble.

People who have **gambling disorder** are unable to resist recurrent urges to gamble despite knowing that it will bring negative consequences to themselves or others. In *DSM-5-TR*, it is included with substance use disorders because it is conceptualized as showing many of the same behaviors, such as cravings, increasing needs to engage in the behavior, and negative social consequences. The unique features of gambling disorder include behaviors such as chasing a bad bet, lying about how much has been lost, searching for financial bailouts, and committing crimes to support gambling.

People who live in areas near casinos and electronic gambling venues are at higher risk of becoming problem gamblers, as indicated by the relationship between financial insolvencies and the number of such venues (Badji, Black, & Johnston, 2020). As legalized online gambling has become more prevalent, and even promoted, it is even more likely that individuals will develop gambling disorder (Chóliz, Marcos, & Lázaro-Mateo, 2019).

Gambling disorder often co-occurs with other psychological disorders (Rodriguez-Monguio, Brand, & Volberg, 2018). These include nicotine dependence (60 percent), dependence on other substances (58 percent), mood disorder (38 percent), and anxiety disorder (37 percent). Individuals with comorbid depressive and gambling disorder have nearly twice the mortality rates of age-matched controls and a 15-fold increase in the number of suicides (Karlsson & Håkansson, 2018).

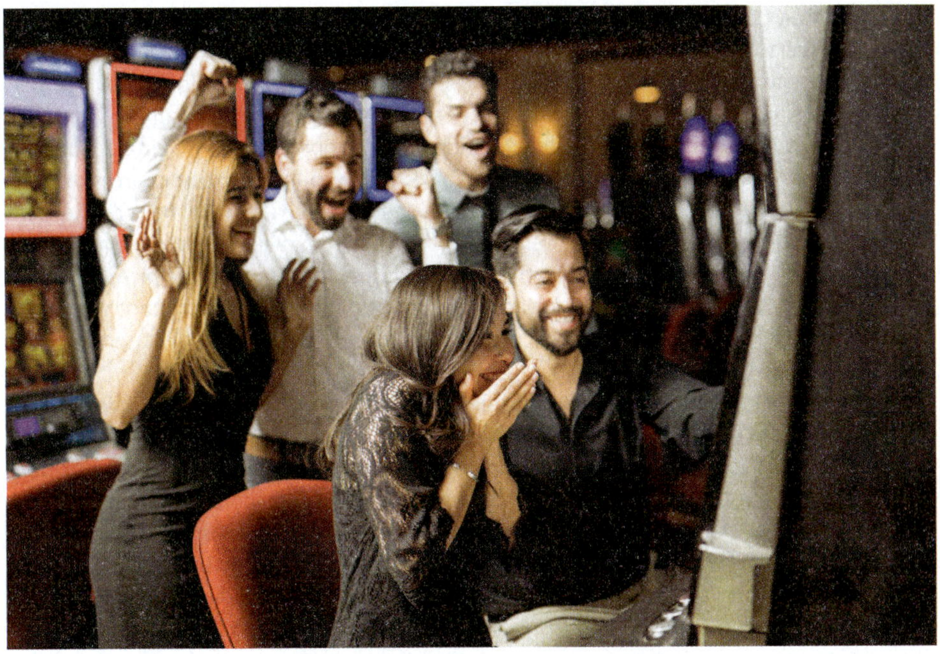

A "big win" may lead individuals to develop gambling problems as they seek to repeat the experience.

antoniodiaz/Shutterstock

Older adults are less likely than younger adults to have gambling disorder, but they are nevertheless at risk, particularly if they have experienced recent stressful life events such as severe financial problems, sexual problems (including extramarital affairs), and problems with substance use (Granaro et al., 2022). Older individuals, additionally may be motivated by a materialistic motives, in part as a way to reduce negative emotions associated with these stressful life events (Estévez et al., 2021).

By definition, people with gambling disorder are unable to control their behavior. A longitudinal study of self-identified characteristics that predict problem gambling in a Canadian sample confirmed that problem gamblers define themselves as high on the trait of impulsivity and a desire for excitement. Additional demographic risk factors identified in this study include being of male gender, South Asian heritage, and Middle Eastern/Arab heritage. Low income is another strong predictor, which is consistent with the self-identified reasons for gambling noted by the people in the study, who saw gambling as a way to earn money. Gambling to escape was another self-identified reason for their behavior, as was presence of a mood disorder. Other contributing factors included adverse childhood experiences, antisociality, substance use/abuse, stress, a family history of problem gambling, and belief in gambling fallacies such as the idea that their behavior can control the outcome of a bet. The availability of electronic gambling machines and online gambling further heightens the risk of developing gambling disorder. However, as the authors note, it can be difficult, even in a longitudinal study, to tease apart factors that cause and those that result from problem gambling (Williams et al., 2023).

From a behavioral perspective, gambling disorder may develop in part because gambling follows a variable-ratio reinforcement schedule in which rewards occur a varying number of times. This pattern of reinforcement produces behaviors that are highly resistant to extinction. Slot machines, in particular, produce payoffs on this type of schedule, maintaining high rates of response by gamblers. Classical conditioning also operates to maintain this behavior, because gamblers learn to associate certain cues with gambling, including their internal states or moods and external stimuli such as advertisements for gambling.

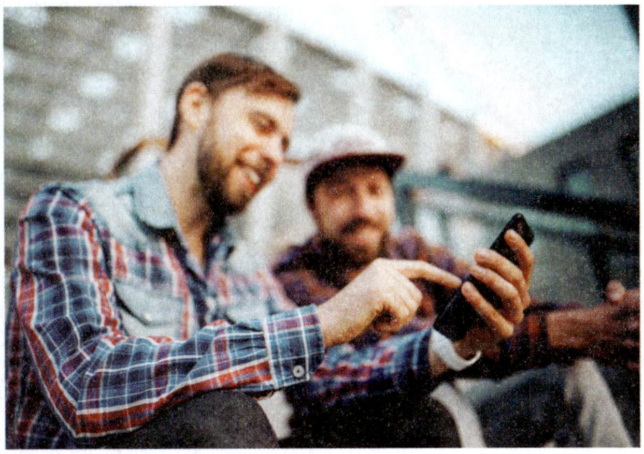

Individuals with gambling disorder may become involved with widely available smartphone-based gaming mobile applications.

Wpadington/Shutterstock

pathways model
Approach to gambling disorder that predicts there are three main developmental paths leading to three distinct subtypes.

The **pathways model** approaches gambling disorder from a developmental perspective, proposing that three main paths lead to three distinct subtypes of people with gambling disorder (Valleur et al., 2016). The person with the behaviorally conditioned subtype had few symptoms prior to developing the disorder but, through frequent exposure to gambling, develops positive associations, distorted cognitions, and poor decision making about gambling. The individual in the emotionally vulnerable subtype had pre-existing depression, anxiety, and perhaps a history of trauma; gambling helps this individual feel better. The third type of person with pathological gambling has pre-existing impulsivity, attentional difficulties, and antisocial characteristics. For this individual, the risk of gambling provides thrills and excitement. This third pathway toward problem gambling may also be motivated by a desire for meaning and purpose, as well as a way to reduce stress (Nower, Blaszczynski, & Anthony, 2022).

The pathways model suggests that differing therapeutic approaches may work for each of the three subtypes of gambling disorder, but cognitive behavioral therapy has the greatest empirical support. The clinician begins teaching clients to understand the triggers for their gambling by having them describe their pattern of gambling behaviors. For example, common triggers include unstructured or free time, negative emotional states, reminders such as sports broadcasts or advertisements, and available money. Using this information to help clients analyze when they gamble and when they do not, the clinician then helps them increase pleasant activities, think of ways to handle cravings or urges, become more assertive, and correct their irrational cognitions. At the end of treatment, the clinician helps prepare clients for setbacks using relapse-prevention methods in which the goal is not complete abstinence but a reduction to a point below pretreatment levels. The individual who shows positive effects may also show personality changes that will serve to protect against relapse (Müller et al., 2017). Other beneficial factors to add to interventions include helping clients discontinue tobacco use and promoting greater involvement in leisure activities (Allami et al., 2023).

Brief motivational interviewing may also be a beneficial treatment for individuals with problem gambling. The individual may choose to pursue complete abstinence or moderation as a goal of this treatment; both can be equally effective in reducing the amount of money gambled, the number of days the individual gambles, as well as the individual's perception of having achieved treatment-related goals (Stea, Hodgins, & Fung, 2015).

Other Non-Substance-Related Disorders

Although Internet-gaming disorder may seem similar to gambling disorder, its proposed criteria are in Section III of the *DSM-5-TR* as a disorder requiring further study. Although there is ample evidence to indicate that Internet gaming is becoming a problematic behavior in its own right, the available research was not considered sufficiently well developed yet to justify inclusion in the diagnostic system despite its significant public health importance. Much of the data in support of this condition was produced by studies conducted in Asia that used inconsistent definitions of the phenomenon. After extensive review, the *DSM-5-TR* work group believed further investigations are required to produce reliable prevalence estimates. Other disorders the work group considered adding were "sex addiction," "exercise addiction," and "shopping addiction," to name a few. However, the group believed there were even fewer empirical studies in peer-reviewed articles to justify their inclusion even in Section III.

12.4 Substance Disorders: The Biopsychosocial Perspective

The biopsychosocial model provides an extremely useful approach for understanding substance use disorders and approaches to treatment. Genetics clearly plays a role in the development of these disorders, and the action of substances on the central nervous system also operates to maintain dependence. Developmental issues in particular are critical for understanding the nature of these disorders, which often have their origins during late childhood and early adolescence. Moreover, because alcohol, drugs, and medications with high abuse potential continue to be widely available, sociocultural factors play a strong role in maintaining dependence among users. Integrated approaches that combine medical treatment (where indicated) with psychotherapy appear to have the most promise for helping individuals overcome these highly debilitating disorders.

Return to the Case: Carl Wadsworth

Carl initially had some difficulties in finding an AA meeting in which he felt comfortable, although once he found the right group for him, he looked forward to attending on a daily basis and remained highly motivated to refrain from drinking. He connected with many members of the group and felt, for the first time in his life, that he had a supportive group of friends. He also began a course of mood-stabilizing medication that did not require weekly blood tests and that resulted in significantly lower side effects than lithium, which was helpful in encouraging him to continue taking his medication regularly. In psychotherapy, Carl and his therapist focused on processing what he was learning in AA as well as on mood-monitoring skills for managing his bipolar disorder. Carl will continue to live with Sharon until he feels stable enough to look for a job and begin to support himself again.

Dr. Tobin's reflections: Carl's case is somewhat unusual in that many individuals who experience substance abuse and/or dependence begin abusing substances earlier in life. Carl, on the other hand, had been able to refrain from drinking for many years until he was tempted by his boss. Until that point, he showed good insight in his awareness that he may be genetically predisposed to alcohol use disorder, based on his parents' history. In therapy, he can explore the reasons he began drinking in order to gain approval from his boss.

Carl's case is also a good example of the destructive combination of alcohol use disorder and a psychological disorder. Such comorbidity is not rare, especially among those suffering from mood disorders, due to the self-medicating effects that alcohol sometimes offers. Fortunately, alcohol use disorders typically have a good prognosis after appropriate intervention, and they are not incurable.

Carl will have to work hard at staying sober and monitoring his bipolar disorder. Much of the focus of his treatment will be on keeping his mood stable in order to prevent relapsing into alcohol abuse in the future. Fortunately, he appears highly motivated to remain abstinent from alcohol and get his life back in order. Finding a supportive AA group in which he feels he can trust the other members is a crucial aspect of his treatment and will be a wonderful source of support that will help him through his recovery.

SUMMARY

- A substance is a chemical that alters a person's mood or behavior when smoked, injected, drunk, inhaled, or ingested. Substance use disorder is a cluster of cognitive, behavioral, and physiological symptoms indicating that the individual uses a substance despite significant substance-related problems. Specifiers indicate such factors as whether use occurs in a controlled environment.
- Substance intoxication is the temporary maladaptive experience of behavioral or psychological changes that are due to the accumulation of a substance in the body. When some substances are discontinued, people may experience symptoms of substance withdrawal that involve a set of physical and psychological disturbances. Tolerance occurs when an individual requires increasingly greater amounts of the substance in order to achieve its desired effects or when the person feels less of an effect after using the same amount of the substance.
- The short-term effects of alcohol use are appealing to many people because of the sedating qualities of this substance, although side effects such as hangovers cause distress. The long-term effects of heavy use are worrisome and include serious harm to many organs of the body, resulting in medical problems and possibly dementia.
- In the realm of biological contributors to alcohol use disorder, researchers have focused on the role of genetics in light of the fact that dependence runs in families. This line of research has focused on markers and genetic mapping. Psychological theories focus on concepts derived from behavioral theory, as well as cognitive behavioral and social learning perspectives. For example, according to the widely accepted alcohol expectancy model, people with alcohol use disorder develop problematic beliefs about alcohol early in life through reinforcement and observational learning. Researchers and theorists working within the sociocultural perspective regard

stressors within the family, community, and culture as factors that lead the person to develop alcohol use disorder.

- Clinicians may derive treatment for alcohol problems in varying degrees from each of the three perspectives. In biological terms, medications may be used to control symptoms of withdrawal, to control symptoms associated with coexisting conditions, or to provoke nausea following alcohol ingestion. Clinicians use various psychological interventions, the most effective of which are based on behavioral and cognitive behavioral techniques.
- Stimulants have an activating effect on the nervous system. Amphetamines in moderate amounts cause euphoria, increased confidence, talkativeness, and energy. In higher doses, the user has more intense reactions and over time can become addicted and develop psychotic symptoms. Cocaine users experience stimulating effects for a shorter period of time that are nevertheless quite intense. In moderate doses, cocaine leads to euphoria, sexual excitement, potency, energy, and talkativeness. At higher doses, psychotic symptoms may develop. In addition to disturbing psychological symptoms, serious medical problems can arise from the use of cocaine.
- Cannabis, or marijuana, causes altered perception and bodily sensations, as well as maladaptive behavioral and psychological reactions. Most of the acute effects of cannabis intoxication are reversible, but a long period of abuse is likely to lead to dependence and adverse psychological and physical effects.
- Hallucinogens cause unusual perceptual experiences in the form of illusions and hallucinations. Opioids include naturally occurring substances (morphine and opium) as well as semi-synthetic drugs (heroin) and synthetic drugs (methadone). Opioid users experience a rush characterized by a range of psychological reactions as well as intense bodily sensations, some of which reflect life-threatening symptoms, particularly during episodes of withdrawal. Sedatives, hypnotics, and anxiolytics are substances that induce relaxation, sleep, tranquility, and reduced awareness. Although not typically regarded as an abused substance, caffeine in high doses can cause a number of psychological and physical problems. Nicotine, the psychoactive chemical found in tobacco, is highly addictive. Withdrawal from nicotine can result in mood and behavior disturbances.
- Various treatment programs for people with substance-related disorders have emerged within the biopsychosocial perspective. Biological treatment may include the prescription of substances that block or reduce cravings. Behavioral treatment relies on techniques such as contingency management, while clinicians utilize cognitive behavioral techniques to help clients modify their thoughts, expectancies, and behaviors associated with drug use. Detailedrelapse-prevention plans are an important part of alcohol treatment programs.
- Gambling disorder is characterized by the persistent urge to gamble. Individuals with this disorder may feel unable to stop themselves from participating in gambling events or games, even after they have experienced significant financial and material losses. The pathways model of gambling disorder provides a model for understanding and treatment of this widespread and debilitating disorder.

KEY TERMS

Acamprosate
Alcohol myopia theory
Alcohol expectancy theory
Amphetamine
Anterograde amnesia
Anxiolytic
Binge alcohol use
Buprenorphine
Caffeine
Cocaine
Depressant
Disulfiram
Dual-process theory
Ecstasy (MDMA)
Gambling disorder
Hallucinogens
Heavy alcohol use
Heroin
Hypnotic
Inhalants
Korsakoff's syndrome
Lysergic acid diethylamide (LSD)
Marijuana
Methadone
Methamphetamine
Naltrexone
Nicotine
Opioid
Pathways model
Peyote
Phencyclidine (PCP)
Potentiation
Psilocybin
Relapse prevention
Retrograde amnesia
Sedative
Stimulant
Substance
Substance intoxication
Substance use disorder
Substance-induced disorders
Tolerance
Wernicke's disease
Withdrawal

Neurocognitive Disorders

CHAPTER 13

OUTLINE

Learning Objectives

13.1 Describe characteristics of neurocognitive disorders.

13.2 Identify the symptoms of delirium.

13.3 Understand the symptoms, theories, and treatment of neurocognitive disorder due to Alzheimer's disease.

13.4 Explain the differences among neurocognitive disorders that are unrelated to Alzheimer's disease.

13.5 Identify neurocognitive disorders due to traumatic brain injury (TBI).

13.6 Describe neurocognitive disorders due to substances/medications and HIV infection.

13.7 Explain neurocognitive disorders due to another general medical condition.

13.8 Analyze neurocognitive disorders through the biopsychosocial perspective.

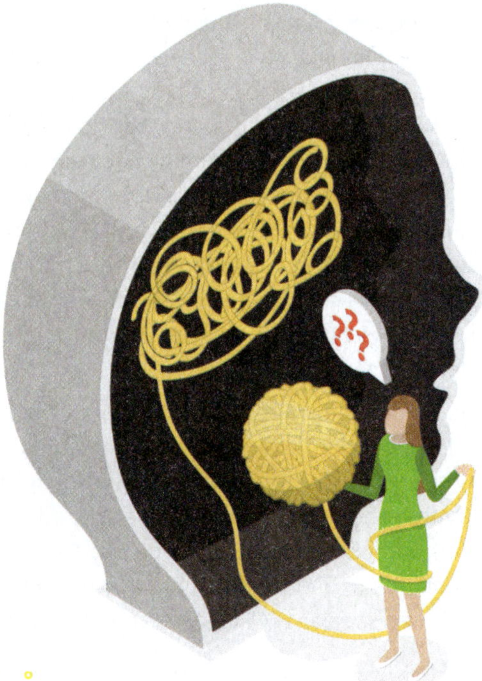

TarikVision/Shutterstock

Case Report

Irene Heller

Demographic information: 76-year-old White heterosexual cisgender woman. Irene's pronouns are she/her/hers.

History of present illness: Irene was referred to a private specialty practice for neuropsychological testing by her primary care physician, who noted a significant decline in Irene's memory and motor functioning from the previous year.

During the initial interview before neuropsychological testing was conducted, Irene was asked about her cognitive functioning. She had difficulty answering some of the questions, and her daughter Jillian, who had accompanied her, provided most of the information. Jillian reported that her mother's visit to the doctor was not the first sign of changes in her recent behavior, and that over the past month she and her brother Steve had noticed their mother was acting strangely. Irene currently lives by herself in the town where her two grown children live. On two separate occasions, neighbors have reported finding her in the parking lot of her apartment complex late at night, wearing her nightgown and looking "totally out of it." The neighbors brought her home, though Irene did not recall these incidents.

When asked about any physical changes she had noticed recently, Irene stated that she was having difficulty writing because she was unable to grasp pens or other writing instruments. As a result, she hadn't been able to pay her bills and sometimes had trouble preparing food for herself. In fact, she noted that she had lost about 10 pounds over the past 2 months because of this. Jillian also reported that she had noticed her mother was having significant walking difficulties recently. Irene preferred to stay at home as a result and had begun to miss out on many activities she had previously enjoyed, including spending time with her family and going to weekly bridge games.

Jillian added that Irene typically called either her or her brother at least once per day, and that they had family meals together once or twice every week. During the past 2 months when she or her brother called their mother on the phone, Jillian said, Irene's speech was sometimes difficult to understand, and she would forget to whom she was speaking. All this was very troubling to Jillian, though Irene wasn't able to acknowledge much of what Jillian was reporting. "I guess I sometimes have a hard time paying my bills or calling my children. I guess I just don't feel like it these days."

Jillian stated that she and her brother thought Irene's behavior might be due to medical reasons. Irene has been diagnosed with type II diabetes and according to Jillian had forgotten to check her blood sugar and take insulin for 2 consecutive days. When they didn't hear from her, Jillian and Steve went to Irene's house to check on her and found her nearly unconscious in her living room. After giving her insulin, the siblings made an appointment with Irene's primary care physician for the next day.

After the clinical interview, Irene completed neuropsychological testing, which consisted of a battery of cognitive tests aimed at measuring her overall cognitive functioning.

Psychiatric history: Irene reported that she has remained relatively healthy in terms of physical and mental health throughout her life and that she has never experienced any major medical, emotional, or cognitive problems. Jillian stated that her mother was diagnosed with type II diabetes 2 years ago and has been taking insulin to regulate her blood sugar. Jillian also reported that until her recent decline, Irene had remained quite active and participated in many social activities, carrying out all her activities of daily living without difficulty.

Case formulation: The sudden onset of Irene's symptoms is typical of neurocognitive disorder due to vascular disease. Since Irene had stopped taking her medication, she was putting herself at significant medical risk. Further, consistent with diagnostic criteria, Irene's functioning was significantly impaired—she had ceased her previous activities and had even stopped paying her bills due to her motor difficulties.

The results of the neuropsychological testing indicated that Irene indeed was experiencing a significant impairment in her short-term memory and her ability to speak fluently and coherently. She also evidenced difficulties in her executive functioning, including organizing and sequencing information presented to her. Taking this together with the physical examination by her doctor, Irene is given a diagnosis of major vascular neurocognitive disorder with

Case Report *continued*

behavioral disturbance, although until she has an MRI to confirm the existence of brain lesions, the diagnosis will be tentative.

Risk level: Low risk. Irene has no current suicidal ideation and no history of suicide attempts.

Treatment plan: Irene will be referred for an MRI to confirm her diagnosis, upon which she will be given a referral for medication and follow-up home care, if needed.

Sarah Tobin, PhD

13.1 Characteristics of Neurocognitive Disorders

The human brain is a sensitive organ which can be significantly impacted by a number of events or injuries, such as trauma, disease, and exposure to toxic substances including drugs. People can develop delusions, hallucinations, mood disturbances, and extreme personality changes as a result of these influences on the brain. The **neurocognitive disorders** specifically describe decline acquired in one or more domains of cognition or other psychological functions associated with alterations in the brain.

neurocognitive disorder
Disorders involving decline acquired in life in one or more domains of cognition associated with alterations in the brain.

Healthcare professionals use neuropsychological testing and neuroimaging techniques, as well as an individual's medical history, to obtain the diagnostic information needed to determine whether that individual's symptoms fall into the category of a neurocognitive disorder. Neuropsychologists who conduct this testing seek to identify specific patterns of responses that appear to match known disease profiles. Combining this knowledge with their client's medical history allows clinicians to examine the possibility that a specific event triggered the symptoms. In addition, neuroimaging provides clinicians with an inside look at the brain to help them connect symptoms with specific illnesses or injuries. Both forms of assessment are required for an individual to receive a diagnosis of one of these disorders.

Table 1 shows the domains covered in the neurocognitive disorders and types of abilities included in each. Clinicians incorporate particular tests from neuropsychological batteries as needed to help assess the client's level of functioning in each of these domains. Using interviews with the client and family members or significant others, they also rate the client as showing major or mild neurocognitive disorder based on criteria indicated within each domain. For example, a mild level of memory impairment might be suggested if the individual relies on notes or reminders in everyday tasks. Major impairment is more likely to be diagnosed if the individual is unable to keep track of short lists or complete a task in a single sitting.

The term *neurocognitive disorders* is intended to signify that fact that these are syndromes whose underlying cause can be traced to changes in the brain. Although the term *dementia* is somewhat imprecise and may have stereotypes associated with it, the *DSM-5-TR* authors recommend that it be retained for use in medical and other health care settings. The term dementia implies, according to the authors, that the individual displaying its symptoms is an older adult rather than a younger person whose impairment is due to brain injury although the distinction is not always made quite so clearly. You will therefore see both terms used in this chapter.

major neurocognitive disorders
Disorders involving significant cognitive decline from a previous level of performance.

mild neurocognitive disorders
Disorders involving modest cognitive decline from a previous level of performance.

mild cognitive impairment
A form of neurocognitive disorder referred to as "mild," meaning that the symptoms have not progressed to the level of severity in the more severe form.

Major neurocognitive disorders are diagnosed when individuals show significant cognitive decline from a previous level of performance in the six domains of Table 1 based on a standardized neuropsychological or other quantified clinical assessment. To be considered diagnosable, these cognitive deficits must interfere with the individual's ability to perform necessary tasks in everyday living, not occur exclusively with delirium, and lack a better explanation as another psychological disorder. The diagnosis of **mild neurocognitive disorder** is applied when the individual shows modest levels of cognitive decline. These declines are not severe enough to interfere with the individual's capacity for living independently. Another term used for this less severe form is **mild cognitive impairment.**

TABLE 1 **Neurocognitive Domains in *DSM-5-TR***

Domain	Examples of Relevant Abilities	Assessment Task Examples
Complex attention	Sustained attention	Maintaining attention over time
	Selective attention	Separating signals from distractors
	Divided attention	Attending to two or more tasks at once
Executive function	Planning	Deciding on a sequence of actions
	Decision making	Performing tasks that require choosing between alternatives
	Working memory	Being able to hold information in memory while manipulating stimuli
	Mental/cognitive flexibility	Switching between two concepts, tasks, or response rules (e.g., picking odd numbers, then picking even numbers)
Learning and memory	Immediate memory span	Remembering a series of digits or words
	Recent memory	Encoding new information such as word lists or a short story
Language	Expressive language	Being able to name objects
	Grammar and syntax	Speaking without errors while performing other tasks
	Receptive language	Being able to understand word definitions and instructions
Perceptual-motor	Visual perception	Assessing whether a figure can be "real" based on its depiction in two-dimensional space
	Visuoconstructional	Assembling items requiring hand–eye coordination
	Praxis	Being able to engage in common motor skills, use common tools, imitate the use of tools, and imitate gestures
	Gnosis	Recognizing faces and colors
Social cognition	Recognition of emotions	Identifying emotions in images of faces
	Theory of mind	Being able to consider another person's mental state based on pictures or stories

SOURCE: American Psychiatric Association. (2022). *Diagnostic and Statistical Manual of Mental Disorders (DSM-5-TR®)*. American Psychiatric Publishing.

After diagnosing the level of cognitive impairment, the clinician next must take on the challenging process of specifying which disease appears to be responsible for the cognitive symptoms. When one specific disease cannot be diagnosed, the clinician can indicate this or suggest that multiple diseases may contribute to the symptoms.

13.2 Delirium

delirium
A neurocognitive disorder that is temporary in nature involving disturbances in attention and awareness.

People diagnosed with **delirium** temporarily experience disturbances in their attention and awareness. The symptoms tend to appear abruptly and fluctuate over the duration of the disorder. The core of delirium is an acute state of confusion or impairment in cognitive processing that affects memory, orientation, executive functioning, ability to use language, visual perception, and learning.

To receive a diagnosis of delirium, the individual must show these changes in consciousness or awareness over a very short period of time, on the order of hours or days. The diagnosis also requires that a general medical condition must cause the disturbance. The healthcare professional therefore specifies whether the delirium results from substance intoxication, substance withdrawal, a medication, or other medical condition(s). The delirium is then rated as acute (occurring in a few hours or days) or persistent (occurring over weeks or months).

Delirium can develop for a variety of reasons, including substance intoxication or withdrawal, head injury, high fever, and vitamin deficiency. People of any age can experience delirium, but it is more common among older adults who have been hospitalized for medical or psychiatric reasons.

MINI CASE

Delirium Due to Another Medical Condition, Acute

Jack is a 23-year-old Afro-Caribbean heterosexual cisgender man. He works as a contractor, and one day toward the end of his shift he collapsed with a high fever accompanied by chills. Luckily, his co-workers saw him. When they told him he would be rushed to the hospital, Jack repeatedly responded with the nonsensical answer, "The hammer's no good." Jack's co-workers were then startled by his suggestions that they were trying to steal his tools. Grabbing at things in the air, he also insisted that people were throwing objects at him. He couldn't remember the name of anyone at the site; in fact, he was unsure where he was. Initially, he resisted his co-workers' attempts to take him to the hospital because of his concern that they had formed a plot to harm him.

In addition to age, the risk factors for delirium include neurocognitive disorder, sensory impairment, a previous history of stroke, and **polypharmacy**, the use of multiple prescription medications (Hein et al., 2014). Infection is another precipitating factor in at-risk individuals. During the COVID-19 pandemic, over half of the patients admitted to intensive care units were affected by delirium (Hawkins et al., 2021). Urinary tract and kidney infections, found to occur particularly in older adults with compromised bladder function, are another source of delirium (Mayne, Bowden, Sundvall, & Gunnarsson, 2019).

polypharmacy
The use of multiple prescription medications.

Diagnosing delirium accurately, given these many possible contributing conditions, presents a challenge for clinicians, with as many as 60 percent missing the diagnosis altogether (Oh, Fong, Hshieh, & Inouye, 2017). Complicating the diagnosis further is the fact that, in addition to the cognitive symptoms of inattention and memory loss, individuals experiencing delirium may also have hallucinations, delusions, atypical sleep/wake cycles, changes in mood, and unusual movement (Tieges, Evans, Neufeld, & MacLullich, 2018).

There are several specialized tests to assess delirium. The Delirium Rating Scale-Revised (DRS-R-98) (Trzepacz et al., 2001) is a widely used measure that has been translated into several languages (Table 2) and has well-established validity and reliability (Gross et al., 2018). The advantage of this scale is that although it was designed for psychiatrists, other professionals (physicians, nurses, psychologists) and researchers can also use it. When completing the instrument, the clinician can use information gathered from family members, visitors, hospital staff, physicians, medical charts, and even hospital roommates.

Treatment of delirium often includes a routine pharmacological approach that relies on antipsychotics including haloperidol and risperidone. However, the appropriateness of this treatment was called into question by a large, double-blind, placebo-controlled trial of patients admitted to hospitals with delirium. Follow-ups with these patients for as long as 90 days after hospitalization revealed no benefits to antipsychotics in survival or in time to discharge (Girard et al., 2018).

Rather than waiting until high-risk individuals develop delirium, clinicians can instead provide high-risk patients with cognitively stimulating activities such as discussions of current events or word games. In this approach, multidisciplinary staff addresses the risk factors of delirium as soon as a patient is admitted to an acute care facility for rehabilitation (after, for example, a hip fracture) rather than wait for delirium to develop (Oberai et al., 2018). It is also important for healthcare professionals to conduct thorough preoperative assessments that can reduce the chances of delirium occurring as the result of the administration of anesthetics (Eschweiler et al., 2021).

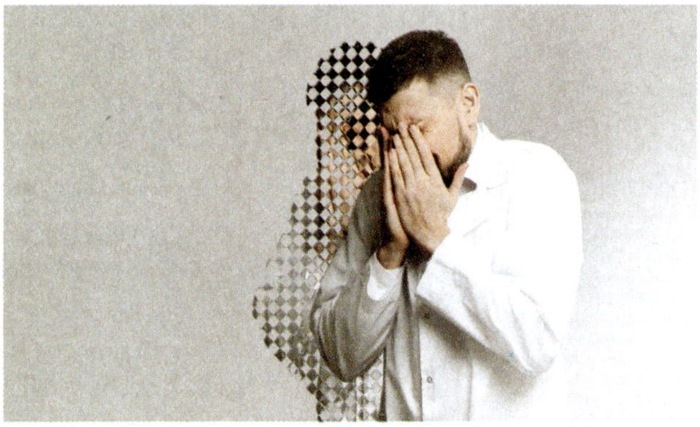

People who experience delirium may have an altered sense of reality, as well as an acute state of confusion.

New Africa/Shutterstock

TABLE 2 Delirium Rating Scale Items

The following items are used to rate the presence of delirium using rating scales developed within each area of functioning:

1. Presence of sleep/wake cycle disturbance
2. Perceptual disturbances and hallucinations
3. Delusions
4. Outward presentation of emotions reflecting instability, lack of self-control, or inappropriate responses to a situation
5. Language impairment
6. Atypical thought processes such as loose associations
7. Motor agitation such as pacing, fidgeting, or restlessness
8. Slowing or loss of spontaneity of motor movements
9. Lack of orientation to person, place, and time
10. Loss of attentional focus and ability to sustain attention
11. Loss of short-term memory
12. Loss of long-term memory
13. Difficulty in navigating one's living area or environment

SOURCE: Trzepacz, P. T., Mittal, D., Torres, R., Kanary, K., Norton, J., & Jimerson, N. (2001). Validation of the Delirium Rating Scale-Revised–98: Comparison with the Delirium Rating Scale and the Cognitive Test for Delirium. *The Journal of Neuropsychiatry and Clinical Neurosciences, 13,* 229–242.

13.3 Neurocognitive Disorder Due to Alzheimer's Disease

neurocognitive disorder due to Alzheimer's disease
A neurocognitive disorder associated with progressive, gradual declines in memory, learning, and at least one other cognitive domain.

Neurocognitive disorder due to Alzheimer's disease is a disorder associated with progressive, gradual declines in memory, learning, and at least one other cognitive domain (see Table 3). The first symptoms of memory loss precede a cascade of changes that eventually ends in death due to the development of medical illness resulting from infection or failure of vital bodily organs. This complex disorder is considered the most prevalent form of neurocognitive disorder, but as you will learn later, may be difficult clinically to distinguish from other neurocognitive disorders. Figure 1 illustrates the progression of the disease in the brain.

TABLE 3 Diagnostic Criteria for Neurocognitive Disorder Due to Alzheimer's Disease

The diagnostic criteria for neurocognitive disorder due to Alzheimer's disease include the diagnostic criteria for major or mild neurocognitive disorder as well as the following:

For major neurocognitive disorder, because Alzheimer's disease cannot be definitively diagnosed until autopsy, clinicians can assign the diagnosis as either "probable" (when both 1 and 2 are met) or "possible" (when only one of the two is met):

1. Evidence of a genetic mutation known to be associated with Alzheimer's disease from family history or genetic testing
2. All three of these symptoms:
   A. Clear evidence of decline in memory and learning and at least one other cognitive domain
   B. Steadily progressive, gradual decline in cognitive functions
   C. No evidence of another neurodegenerative disease or other disease that can contribute to cognitive decline

For minor neurocognitive disorder, "probable" is diagnosed if either genetic testing or family history provide evidence of a genetic mutation, and "possible" if there is no genetic indication, but all three of the above symptoms in criterion 2 are present.

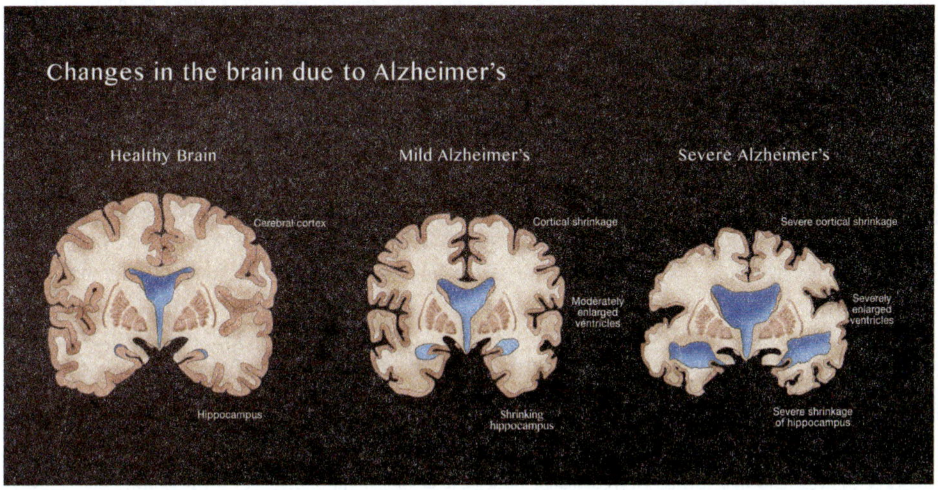

FIGURE 1 The Progression of Alzheimer's Disease

On the left is a healthy brain. The middle brain displays cortical shrinkage, moderately enlarged ventricles, and a shrinking hippocampus, symptoms of mild Alzheimer's. The right brain shows severe cortical shrinkage, severely enlarged ventricles, and severe shrinkage of the hippocampus, indicative of severe Alzheimer's.

Science History Images/Alamy Stock Photo

Alzheimer's disease was first reported in 1907 by a German psychiatrist and neuropathologist, Alois Alzheimer (1864–1915), who documented the case of "Auguste D.," a 51-year-old woman complaining of poor memory and disorientation regarding time and place (Alzheimer, 1907/1987). Eventually, Auguste D. became depressed and began to hallucinate. She showed the classic cognitive symptoms now understood as part of the diagnostic criteria for the disorder. Alzheimer was unable to explain this process of deterioration until after the patient had died, when an autopsy revealed that most of the tissue in her cerebral cortex had undergone severe degeneration. Upon examining the brain tissue under a microscope, Alzheimer also found that individual neurons had degenerated and formed unexplainable clumps of neural tissue. Ninety years later, a discovery of brain slides from this famous case confirmed that the changes seen in Auguste D.'s brain were those of what now is known as Alzheimer's disease (Enserink, 1998). It was actually Emil Kraepelin, a friend and colleague of Alzheimer, who gave the disease its name.

Prevalence of Alzheimer's Disease

To understand the prevalence of this devastating disease, it is important to note that there are many underlying brain changes that can produce similar behavioral symptoms, including memory loss. Researchers recognize that there are large individual variations in aging brains, that more than one factor may be contributing to memory loss in any given individual, and greater sensitivity is therefore needed in order to establish reliable prevalence statistics (Nelson et al., 2019).

Yet, it is important to provide some estimates of the prevalence of Alzheimer's disease, as well as the risk factors that can increase an individual's likelihood of developing the disease. Even if the neurocognitive disorder is caused by factors other than those specific to Alzheimer's, it remains the case that care for individuals who develop a neurocognitive disorder affects them and their families, as well as society as a whole. If there is someone in your life who has this diagnosis, you are certainly aware of the many challenges it can present.

Looking now at the prevalence statistics, the global estimates of Alzheimer's disease prevalence are considerably higher than those from the United States. The World Health Organization (2021) estimates the prevalence of all forms of neurocognitive disease at 5 to 8 percent, with 60 to 70 percent due to Alzheimer's disease. Slightly over half of these cases (58 percent) live in low- to middle-income countries. In the United States, prevalence estimates average 10.8 percent across the 65 and older population (Rajan et al., 2021).

DSM-5-TR notes that detection may vary by culture and settings where older adults face fewer cognitive demands in everyday life. Such variations may contribute to some of the differences in prevalence rate estimates.

What's in the *DSM-5-TR*

Recategorization of Neurocognitive Disorders

Revisions in the *DSM-5* resulted in major categorization changes in the set of disorders that formerly included delirium and dementia. This regrouping is retained in the *DSM-5-TR*. The revisions divided the disorders into two broad groups consisting of major and mild neurocognitive disorders. Among the many controversies pertaining to new diagnoses, mild neurocognitive disorder due to Alzheimer's disease was one of the most heavily criticized. Mild neurocognitive disorder includes an insidious onset or gradual decline from previous functioning but is not so severe as to interfere with an individual's ability to live independently although it may require compensatory strategies in response.

Critics of this category argue that it applies a diagnostic label to behaviors that clinicians would not otherwise consider diagnosable. Moreover, if the deficits do not affect an individual's ability to live independently in the community, the benefits of assigning a diagnosis are not all that clear. An additional problem pertains to lack of accuracy of early diagnosis in Alzheimer's disease, meaning that an individual may believe that they "have" Alzheimer's disease rather than ordinary age-related cognitive changes that may occur.

Another issue pertains to the term *probable* to be applied in the absence of any deficits in memory and learning, but only some loss of abilities and a family history of Alzheimer's disease. The distinction between *probable* and *possible* may be a difficult one for the general public, if not professionals, to grasp. Individuals hearing the terms out of context may not discern the nuance and come to the wrong conclusion about their own, or a relative's, condition.

Stages of Alzheimer's Disease

By definition, the symptoms of Alzheimer's disease become progressively worse over time. However, not all people who show early symptoms of Alzheimer's disease actually have this disease. Figure 2 shows the progression from normal aging through the total loss of independent function in those individuals who develop Alzheimer's disease. There is only minimal loss in cognition in individuals who never go on to develop the disorder. This relatively healthy group may experience memory problems (referred to here as "amnestic mild neurocognitive disorder") but they are able to compensate for them and never develop Alzheimer's disease.

The National Institute on Aging provides a useful summary of the specific stages of Alzheimer's disease (2023a). As you can see, these stages would correspond to those shown in the blue-green line of Figure 2.

Diagnosis of Alzheimer's Disease

Because of the need for early diagnosis to rule out treatable neurocognitive disorders, researchers and clinicians devote significant energy and attention to the development of behavioral tests for diagnosing Alzheimer's disease in its initial stages. An incorrect diagnosis would be a fatal mistake if the person had a neurocognitive disorder that would have been reversible if the clinician had applied proper treatment when the symptoms first became evident. Similarly, if the individual had a disorder with a strictly psychological basis,

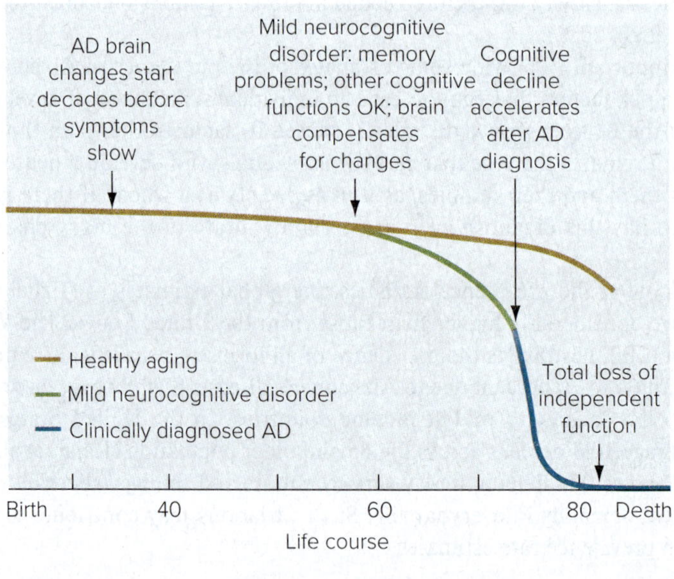

FIGURE 2 Charting the Course of Healthy Aging, Mild Neurocognitive Disorder, and Alzheimer's Disease (AD)

Progress Report on Alzheimer's Disease 2004–2005, U.S. Department of Health and Human Services.

Early stage:
Memory problems that do not interfere with daily life (MCI)
Problems in word-finding
Visual/spatial confusion
Impaired reasoning or judgment

Mild stage:
Greater memory loss
Wandering and getting lost
Trouble handling money and paying bills
Repeating questions
Taking longer to complete daily tasks
Personality and behavior changes

Moderate stage:
Memory loss and confusion grow worse
Inability to learn new things
Difficulty getting dressed
Problems in coping with new situations
Potential for hallucinations, delusions, and paranoia
Behavioral impulsivity

Severe stage:
Unable to communicate
Completely dependent on others for care
Near end of life, cannot get out of bed

the clinician would have missed a crucial opportunity to intervene. Unfortunately, the early symptoms of Alzheimer's do not provide a sufficient basis for diagnosis.

One question that many individuals have is whether the memory changes an individual shows are the result of "normal" aging (i.e., non-disease-related) or a sign of Alzheimer's disease. Figure 3 is an infographic developed by the National Institute on Aging (2023b) that provides a useful set of evidence-based distinctions. Anyone of any age can show one or two of the signs of age-related forgetfulness, but they do become more probable in later adulthood. However, signs of dementia clearly present a greater risk and, if present, would constitute reasons for an individual or their family seeking further diagnostic testing.

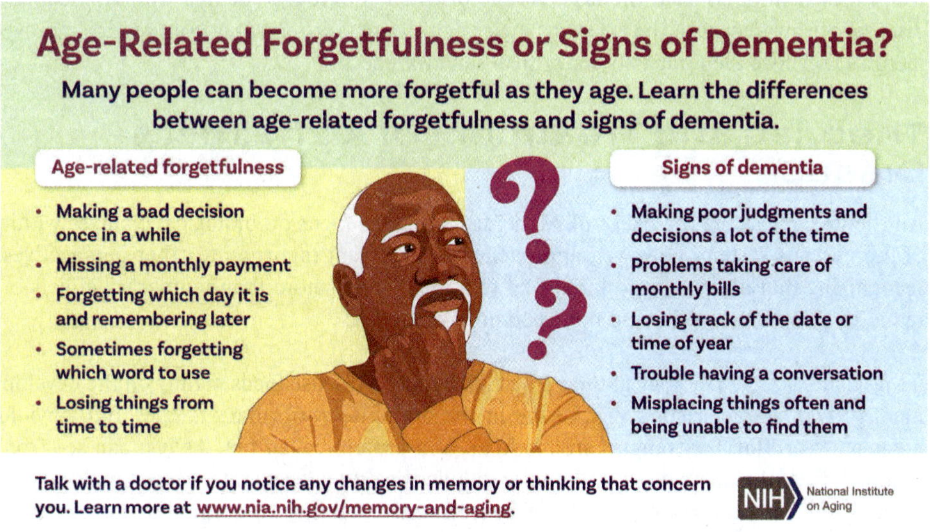

FIGURE 3 Age-related forgetfulness or signs of dementia?

SOURCE: National Institute on Aging. (2023b). https://www.nia.nih.gov/health/infographics/age-related-forgetfulness-or-signs-dementia

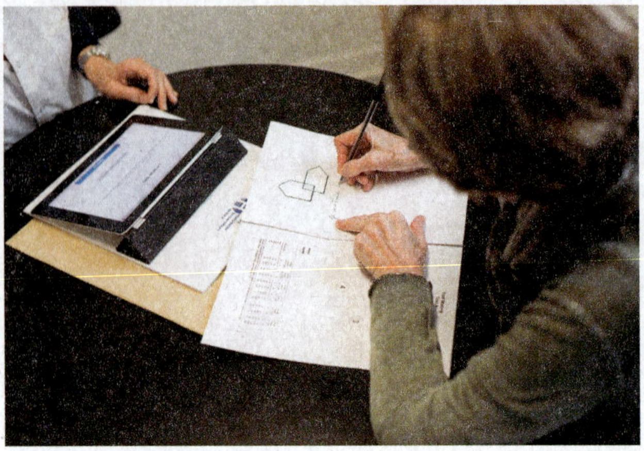

Neuropsychological testing is an important feature of a thorough assessment for Alzheimer's disease and other neurocognitive disorders.

BSIP/Getty Images

Technically, only an autopsy can produce a diagnosis of Alzheimer's disease because it is the only way that pathologists can observe the characteristic changes in brain tissue and structure. However, even though pathologic diagnosis is the "gold standard," it does not completely rule out other diseases or even changes due to normal aging. In one large-scale study of brains donated to the Mayo Clinic Brain Bank, individuals diagnosed in life as having Alzheimer's disease were found, upon autopsy, to have other clinical syndromes that could masquerade as the disease (DeTure & Dickson, 2019).

Although none can guarantee complete certainty in the diagnosis, there are a set of procedures that health care professionals can use to guide the process of differential diagnosis to separate Alzheimer's disease from other forms of neurocognitive disorders. These methods are important for treatment planning, and particularly to detect neurocognitive disorders that may be treatable with approaches other than those currently available for Alzheimer's disease.

As you read in Chapter 3, clinicians can use brief screening instruments to assess the need for further neurocognitive disorder testing. These can be of some value, but clinicians also need to ensure that the instrument is culturally tailored for racial and ethnic minorities (Chodosh, Thorpe, & Trinh-Shevrin, 2018).

Other available assessment measures rely on a multi-faceted approach that incorporates psychological testing with identification of biochemical markers and brain scans. Rather rely solely on family member reports, health professional impressions, or even neuropsychological testing, it is important that the individual receive this set of comprehensive diagnostic procedures. These can include blood and urine tests, collection of cerebrospinal fluid, and CT, MRI, or PET scans. It is important, also, for clinicians to recognize that Alzheimer's disease may co-occur with other brain pathologies, making detection that much more difficult (Devi, 2023). These tests can also help rule out other contributors to neurocognitive disorder, including Lyme disease, traumatic brain injury, sleep apnea, thyroid problems, certain vitamin deficiencies, and excessive alcohol consumption (Alzheimer's Association, 2023).

Adding to the complexity of separating the causes of neurocognitive disorder in disorders other than Alzheimer's is the fact that depression can lead to symptoms similar to those apparent in the early stages of Alzheimer's disease such as apathy (Connors et al., 2023). The condition known as **pseudodementia**, or false neurocognitive disorder, is a severe form of depression that has primarily cognitive symptoms.

pseudodementia
Literally, false neurocognitive disorder, or a set of symptoms caused by depression that mimic those apparent in the early stages of Alzheimer's disease.

Several indicators can help the clinician differentiate depression from neurocognitive disorder. For example, depressed individuals are more keenly aware of their impaired cognition and frequently complain about their faulty memory. In contrast, individuals with Alzheimer's usually try to hide or minimize the extent of impairment or explain it away when they cannot conceal the loss. As the disorder progresses, people with Alzheimer's disease lose awareness of the extent of their cognitive deficits and may even report improvement as they lose their capacity for critical self-awareness.

Theories and Treatment of Alzheimer's Disease

All theories regarding the cause of Alzheimer's disease focus on biological changes within of the nervous system. However, approaches to treatment incorporate other perspectives, recognizing that at present no biological treatments have more than temporary effects on reducing symptom severity and none can provide a cure.

neurofibrillary tangles
A characteristic of Alzheimer's disease in which the material within the cell bodies of neurons becomes filled with densely packed, twisted protein microfibrils, or tiny strands.

tau
A protein that normally helps maintain the internal support structure of the axons.

Theories

The biological theories of Alzheimer's disease focus mainly on the development of two characteristic *irregularities* in the brain: neurofibrillary tangles and amyloid plaques. **Neurofibrillary tangles** are made up of a protein called **tau**. As you can see from Figure 4, in Alzheimer's disease, the microtubules begin to degenerate. Microtubules play a critical role in the functioning of the neuron and its ability to communicate. As these

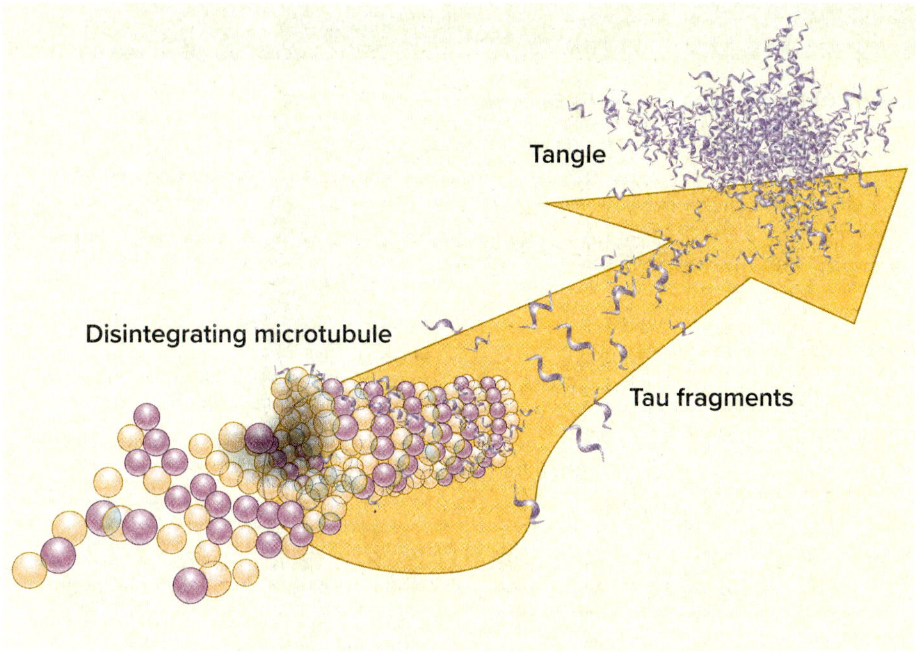

FIGURE 4 Neurofibrillary Tangle Develops over Time

disintegrate, they release fragments of tau, which become tangled among each other. The development of neurofibrillary tangles appears to occur early in the disease process and may progress quite substantially before the individual shows any behavioral symptoms.

A second significant change associated with Alzheimer's disease is the formation of **amyloid plaques**, which are clusters of dead or dying neurons that become mixed together with fragments of protein molecules. Amyloid is a generic name for protein fragments that can form insoluble deposits. The formation of amyloid plaques occurs when a substance found in the brain known as amyloid precursor protein (APP) embeds itself in the neuron's membrane. A small piece of APP lodges inside the neuron, and a larger part of it remains outside. In healthy aging, enzymes called **secretases** harmlessly trim away the extra length of the APP. In Alzheimer's disease, something goes wrong with this process so that the APP is snipped in two places, releasing the beta amyloid. The cut-off fragments of beta amyloid eventually clump together into beta amyloid plaques that the body cannot dispose of or recycle (Figure 5).

amyloid plaques
A characteristic of Alzheimer's disease in which clusters of dead or dying neurons become mixed together with fragments of protein molecules.

secretases
Enzymes that trim part of the APP remaining outside the neuron so that it is flush with the neuron's outer membrane.

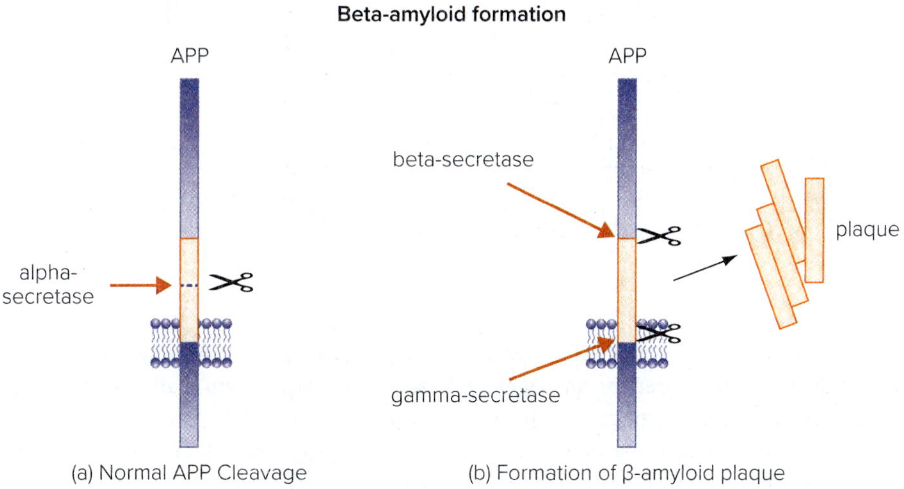

FIGURE 5 Beta-amyloid formation.

Normal cleavage of APP (a) occurs when it is snipped by α-secretase, releasing a neuroprotective fragment along with the snipped APP. In the formation of a plaque (b), the snipping by β-secretase and γ-secretase results in abnormal cleavage and the production of plaques.

You Be the Judge

Early Diagnosis of Alzheimer's Disease

As you've learned there are no treatments of Alzheimer's disease for anything other than its symptoms, and even these treatments can stave off decline for only a matter of months. These problems raise the question whether early diagnosis of Alzheimer's disease through potentially invasive methods such as spinal taps and brain scans would be worth the expense and effort.

On one hand, early diagnosis that rules out Alzheimer's disease is beneficial to individuals who have a treatable form of a neurocognitive disorder. By identifying one of the many other conditions that can lead to severe cognitive changes, clinicians can diagnose surgical, medical, or other rehabilitative procedures to allow these individuals to resume their previous levels of activity and engagement in work, family, and social roles. On the other hand, because the methods of diagnosis are not 100 percent accurate, clinicians might incorrectly tell people who do not have Alzheimer's disease that their condition is untreatable.

Genetic testing can also identify those at risk of developing Alzheimer's disease. But if a person is asymptomatic, what might be the benefits of informing them of a genetic risk for which there are no treatments? The individual could try interventions that seem to have some benefits, such as physical exercise, mentally challenging activities, or avoidance of potentially harmful environmental toxins. There is no harm in engaging in these behaviors, as they benefit most older individuals, not just those with a genetic marker for Alzheimer's disease.

Advocates of early diagnosis argue that knowledge gained from genetic testing can allow individuals and their families to make plans for the future. But if the information were available to insurance companies and programs, including those administered by the government, at-risk individuals could face increases in their premiums or restrictions on how they could spend their assets. For example, if you knew you were going to develop Alzheimer's disease and would therefore require expensive private care, you might divest yourself of your assets by putting money into a trust fund for your children in order to qualify for government assistance with your medical bills.

Pharmaceutical companies advocate for providing medications to people with no symptoms but who show evidence of biomarkers such as high amyloid in the blood, creating another set of ethical dilemmas. These companies stand to benefit from the expansion of diagnostic criteria for the disease, which would increase the potential market for new medications that they are currently testing. However, the National Institute on Aging believes that there is no scientific support for diagnosing people with Alzheimer's disease who show no cognitive symptoms, particularly since the newest medications that would be used for these asymptomatic individuals lack demonstrated effectiveness (Sperling et al., 2023).

These are only a few of the practical and ethical dilemmas raised by the question of whether individuals should receive a diagnosis that can only be "probable" at best for a disease that has no known treatment at worst.

Q: *You be the judge:* Under these conditions, would you want to know whether you were at risk for developing Alzheimer's disease?

These and other microscopic changes within brain tissue do not necessarily result in neuronal death or as influences on cognitive functioning. More significant is the loss of synapses, or the routes through which neurons communicate in the brain. Researchers believe that synaptic loss in parts of the brain responsible for memory and verbal fluency are more significant contributors to symptoms of neurocognitive disorders including, but not limited to, Alzheimer's disease (Overk & Masliah, 2014).

Although researchers are testing various theories to identify the causes of Alzheimer's disease, the most probable is that an underlying defect in the genetic programming of proteins, resulting in the formation of tangles and plaques. The genetic theory was given impetus with the discovery that a form of the disease occurs with higher than expected prevalence in certain families. This form is called **early-onset familial Alzheimer's disease**, and it begins in the unusually young age range of 40 to 50. Other genes appear to be involved in a form of late-onset familial Alzheimer's disease that starts at the more expected age of 60 to 65.

With the discovery of familial patterns of early-onset Alzheimer's disease along with advances in genetic engineering, researchers have identified several genes that may hold the key to understanding the cause of the disease. One particular candidate is the ***APOE* gene** on chromosome 19. *APOE* is a protein involved in cholesterol metabolism but also binds to beta amyloid. Individuals who carry the form of these gene known as the E4 allele are considered to be at higher genetic risk for developing the **late-onset form of Alzheimer's disease**, which starts at the more conventional age of 65 or later.

A number of other genes are being considered in efforts at understanding the genetics of the disease, but rather than examining individual genes as contributors, researchers are taking advantage of the technology available in genome-wide association studies. In this method, individuals with Alzheimer's disease are compared to cognitively healthy older adults matched on age to identify differences in specific gene sequences (Kim, Nho, & Lee, 2021).

The genetic theory is compelling, but it accounts for at most 50 percent of cases of people who develop Alzheimer's disease. The remainder have no known genetic risk, so behavioral factors would appear to be implicated. These include cigarette smoking (Durazzo, Meyerhoff, & Yoder, 2018) and a sedentary lifestyle (Rody, De Amorim, & De Felice, 2022). Conversely, people who eat healthy diets have a lower risk of Alzheimer's disease. The Mediterranean diet includes foods that are high in tomatoes and olive oil, leafy vegetables, low amounts of red meat and an occasional glass of red wine. This can be particularly effective when combined with the "DASH" (Dietary Approaches to Stop Hypertension) diet, which also addresses cardiovascular disease and diabetes (Agarwal et al., 2023). Finally, education interacts with genetic risk for the disease, with more years of education serving as a protective factor (Ferrari et al., 2018).

All of these risk factors are shared with other causes of neurocognitive disorders, particularly those related to disease processes in the cardiovascular system. These common risk factors, and methods of prevention, reinforce the likelihood that the cognitive changes associated with Alzheimer's disease may have other contributing causes than the accumulation of plaques and tangles.

There are two other important implications of research documenting the behavioral risk factors for Alzheimer's disease. First, people can reduce their risk of Alzheimer's disease by avoiding behaviors that contribute to its development. Second, these risk factors also increase the likelihood of an individual's developing cerebrovascular disease, depression, and other causes of neurocognitive disorder. Advances in public health efforts intended to reduce obesity, diabetes, and smoking seem already to be contributing to a slight decrease in the prevalence of the disorder (Knopman, 2020).

early-onset familial Alzheimer's disease
A form of Alzheimer's disease that begins at the unusually young ages of 40 to 50 years old and is more likely to cluster in families.

***APOE* gene**
A gene located on chromosome 19 thought to be involved in the late-onset form of Alzheimer's disease.

late-onset form of Alzheimer's disease
The form of Alzheimer's disease that starts at the age of 65 years old or later.

Treatment

Clearly, the ultimate goal of the intense research on Alzheimer's disease is to find effective treatment, if not a prevention or cure. There is a great deal of optimism in the scientific community that this treatment, when discovered, will also benefit those with other degenerative brain diseases. As the search for the cause of Alzheimer's disease proceeds, researchers are attempting to find medications that will alleviate its symptoms.

The U.S. Food and Drug Administration-approved medications for treating mild to moderate Alzheimer's disease are shown in Table 4 and include galantamine (Razadyne®), rivastigmine (Exelon®), and donepezil (Aricept®), and the potentially disease-modifying monoclonal antibody known as and lecanemab (Lequembi®). Another monoclonal antibody initially approved by the FDA, aducanumab (Aduhelm®), was discontinued following controversy regarding its effectiveness and low sales performance. Another medication, tacrine (Cognex®), also has lost favor as a treatment due to concerns about its safety and limited effectiveness. However, as you can see from the list of side effects, all present significant side effects, particularly the monoclonal antibodies. This category of medications also come at a high price (Leqembi is $5300 per year, with insurance), and their clinically significant effectiveness is moderate at best (Qiao, Chi, Zhang, & Ma, 2023).

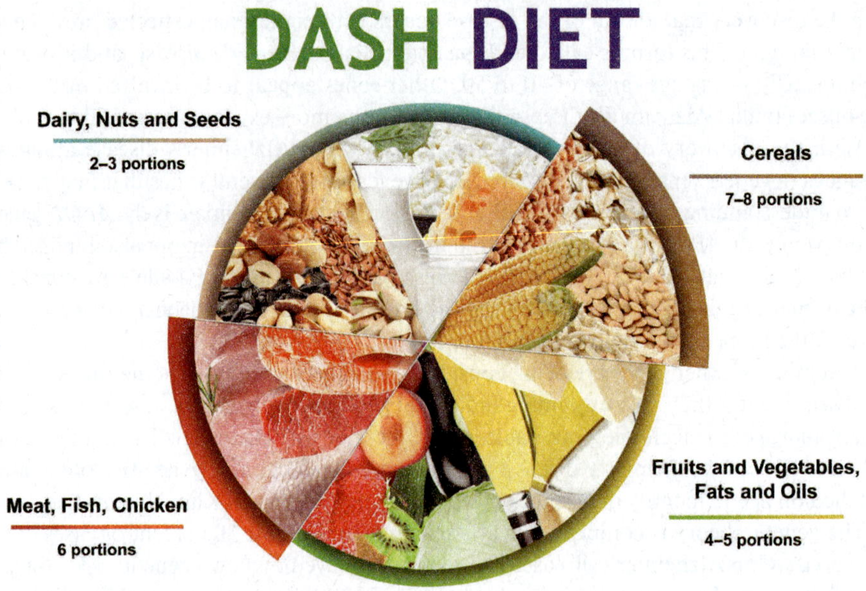

The DASH diet can help to prevent Alzheimer's disease as well as diabetes and changes in the cardiovascular system that can affect cognitive functioning, particularly in middle-aged and older adults.

New Africa/Shutterstock

Side effects: dizziness, headache, visual changes, worsening confusion, brain swelling or bleeding, rare cases of death.

Health care professionals must, for all of these medications, weigh benefits against side effects when prescribing these medications, which themselves may interact with those the individual is receiving for other health conditions, such as aspirin and nonsteroidal anti-inflammatory drugs (NSAIDs), Tagamet (used to treat heartburn), certain antibiotics, antidepressants, and medications that improve breathing.

As encouraging as is the idea that the progressive changes in Alzheimer's disease could be modified by the monoclonal antibodies (the only disease-targeting therapies), individuals with the disease and their families must still confront the limitations of their demonstrated

TABLE 4 Mechanism of Action and Side Effects of Alzheimer's Medications

Drug Name	Drug Type and Use	How It Works	Side Effects
Namenda® (memantine)	N-methyl D-aspartate (NMDA) antagonist prescribed to treat symptoms of moderate to severe AD	Blocks the toxic effects associated with excess glutamate and regulates glutamate activation	Dizziness, headache, constipation, confusion
Razadyne® (galantamine)	Cholinesterase inhibitor prescribed to treat symptoms of mild to moderate AD	Prevents the breakdown of acetylcholine and stimulates nicotinic receptors to release more acetylcholine in the brain	Nausea, vomiting, diarrhea, weight loss, loss of appetite
Exelon® (rivastigmine)	Cholinesterase inhibitor prescribed to treat symptoms of mild to moderate AD	Prevents the breakdown of acetylcholine and butyrylcholine (a brain chemical similar to acetylcholine) in the brain	Nausea, vomiting, diarrhea, weight loss, loss of appetite, muscle weakness
Aricept® (donepezil)	Cholinesterase inhibitor prescribed to treat symptoms of mild to moderate, and moderate to severe AD	Prevents the breakdown of acetylcholine in the brain	Nausea, vomiting, diarrhea
Lecanemab	Monoclonal antibody	Targets amyloid plaques	Headache, confusion, delirium, disorientation, visual disturbances, nausea, and brain bleeding.

SOURCE: "Evaluating Prescription Drugs Used to Treat: Alzheimer's Disease," Consumer Reports Best Buy Drugs, updated May, 2012.

effectiveness thus far compared to the risk (Villain, Planche, & Levy, 2022). In addition to the expense, the monoclonal antibodies require monthly infusions which can only be provided in certain clinics and hospitals. Researchers are hopeful that these drugs may pave the way for further advances that could provide safer and more effective ways to target both tau and amyloid but at present there still remain serious concerns (Imbimbo, Ippati, Watling, & Balducci, 2022).

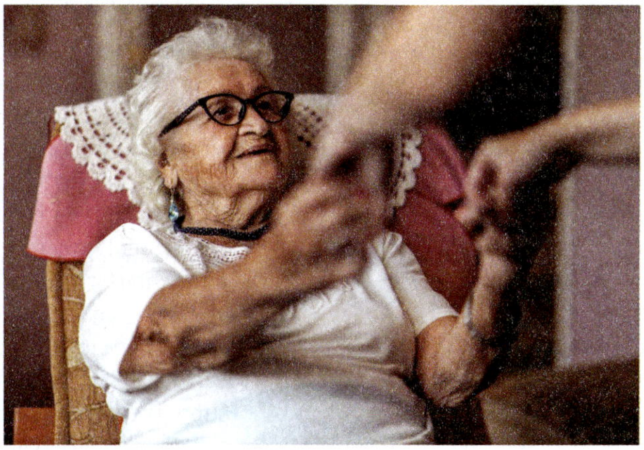

Caregivers can implement a number of strategies to maximize the functioning of older adults with Alzheimer's disease.

pikselstock/Shutterstock

Other approaches to treating neurocognitive disorder due to Alzheimer's disease target the free radicals, which are molecules that form when beta amyloid breaks into fragments. Free radicals can damage neurons in the surrounding brain tissue (Wani et al., 2017). Antioxidants can disarm free radicals and therefore may be another treatment for Alzheimer's disease. Bioflavonoid, a substance that occurs naturally in wine, tea, fruits, and vegetables, is one such antioxidant that can serve to counteract the effect of free radicals on the central nervous system (de Andrade Teles et al., 2018).

Given that no medical treatments exist to cure the disease, behavioral psychologists continue to develop strategies to maximize the daily functioning of people with Alzheimer's disease. They often target these efforts at the caregivers, who are the people (usually family members) primarily responsible for caring for the person with the disease. Caregivers often suffer adverse effects from the constant demands placed on them, effects referred to as "caregiver burden." However, caregivers can learn behavioral strategies that promote the independence of their loved ones while also reducing the frequency of their distressing behaviors. Support groups can also provide a forum in which caregivers learn ways to manage the emotional stress that occurs with their role.

Behavioral strategies aimed at increasing the patient's independence include giving prompts, cues, and guidance for self-maintenance. For example, the clinician can encourage the patient to relearn the steps in getting dressed and then provide positive rewards such as praise and attention for having completed them. Through modeling, the patient relearns old skills through imitation. The caregiver can also learn time management, which encourages following a strict daily schedule. As a result, the patient is more likely to fall into a regular routine of everyday activities. All these methods benefit both the patient and the caregiver. The patient regains some measure of independence, which reduces the caregiver's burden to the extent that the patient can engage in self-care tasks.

Behavioral strategies can also eliminate, or at least reduce the frequency of, wandering and aggression in an Alzheimer's patient. One possible approach, which is not always practical, is extinction. The caregiver ignores certain disruptive behaviors, with the intention of eliminating the reinforcement that has helped maintain them. Extinction is not practical for behaviors that may lead to patient harm, however, such as leaving the house and wandering

MINI CASE

Major Neurocognitive Disorder Due to Alzheimer's Disease, Probable

Ellen is a 69-year-old White lesbian cisgender woman. Her wife took her to her family physician after becoming increasingly concerned by Ellen's failing memory and strange behavior, such as her not being able to remember the names of basic household items like *spoon* and *dishwasher*. Her day-to-day forgetfulness had become so problematic that she would repeatedly forget to feed or walk the dog. As the weeks went by, Ellen seemed to get worse. She would leave food burning on the stove and water overflowing the bathtub. However, she had no family history of relatives diagnosed with early-onset Alzheimer's disease. Ellen's physician sought consultation from a neuropsychologist, who determined that Ellen showed significant impairments in memory, learning, and language. In addition, a complete medical examination identified no other possible causes for her cognitive symptoms, and she did not meet the criteria for major depressive disorder.

into the street. One possibility is to give the patient positive reinforcement for staying within certain boundaries; however, this may not be sufficient, and at that point the caregiver needs to install protective barriers.

Another possible approach is for the caregiver to identify situations that are particularly problematic for the patient, such as the bathtub or the dining table. The caregiver can then use behavioral methods in these circumstances. For example, if the problem occurs while eating, it may be that the caretaker can encourage the patient to relearn how to use a knife and fork, rather than feeding him or her. In one study of nursing home staff, the use of positively reinforcing verbal interactions was found to be related to fewer eating problems among residents (Liu et al., 2021).

The caregiver can implement behavioral interventions through individual therapy or in a support group. The support group facilitator can teach these methods to participants, and caregivers can share strategies among themselves based on their experiences. The emotional support caregivers can provide for each other can be just as valuable as the actual instruction they receive. Ultimately, the Alzheimer's patient receives better-quality care when caregiver burden is minimized.

You can see, then, that although the prospect of Alzheimer's is frightening and painful for all those concerned about the individual, a number of interventions are available. Until researchers find a cure for the disorder, however, clinicians must be content to measure their gains less as progress toward a cure and more as success in prolonging the period of maximum functioning for the individual and the family.

13.4 Neurocognitive Disorders Due to Neurological Disorders Other Than Alzheimer's Disease

The symptoms of neurocognitive disorder can have a number of causes that include degenerative neurological conditions other than Alzheimer's disease. Each of these disorders has a separate diagnosis associated with it in *DSM-5-TR*. Figure 6 shows the overlap among symptoms of these neurological disorders. As you can see, Alzheimer's disease (AD) still receives the majority of diagnoses but also shows overlap with other neurocognitive disorders.

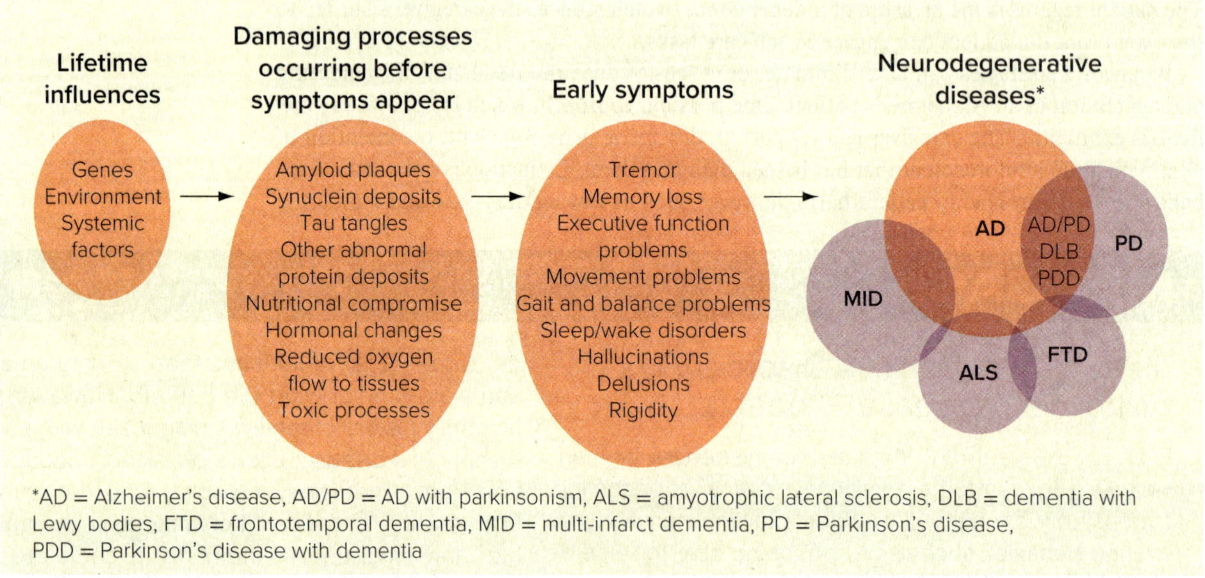

FIGURE 6 Other Diseases That Can Cause Deterioration in Cognitive Function

As shown here, a variety of lifetime influences and damaging processes ranging from nutritional influences to toxins can lead to symptoms that appear to mimic Alzheimer's disease. These disorders may occur along with Alzheimer's disease (shown in the overlapping circles) or may occur independently of it.

SOURCE: *Progress report on Alzheimer's disease 2004–2005.* U.S. Department of Health and Human Services.

Frontotemporal neurocognitive disorder (FTD) is the result of a disease in the frontal and temporal lobes of the brain, damage that leads to personality changes that include apathy, lack of inhibition, obsessiveness, and loss of judgment. The onset of the disorder is slow and insidious, and as it progresses, the individual becomes neglectful of personal habits and loses the ability to communicate.

Neurocognitive disorder with Lewy bodies is characterized by progressive loss of memory, language, calculation, and reasoning, as well as other higher mental functions. The disorder gets its name from the presence in the brain of *Lewy bodies*, atypical deposits of a protein called alpha-synuclein. These deposits affect dopamine and norepinephrine, which in turn affect motor functioning and memory. Individuals with neurocognitive disorder with Lewy bodies experience alterations in mood and movement in addition to cognitive changes.

Cardiovascular disease affecting the supply of blood to the brain can cause **vascular neurocognitive disorder** also known as **multi-infarct dementia (MID)**. In this disorder, temporary or transient blockages develop in blood flow to the brain due to a clogged or burst artery. The damage to the artery deprives the surrounding neurons of blood and oxygen, which causes the neurons to die. Although each infarct is too small to be noticed at first, over time the progressive damage caused by the infarcts leads the individual to lose cognitive abilities. People with vascular neurocognitive disorder show a particular set of physical variations, such as walking difficulties and weakness in the arms and legs, and the pattern of cognitive functioning they experience is distinctly different from that in people with Alzheimer's.

In the typical clinical picture of vascular neurocognitive disorder, certain cognitive functions remain intact and others show significant loss, a pattern neuropsychologists call *patchy deterioration*. Another unique feature of vascular neurocognitive disorder is that the deterioration in cognitive functioning occurs in a *step-wise* rather than gradual progression. A function that was relatively unimpaired is suddenly lost or severely deteriorates.

As is true for Alzheimer's disease, there is no treatment to reverse the cognitive losses in vascular neurocognitive disorder. However, individuals can take preventive actions throughout adulthood to protect themselves from the subsequent onset of this disease. These include management of diet to prevent diabetes mellitus (Type 2) (Sherzai et al., 2016) and obesity (Arnoldussen et al., 2018). The DASH diet referred to earlier therefore applies to prevention of this neurocognitive disorder as well.

Pick's disease is a relatively rare, progressive degenerative disease that affects the frontal and temporal lobes of the cerebral cortex. It is caused by the accumulation in neurons of unusual protein deposits called Pick bodies. In addition to having memory problems, people with this disorder become socially disinhibited, either acting inappropriately and impulsively or appearing apathetic and unmotivated. In contrast to the sequence of changes that occur in Alzheimer's disease, Pick's disease leads to personality alterations prior to the development of memory loss. These personality changes include deterioration in social skills, language deficits, flat emotionality, and a loss of inhibition.

Neurocognitive disorder due to Parkinson's disease is the result of neuronal degeneration of the basal ganglia, the subcortical structures that control motor movements. For example, at rest, the person's hands, legs, or head may shake involuntarily. The muscles become rigid, and it is difficult for the person to initiate movement, a symptom called **akinesia**. A general slowing of motor activity, known as **bradykinesia**, also occurs, as does a loss of fine motor coordination. Cognitive changes occur late in the progression of the disease, but depressive symptoms

frontotemporal neurocognitive disorder (FTD)
Neurocognitive disorder that involves the frontotemporal area of the brain.

neurocognitive disorder with Lewy bodies
A form of neurocognitive disorder with progressive loss of memory, language, calculation, and reasoning, as well as other higher mental functions resulting from the atypical deposits called Lewy bodies throughout the brain.

vascular neurocognitive disorder
A form of neurocognitive disorder resulting from a vascular disease that causes deprivation of the blood supply to the brain.

multi-infarct dementia (MID)
A form of neurocognitive disorder caused by transient attacks in which blood flow to the brain is interrupted by a clogged or burst artery.

Pick's disease
A relatively rare degenerative disease that affects the frontal and temporal lobes of the cerebral cortex and that can cause neurocognitive disorders.

neurocognitive disorder due to Parkinson's disease
A neurocognitive disorder that involves degeneration of neurons in the subcortical structures that control motor movements.

akinesia
A motor disturbance in which a person's muscles become rigid and movement is difficult to initiate.

bradykinesia
A motor disturbance involving a general slowing of motor activity.

REAL STORIES

Michael J. Fox (1961–Present)

At the age of 30, in the midst of a successful comedic acting career, Michael J. Fox revealed that he had been diagnosed with Parkinson's disease. Fox had been a star of television and film for nearly two decades, headlining multiple successful franchises including *Family Ties, Back to the Future,* and *Spin City,* which he was still shooting when he opened up about his diagnosis in 1998. He had been diagnosed several years before, but he had struggled to accept the reality of his condition and continued to work despite mounting physical limitations.

Following his revelation, Fox continued to appear in film and television shows until formally retiring from acting in 2020. Throughout that time, he wrote and published four memoirs, the last which was released in 2020 and became a *New York Times* bestseller. Throughout his memoirs, Fox has been candid about his experiences with Parkinson's, which was diagnosed at a much earlier age than is typical for the disease, and has reflected back on his struggles with optimism and humor.

In Fox's first book, *Lucky Man: A Memoir* (2002), he recalls the first faint signs of the diagnosis he felt in 1990. ". . . I noticed my pinkie. It was trembling, twitching, auto-animated. How long had this been going on I wasn't exactly sure. But now that I noticed it, I was surprised to discover that I couldn't stop it. . . . Throughout the course of the morning, the twitching would intensify, as would my search for a cause–not just for the rest of that day, but for months to follow. The true answer was elusive, and in fact wouldn't reveal itself for another full year."

Fox underwent neurological evaluation soon after noticing these early signs and was told that his concerns did not point to any serious issues. However, he continued to experience more unexplained twitching throughout his body, until a mysterious muscular issue hit him while running on vacation in Martha's Vineyard. After examination, doctors believed his symptoms were related to a botched stunt while filming a recent movie. Following an MRI, however, he was sent to a neurologist and was then formally diagnosed with Parkinson's disease.

At the time, Fox and his wife had a young son (they went on to have three more children together), and following the diagnosis he started drinking heavily and fell into a deep depression. He eventually started seeing a therapist and quit drinking, while working with doctors to find the best treatment and medical procedures necessary to fight the disease. In 1998, he underwent brain surgery to help with a tremor on his left side. Fox continued to work on the show *Spin City*, despite often running into challenges while trying to manage his Parkinson's disease.

In his 2009 memoir *Always Looking Up* (Fox, 2009), he writes, "In a futile attempt to be 'on' at the optimal times–that is, when I was performing–I would try to get through my producing duties with as little levodopa [or L-Dopa, the synthetic dopamine that Parkinson's patients take to control symptoms] in my system as possible, so that when I had to act, I could up the dose and be steady in front of the cameras. Rarely, if ever, did I get it right. Getting it wrong–erring on the side of too much levodopa–brought on a torrent of dyskinesias; uncontrollable movements like undulating, weaving, rocking, and bobbing. The cruel joke was that I didn't notice it as much going through my paces as I did afterward when I watched the footage in the editing room." Despite his best efforts to mask his symptoms while shooting, Fox worried about his character not having the diagnosis and his being able to "believably pass as physically uncompromised." Eventually he made the difficult decision to leave the show in 2000, believing his career was over due to the worsening of his Parkinson's. He worked with a professional team to find medications and health routines that helped him keep his symptoms at bay. Fortunately, after leaving the show he was able to perform in some acting roles because the disease took unexpected turns, though he never returned to full-time series work.

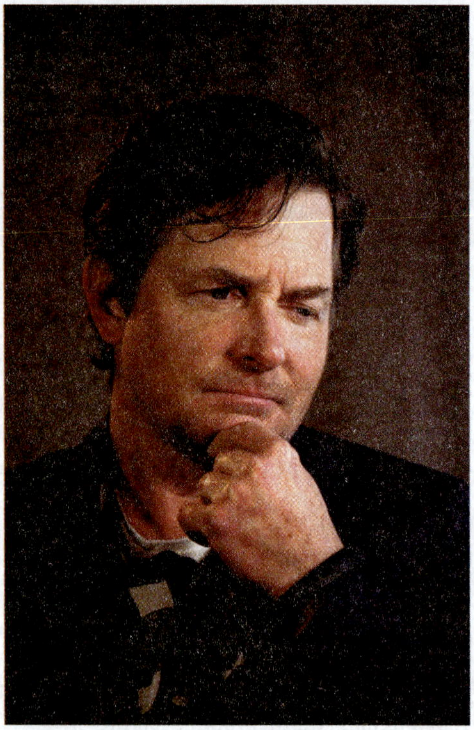

Michael J. Fox, in a 2012 interview.
Trevor Collens/Alamy Stock Photo

In *Always Looking Up*, Fox recalled the impact on his marriage of his struggle to accept his diagnosis, and how he and his wife, Tracy Pollan, grew together through the experience. "Confronted with a complication as seemingly dire as my PD diagnosis, so early on in our marriage, could have left us undone. I, for one, was not a willing supplicant to reality. I was a big believer in my own press: a happy-go-lucky lottery winner who'd had it all–a great career, a beautiful wife, a healthy son. I was struggling, though, with figuring out how to keep it all going. I was working more than I needed to, worrying more than I liked to admit, and drinking more than anyone should. I was, to put it mildly, not well positioned to deal with what was coming. . . . The change that Parkinson's itself has forced upon me and, by extension, Tracy and the family pales in comparison to the changes we have brought upon ourselves. We give more to each other than Parkinson's could ever take away."

In addition to writing about his experiences, Fox has been an active advocate of research funding for Parkinson's disease and has contributed over $1 billion to research through the Michael J. Fox research fund, which he founded in 2000 shortly after opening up about his diagnosis.

In his most recent memoir (2020), Fox shared his thoughts on the recipe for his ongoing optimism in the face of a degenerative disease that has kept him from the profession he loves. Part of it has come from having to deal with other major life setbacks, such as a series of tragedies in 2018 when he unexpectedly lost his beloved father-in-law and had to undergo surgery for a spinal tumor (unrelated to his Parkinson's), which severely affected his ability to walk. Surprisingly enough, a turning point came that year when he broke his arm after a fall. He recalls feeling ready to just give up on life and on the trademark optimism that he had written about in his previous memoirs. But as he had done for most of his life, he kept going and was able to tap into new ways of thinking about how to stay optimistic.

In a 2021 interview (Kennedy, 2021), Fox recalls that this shift came when "I started to work gratitude into all my scenarios. . . . And it hit me, summing it all up: with gratitude, optimism is sustainable."

and loss of ability to perform speeded tasks may develop at very early stages, perhaps even 2 years prior to an individual's receiving the diagnosis (Foubert-Samier et al., 2020).

Neurocognitive disorder due to Huntington's disease is a degenerative neurological disorder targeting motor functioning that can also affect personality and cognition. Following an autosomal dominant pattern, Huntington's disease is caused by a variation on chromosome 4 that causes huntingtin (a protein) to accumulate and reach toxic levels. These cellular changes contribute to the development of uncontrolled motor movements that can interfere with sustained performance of any behavior, even maintaining an upright posture. Eventually most people with Huntington's disease become bedridden. The symptoms first appear during adulthood, between ages 30 and 50.

neurocognitive disorder due to Huntington's disease
A hereditary condition causing neurocognitive disorder that involves a widespread deterioration of the subcortical brain structures and parts of the frontal cortex that control motor movements.

The personality changes associated with Huntington's disease include mood disturbances, irritability, and explosiveness. People with Huntington's disease can also appear apathetic because of their decreased ability to plan, initiate, or carry out complex activities. They may become suicidal. The presence of these symptoms may lead clinicians to incorrectly diagnose the disorder as schizophrenia or a mood disorder, even if the individual has no history suggestive of these disorders.

Neurocognitive disorder due to prion disease, also known as **Creutzfeldt-Jakob disease**, is a rare neurological disorder known as a **prion disease**, which researchers believe is caused by an infectious agent and that results in atypical protein accumulations in the brain. Initial symptoms include fatigue, appetite disturbance, sleep problems, and concentration difficulties. As the disease progresses, the individual shows increasing signs of neurocognitive loss and eventually dies. Underlying these symptoms is widespread damage known as spongiform encephalopathy, meaning that large holes develop in brain tissue. The diseasc appears to be transmitted to humans from cattle that have eaten the body parts of dead farm animals infected with the disease (particularly sheep, in which the disease is known as scrapie). In 1996, an epidemic in England of "mad cow disease" (bovine spongiform encephalitis), along with reported cases of the disease in humans, led to a ban on importation of British beef. Even though the epidemic subsided, outbreaks of the disease in animals can occur, presenting renewed threats to humans (Quimby & Shamy, 2015).

neurocognitive disorder due to prion disease (Creutzfeldt-Jakob disease)
A neurological disease transmitted from animals to humans that leads to neurocognitive disorder and death resulting from atypical protein accumulations in the brain.

prion disease
A disease caused by an atypical protein particle that infects brain tissue.

Another form of dementia that may resemble Alzheimer's disease is limbic-predominant age-related TDP-43 proteinopathy (Nelson, 2019). This disease occurs as a result of dysfunction of the TDP-43 protein, which is critical for normal neurological development and functioning and is involved in other dementias, including FTD (Boer et al., 2021).

13.5 Neurocognitive Disorder Due to Traumatic Brain Injury

Trauma to the head that results in an alteration or loss of consciousness, or post-traumatic amnesia, is called **traumatic brain injury (TBI)**. The diagnostic criteria for **neurocognitive disorder due to traumatic brain injury** require evidence of impact to the head along with loss of consciousness, amnesia following the trauma, disorientation and confusion, and neurological conditions such as seizures. The symptoms must occur immediately after the trauma or after recovery of consciousness, and past the acute postinjury period.

traumatic brain injury (TBI)
Damage to the brain caused by exposure to trauma.

neurocognitive disorder due to traumatic brain injury
A disorder in which there is evidence of impact to the head along with cognitive and neurological symptoms that persist past the acute postinjury period.

In 2020, there were an estimated 214,110 TBI-related hospitalizations and, in 2020, 69,473 deaths. These numbers do not reflect, however, emergency room, primary care, or urgent care visits, or injuries that remain untreated. About one-third of TBI's occur in adults 75 and older, and are associated with falls (Centers for Disease Control and Prevention, 2023).

Nearly 414,000 cases of TBIs were reported in U.S. service members worldwide between 2000 and late 2019, as estimated by the Veterans Administration. Although most cases are mild, TBI carries significant health risks and is a major source of disability (Veterans Administration Office of Research and Development, 2021). Veterans who experienced it are also at higher risk of developing PTSD as well as low quality of life (Jackson et al., 2021).

People undergoing mild TBI may experience a related condition known as **postconcussion syndrome (PCS)** in which they continue to have symptoms such as fatigue, dizziness, poor concentration, memory problems, headache, insomnia, and irritability. These symptoms may persist for years, having a long-term effect on quality of life (Doroszkiewicz et al., 2021).

postconcussion syndrome (PCS)
A disorder in which a constellation of physical, emotional, and cognitive symptoms persists from weeks to years.

MINI CASE

Neurocognitive Disorder Due to Traumatic Brain Injury

Stephen is a 28-year-old biracial heterosexual cisgender man and has been a running back in the National Football League since graduating college 6 years ago. During a game, he suffered a particularly hard hit when another player tackled him. Stephen's helmet came off, and he suffered a traumatic brain injury as a result. He was taken off the field and assessed by the team's medical staff. During the assessment, he was unable to remember how old he was, where he was born, whether he was married, or anything that had happened during the preceding 2 weeks. This inability to remember his personal past was a source of great distress to Stephen. In contrast, he had no trouble remembering the ambulance ride to the hospital or the name of the team physician who first examined him. Following a 3-day hospital stay, Stephen was transferred to a rehabilitation facility for 3 months, where memory therapy helped him learn mnemonic strategies for recalling important information.

Repeated injuries over time, such as those experienced by college and professional football players, may lead to chronic traumatic encephalography (CTE), which causes a form of neurocognitive disorder and can lead to premature death. Football players with a history of repeated head injury appear to be most at risk for development of this form of brain damage (Alosco et al., 2020). CTE's effects appear to be attributable, at least in part, to alterations in tau proteins, leading to the development of neurofibrillary tangles in areas of the brain active in both motor control and cognitive functioning (Mufson et al., 2016).

There are sociocultural contributions to TBI's as well in terms of availability of treatment. The Centers of Disease Control and Prevention (2023) notes that members of marginalized communities, particularly those who identify as non-Hispanic Black and Hispanic, are less likely to receive care, including rehabilitation, compared to non-Hispanic white adults. As a result, they are more likely to suffer adverse psychosocial, functional, and employment outcomes.

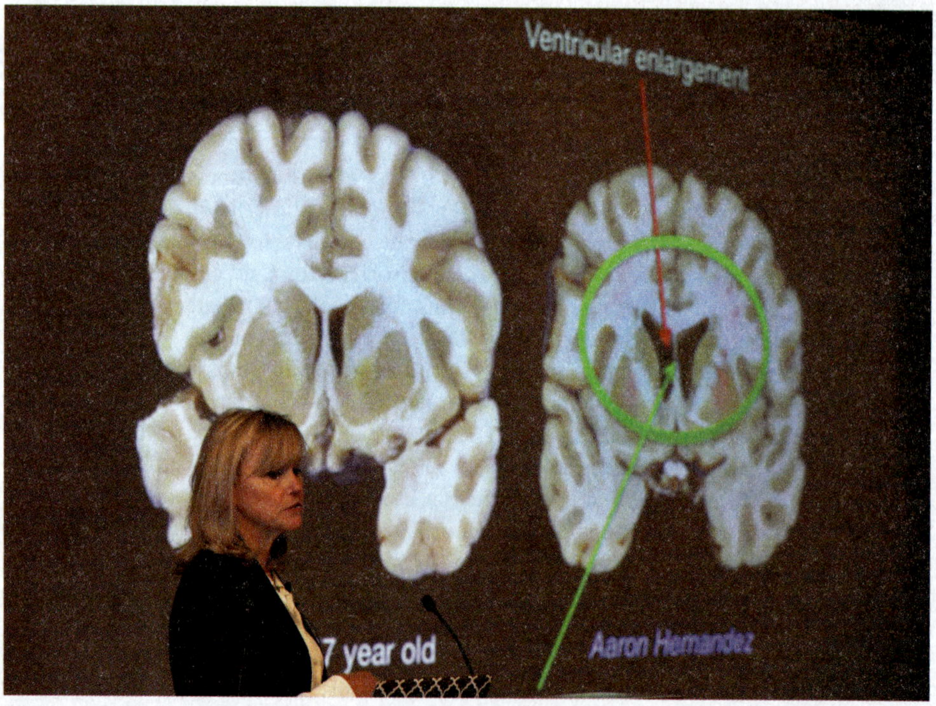

Dr. Ann McKee addresses an audience at Boston University in 2017 about the study of CTE in former NFL star Aaron Hernandez's brain.

Boston Globe/Getty Images

13.6 Neurocognitive Disorders Due to Substances/Medications and HIV Infection

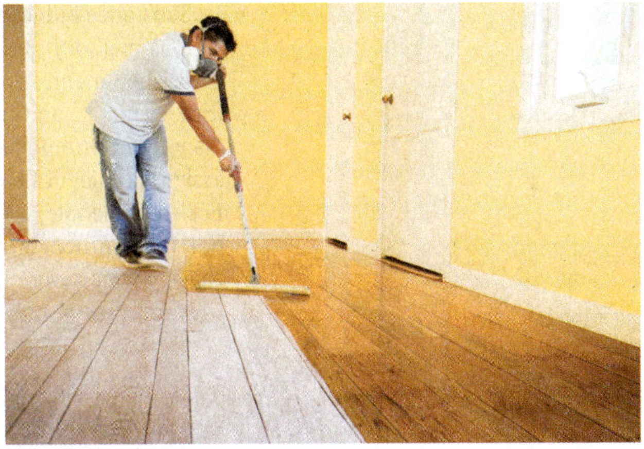

Exposure to environmental toxins can increase the risk of an individual's development of a substance-induced neurocognitive disorder.

Sollina Images/Blend Images LLC

A wide range of infectious diseases can cause the changes that occur with neurocognitive disorder. These include neurosyphilis, encephalitis, tuberculosis, meningitis, human immunodeficiency virus (HIV), and localized infections in the brain. People who experience kidney failure may have symptoms of neurocognitive disorder as a result of the toxic accumulation of substances that the kidneys cannot cleanse from the blood. Brain tumors can also result in cognitive impairments and other symptoms of neurocognitive disorder.

The individual's cognitive functioning can also be negatively affected by **anoxia**, or oxygen deprivation to the brain, which may occur during surgery under general anesthesia or as a result of carbon monoxide poisoning. Anoxia can have severe effects on many brain functions because neurons die quickly if they are deprived of oxygen. Because brain neurons do not replace themselves, significant neuron loss can lead to impairments in concrete thinking and functions such as new learning ability, attention, concentration, and tracking. The emotional effects of brain damage due to anoxia can include affective dulling and disinhibition, as well as depression. These changes can drastically reduce the person's ability to plan, initiate, and carry out activities.

anoxia
Oxygen deprivation to the brain.

Exposure to certain drugs and environmental toxins can cause brain damage and result in a condition called substance/medication-induced neurocognitive disorder. Such toxins can come from intense fumes from house paint, styrene used in plastics manufacturing, and fuels distilled from petroleum.

In the early research on COVID-19 collected in its first year (2020), researchers began to identify potential long-term cognitive consequences (Riederer & ter Meulen, 2020). Studies conducted in 2021 on adults ranging from 18 to 85 years old confirmed that even those who did not report cognitive impairments performed more poorly on a number of neuropsychological tests, potentially creating significant disability and poorer quality of life (Ariza et al., 2022).

Another source of cognitive decline is malnutrition. People who are severely undernourished are prone to develop a deficiency of folate, a critical nutrient, leading to progressive cerebral atrophy. If the deficiency is not corrected by dietary improvements, the individual can become depressed and show various cognitive impairments, such as poor memory and impaired abstract reasoning.

The cognitive losses that occur with physical disorders and toxic reactions may be reversible if the person receives prompt and appropriate medical treatment. However, if intervention for a treatable neurocognitive disorder is not introduced in the early stages, the brain damage becomes irreversible. The more widespread the structural damage to the brain, the lower the chance that the person will ever regain lost functions.

Prior to the introduction of antiretroviral therapies for acquired immune deficiency syndrome (AIDS), the disease that can result from HIV, neurocognitive disorder in the late stages of the disease was a common and devastating complication (Gisslen et al., 2007). With improvements in treatment, this condition, known as AIDS dementia complex, has become less prevalent; however, cases continue to rise among people who go undiagnosed and untreated, a situation particularly common in developing countries (Zhao et al., 2015).

13.7 Neurocognitive Disorders Due to Another General Medical Condition

Amnesia is the inability to recall information that was previously learned or to register new memories. In *DSM-5-TR*, people with amnesia receive a diagnosis of **major neurocognitive disorder due to another general medical condition**. Their memory loss can result from a wide variety of medical problems, including head trauma, loss of oxygen, and herpes simplex.

amnesia
Inability to recall information that was previously learned or to register new memories.

major neurocognitive disorder due to another medical condition
Cognitive disorders involving the inability to recall previously learned information or to register new memories.

Substance-induced persisting amnestic disorder occurs when drugs or medications cause serious memory impairment. An array of substances may cause this condition, including prescribed medications, illicit drugs, industrial solvents, and environmental toxins such as lead, mercury, and insecticides. The most common cause of this form of neurocognitive disorder is chronic alcohol use. The memory loss must persist over time for the clinician to assign the diagnosis of neurocognitive disorder due to another general medical condition. For some people, especially those who chronically abuse alcohol, chronic abusers of alcohol, the neurocognitive disorder due to another general medical condition persists for life, causing such severe impairment that the individual may require custodial care. For others, such as those whose condition results from medications, full recovery is possible.

13.8 Neurocognitive Disorders: The Biopsychosocial Perspective

The cognitive impairments that occur with the disorders discussed in this chapter have known biological causes and are, by definition, linked to neurological changes affecting the brain. However, the biological perspective has not yet produced a viable treatment for one of the most devastating of these disorders, Alzheimer's disease. Until researchers find a cure, individuals and their families whose lives are touched by the disease must be willing to try a variety of approaches to alleviate the suffering. Many research programs are currently underway to explore strategies for reducing the stress placed on caregivers. Some of these strategies make use of innovative, high-tech methods such as computer networks. Others take the more traditional approach of providing emotional support to individuals with Alzheimer's disease and their families. The application of cognitive behavioral and other methods of therapy to help people cope with Alzheimer's is another useful approach. It seems that the bottom line in all this research on understanding and treating those affected by Alzheimer's disease is that it is not necessary for psychologists to wait until biomedical researchers discover a cure. They can do a considerable amount to improve the quality of life for people with Alzheimer's and to help them maintain their functioning and dignity for as long as possible.

With respect to other neurocognitive disorders, such as those that have another medical cause or are the result of injury or malnutrition, the biopsychosocial perspective also provides valuable insights, particularly into the prevention of these disorders. In the case of other degenerative disorders, such as Parkinson's disease, that do not appear to be preventable, clients and their families can nevertheless work toward finding behavioral interventions that can maximize the individual's functioning for as long as possible.

Return to the Case: Irene Heller

Irene's MRI showed multiple vascular legions on her cerebral cortex and the subcortical structures of her brain, confirming her diagnosis of neurocognitive disorder due to vascular disease. The qualifier of "with behavioral disturbance" was added to her diagnosis due to her history of wandering spells that had occurred with the onset of her symptoms.

Following her diagnosis, Irene was immediately started on medication, and after a few weeks she and her family began noticing that she had returned to her "premorbid" (previous) level of functioning. Upon a recommendation made by the neuropsychologist she saw for testing, Irene began to attend a support group for those who have been diagnosed with neurocognitive disorder due to vascular disease, offered in a community center in her town. Irene avidly attends every week and has reported benefiting from the social support of the group as well as learning more about the disease and how it affects each person differently. The support group has also educated Irene to be mindful of any changes in her cognition or motor movements and to immediately seek consultation with her physician should any new difficulties arise. Due to her improved memory, Irene's health remained stable because she was now remembering to take her insulin as prescribed. Irene enjoyed taking part in her regular activities again and spending time with her family, no longer burdened by motor difficulties. Irene will undergo a brief battery of neuropsychological testing every 6 months to monitor for any further deterioration in her cognition and to assess the efficacy of her treatment regimen.

Dr. Tobin's reflections: Neurocognitive disorder due to vascular disease can result from a stroke. Due to the patchy and irregular deterioration of Irene's symptoms, it is more likely that her symptoms resulted from a more gradual process of cerebrovascular disease. In many cases, adults live for some time with mild symptoms of neurocognitive disorder. Irene was fortunate to have attentive children who noticed her symptoms relatively soon after they arose, and she was able to seek treatment that I hope will slow the development of this disorder. She was also fortunate that her diagnosis was based on careful consideration of multiple sources of testing, because many older adults with neurocognitive disorder due to vascular disease are incorrectly diagnosed with Alzheimer's disease, which is irreversible and requires a different course of treatment and case planning.

SUMMARY

- Neurocognitive disorders (former called "delirium, dementia, amnestic, and other cognitive disorders") are those in which the central characteristic is cognitive impairment that results from causes such as brain trauma, disease, or exposure to toxic substances.
- Delirium is a temporary state with rapid onset in which individuals experience a clouding of consciousness during which they are unaware of what is happening and are unable to focus or pay attention. They may have various other symptoms, such as rambling speech, delusions, hallucinations, and emotional disturbances. A number of conditions can produce delirium, including substance intoxication or withdrawal, head injury, high fever, and vitamin deficiency.
- In neurocognitive disorder due to Alzheimer's disease, individuals experience progressive cognitive impairment involving a person's memory, communication abilities, judgment skills, motor coordination, and ability to learn new information. In addition to experiencing cognitive changes, individuals with this condition undergo changes in their personality and emotional state. It is challenging to make this diagnosis due to the fact that some conditions, such as vascular neurocognitive disorder and major depressive disorder, mimic the symptoms of Alzheimer's disease.
- The biological perspective is predominant among theories regarding the cause of Alzheimer's. Current research focuses on variations in the nervous system—specifically, two types of structure changes in the brain. The first is the formation of neurofibrillary tangles, in which the cellular material within the cell bodies of neurons becomes replaced by densely packed, twisted microfibrils, or tiny strands, of protein. The second change is the development of amyloid plaques, which are clusters of dead or dying neurons mixed with fragments of protein molecules. There is no cure for this disease and current medications have yet to produce safe and effective ways to reverse or slow its progression. In the absence of a biological cure, psychological perspectives focus on behavioral interventions, particularly those involving caregivers. Researchers are also exploring the role of certain behaviors in preventing the development of the disease such as exercise and control over diet.
- Neurocognitive disorders can also occur as the result of other disease processes as well as substances or medication. They may also be associated with infectious diseases, including AIDS, which is a disease that can result from HIV infection.
- Researchers are increasingly recognizing traumatic brain injury (TBI) as an important cause of mental and physical dysfunction. Chronic traumatic encephalitis (CTE) is a form of TBI observed in athletes who suffer repeated head injuries.
- Major neurocognitive disorder due to another medical condition is a disorder in which people are unable to recall previously learned information or to register new memories due either to substance use or medical problems, including head trauma, loss of oxygen, and herpes simplex.

KEY TERMS

Aducanumab
Akinesia
Amnesia
Amyloid plaques
Anoxia
APOE gene
Bradykinesia
Delirium
Early-onset familial Alzheimer's disease
Frontotemporal neurocognitive disorder (FTD)
Late-onset form of Alzheimer's disease
Major neurocognitive disorder due to another medical condition
Major neurocognitive disorders
Mild cognitive impairment
Mild neurocognitive disorders
Multi-infarct dementia (MID)
Neurocognitive disorder
Neurocognitive disorder due to Alzheimer's disease
Neurocognitive disorder due to Huntington's disease
Neurocognitive disorder due to Parkinson's disease
Neurocognitive disorder due to prion disease (Creutzfeld-Jakob disease)
Neurocognitive disorder due to traumatic brain injury
Neurocognitive disorder with Lewy bodies
Neurofibrillary tangles
Pick's disease
Polypharmacy
Postconcussion syndrome (PCS)
Prion disease
Pseudodementia
Secretases
Tau
Traumatic brain injury (TBI)
Vascular neurocognitive disorder

CHAPTER 14

Personality Disorders

OUTLINE

Learning Objectives

14.1 Describe the nature of personality disorders and the alternative diagnostic system in the *DSM-5-TR*.

14.2 Identify the characteristics, theories, and treatments of Cluster A personality disorders.

14.3 Identify the characteristics, theories, and treatments of Cluster B personality disorders.

14.4 Identify the characteristics, theories, and treatments of Cluster C personality disorders.

14.5 Analyze the biopsychosocial perspective on personality disorders.

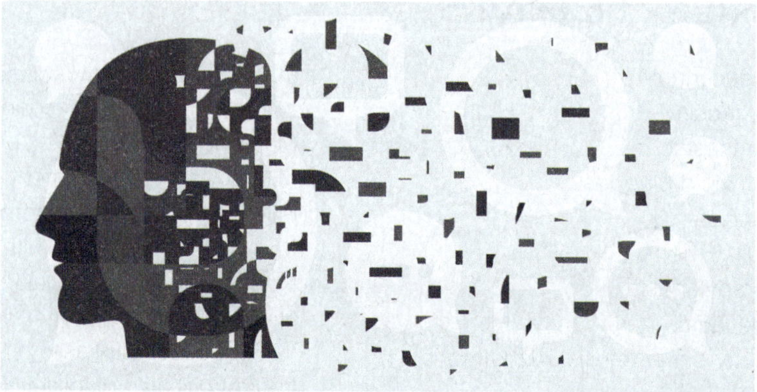

magic pictures/Shutterstock

Case Report

Saman Ahmadi

Demographic information: Saman is a 21-year-old Iranian heterosexual cisgender man. Saman's pronouns are he/him/his.

History of present illness: Saman presented for an emergency intake evaluation at his university's counseling center due to self-reported suicidal ideation in the form of a strong, pervasive desire to kill himself. He presented as angry and emotionally distraught, and he easily grew frustrated with the counselor several times throughout the interview. Saman reported that this was not the first time he had wanted to kill himself, and without being prompted he showed the counselor a large, vertical scar down his left forearm indicating a previous suicide attempt. He said he was 17 at the time he slit his wrist, and that he barely remembered the incident. Following this suicide attempt, Saman had been admitted to an inpatient psychiatric unit and was stabilized on medication, though he discontinued the medication on his own once he was discharged, against the recommendations of his doctors.

During the evaluation, Saman became highly agitated when asked questions about his past, at one point yelling at the counselor and threatening to storm out of the room. Once the counselor was able to calm him down, Saman said tearfully, "I'm just so sick of feeling this way," and agreed to continue with the evaluation.

Saman reported having few close interpersonal relationships. He said he didn't have any close friends at school and had switched dormitories four times during his freshman year alone. He was vague in describing the reason, remarking only that "all my roommates have been total jerks." He denied that any of the roommates had engaged in discriminatory or racist behavior due to his status as a Muslim international student. Saman went on to discuss his history of romantic relationships throughout the past 4 years. Each relationship lasted a few weeks, the longest for 2 months, and they usually ended due to "blow out" arguments. When asked about the nature of the arguments, Saman said in each case he had accused the woman of infidelity and immediately ended the relationship. He described feeling that "no one could ever make me happy. I don't know why I even try. Nothing that I ever do makes me feel better, so I keep trying new things and looking for new people. But none of it works." He related this to his recurrent thoughts of suicide and past suicide attempts. When asked about his family, Saman reported that he was "disgusted" with them and the way they treated him as a child (see "Psychiatric History" section). His parents are living in his home country of Iran, and he reports he has not seen them since he moved to the United States for college. He rarely speaks to them or anyone else in his family.

Saman reported that he frequently abuses alcohol—despite the fact that he identifies as Muslim. He states that he began drinking in college where it was a normal part of the culture. He currently drinks as many as 7 days per week—and typically to the point of blacking out. He explained that he mostly enjoys going to bars and did so with a fake ID before he turned 21. He said he enjoys meeting new people, and drinking "helps me to not be so bored all the time." Saman also reported a history of abusing drugs including marijuana, cocaine, and ecstasy since the age of 13. He had been caught with substances by the police on campus, though he had avoided being arrested. He was arrested for DUI during his freshman year and attended alcohol education classes, which he called "a complete waste of my time." Following the arrest, Saman lost his driver's license, which greatly upset him because he typically enjoyed driving to bars in other towns when he was feeling tired of his own town. He regained his license and had been frequenting bars and drinking heavily until 3 weeks prior to the current intake evaluation.

Saman explained that for the past 3 weeks he had been spending most of his time alone in his room, saying, "Why would anyone want to spend time with such a lousy person? That's why I wanted to die." He had also quit his part-time job at a grocery store and was attending only a few classes per week. He was unable to recall a specific event that had brought on his current depression, and when asked about it, he burst into tears and pleaded with the clinician for help. "I just know I'm going to kill myself." He revealed burn marks on his legs that appeared to be recently inflicted. The clinician asked Saman about his current suicidal ideation, and he was able to contract for safety, meaning he agreed not to hurt himself and affirmed that if his thoughts about death grew stronger he would call the emergency room or the counseling

Case Report *continued*

center. Then Saman asked the clinician whether she could be his therapist. She described the counseling center's policy, that as the intake clinician she could not see clients being evaluated for psychotherapy. "Just like a typical woman," he retorted. "You don't want to be with me. I think you're terrible at your job, anyway."

Psychiatric history: Saman stated that he had attended psychotherapy sessions in the past but had "hated every single one of them," referring to his therapists, when describing why he never stayed in therapy long. He had seen about five different therapists since the age of 14 but described the experiences as "uncomfortable and just weird. They didn't get me." When the clinician asked Saman why he had gone to therapy as an adolescent, he stated, "I think my mom thought I was messed up. I didn't think I needed it." He described his childhood as "a disaster" and his father as emotionally and sometimes physically abusive. He reported that both parents were often very busy with their careers, and so as a child he spent much of his time alone.

Case formulation: Saman's behaviors and reported history during the evaluation match the criteria for a personality disorder as defined by the *DSM-5-TR*, and his symptoms meet criteria for borderline personality disorder. Although he often abused substances, Saman's personality disorder was not a result of substance use and instead was a reflection of the impulsivity and inability to cope with strong emotions that are typical of borderline individuals.

His symptoms of depression for the past 3 weeks meet criteria for a major depressive episode, though it is unknown whether these have been recurrent or whether this was a discrete, severe episode. Given his prior suicide attempts, it is possible that he has had recurrent depressive episodes, though these may be more closely related to the instability that is a feature of his borderline personality disorder. Thus, major depressive disorder was ruled out as a diagnosis.

Risk level: Moderate-high, due to presence of pervasive suicidal ideation, history of self-harm, and past history of suicide attempt. Other risk factors include recent substance abuse and lack of social supports. Protective factors include willingness to engage in treatment and ability to contract for safety.

Treatment plan: Dialectical behavior therapy (DBT) is currently the preferred treatment for borderline personality disorder. It consists of a combination of intensive individual psychotherapy and group therapy. Once Saman had made a safety plan with the counselor, he was referred to a private DBT outpatient program 2 miles from his college campus. Saman was also referred to the psychiatrist on campus for a medication consultation.

Sarah Tobin, PhD

In this chapter, our focus shifts to the set of disorders that represent long-standing patterns of impairments in an individual's self-understanding, ways of relating to others, and personality traits. As we discussed in the chapter "Theoretical Perspectives," a personality trait is an enduring pattern of perceiving, relating to, and thinking about the environment and others, a pattern that characterizes the majority of a person's interactions and experiences. Most people are able to draw upon their personality traits in a flexible manner, adjusting their responses to the needs of the situation. When people become rigidly fixed on one particular trait or set of traits, however, they may place themselves at risk for developing a personality disorder.

14.1 The Nature of Personality Disorders

When does a personality trait become a disorder? When does an individual's characteristic way of responding develop into behavior that may be considered a "disorder?" Perhaps you like to have your living space look "just so." If a roommate or family member moves the furniture around without telling you first, you feel annoyed. However, what if you become angry and insist on returning the furniture to its original position? At what point does your reaction become so problematic that you have crossed over from a being a little picky to showing signs of a personality disorder characterized by extreme rigidity? Should this behavioral pattern place you in a diagnostic category with a distinct set of criteria that separates you from people with other personality traits and related behaviors? These are the questions raised in the diagnosis of the disorders you will read about in this chapter.

What's in the *DSM-5-TR*

Dimensionalizing the Personality Disorders

The history of personality disorders, which are not so much illnesses as characteristics of an individual's core ways of relating to others and experiencing the self, reflects the tension between those who support categorical diagnoses and those who prefer a system of personality trait ratings. Proponents of the dimensional approach argue that we cannot summarize the many complex facets of personality into a discrete set of units. However, clinicians are used to thinking of these disorders in terms of categories. It is more convenient to describe a client as fitting into the "borderline" diagnostic category rather than to list all the personality traits that particular individual displays. Therefore, proponents of the categorical system argue that these diagnoses are a more legitimate way to capture the essence of a personality disorder.

Reflecting these debates, the area of personality disorders received perhaps the greatest attention from clinicians and researchers as they awaited the unveiling of the final revisions to the *DSM-5* in the spring of 2013. To satisfy proponents of both approaches, the *DSM-5* authors initially proposed a compromise that would have included categorical diagnoses for six of the personality disorders as well as a dimensional rating system of pathological personality traits. However, these changes were not implemented.

The *DSM-5-TR* does contain updates to the prior manual, but retains the categorical diagnoses of the ten major personality disorders in its Section II. An "Alternate Model for Personality Disorders (AMPD)" appears in Section III and researchers continue to evaluate, on an empirical basis, whether the AMPD alone provides better diagnostic specificity and validity than the current system.

Personality Disorders in *DSM-5-TR*

A **personality disorder** is a characteristic way of relating to other people, situations, and events, that becomes a rigid and maladaptive pattern of inner experience and behavior, dating back to adolescence or early adulthood. As conceptualized in the *DSM-5-TR,* the personality disorders represent a collection of distinguishable sets of behavior falling into 10 distinct categories (plus one additional "not otherwise specified" diagnosis). Fitting the general definition of a psychological disorder, a personality disorder deviates markedly from the individual's culture and leads to distress or impairment. To fit the current diagnostic criteria, these behaviors must manifest themselves in at least two of four areas: (1) cognition, (2) affectivity, (3) interpersonal functioning, and (4) impulse control. Moreover, as a result of these behaviors, the individual experiences distress or impairment.

personality disorder
A characteristic way of relating to other people, situations, and events involving a rigid and maladaptive pattern of inner experience and behavior, dating back to adolescence or early adulthood.

The 10 diagnoses appear in three clusters based on what the *DSM-5* authors consider shared fundamental characteristics. Cluster A includes paranoid, schizoid, and schizotypal personality disorders, all of which share features of odd and eccentric behavior. Cluster B includes antisocial, borderline, histrionic, and narcissistic personality disorders, marked by overdramatic, emotional, and erratic or unpredictable attitudes and behaviors. Cluster C includes avoidant, dependent, and obsessive-compulsive personality disorders, which have anxious and fearful behaviors in common. The final, 11th, personality disorder is reserved for individuals who do not clearly meet one of the other 10 diagnostic criteria, which is why it receives the label "not otherwise specified."

Clinicians evaluating individuals for a possible diagnosis must decide how many of the criteria a client meets within each category and assign the diagnosis on that basis. In addition to noting the presence of symptoms, as suggested in *DSM-5-TR*, clinicians should take into account a client's ethnic, cultural, and social background which potentially represent adaptive responses to constraints presented by their culture or community. Each personality disorder's diagnostic criteria provide specific considerations for these sociocultural factors.

The prevalence of personality disorders in the adult population, worldwide, is estimated at 3.8 percent (Cluster A), 2.8 percent (Cluster B), and 5 percent (Cluster C). Overall, the global prevalence rate of personality disorders is estimated at 7.8 percent, with higher prevalence rates reported in studies carried out in high-income countries (Winsper et al., 2020).

Alternative Model for Personality Disorders (AMPD) in Section III of the *DSM-5-TR*

Alternative Model for Personality Disorders (AMPD)
A dimensional approach for personality disorders along the dimensions of self and interpersonal functioning.

As you read about in the "What's in the *DSM-5-TR*" box, the categorical diagnostic system as applied to personality disorders has faced serious criticism, dating back to the release of its predecessor, the *DSM-5*. With the **Alternative Model for Personality Disorder (AMPD)** in Section III, clinicians can take advantage of a dimensional approach for enhancing their diagnoses along the dimensions of self and interpersonal functioning (see Table 1).

Because it focuses attention on multiple areas of personality variation in each client, the AMPD allows clinicians to broaden their scope from focusing on a single categorical rating to a more systematic understanding of their client's functioning. Using the trait model makes it possible for the personality "disorder" to be understood along the continuum of the major personality traits. Additionally, the dimensional ratings of self and personality can lead the clinician to ask such questions as how well their clients understand themselves and what challenges might they face in their close relationships.

The authors of the AMPD hope that through this approach, clinicians can make more informed decisions about the functional impairment, potential risks for self-harm, violence, and criminality, and recommended treatment approaches and prognosis. Even if a client does not meet the criteria for a personality disorder, such information can prove invaluable.

TABLE 1 **Dimensional Ratings of *DSM-5-TR* Personality Disorders from Section III**

Personality Disorder	Self		Interpersonal		Personality Traits
	Identity	Self-direction	Empathy	Intimacy	
Antisocial	Egocentrism with self-esteem based on being able to get power	Sets goals based on personal needs; fails to comply with laws or ethical standards	Lacks ability to understand feelings and needs of others	Unable to engage in mutually intimate relationships	Antagonism Disinhibition
Avoidant	Low self-esteem and sees self as socially inferior	Unable to take risks or engage in new activities involving contact with others	Preoccupied with being criticized or rejected	Difficulty forming close relationships unless sure of being liked	Negative affectivity Detachment
Borderline	Poorly developed and unstable self-image; chronic feelings of emptiness	Unstable goals, aspirations, and plans	Unable to understand how others may be feeling	Intense, conflicted, and unstable relationships	Negative affectivity Disinhibition Antagonism
Narcissistic	Excessively dependent on being appreciated by others	Sets either unrealistically high or low standards	Unable to gauge how others are feeling due to extreme self-preoccupation	Superficial relationships; sees others as relevant only in terms of own self-esteem	Antagonism
Obsessive-compulsive	Identity derived primarily from work or being productive	Difficulty completing tasks due to excessively high standards	Difficulty understanding feelings of others	Work seen as more important than relationships	Extreme conscientiousness Negative affectivity Detachment
Schizotypal	Unable to distinguish boundaries between self and others	No clear set of goals	Misunderstands how others are feeling	Mistrustful and anxious about close relationships	Psychoticism Detachment

SOURCE: Livesley, W. J. (2011). An empirically-based classification of personality disorder. *Journal of Personality Disorders, 25*, 397–420.

TABLE 2 General Criteria for a Personality Disorder in Section III

This description summarizes the Section III personality trait criteria from *DSM-5-TR*.

- Moderate or greater impairment in personality as reflected in self and interpersonal functioning (Table 1).
- One or more pathological personality traits (Table 3).
- These impairments are relatively inflexible, pervasive across a range of situations, stable across time, and can be traced back at least to adolescence or early adulthood.
- Another psychological disorder does not better explain these impairments, nor are they attributable to the physiological effects of a substance or another medical condition.
- The impairments are not better understood as normal for an individual's developmental level or social and cultural context.

TABLE 3 Personality Domains in the *DSM-5-TR* Section III Rating System

Negative Affectivity: Experiencing negative emotions frequently and intensely.

Detachment: Withdrawal from other people and from social interactions.

Antagonism: Behaviors that put the person at odds with other people.

Disinhibition: Engaging in behaviors on impulse, without reflecting on potential future consequences.

Psychoticism: Having unusual and bizarre experiences.

SOURCE: Few, L. R., et al. (2013). Examination of the Section III *DSM-5* diagnostic system for personality disorders in an outpatient clinical sample. *Journal of Abnormal Psychology, 122,* 1057–1069.

To use the Section III dimensional ratings, clinicians assign one of six personality disorder diagnoses included in this section and then evaluate the client on the five dimensions described (divided into three groups). The first group of dimensions reflects "personality functioning," defined as the individual's sense of identity and self-direction. The second group includes two ratings of "interpersonal functioning" that tap the client's ability to understand other people's perspectives (empathy) and form close relationships (intimacy). Clinicians rate individuals from mild to extreme in these domains. The third group is actually a single rating of the client on traits related to each of the six personality disorders.

Table 2 summarizes in brief how personality disorders would be diagnosed using the dimensional criteria, and Table 3 defines each of the personality traits listed in Table 1. Keep in mind that this system is not yet in place but is being actively investigated as an alternative to the categorization system in *DSM-5-TR* currently in use, you will read more specifics about the status of the AMPD along with its relevance to specific disorders.

Although these ratings remain provisional in *DSM-5-TR*, the *ICD-11* has moved almost entirely to a dimensional system. Clinicians using the *ICD-11* provide ratings of traits based on the Five Factor Model on negative affectivity, detachment, dissociality (antagonism in *DSM-5*), disinhibition, and anankastia (rigid perfectionism), but they also include a qualifier for borderline personality disorder (Bagby & Widiger, 2020).

As you read about the personality disorders in *DSM-5-TR* as currently structured, think about this alternative system and consider whether you believe the dimensional ratings would help or hinder the accurate diagnosis of individuals with these long-standing maladaptive qualities.

14.2 Cluster A Personality Disorders

Cluster A of the personality disorders in *DSM-5-TR* include those disorders characterized by odd and eccentric behavior. People with these disorders have qualities suggesting they feel different, unlikable, and unable to fit into the social world of their friends, families, fellow students, and co-workers, leaving them with a preference for avoiding interpersonal relationships.

Paranoid Personality Disorder

paranoid personality disorder
A personality disorder whose outstanding feature is that the individual is unduly suspicious of others and is always on guard against potential danger or harm.

People with **paranoid personality disorder** are extremely suspicious of others and are always on guard against potential danger or harm. Their view of the world is narrowly focused, in that they seek to confirm their expectations that other people will take advantage of them, making it virtually impossible for them to trust even their friends and associates.

As an example, consider an individual with this disorder who believes a spouse or partner to be unfaithful, even if no substantiating evidence exists. Seeing an unexplained text on a partner's phone, such an individual will regard this as proof that the partner is having an affair. Indeed, with their guarded behavior and suspiciousness, those with paranoid personality disorder have difficulty establishing the type of interpersonal closeness that helps maintain the quality of a long-term intimate relationship (Disney, Weinstein, & Oltmanns, 2012).

Another manifestation of paranoid personality disorder is the inability to take blame for mistakes, seeing others as being at fault instead. The disorder also shows up as the perception that there is hidden meaning in innocent comments or glances. A real or imagined slight leads to years of resentment.

On the positive side, individuals with this disorder may be relatively successful in certain kinds of jobs requiring that they be on the lookout for threats to themselves, co-workers, or the public. As pointed out in the *DSM-5-TR*, these traits can be adaptive in dangerous political climates in which people must be on guard just to stay alive, or situations where individuals experience oppression or discrimination based on their minoritized status. During the early days of the COVID-19 pandemic, for instance, such watchfulness could have been an adaptive mechanism used to avoid becoming infected with the virus. However, in ordinary circumstances, excessive caution and a high level of suspicion can make it difficult to place trust in other people, even those who love and care about the individual.

Because people with paranoid personality disorder do not see themselves as the source of their problems, they resist seeking professional help. In the unlikely event they do seek therapy, their rigidity and defensiveness make it difficult for the clinician to form the kind of working relationship needed to make progress and work toward any kind of lasting change.

Schizoid Personality Disorder

schizoid personality disorder
A personality disorder primarily characterized by an indifference to social relationships, as well as a limited range of emotional experience and expression.

An indifference to social and sexual relationships characterizes **schizoid personality disorder**. With a limited range of emotional experience and expression, individuals with this disorder prefer to be by themselves rather than with others, and they appear to lack any desire for

MINI CASE

Paranoid Personality Disorder

Laura is a 34-year-old White gay cisgender woman. She is a computer programmer who constantly worries that other people will exploit her knowledge. She regards as "top secret" the new database management program she is writing and even fears that, when she leaves the office at night, someone will sneak into her desk and steal her notes. Laura's distrust of others pervades all her interpersonal dealings, with suspicions that she is being cheated tainting even routine transactions in banks and stores. Laura likes to think of herself as rational and able to make objective decisions; she regards her inability to trust other people as a natural reaction to a world filled with what she calls "opportunistic and insincere corporate ladder climbers."

acceptance or love, even by their families. They are not interested in becoming sexually involved with others. In turn, others perceive them as cold, reserved, withdrawn, and seclusive.

Throughout their lives, people with schizoid personality disorder seek out situations that require only minimal interaction with others. Those who are able to tolerate work are drawn to jobs in which they spend all their work hours alone. They choose to live alone, guarding their privacy and avoiding any but the most superficial dealings with neighbors.

Both paranoid and schizoid personality disorders would have been eliminated in the AMPD. Researchers believe that existing research does not support their continued inclusion in the psychiatric nomenclature because they cannot be uniquely identified (Hummelen, Pedersen, Wilberg, & Karterud, 2015). Furthermore, their names are also somewhat misleading in that they sound as if they refer to a variant of schizophrenia, when in fact individuals with these qualities have not lost touch with reality.

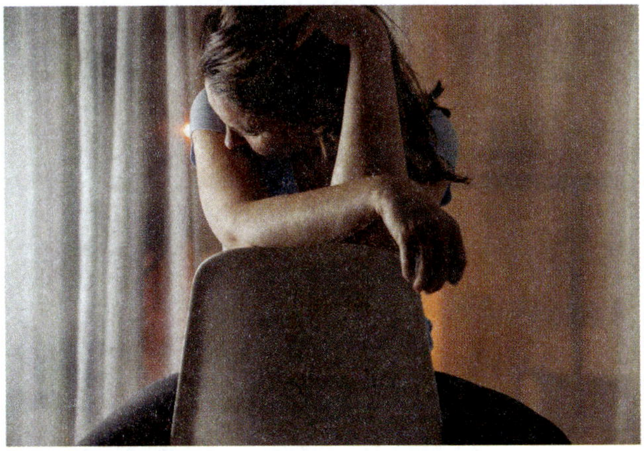

Individuals with schizoid personality disorder prefer to be by themselves, seemingly indifferent to establishing relations with other people.

Small365/Shutterstock

Schizotypal Personality Disorder

Individuals with **schizotypal personality disorder** have odd if not eccentric beliefs, behavior, appearance, and interpersonal style. Unlike the term *schizoid*, the term *schizotypal* implies a connection with schizophrenia, and people who fit this diagnosis are vulnerable to developing a full-blown psychosis if exposed to difficult life circumstances that challenge their coping ability.

The pathological personality traits of people with schizotypal personality disorder fall along the extremely maladaptive end of the psychoticism dimension (Balaratnasingam & Janca, 2015). Thus, individuals with this disorder may hold eccentric ideas, have unusual beliefs and experiences, and have difficulty forming accurate perceptions and cognitions about their world, leading to more negative views about themselves than are warranted by objective data (Cohen, Auster, MacAulay, & McGovern, 2014). They also show a tendency to be high on the personality trait of openness to experience, and at the positive end of schizotypy, individuals have high scores on a factor called "oddity" (Straub & Kerns, 2021). As you saw in Table 1, people with schizotypal personality disorder also have restricted affect and withdrawal tendencies, which reflect the pathological personality trait of detachment.

schizotypal personality disorder
A personality disorder that primarily involves odd beliefs, behavior, appearance, and interpersonal style. People with this disorder may have bizarre ideas or preoccupations, such as magical thinking and beliefs in psychic phenomena.

MINI CASE

Schizoid Personality Disorder

Demetrios is a single 45-year-old Greek American heterosexual cisgender man. He works as a night security guard at a bank and likes his job because he can enter the private world of his thoughts without interruptions from other people. Even though his long years of service make him eligible for a daytime security position, Demetrios has repeatedly turned down these opportunities because daytime work would require him to deal with bank employees and customers. Demetrios has resided for more than 20 years in a small apartment. He has no cellphone or internet, and he has resisted any attempts by other house residents to include him in social activities. He has made it clear he is not interested in small talk and prefers to be left alone. Neighbors, co-workers, and even his family members (whom he also avoids) perceive him as a peculiar person who seems strikingly cold and detached. When his brother died, Demetrios decided not to attend the funeral because he did not want to be bothered by all the carrying on and sympathetic wishes of relatives and others.

MINI CASE

Schizotypal Personality Disorder

Ronan is a single 21-year-old White asexual cisgender man. He is a college junior who has devised an elaborate system for deciding which courses to take, depending on the course number. He will not take a course with the number 5 in it because he believes that if he does so, he might have to "plead the Fifth Amendment." Rarely does he talk to people in his dormitory, believing that others are intent on stealing his term paper ideas. He has acquired a reputation for being somewhat of a "flake" because of his odd manner of dress, his reclusive tendencies, and the ominous drawings of sinister animals displayed on the door of his room. The sound of the nearby elevator, he claims, is actually a set of voices singing a monastic chant.

antisocial personality disorder
A personality disorder characterized by a lack of regard for society's moral or legal standards and an impulsive and risky lifestyle.

psychopathy
A cluster of traits that includes lack of empathy, lack of remorse, tendency to manipulate other people, superficial charm, egocentricity, deception, and a grandiosely high sense of self-worth.

antisocial behavior
The tendency to engage in impulsive and aggressive acts, take risks despite experiencing negative consequences, fail to conform to social or ethical norms, and a history of early behavioral problems or juvenile delinquency.

14.3 Cluster B Personality Disorders

People with Cluster B personality disorders behave in ways that are best described as dramatic, emotional, or erratic. These individuals act impulsively, seem to have an inflated view of their own importance or self-esteem, and are high in the desire to seek stimulation.

Antisocial Personality Disorder

Synonymous in the past with *psychopath* or *sociopath*, the *DSM-5-TR* term **antisocial personality disorder** describes a personality disorder characterized by a lack of regard for society's moral or legal standards and an impulsive and risky lifestyle. One component of the diagnostic criteria includes the presence of **psychopathy**, meaning a lack of empathy and remorse, tendency to manipulate other people, glibness, egocentrism, grandiosely high sense of self-worth, and proneness to deception. The **antisocial behavior** component is reflected in impulsivity, aggression, high-stakes risk-taking, and failure to conform to social or ethical norms. The antisocial lifestyle may also include a history of early behavioral problems or juvenile delinquency. However, as *DSM-5-TR* notes, an individual's social and economic context may render antisocial traits as adaptive.

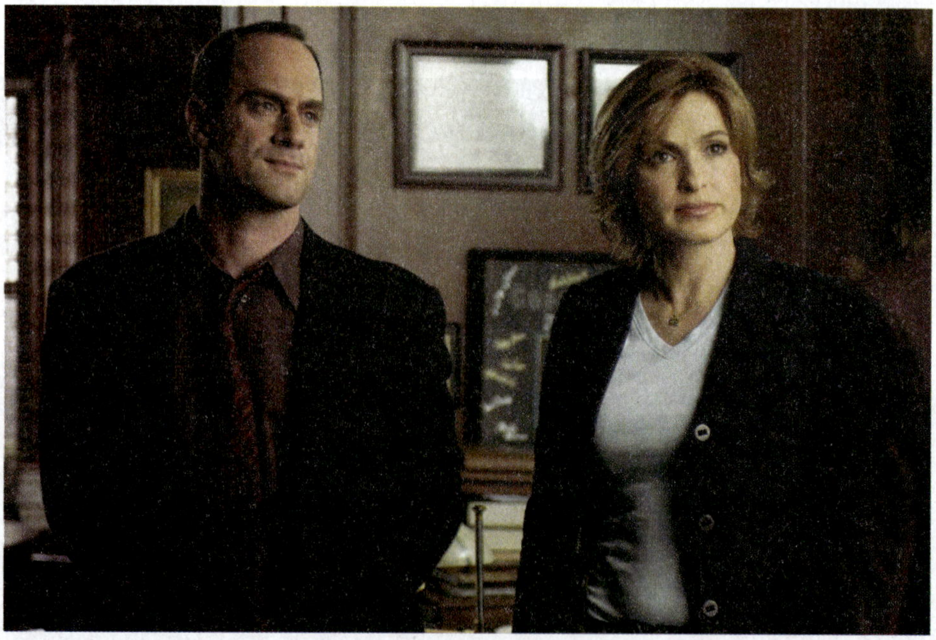

Television crime dramas, such as *Law and Order: Special Victims Unit*, often portray characters who meet the criteria for antisocial personality disorder.
Universal Tv/Kobal/Shutterstock

MINI CASE

Antisocial Personality Disorder

Tommy is a 38-year-old White heterosexual cisgender man. He grew up in a chaotic home atmosphere, his mother having lived with a series of violent men who were heavily involved in drug dealing and sex work. At age 18, Tommy was jailed for brutally mugging and stabbing an older woman. This was the first in a long series of arrests for offenses ranging from drug trafficking to car thefts to counterfeiting. At one point, between jail terms, he met a woman at a bar and married her the next day. Two weeks later, he physically assaulted her when she expressed concern about his incessant drinking and involvement with people she felt seemed "shady." Tommy left his wife when she became pregnant, and he refused to pay child support. From his vantage point now, as a drug trafficker and leader of a child sex trafficking ring, Tommy shows no regret for what he has done, claiming that life has "sure given me a bum steer."

It's possible that a person with antisocial personality disorder may not be all that easy to detect in everyday life. They can feign their regret for harming others to get themselves out of difficult situations when they get caught. You might also find them to be quite charming and likeable, because they know how to present themselves in as favorable a light as possible. "Smooth talkers," they are able to con anyone out of anything, such as asking for money or favors they have no intention of repaying.

The AMPD proposes that antisocial personality disorder be diagnosed on the basis of the personality dimensions, or traits, of manipulativeness, deceitfulness, callousness, hostility, irresponsibility, and risk taking along with the current *DSM-5* inclusion of evidence of antisocial behavior. Individuals who are high in psychopathic traits of a bold interpersonal style that may mask maladaptive behaviors. but do not meet the behavioral criteria would receive a "psychopathy specifier," meaning that their disorder is limited to this set of personality traits alone. However, subsequent research suggests that the psychopathy specifier may not be a valid diagnostic entity (Fuller, Gatner, & Douglas, 2023) and adding boldness does not appear to improve upon the current AMPD traits in terms of diagnostic utility (McCabe, Smith, & Widiger, 2023).

Setting aside these diagnostic considerations, another characteristic that personality researchers regard as important to understanding people who show antisocial behavior bears the fitting term **dark triad** and includes the traits of high levels of psychopathy as well as grandiosity ("narcissism") and manipulativeness toward others ("Machiavellianism") (Jonason et al., 2015). In daily life, such as in the workplace, individuals who have these traits are also highly likely to engage in deviant behaviors that cause deliberate harm to the organization, such as bullying and sexual harassment (Ellen et al., 2021). Another variant of the dark triad is the "dark tetrad," which adds the quality of sadism, which can also be a component of antisocial personality disorder (Wertag, Ribar, & Sučić, 2023).

dark triad
Personality traits that include psychopathy, extreme self-centeredness, and a tendency to regard other people as objects to be used.

The accepted wisdom for many years in the field of clinical psychology was that people with antisocial personality disorder are untreatable (e.g., Wilson, 2014) because they seem unable to experience empathy and do not learn from the negative consequences of their behaviors, they are resistant to approaches using either insight or behavioral interventions. Indeed, the problems of working with these individuals include the very characteristics of the disorder itself: a seeming lack of motivation to change, a tendency toward deception and manipulation, inability to see the world from the perspective of other people, and a lack of deep or lasting emotion (Newbury-Helps, Feigenbaum, & Fonagy, 2017).

What, then, are reasonable treatment goals? Should researchers measure the effectiveness of therapy in terms of rearrest or recidivism (return of symptoms), or should they focus instead on changes in job performance, relationships with others, and engagement in noncriminal activities (such as sports or hobbies) (Salekin, Worley, & Grimes, 2010)?

Reflecting the many difficulties of both working with the population and defining reasonable goals of therapy, at present no one accepted method of treatment has been shown

You Be the Judge

Antisocial Personality Disorder and Moral Culpability

If antisocial personality disorder is a psychological disorder, should people who meet the diagnosis be held responsible for criminal acts they may commit? What about people who have the personality trait of psychopathy? Are they somehow more or less culpable than others? The question of criminal responsibility permeates the ethical literature on antisocial personality disorder and the related personality trait of psychopathy. According to Robert Hare (1997), when the judicial system applies the term *psychopathy* rather than *antisocial personality disorder* to an offender, that offender is likely to receive a harsher sentence because the court perceives the person (usually a male) as lacking any redeeming qualities. Canadian philosopher Ishtiyaque Haji (2010) challenges the idea that people high in psychopathy are mentally healthy and thus responsible for their crimes. He suggests that these individuals have less moral responsibility for their crimes than do people who are not high in the psychopathy trait. According to Haji, the emotional insensitivity that is a hallmark of psychopathy makes an individual less able to appreciate the moral consequences of his or her actions.

Carrying this argument further, consider the factors that may lead individuals to develop high levels of the psychopathy trait. Perhaps their lack of emotional sensitivity relates to a variation in brain development, as some researchers suggest. If they truly cannot experience empathy, how can they relate to the harm they may be causing a victim? Similarly, if they lack the neurological basis for learning fear and thus are less likely to avoid the negative consequences of criminal activity, does this flaw of brain development make them similar to people who have a physical illness? Without the ability to appreciate the punishment that may follow a crime, people high in psychopathy cannot learn from their experiences and seem doomed to continue being "emotionally depraved" (in Haji's words).

The question whether people high in psychopathy have a true impairment that prevents them from recognizing the moral implications of their actions will, no doubt, continue to be debated. Each serial murderer with antisocial personality disorder or psychopathy seems to raise the issue all over again. With increasingly sophisticated evidence on the neurodevelopmental factors that predispose individuals to developing this disorder, we may eventually understand the issue with greater clarity.

Q: *You be the judge:* Should people with antisocial personality disorder be considered responsible for their illegal behaviors? Why or why not?

to be effective in reducing the core features of the disorder (Hatchett, 2015). Nevertheless, clinicians can take a pragmatic approach to helping clients satisfy their needs through prosocial ways, such as cooperation rather than exploitation and manipulation. Motivational interviewing, focused on providing clients with opportunities to connect to core values and the need for fulfillment, can also be of value as a means to help these clients make better life decisions (Mitchell, Tafrate, & Freeman, 2015). Underlying any approach with individuals who have this disorder is the establishment of a strong therapeutic alliance based on the therapist's being firm, authentic, non-judgmental, and attentive (Aerts, Rijckmans, Bogaerts, & van Dam, 2023).

Borderline Personality Disorder

borderline personality disorder (BPD)
A personality disorder characterized by a pervasive pattern of poor impulse control and instability in mood, interpersonal relationships, and sense of self.

The central quality of instability of self and relationships forms the key diagnostic feature of **borderline personality disorder (BPD)**. Diagnosis of BPD rests on the individual's demonstration of at least five of nine possible behaviors: frantic efforts to avoid abandonment; unstable and intense relationships; identity disturbance; impulsivity in areas such as sexuality, spending , or driving; recurrent suicidal behavior; unstable affect; chronic feelings of emptiness; difficulty controlling anger; and occasional feelings of paranoia or dissociative symptoms.

MINI CASE

Borderline Personality Disorder

Deepa is a single 28-year-old South Asian heterosexual cisgender woman. She works as an account executive, and at the office her co-workers view her as intensely moody and unpredictable. On some days she is pleasant and high spirited, but on other days she exhibits uncontrollable anger. People are often struck by her inconsistent attitudes toward her supervisors. She may boast about the brilliance of a supervisor one day, only to deliver a burning criticism the next. Her co-workers keep their distance from her because they have become annoyed with her constant demands for attention. Deepa has also gained a reputation in the office for her seemingly impulsive sexual relationships with several of her co-workers. On several occasions, colleagues have reprimanded her for becoming inappropriately entangled in the personal lives of her clients. One day, after losing one of her accounts, she became so distraught that she slashed her wrists. This incident prompted her supervisor to insist that Deepa obtain professional help.

The symptoms of BPD influence the lives of people with the disorder in a number of significant ways. Their insecurity reaches such an extreme that they rely on other people to help them feel "whole." Even after they have passed through the customary time of identity questioning that most people experience in adolescence, these individuals remain unsure and conflicted about their life's goals. Their chronic feelings of emptiness also lead them to almost merge their identities into those of the people to whom they are close. Unfortunately for them, the more they seek the reassurance and closeness of others, the more they drive these people away. As a result, their disturbed feelings only become more intense, and they become more and more demanding, moody, and reckless. In this way, the symptoms of the disorder become cyclical and self-perpetuating, often escalating to the point at which the individual requires hospitalization.

A term that aptly describes the way people with BPD often relate to others is **splitting**. This means their preoccupation with feelings of love for the object of their desire and attention can readily turn to extreme rage and hatred when that love object rejects them. They may apply this all-good versus all-bad dichotomy to other experiences and people as well. Adding to their difficulties in relating to people are limitations in their ability to read others' thoughts and emotions and poor understanding of the way their own limits affect their relationships (Colle et al., 2019).

splitting
A defense, common in people with borderline personality disorder, in which individuals perceive others, or themselves, as being all good or all bad, usually resulting in disturbed interpersonal relationships.

The intense despair into which they can be thrust may also lead them to perform suicidal gestures, as a way to either gain attention or derive feelings of reality from the physical pain the action causes. These so-called **parasuicides** may lead to hospitalization, where clinicians detect that the act was, in fact, a gesture and not a true desire to end their lives.

parasuicide
Attempted suicide, often a call for help.

DSM-5-TR points out that sociocultural factors should be evaluated when clinicians diagnose BPD, including sex- and gender-related diagnostic issues. Men with BPD are more likely to have substance use disorder and antisocial personality disorder. Women with BPD have higher rates of mood and anxiety disorders, eating disorders, and post-traumatic stress disorder. These differences may account for the previous estimates of higher rates of the disorder in women, whom clinicians more likely encountered in mental health settings. In contrast, clinicians are more likely to see men in substance use disorder programs (Sansone, Dittoe, Hahn, & Wiederman, 2011).

A diagnosis of BPD prior to the age of 19 may signify that the individual may struggle with the disorder throughout their lifespan. In a review of 18 studies on long-term outcomes of BPD among children and adolescents, researchers found evidence that diagnosis prior to adulthood predicted significant social, educational, work, and financial impairment in the years to come (Winsper et al., 2015). Later in adulthood, individuals with BPD may retain certain core personality features, including instability, feelings of emptiness, and constant demands to have their needs met, buy may be less likely to act in impulsive ways. As a result, clinicians need to be aware of different presentations of the disorder in older individuals (D'Agostino, Pepi, & Starcevic, 2022).

Early childhood experiences play an important role in the development of BPD. These include childhood neglect, traumatic experiences, and marital or psychiatric difficulties in the home. The insecure attachment people with BPD have experienced is marked by fear of abandonment, along with the belief that they lack the ability to have close and loving relationships (Smith & South, 2020).

stress generation
The tendency of people with borderline personality disorder to create stressful situations in their lives as a function of their instability and interpersonal difficulties.

emotional dysregulation
Lack of awareness, understanding, or acceptance of emotions; inability to control the intensity or duration of emotions; unwillingness to experience emotional distress as an aspect of pursuing goals; and inability to engage in goal-directed behaviors when experiencing distress.

As they progress through their adult years, people with BPD may face challenges as the result of **stress generation**, their tendency to create stressful situations in their lives as a function of their instability and interpersonal difficulties (Allen, Dombrovski, Soloff, & Hallquist, 2020). Their inability to regulate emotions, known as **emotional dysregulation**, creates limitations in their ability to withstand distress (distress tolerance), as well as avoidance of emotionally uncomfortable situations and feelings (experiential avoidance) (Chapman, 2019). It may actually be this quality of emotion dysregulation that contributes the challenges to clinicians who work with these individuals, as clients high on this quality are particularly likely to drop out of treatment prematurely (Doyle et al., 2023). People with BPD also have a fragmented sense of personal identity, leading them to view the events in their lives as having less coherence (Sajjadi, Gross, Sellbom, & Hayne, 2021). These are all factors that can add to the challenges that these individuals face in finding ways to navigate the adult years.

Nevertheless, treatment for BPD, though challenging, is possible. The treatment with the greatest demonstrated effectiveness is dialectical behavior therapy (DBT), a form of behavioral therapy. Psychologist Marsha Linehan developed DBT specifically to treat individuals with BPD who might otherwise not respond to conventional psychotherapy (Linehan, Cochran, & Kehrer, 2001). In DBT, the clinician integrates supportive and cognitive behavioral treatments with the goal of reducing the frequency of the client's self-destructive acts and increasing his or her ability to handle emotional distress.

Using a process called core mindfulness, DBT clinicians teach their clients to balance their emotions, reason, and intuition as they approach life's problems. Although important for any type of psychotherapy, the building of the therapeutic alliance seems particularly crucial in DBT, and specifically in reducing the likelihood of suicide attempts (Bedics, Atkins, Harned, & Linehan, 2015).

transference-focused psychotherapy
A treatment for borderline personality disorder that uses the client–clinician relationship as the framework for helping clients achieve greater understanding of their unconscious feelings and motives.

Mentalization therapy can help individuals with BPD gain control over their dysfunctional thoughts and corresponding emotions (Caligor, Levy, & Yeomans, 2015). As therapy proceeds, these individuals can apply what they learned in treatment to their outside relationships (Daubney & Bateman, 2015). Another evidence-based psychodynamic treatment for BPD, **transference-focused psychotherapy**, uses the client–clinician relationship as the framework for helping clients achieve greater understanding of their unconscious feelings and motives and can be particularly effective when combined with mentalization therapy (Keefe et al., 2023).

Another approach, known as "BPD Compass Therapy," provides clients with concrete ways to improve on the key personality traits of low agreeableness, high neuroticism, and low conscientiousness. Based on principles of cognitive behavioral therapy, BPD Compass combines principles of third-wave therapies as well as reducing these maladaptive traits as well as the frequency of BPD-type behaviors (Sauer- Zavala et al., 2023).

Regardless of the specific treatment approach they use, clinicians have the greatest success if they follow a set of basic principles (Table 4). These principles set the stage for the clinician to help the client because they focus on providing key features that can be therapeutic for people with this specific disorder. Although many of these principles could generalize beyond clients with BPD, the need to establish clear boundaries, expectations, structure, and support is particularly important for individuals with this diagnosis.

The last principle encourages clinicians to seek support themselves when the client's symptoms lead to difficulties within therapy. For example, the symptom of splitting shown by individuals with BPD may lead them alternatively to devalue and idealize the clinician. In these cases, the clinician may experience complicated reactions and may benefit from the outside perspective of a supervisor or consultant.

TABLE 4 **Needs Involved in Basic Principles of Effective Treatment for Clients with BPD**

Need for Clinicians to:	Explanation
Take over a primary role in treatment	One clinician discusses diagnosis, assesses progress, monitors safety, and oversees communication with other practitioners and family.
Provide a therapeutic structure	The clinician establishes and maintains goals and roles, particularly outlining limits on his or her availability and a plan to manage the client's possible suicidal impulses or other emergencies.
Support the client	The clinician validates the client's emotions of distress and desperation, providing hopeful statements that change is possible.
Involve the client in the therapeutic process	The clinician recognizes that progress depends on the client's active efforts to take control over his or her behavior.
Take an active role in treatment	The clinician is active in therapy, focuses on situations in the here-and-now, and helps the client connect his or her feelings to events in the past.
Deal with the client's suicidal threats or self-harming acts	The clinician expresses concern about and listens patiently to threats, but behaves judiciously (i.e., not always recommending hospitalization).
Be self-aware and ready to consult with colleagues	The clinician may require consultation when the client–clinician relationship becomes problematic.

SOURCE: Gunderson, J. G. (2011). Clinical practice: Borderline personality disorder. *New England Journal of Medicine, 364,* 2037–2042.

Histrionic Personality Disorder

Clinicians diagnose **histrionic personality disorder** in people who show extreme pleasure at being the center of attention and who behave however necessary to ensure that this happens. The diagnostic criteria include excessive concern with physical appearance and constant and extreme efforts to draw attention to self. Flirtatious and seductive, they become furious if they don't get the attention they seek. They want immediate gratification of their wishes and can overreact to minor provocations in an exaggerated way such as by weeping or fainting. As noted in *DSM-5-TR*, these behaviors, to be considered evidence of a diagnosis, should cause clinically significant impairments or stress, and not constitute a reaction to sociocultural factors.

histrionic personality disorder
A personality disorder characterized by exaggerated emotional reactions, approaching theatricality, in everyday behavior.

Their relationships may be superficial, but people with histrionic personality disorder interpret them as being close and intimate. Even their casual acquaintances are "good friends" in their eyes. Their cognitive style is vague and impressionistic, making them easily influenced by others and unable to solve problems on their own. To some extent, individuals with these traits may be successful because of their outward self-confidence and attention-grabbing behavior, but in the long run their flightiness, tendency to flirt, and shallowness lead to instability in close relationships, including higher divorce rates (Disney, Weinstein, & Oltmanns, 2012).

Histrionic personality disorder was once regarded as synonymous with Freud's characterization of the "hysteric" individual (typically a woman). With the decline in psychoanalytic thinking, it has fallen out of use (Blashfield, Reynolds, & Stennett, 2012), and indeed it is considered

REAL STORIES

Brandon Marshall (1984–Present)

Early in his NFL career, football wide receiver Brandon Marshall started to exhibit erratic, emotional, and volatile behavior on and off the field. His legal troubles started in 2004 when he was still an undergraduate at the University of Central Florida, following an arrest on Halloween for assaulting a law enforcement officer and disorderly conduct. As his career in the NFL took off, behavioral and legal issues continued to spiral. In 2007 Marshall was arrested following an incident in which he blocked his girlfriend from leaving his house in a taxi and then broke the window of the vehicle while yelling at her. The charges were dropped after he completed an anger management course (Associated Press, 2007). In 2008, he was arrested for both a DUI and domestic violence, resulting in a fine and brief suspension from the NFL.

At 27 years old, Marshall was gaining acclaim as a player and amassing fame and fortune. He played in six Pro Bowls and was regarded as one of the best receivers in the league. He was never able to enjoy his success, however, because his undiagnosed mental health struggles continued to play out in the form of anger and aggression, especially in his life off the field. In early 2011 during a fight with his wife, Michi Nogami-Marshall, she stabbed him in self-defense. At this point in his career, he often made more headlines due to his erratic behavior and legal troubles, which damaged his reputation within the NFL and signaled larger concerns about his mental health and well-being (Carrollo, 2011).

Due to mounting concerns, in 2011 his agent convinced Marshall to fly to Boston to seek help at McLean Hospital, where he saw Dr. John Gunderson, who had been at the forefront of treatment for borderline personality disorder at the acclaimed psychiatric hospital. Marshall was diagnosed with BPD and completed a 3-month intensive outpatient program, during which he started to develop tools and skills for managing his rapidly shifting emotional states.

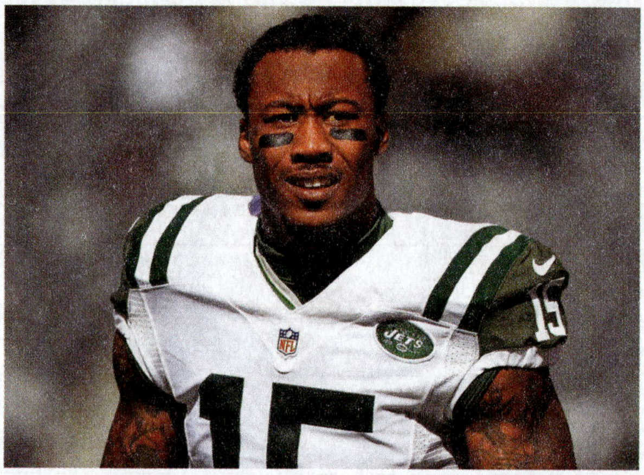

Brandon Marshall of the New York Jets looks on before a game against the Washington Redskins at MetLife Stadium in October 2015.
Alex Goodlett/Getty Images

Of his time in treatment at McLean, Marshall has reflected on how building skills through dialectical behavioral therapy and cognitive behavioral therapy provided him with hope and felt to him like a complete transformation (Associated Press, 2020). Around this time, Marshall also started opening up to the press about his BPD diagnosis, in part to help address his past behavior publicly and to acknowledge that he was making positive changes in his life. He also wanted to send a meaningful message to the world about the prevalence of mental health struggles, particularly for young Black men.

"Nobody thinks of an African American male who plays football as having mental health issues." Nogami-Marshall says. "It's difficult to say 'I need help. I am suffering.'" Brandon Marshall also drew a connection between his social-emotional environment and his difficulties managing his emotions: "It was embedded in me as a kid to never show any signs of weakness" (Young, 2017).

Marshall grew up in Florida and Georgia, and in interviews he has discussed how he assumed that he had to continue repeating the patterns of anger and violence throughout his life, not realizing that emotional issues beyond his control were at play. "I definitely think there were signs when I was younger, but I was a product of a very volatile neighborhood with a lot of violence, drugs and unhealthy living. . . . What I was dealing with was nothing different than the rest of the kids in school. You have kids with emotional issues, kids with anger issues and kids that have many challenges–and I was one of them" (Young, 2017).

After his initial diagnosis and treatment, Marshall remained in the NFL and went on to play a total of 13 seasons. Following his retirement from football, with Nogami-Marshall he created Project 375 Foundation, a nonprofit advocacy center for mental health that in part helps to fund free trainings for Mental Health First Aid. Marshall later recalled on how this work felt uniquely meaningful to him, compared with his experiences in the NFL: ". . . when you are in a position to potentially save a life, that's a phenomenal experience."

In addition to their foundation, Marshall and his wife focus on teaching their children communication, validation, and meditation to help manage emotions, which they refer to as "superpowers" (McAshan, 2017).

In a 2020 interview, Marshall reflected on the importance of ongoing treatment, healthy routines, and taking the time for his mental health. As he notes, these have been invaluable to him, particularly during the COVID-19 pandemic. Through his advocacy he has worked on ensuring that others who are also struggling with mental health issues, and especially those with no treatment background, can find the resources and tools that have been life changing for him (Associated Press, 2020).

a modern-day relic of the history of psychiatry (Tripathi, Messias, Spollen, & Salomon, 2019). Rarely diagnosed and difficult to distinguish reliably from other personality disorders, it was almost eliminated when *DSM-5* was written. Indeed, among all possible diagnoses that clinicians use to describe psychological disorders, one survey found that histrionic ranks among the least-frequently used (8 percent), compared to borderline (36 percent) (Cohen et al., 2022).

MINI CASE

Histrionic Personality Disorder

Lynnette is a 44-year-old White bisexual cisgender woman. She works as an administrator at a local college and has gained a reputation for outlandish behavior and inappropriate flirtatiousness. She often greets students with overwhelming warmth and apparent concern over their welfare, which leads some to find her appealing and engaging at first; however, they invariably become disenchanted when they realize her shallowness. To her colleagues, she brags about her minor accomplishments as if they were major victories, yet if she fails to achieve a desired objective, she sulks and breaks down into tears. She is so desperate for the approval of others that she will change her story to suit whomever she is talking to at the time. Because she is always creating crises and never reciprocates the concern of others, people have become immune and unresponsive to her frequent pleas for help and attention.

Despite questions about its validity as a diagnosis, researchers continue to investigate personality traits associated with this disorder. For example, the "colorful" personality includes people who would not receive the diagnosis but who enjoy expressing themselves in a dramatic fashion, have difficulty listening to others, tend to interrupt, and enjoy being the focus of attention (Furnham, 2014).

Narcissistic Personality Disorder

People who meet the criteria for the diagnosis of **narcissistic personality disorder (NPD)** have as their core characteristic an extreme form of egocentrism in which they see themselves as the center of the universe. A term now in widespread popular use, *narcissism* refers to the excessive self-love and grandiosity (Krizan & Herlache, 2018) believed to be a predominant feature of NPD. Anyone in a relationship with a person who has a true diagnosis of NPD (versus being highly narcissistic) knows how difficult such a person can be to tolerate. Entitled, haughty, and unable to see the world from anyone's perspective but their own, people with NPD seem to show little regard for the people who care about them. Ironically, however, they are highly dependent on the way they believe others perceive them, and as a result they need constant flattery, attention, and reassurance.

The sense of entitlement is one of NPD's most prominent symptoms, but it is a sword that can cut both ways. Because individuals with this disorder see themselves as exceptional, they may set their personal standards unrealistically high, being satisfied with nothing less than perfection. Indeed, as *DSM-5-TR* points out, this perfectionism may place them at risk for suicidal thoughts or behavior. Conversely, they may regard themselves as deserving of whatever they want and therefore not push themselves as hard as they could, setting their personal standards far too low while believing they merit the best others can offer them.

The greatest paradox in NPD is the combination of grandiosity and vulnerability in the individual's sense of self. Some individuals with NPD seem to think of themselves entirely in an inflated and self-aggrandizing way. These are the NPD individuals clinicians refer to as high in **grandiose narcissism**. Those high in **vulnerable narcissism**, in contrast, have an internally weak sense of self and so become despondent when they feel someone important to them is humiliating or betraying them (Besser & Priel, 2010). The *DSM-5-TR* does not explicitly make this distinction, but clinicians and researchers maintain that it is an important differentiation (Jauk et al., 2022).

If you know someone high in narcissism or diagnosed with NPD, you are undoubtedly aware of how difficult it is to maintain a close relationship. Although such individuals may at first appear to

narcissistic personality disorder (NPD)
A personality disorder primarily characterized by an unrealistic, inflated sense of self-importance and a lack of sensitivity to the needs of other people.

grandiose narcissism
The form of narcissistic personality disorder in which individuals think of themselves entirely in an inflated and self-aggrandizing way.

vulnerable narcissism
The form of narcissistic personality disorder in which individuals have an internally weak sense of self and so become despondent when they feel that someone who is important to them is humiliating or betraying them.

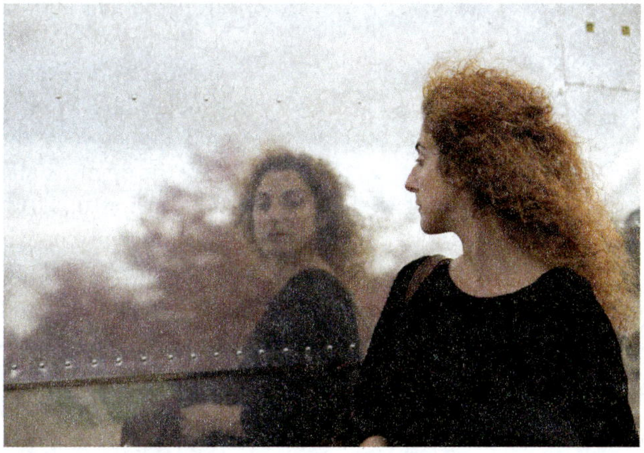

People with narcissistic personality disorder are excessively preoccupied with the outward image they present to the world.
paul rushton/Shutterstock

MINI CASE

Narcissistic Personality Disorder

Chad is a single 26-year-old White heterosexual cisgender man. For the past few years, he has been desperately trying to find success as an actor. However, he has had only minor acting jobs and has been forced to support himself by working as a server in a restaurant. Despite his lack of success, he brags to others about all the roles he rejects because they aren't good enough for him. Trying to break into acting, he has been selfishly exploitative of any person he sees as a possible connection. He intensely resents acquaintances who have obtained acting roles and devalues their achievements by commenting that they are just lucky. Yet if anyone tries to give him constructive criticism, Chad reacts with outrage, refusing to talk to the person for weeks. Because of what he regards as his terrific looks, he thinks he deserves special treatment from everyone. At the restaurant, he has recurrent arguments with his supervisor because he insists he is a "professional" who should not have to demean himself by clearing dirty dishes from the tables. He annoys others because he always seeks compliments on his clothes, hair, intelligence, and wit. He is so caught up in himself that he barely notices other people and is grossly insensitive to their needs and problems.

be highly attractive and desirable, they lose their appeal as romantic partners due to their unwavering demands for attention, insistence on being admired and even revered, and constant complaints about the inferiority of other people, including you. These so-called noxious behaviors eventually lead you to try to leave such relationships. In turn, individuals high in narcissism ultimately may experience lower quality of life (Ellison et al., 2020). Perhaps somewhat ironically, they also have better health across adulthood because, by valuing their physical appearance, they also put significant effort into caring for their bodies (Wetzel, Grijalva, Robins, & Roberts, 2020).

Claims in the popular press propose that the current generation of college students and young adults are higher in narcissism than any previous generation, based on the ubiquity of social media and opportunities to post steady streams of photos, videos, and updates. However, research comparing narcissism trends across recent past cohorts of young adults paints the opposite picture. Scores on standard narcissism inventories have actually dropped between the 1990s and the 2010s, particularly in the qualities of vanity and entitlement (Wetzel et al., 2017).

Theorists operating within the object relations approach regard the narcissistic individual as having failed to form a cohesive, integrated sense of self. The narcissistic individual expresses insecurity, paradoxically, in an inflated sense of self-importance as he or she tries to make up for early parental support (Kohut, 1966, 1971). Lacking the firm foundation of a healthy self, such a person develops a false self precariously based on grandiose and unrealistic notions about his or her competence and desirability (Masterson, 1981).

People with NPD are difficult to treat because they tend not to have insight into their disorder. Moreover, the clinicians who treat them can be challenged by the same behaviors people with NPD show outside therapy (Kealy et al., 2017). Even nontraditional approaches that employ yoga and other mind-body practices have only limited benefit, and they may have the opposite effect of enhancing, rather than quieting, the individual's focus on the self (Gebauer et al., 2018).

Current psychodynamic perspectives incorporate the object relations view in seeing narcissistic personality disorder as the adult's expression of childhood insecurity and need for attention. Transference-focused psychotherapy attempts to diminish the individual's sense of grandiosity and dysfunctional interpersonal patterns through focusing on the therapeutic interaction (Diamond, Yeomans, & Keefe, 2021). Part of this process may be a form of reparenting in which the clinician works with the client to foster early, unmet needs (Behary & Dieckmann, 2013).

Cognitive behavioral theorists focus on the maladaptive ideas their clients hold, particularly the view held by people with the grandiose variety of the disorder in which they regard themselves as exceptional people who deserve far better treatment than ordinary humans. These beliefs hamper their ability to perceive their experiences realistically, and as a result they encounter problems when their inflated ideas about themselves clash with their experiences of failure in the real world.

Rather than simply confronting them with their erroneous beliefs, clinicians working in the cognitive behavioral perspective structure interventions that work with, rather than against, the client's self-aggrandizing and egocentric tendencies (Freeman & Fox, 2013). This allows the individual to accept the therapist's help because the intervention seems less threatening. For example, rather than try to convince the client to act less selfishly, the clinician might try to show that there are better ways to reach important personal goals. At the same time, the clinician avoids capitulating to the client's demands for special favors and attention. Interestingly, this approach is not all that different from the contemporary psychodynamic perspective, which supports the need to feel recognized and accepted while still helping the client develop a more realistic sense of self.

14.4 Cluster C Personality Disorders

People within the Cluster C personality disorders tend to be extremely restrained and may draw little attention to themselves, in contrast to those individuals with personality disorders in Cluster B. Each disorder in Cluster C has its own unique qualities that distinguish it, but as a group they share this inner directedness.

Avoidant Personality Disorder

As the term implies, people with **avoidant personality disorder** stay away from others, believing they lack social skills and have no desirable qualities that would make others want to be with them. Their symptoms go beyond shyness to feelings of shame and inadequacy so strong that they prefer not to be around others. They stay away almost entirely from social encounters and are especially likely to avoid any situation that could embarrass them. They may set unrealistically high standards for themselves, which in turn lead them to avoid situations in which they feel doomed to fail. Intimate relationships present a severe threat to them because they fear shame or ridicule should they expose their flaws to a partner.

avoidant personality disorder
A personality disorder in which people have low estimation of their social skills and are fearful of disapproval, rejection, and criticism or being ashamed or embarrassed.

The *DSM-5-TR* points out the importance of considering sociocultural factors, such as the result of problems in acculturation following migration. Marked patterns of avoidance may also be the result of culturally-defined social embarrassment or failure to meet life goals.

Although avoidant personality disorder is a highly disabling condition, it is possible for individuals to show improvement with treatment. A longitudinal study of 460 adults with this disorder who were followed for 7 years showed that improvement in social functioning is possible. However, psychotherapy was less likely to be effective in those who lived alone (Kvarstein et al., 2021).

MINI CASE

Avoidant Personality Disorder

Eduard is a single 53-year-old African American gay cisgender man. He works as delivery person for a large equipment corporation. Eduard's co-workers describe him as a loner because he does not spend time in casual conversation and avoids going out to lunch with others. Little do they know that every day he struggles with the desire to interact with them but is too intimidated to follow through. Recently, Eduard turned down a promotion to a manager's job because he realized it would require a considerable amount of day-to-day contact with others. What bothered him most about the prospect was that he might make mistakes others would notice. Eduard has hardly dated, and every time he feels interested in a man, he becomes paralyzed with anxiety over the prospect of talking to him, much less asking him for a date. When co-workers talk to him, he blushes and nervously tries to end the conversation as soon as possible.

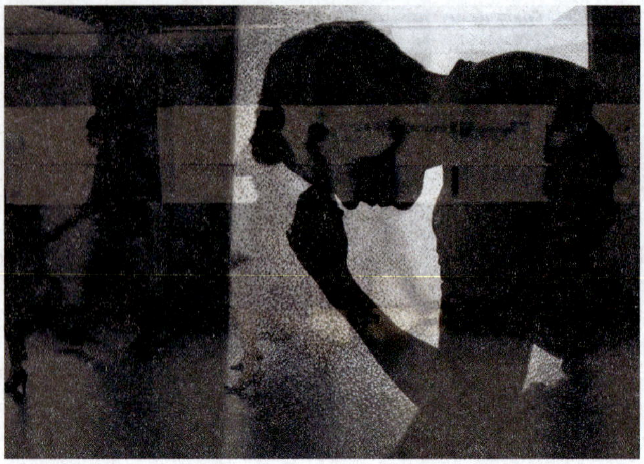

People with avoidant personality disorder stay away from social contact of any kind for a significant portion of the time due to excessive fears of embarrassment or rejection by others.

KieferPix/Shutterstock

Researchers believe avoidant personality disorder exists along a continuum extending from the normal personality trait of shyness to social anxiety disorder (Lampe, 2016). According to this view, avoidant personality disorder is a more severe form of social anxiety disorder. Individuals with the disorder have a long history of difficulties in connecting to others and navigating life transitions, experiencing their personal histories with a sense of being "forlorn" (Sørensen, Wilberg, Berthelsen, & Råbu, 2020).

Contemporary psychodynamic approaches to this disorder regard it as the expression of fear of attachment in close relationships. People with this disorder avoid getting close to others because they fear being abandoned or neglected in the same way they were by their caregiver in early childhood (Levy et al., 2015).

From a cognitive behavioral perspective, avoidant personality disorder may reflect the individual's hypersensitivity to shame (Currie, Katz, & Yovel, 2017). This hypersensitivity causes them to misinterpret seemingly neutral and even positive remarks. Hurt by perceived rejection, they retreat inward, placing further distance between themselves and others. Yet, they continue to long for connection, even while they fear the consequences of becoming closer to others (Sørensen et al., 2019).

The main goal of clinicians working in the cognitive behavioral framework is to break the client's negative cycle of avoidance. Clients learn to articulate the automatic thoughts and dysfunctional attitudes that interfere with their ability to establish relationships with others. Although clinicians point out the irrationality of these beliefs, they do so in a supportive atmosphere. In order for these interventions to be successful, however, clients must learn to trust the therapist rather than see him or her as yet another person who may ridicule or reject them.

Cognitive behavioral clinicians may also use graduated exposure to present the client with social situations that are increasingly more difficult to confront. Clinicians may train the client in specific skills intended to improve the quality of their intimate relationships. However, they also need to address a more general issue for people with avoidant personality disorder who show challenges in the area of metacognition, or the ability to think about their own thoughts and those of others (Sperry & Casteleiro, 2022).

Dependent Personality Disorder

dependent personality disorder
A personality disorder whose main characteristic is that the individual is extremely passive and tends to cling to other people, to the point of being unable to make any decisions or to take independent action.

Individuals with **dependent personality disorder** are strongly drawn to others. However, they are so clinging and passive that they may achieve the opposite of their desires as others become impatient with their lack of autonomy. Convinced of their inadequacy, they cannot make even the most trivial decisions on their own.

Others may characterize individuals with dependent personality disorder as "clingy," and indeed, when alone these clients feel despondent and abandoned. They are likely to throw themselves wholeheartedly into relationships and are therefore devastated when relationships end. Their extreme dependence causes them to urgently seek another relationship to fill the void. Even when with others, they become preoccupied with the fear of being left. They cannot comfortably initiate new activities on their own because they are hampered by worries that they will make mistakes unless others guide their actions. People with this disorder go to extremes to avoid having people dislike them—for example, by stating that they agree with others even when they do not.

DSM-5-TR points out that age and cultural factors should be taken into account when diagnosing this disorder. Dependent behavior should be considered in the context of prevailing social norms, such as a culture's expectations of passivity in women.

Research on the personality traits of individuals with dependent personality disorder suggests that they have unusually high levels of agreeableness. Although you might think of agreeableness as an adaptive trait, at high levels, it can become a tendency to be overly docile, self-sacrificing, and clinging (Samuel & Gore, 2012). Anxiousness, submissiveness, and an insecure attachment style are the pathological traits associated with dependent personality disorder (McClintock & McCarrick, 2017).

MINI CASE

Dependent Personality Disorder

Bridget is a 52-year-old White heterosexual cisgender woman. She has never lived on her own; even while a college student 30 years ago, she commuted from home. Bridget was known by her classmates as someone who was dependent on others. Relying on others to make choices for her, she did whatever her friends advised, whether it was choosing courses or selecting the clothes she should wear each day. The week after graduation, she married Ken, whom she had dated all senior year. Bridget was particularly attracted to Ken because his domineering style relieved her of the responsibility to make decisions. As she has customarily done with all the close people in her life, Bridget goes along with whatever Ken suggests, even if she does not fully agree. She fears that he will become angry with her and leave her if she rocks the boat. Although Bridget wants to get a job outside the home, Ken has insisted that she stay home full-time instead of working, and she has complied with his wishes. However, when she is home alone, she calls friends and desperately pleads with them to come over for coffee. The slightest criticism from Ken, her friends, or anyone else can leave her feeling depressed and upset for the whole day.

Cognitive behavioral treatment for people with dependent personality disorder appears to be effective, particularly if the clinician alternates as needed between changing behaviors and challenging the client's faulty beliefs (Brauer & Reinecke, 2015). Mindfulness training can also be useful in helping individuals with this disorder identify and manage their interpersonal anxiety (McClintock & Anderson, 2015).

Obsessive-Compulsive Personality Disorder

People with **obsessive-compulsive personality disorder (OCPD)** have a set of symptoms that revolve around defining their sense of self and self-worth in terms of their work productivity. Perfectionistic to a fault, people with OCPD find it difficult to complete a task because they can always see a flaw in what they have done. Their work products are never good enough to meet their unrealistic standards. They can also be overly moralistic because they stick to overly conscientious standards that almost anyone would find difficult to meet.

obsessive-compulsive personality disorder (OCPD)
A personality disorder involving intense perfectionism and inflexibility manifested in worrying, indecisiveness, and behavioral rigidity.

The words *obsessive* and *compulsive* as applied to the OCPD personality disorder have a different meaning than in the context of obsessive-compulsive disorder (OCD). Unlike those with OCD, people with OCPD do not experience obsessions and compulsions but instead are rigidly compulsive (such as being fixated on certain routines) and obsessed with the need to be perfect. Critics of the AMPD conceptualization of this disorder argue that it fails to take into account such qualities as workaholism, excessive deliberation in decision-making, and moral scrupulousness (Samuel, Balling, & Bucher, 2022).

The interpersonal relationships of people with OCPD suffer due to their difficulty understanding how others feel, particularly when those feelings differ from their own. Because they have such high standards for themselves, people with OCPD are critical of others who they see as not matching their own expectations. Others, in turn, perceive those with OCPD as rigid and stubborn. Consistent with this profile, individuals scoring high on a symptom measure of OCPD showed high levels of social interaction anxiety and poor coping mechanisms, along with rigid perfectionism (Seretis, Hart, & Maguire, 2023). Not surprisingly, given their extreme conscientiousness, a prospective study of adults followed for nearly 20 years showed that people high in OCPD traits were less likely to develop hypertension. However, the indecisiveness component of OCPD appeared to contribute to a greater probability of developing heart conditions (Morreale, Holingue, Samuels, & Nestadt, 2021).

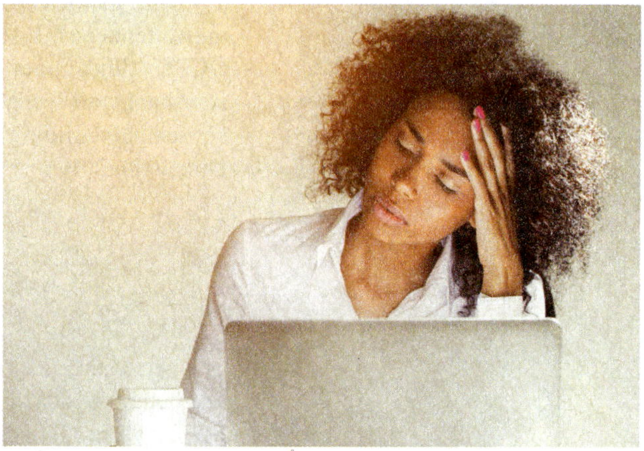

People with obsessive-compulsive personality disorder may struggle with workaholism due to their excessive concern with maintaining their productivity.
ImageFlow/Shutterstock

MINI CASE

Obsessive-Compulsive Personality Disorder

Carmen is a 42-year-old Latina queer transgender woman. For as long as she can remember, Carmen has been preoccupied with neatness and order. As a child, she kept her room meticulously clean. Friends and relatives chided her for excessive organization. For example, she insisted on arranging the toys in her toy closet according to color and category. In college, her rigid housekeeping regimen both amazed and annoyed her roommates. She was overbearing in her insistence on keeping the room orderly and free of clutter. Carmen has continued this pattern into her adult life. Employed as a file clerk, she prides herself on never having missed a day of work, regardless of health problems and family crises. However, her boss will not offer Carmen a promotion because she feels she is overly attentive to details of the filing process, thus slowing the work of the office as she checks and rechecks everything she does. Carmen enhances her sense of self-importance in the office by looking for opportunities to take control. For example, when her co-workers are planning a party, she tends to slow matters because of her concerns about every detail of the event, such as the time it will start, how much food to order, and decorations. More often than not, her co-workers try to avoid letting her get involved because they object to her rigidity in such trivial matters.

From the standpoint of cognitive behavioral theory, people with this disorder have unrealistic expectations about being perfect and avoiding mistakes (Beck, Freeman, & Davis, 2004). Their feelings of self-worth depend on their behaving in ways that conform to an abstract ideal of perfectionism. If they fail to achieve that ideal (which, inevitably, they must), they regard themselves as worthless. In this framework, obsessive-compulsive personality disorder is based on a problematic way of viewing the self.

There may also be cultural factors in the diagnosis of OCPD, as noted in *DSM-5-TR*. Certain cultures place high value on work and productivity, and individuals in certain communities may also feel extreme pressure to conform to codes of conducts or work demands. These behaviors on their own should not be considered diagnostic of OCPD.

Clinicians using cognitive behavioral treatment for clients with OCPD face challenges due to the characteristic features of this personality disorder. The person with OCPD tends to intellectualize, to ruminate over past actions, and to worry about making mistakes. Clients with OCPD who fear violating their overly high moral or religious standards may be particularly hard to treat, because they show lack of insight into their scrupulosity (Siev, Rasmussen, Sullivan, & Wilhelm, 2021). Cognitive behavioral therapy, with its focus on examining the client's thought processes, may reinforce this ruminative tendency. Instead, metacognitive interpersonal therapy can help individuals with OCPD "think about their thinking." In this procedure, clinicians help their clients take a step back and learn to identify their problematic ruminative thinking patterns in the context of building a supportive therapeutic alliance (Gordon-King, Schweitzer, & Dimaggio, 2019).

14.5 Personality Disorders: The Biopsychosocial Perspective

The personality disorders represent a fascinating mix of long-standing personal dispositions and behavior patterns and disturbances in self and relationships. Taking a life-span perspective, in which these disorders are viewed as evolving from childhood throughout adulthood, is important in understanding them, given that they are defined as long-standing personality dimensions. Continued refinement of the *DSM*, particularly because *ICD-11* has already moved to a dimensional system, may help to further this life-span understanding of personality disorders.

Return to the Case: Saman ahmadi

Saman was enrolled in a year-long contract at a local DBT clinic where he attended twice-weekly psychotherapy and three therapy groups per week. The program focused on teaching emotion-regulation skills, mindfulness, interpersonal effectiveness, and distress tolerance. By fostering a supportive relationship with Saman, his therapist was able to model correct emotional regulation and validation of a wide range of emotions, so that Saman would not feel the need to resort to extreme measures in order to gain attention from others.

Dr. Tobin's reflections: Like many individuals with borderline personality disorder, Saman grew up in what is known as an invalidating environment—with parents who were more or less absent in his upbringing. He found that acting in an extreme manner was the only way he was able to get attention from them, so this became the only way for him to connect with others. He even displayed this in the intake evaluation by showing the clinician the marks of his self-mutilation, threatening to storm out of the room, and spontaneously bursting into tears. Further, he showed interpersonal instability in his request of the clinician to be his therapist and then immediately turning on her (or "devaluing" her) when told she could not see him for therapy. Unlike cisgender women with borderline personality disorder, who often present with largely depressed affect, cisgender men tend to present with an angry affect and are more likely to engage in substance abuse as a coping mechanism. Cisgender women might more likely be sexually promiscuous or engage in eating-disordered behaviors in order to cope with their extreme emotions.

It is typical for an individual with borderline personality disorder to present for treatment only after making a suicide attempt or having strong suicidal ideation, because the disorder is ego-syntonic—meaning the individual rarely understands that the behavior is atypical. With the appropriate treatment, Saman's chance of continuing to experience highly unstable and shifting mood and relational patterns greatly decreases.

You may be wondering why Saman was not referred for substance abuse treatment. It was the opinion of the intake clinician that his substance abuse, especially his alcohol use, was secondary to Saman's personality disorder. It is typical for DBT treatment programs to require clients to abstain from abusing substances during the course of treatment. Further, with more appropriate mood-regulation skills, Saman's substance abuse may remit. Should he continue to abuse substances throughout his treatment, he will then be referred for a specific substance use disorder treatment program.

SUMMARY

- A personality disorder is a long-standing pattern of relating to other people, situations, and events with a rigid and maladaptive pattern of inner experience and behavior, dating back to adolescence or early adulthood. In the *DSM-5-TR*, personality disorders represent a collection of distinguishable sets of symptoms, falling into 10 distinct categories. The AMPD included in Section III provides a dimensional rating system whose validity continues to be examined in the personality disorder research community.
- Cluster A includes paranoid, schizoid, and schizotypal personality disorders, which share the features of odd and eccentric behavior.
- Cluster B includes antisocial, borderline, histrionic, and narcissistic personality disorders, which share overdramatic, emotional, and erratic or unpredictable attitudes and behaviors.
- Cluster C includes avoidant, dependent, and obsessive-compulsive personality disorders, which share anxious and fearful behaviors.
- Because the personality disorders are grouped into discrete categories, clinicians evaluating individuals for a possible diagnosis must decide how many of the criteria a client meets within each category and assign a diagnosis on that basis. The client either has the disorder or does not. The clinician may start by trying to match the client's most prominent symptoms with the diagnostic criteria. If the individual does not fit the criteria for that disorder, the clinician may either move to another disorder or decide the client has a personality disorder "not otherwise specified."
- The personality disorders are historically regarded as challenging to treat, but they are proving to respond to cognitive behavioral therapy in which clients are helped to question their long-standing assumptions and change their disturbed behaviors. Psychodynamic therapy can also be efficacious, particularly for those disorders such as borderline and narcissistic personality disorders, which have such strong links to deficits in early childhood relationships. Understanding of these disorders will likely change as *DSM* increasingly moves to a dimensional diagnostic approach, one already in use in the *ICD-11*.

KEY TERMS

Alternative Model for Personality Disorders (AMPD)
Antisocial behavior
Antisocial personality disorder
Avoidant personality disorder
Borderline personality disorder (BPD)
Dark triad
Dependent personality disorder
Emotional dysregulation
Grandiose narcissism
Histrionic personality disorder
Narcissistic personality disorder (NPD)
Obsessive-compulsive personality disorder (OCPD)
Paranoid personality disorder
Parasuicide
Personality disorder
Psychopathy
Schizoid personality disorder
Schizotypal personality disorder
Splitting
Stress generation
Transference-focused psychotherapy
Vulnerable narcissism

Ethical and Legal Issues

CHAPTER 15

OUTLINE

Learning Objectives

15.1 Explain ethical standards including competence, informed consent, confidentiality, relationships with clients/students/research collaborators, and record keeping.

15.2 Explain ethical and legal issues in providing services, including commitment of clients, right to treatment, and refusal of treatment and least restrictive alternatives.

15.3 Understand forensic issues in psychological treatment, such as the insanity defense, competency to stand trial, and the purpose of punishment.

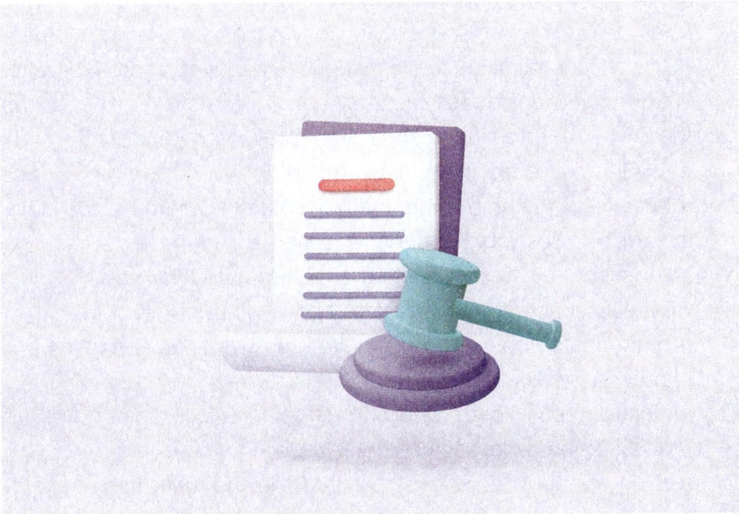

Vector Stock Pro/Shutterstock

Case Report

Allison Yang

Demographic information: 19-year-old Chinese American heterosexual cisgender woman. Allison's pronouns are she/her/hers.

History of present illness: Allison has been attending individual psychotherapy at a private outpatient clinic on a weekly basis for 8 months after initially presenting to treatment following a major depressive episode. Allison had never before received psychiatric treatment, and after she confided to the resident director of her dormitory that she had been having a difficult time with her transition to college, the director gave her information about nearby therapy clinics because the small college had no counseling center of its own. Shortly after Allison began therapy, the clinician referred her to a psychiatrist who prescribed an SSRI. Allison responded well to both therapy and the antidepressant, and her symptoms remitted within about 4 weeks, although she still experienced a persistently low mood. She continued to come for weekly psychotherapy sessions to work on the issues underlying her depression. Her mood has been relatively stable, and she has had few complaints about depressive symptoms for the majority of the time since starting therapy. Allison started to become more engaged in extracurricular activities at school and began attending more social events.

Over the past three sessions, however, she has been presenting with increased depressive symptoms. She reported sleeping about 10 to 12 hours per night and still does not feel rested. She is eating only once per day, has difficulty concentrating, and experiences frequent, unprovoked crying episodes. These symptoms are similar to those she reported when she initially presented for therapy. Allison also admitted that she had not left her dorm room except to come to her therapy session. During her most recent session, her affect was markedly depressed and despondent. She was tearful as she reported that she was feeling increasingly hopeless and was having recurrent thoughts about ending her life. She was unable to identify a particular stressor for this current episode, remarking that "all of a sudden things just feel so . . . pointless." She stated that she had been having thoughts about suicide for about 2 weeks, but that the thoughts had become much more pervasive over the past few days.

During the session, Allison's therapist responded to her report of suicidality by performing a safety evaluation. He asked whether Allison had thought about how she would die by suicide, to which Allison responded that she was in possession of a rope at home and planned on hanging herself from a ceiling beam in her dorm room. The therapist then asked how strong her intention was to follow through with this plan, to which Allison responded that she had planned on hanging herself that morning but decided to come in for one last therapy session and to "say goodbye." She said that she had also written e-mails to friends and family and scheduled them to be delivered later in the day, after the point when she had planned to end her life.

Recently in therapy Allison had been discussing how she felt significant pressure from her family to achieve high grades in college. As a double major in biology and chemistry, she had been finding it difficult to keep up with all her coursework and attain "acceptable" grades. She attributed this in part to her parents, who, as immigrants to the United States from China, often pushed her to excel academically and frequently reminded her of the sacrifices they made for her to be successful.

Much of her work in therapy had focused on the impact of her parents' pushing her, with her low self-image and propensity to undervalue not only her achievements but also her abilities to perform well in school and in other areas. Allison had been working with her therapist to learn strategies to help generate feelings of self-worth and to take pride in her accomplishments so far. She attributed her patterns of low self-worth to her parents and the way, as she explained, "They never think I'm good enough, no matter what I do. I always have to be doing better. They're never satisfied."

Allison has no siblings, which she believes adds to her parents' "excessive nagging." Although she recognized that this was a source of distress, she found it difficult to "fight back" and value herself because she had never learned to do this on her own. Throughout therapy, Allison and her clinician discussed ways to improve her relationship with her family, while also looking through a cultural lens and understanding how some of the pressures her parents had felt as immigrants translated into pushing her constantly to achieve. Allison found this difficult given that she and her parents got into arguments

Case Report *continued*

when they spoke on the phone. Several times she had thought about cutting off contact with them altogether; however, this presented a challenge, given that her parents supported her financially. Due to her intensive focus on schoolwork, Allison had little time in college to make friends and was often by herself in her dorm room. She reported that even when she had down time, she was constantly worrying about schoolwork and found it quite difficult to relax. Further, she explained that she had never told anyone about her mental health struggles, and that she felt extremely uncomfortable at the thought of telling her parents, stating that "they don't believe in mental health."

Psychiatric history: Allison experienced three depressive episodes prior to starting therapy. The first lasted approximately 8 months and remitted without intervention. The other two lasted approximately 2 to 3 months each and also remitted on their own. Although these episodes were much shorter than the first, the time between them was very short. The period between Allison's starting therapy and her current depressive episode was the longest gap between episodes to date. Although she had reported thoughts of suicide during her prior depressive episodes, she had never had a plan or clear intent to die by suicide. Allison reported that she wasn't sure whether her family had any history of depression or mood disorders.

Case formulation: Due to her prior depressive episodes and absence of a manic episode, Allison carries a diagnosis of major depressive disorder, recurrent. In addition, she currently meets criteria for a major depressive episode. We add the qualifier of "severe" to the diagnosis, due to her intent and plan to die by suicide.

Risk level: High, due to current presence of suicidal ideation, current intent, plan (hanging by rope), and means (currently has the rope in her room). Allison is unable to contract for safety at this time and is presenting as a high risk to her own safety. Other risk factors include the writing of suicide notes and current severe depressive symptoms.

Treatment plan: Allison's clinician determined that she posed a significant threat to herself based on her report that she had a plan and intent to die by suicide. The clinician asked Allison whether she could agree to make a contract to protect her safety. He would allow Allison to leave the session only if she agreed to call 911 should she feel an increase in intent to die by suicide. Allison was unable to state that she would be safe should she go home, and the clinician informed Allison that she would have to go to the hospital immediately. The clinician called 911, and an ambulance transported Allison to a nearby psychiatric hospital for stabilization.

Sarah Tobin, PhD

Psychologists are guided in both their clinical and research work by the professional guidelines established by the major professional organization, the American Psychological Association (APA). These guidelines do not hold legal power, but individual states and territories in the United States establish strict codes required for psychologists and other mental health professionals to obtain and keep their licenses. Not only are health professionals required to follow these standards, but they must regularly recertify their ability to provide services by obtaining continuing education to ensure that they are able to practice according to the highest standards. At the same time, when making diagnoses, psychologists and other mental health professionals are required to use the criteria provided by either the *DSM-5-TR* or the *ICD11*.

15.1 Ethical Standards

Many states require that, to be considered a psychologist, an individual must pass a rigid set of licensing requirements. All states in the United States have a board of psychologists that oversees the legal requirements for obtaining and retaining a psychology license. These requirements typically include passing an examination, obtaining a certain number of hours of supervised training, receiving recommendations from other licensed psychologists, and, to remain licensed, participating in a certain number of hours of continuing education.

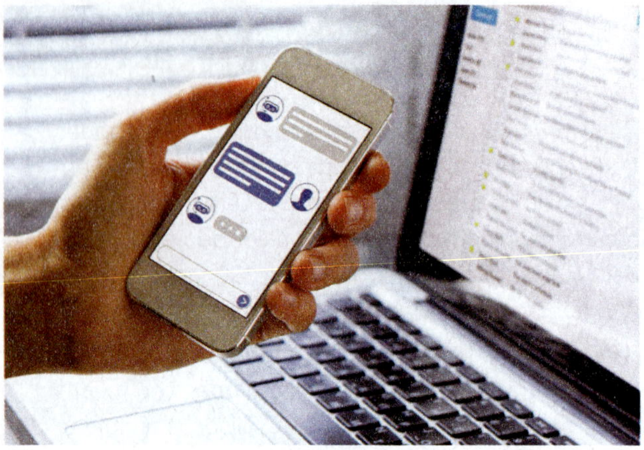

The use of artificial intelligence in providing online therapy raises ethical concerns that the mental health community is just now beginning to address.

NicoElNino/Shutterstock

Psychologists follow the APA Ethical Principles of Psychologists and Code of Conduct (American Psychological Association, 2017). The general principles are not enforceable rules but are intended for psychologists to consider in arriving at an ethical course of action. In contrast, the ethical standards are enforceable rules. Failure to follow them can result in sanctions, including loss of membership in the APA and of a state professional license. In making decisions about their professional behavior, psychologists must consider the Ethics Code as well as any applicable laws and regulations of their state psychology boards.

There are 10 standards contained within the Ethics Code (see Table 1). Since writing the first version in 1953, the APA has rewritten the Ethics Code to keep up with changes in electronic communication and, most recently, to set forth codes that psychologists in the military should follow that prohibit their participation in interrogation of suspected terrorists. As stated in the 2016 amendment (Section 3.04), "Psychologists do not participate in, facilitate, assist,

TABLE 1 **Summary of APA Ethics Code**

Standard	Summary
1: Resolving Ethical Issues	Establishes the way psychologists should resolve ethical conflicts, report ethical violations, and cooperate with professional ethics committees.
2: Competence	Establishes the fact that psychologists must work within their boundaries of competence based on their training, experience, consultation, and supervision; describes what psychologists should do in emergencies; sets forth criteria for delegating work to others; describes how to resolve personal problems and conflicts that might interfere with their ability to provide services.
3: Human Relations	Provides criteria that psychologists must follow when they relate to employees, clients, and trainees; describes how psychologists should avoid conflicts of interest; regulates the nature of informed consent in research, clinical practice, or consulting, including administering psychological services through corporations.
4: Privacy and Confidentiality	Sets forth the principles for protecting research participants and clients; mandates that any public information (such as published research) includes reasonable steps to disguise the person or organization.
5: Advertising and Other Public Statements	Instructs psychologists not to provide false statements through advertising or other public outlets, in media presentations, and in testimonials; sets forth limits to in-person solicitation of potential clients or people in need of care.
6: Record Keeping and Fees	Provides conditions that psychologists must follow in maintaining their records, charging clients for services, and providing reports to payors of service or sources of research funding.
7: Education and Training	Regulates the activities of psychologists in the classroom, as supervisors or trainers, and as developers of education and training programs.
8: Research and Publication	Offers specific guidelines for psychologists who conduct research, including informing participants about their rights, offering inducements for research participation, using deception in research, debriefing participants, providing humane care for animals, reporting research results, avoiding plagiarism, and taking precautions in publishing of research articles.
9: Assessment	Describes the code for psychologists in conducting assessments, including how assessment data should be collected, use of informed consent, release of test data, principles of test construction, scoring and interpretation of test results, and maintenance of test security.
10: Therapy	Sets forth code for psychologists who provide therapy, including obtaining informed consent; conducting therapy with individuals, couples, families, and groups; interrupting and terminating therapy; and avoiding sexual intimacies with clients, relatives of clients, and former clients.

or otherwise engage in torture, defined as any act by which severe pain or suffering, whether physical or mental, is intentionally inflicted on a person, or in any other cruel, inhuman, or degrading behavior that violates 3.04(a)."

Although not yet addressed in APA's Ethical Guidelines, concerns will almost certainly emerge about the role of artificial intelligence and machine learning both in assessment and the provision of psychotherapy. Chatbots can generate messages based on input provided by psychologists, and artificial intelligence could be useful in diagnosis. However, taking the "human" element out of psychological practice could be fraught with dilemmas, particularly if clients are not completely aware that an intervention is guided by computer-generated algorithms. Other ethical issues will involve the handling of client data, integration of these new technologies into training of clinicians, the potential for misuse, and whether by replacing established services, existing health inequities might be exacerbated (Fiske, Henningsen, & Buyx, 2019).

What's in the *DSM-5-TR*

Ethical Implications of the *DSM-5-TR* Diagnostic System

Following release of the *DSM-5* draft in late 2011, a number of mental health professional organizations composed a joint response to what they perceived as the potentially disastrous consequences of adding some diagnoses and removing others. For example, critics contend that eliminating the category of Asperger's syndrome could leave many thousands of individuals who suffer from its symptoms untreated. In the chapter "Neurocognitive Disorders," you read about the potential problems in broadening the dementia diagnosis to include individuals with mild cognitive impairments. Such changes would create the opposite problem, mislabeling individuals who are experiencing normal age-related changes in memory.

The *DSM-5-TR*, which now replaces the *DSM-5,* is written in a manner intended to reflect the latest scientific evidence in the most objective manner possible. Inevitably, however, there will be room for debate as researchers and clinicians examine the available research studies and the evidence they infer from working with their clients. There are also social and political implications of changes in the diagnostic system. If individuals do not receive a diagnosis, as may happen with children formerly diagnosed with autistic disorder, then they cannot qualify for certain types of insurance to cover the costs of their education, treatment, and medications. Politicians then are faced with making decisions about how to allocate public funding for treatment, education, and research.

Another significant change in the *DSM-5-TR* that has widespread implications is the shift to diagnosing prolonged grief disorder in the cases of people who are suffering bereavement after the loss of a loved one. Previously, people who suffered the symptoms of bereavement were excluded from the diagnosis of major depressive disorder, a situation called the bereavement exclusion. The elimination of the bereavement exclusion means that after the death of a person close to them, an individual will now have a psychiatric diagnosis that could interfere with their ability to find employment in certain sectors.

However, if practitioners don't assign a diagnosis to a client with clinically significant symptoms, does this mean the clients will be unable to obtain medication to treat their symptoms? Conversely, in order to continue to provide services to their clients who may no longer qualify for a diagnosis, should clinicians find ways around the changing guidelines to ensure their clients do receive the diagnosis?

Unfortunately, because in many cases psychological symptoms are more difficult to identify than are physical symptoms, the debate about appropriate diagnostic categories and criteria will no doubt continue throughout each subsequent edition of the *DSM.* Maintaining your awareness of these continued debates can ultimately help you and the people you know receive the best care possible. If you continue in a professional career in mental health, it will be vital for you to stay on top of both the latest literature and the latest diagnostic issues to provide the best treatment possible for your own clients.

Competence

Standard 2 specifies that psychologists are expected to have appropriate competence to carry out therapy, consulting, teaching, and research. They achieve this competence, first of all, in their postbaccalaureate training. The APA provides accreditation to clinical doctoral training programs in the United States to ensure that these programs provide future psychologists with sufficient breadth and depth to form the basis for their career in providing mental health services. As you read in the chapter"Diagnosis and Treatment," upon completing their coursework, PhD and PsyD (Doctor of Psychology) graduates must obtain intensive supervision as interns and postdoctoral trainees. They must then pass a nationally administered licensing exam and complete any additional requirements of their particular state. To maintain their license, they must take and complete a required number of continuing education courses within each year or two after licensure and be able to document this participation.

The result of this intensive training is that psychologists have the competence to assess, conceptualize, and provide interventions for clients whom they accept into treatment. On a related note, Standard 5 also instructs psychologists to be truthful about their areas of expertise. Clinicians who claim to be, for example, sports psychologists should have received training in this field, preferably with supervision under a professional with appropriate training credentials. When clinicians advertise their specialty, they should have suitable expertise, including current familiarity with a field, in order to be able to offer those services.

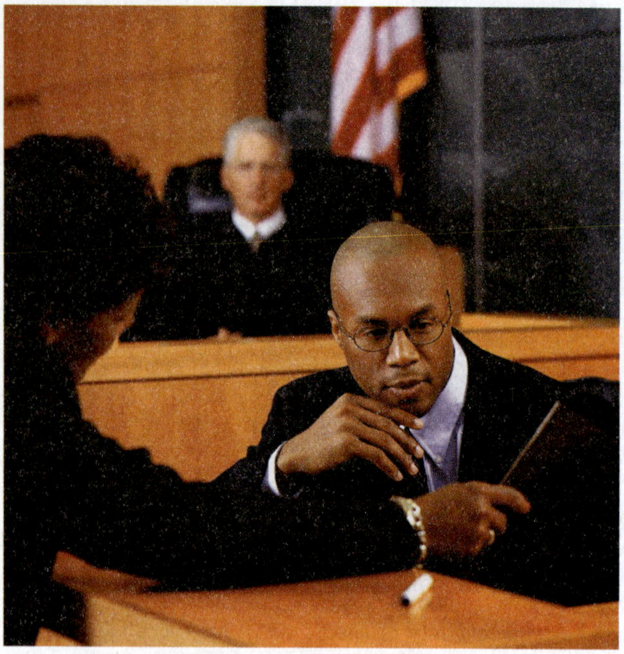

A psychologist may serve as an expert witness in forensic cases.
CORBIS Premium RF/Alamy Stock Photo

Turning to other requirements of professional training, clinicians should also have the **emotional competence** to be able to provide services to their clients. This means that, within a range of acceptable variations, they should be free of a diagnosable psychological disorder. Should they develop such a disorder, they should receive treatment and consider suspending their practice until their symptoms are in remission or at least under control. To ensure that mental health professionals meet these standards of competence, they are expected to conduct regular self-scrutiny, in which they objectively evaluate their competence to carry out their work. They can also benefit from seeking supervision or consultation from another professional, perhaps one with more experience or expertise.

In a court of law, counsel often asks psychologists to give expert testimony, such as outlining the limits of eyewitness memory or explaining the nature of a psychiatric diagnosis. If they do, they must make clear the limits of their areas of expertise. If they do not have expertise in a particular area, they must obtain consultation from an expert who does.

Even more complicated than the role of expert witness is the task of conducting evaluations in child protection cases. Such evaluations are necessary in situations in which there are concerns about the child's welfare. For example, if there has been evidence of or charges of abuse, a court might call a mental health professional to make recommendations about the child's care. A judge might appoint a clinician as an agent of the court or a child protection agency, or one of the parents might hire the clinician. In some instances, the clinician is a **guardian *ad litem***, a person whom the court appoints to represent or make decisions for a minor or incapacitated adult who is legally incapable of doing so in a civil legal proceeding.

emotional competence
A quality desired in clinicians in which they are free of a diagnosable psychological disorder.

guardian *ad litem*
A person appointed by the court to represent or make decisions for a minor or an incapacitated adult who is legally incapable of doing so in a civil legal proceeding.

A related issue involves the assessments that clinicians may conduct of parents whose children are being seen in mental health settings. Such assessments can assist clinicians in diagnosis and treatment planning by providing an understanding of how anxiety, depression, or parenting stress are affecting the child. Adopting APA Ethics Code principles, steps would need to be taken to ensure that such assessments are relevant to the child's care, would not present harm to the parents or family, would respect the autonomy of parents and their rights to refusal, and include provision of any resources the parents may need that become evident as a result of the assessment. As you can imagine, these assessments could benefit the child's treatment, but appropriate protections must be in place (Molitor & LeNoble, 2023).

Involving parents in the treatment of adolescents who are under the age of consent also presents another issue. Due to the increasing numbers of youth suicides in Colorado, the legislature passed a law that would lower the age of consent for psychotherapy from 15 to 12 years old. This means that a teenager can now seek treatment without parental permission. Although this legislation could potentially result in fewer suicides in this age group, it raises tough questions for clinicians, particularly if they feel that it would be helpful to involve the parents in the therapeutic process (McNamara, 2023).

Other challenges present themselves when clients seeking the services of clinicians have needs beyond the clinician's area of competence. In these cases, the clinician should either make a referral or obtain appropriate supervision. For example, a clinician who does not treat older adults with neurocognitive disorder may receive a referral from a middle-aged client seeking help with her mother who is experiencing memory problems. Unless the clinician is qualified to provide psychological assessments of older adults, they should recommend that someone else evaluate the mother.

To assist psychologists in evaluating their competencies in areas that may be outside their areas of expertise, APA has developed guidelines in specific areas of treatment. APA has approved a variety of practice guidelines and related criteria as policy in such areas as

TABLE 2 Guidelines for Psychotherapy with Lesbian, Gay, and Bisexual Clients

1. Psychologists understand that homosexuality and bisexuality are not indicative of mental illness.
2. Psychologists are encouraged to recognize how their attitudes and knowledge about lesbian, gay, and bisexual issues may be relevant to assessment and treatment and seek consultation or make appropriate referrals when indicated.
3. Psychologists strive to understand the ways in which social stigmatization (i.e., prejudice, discrimination, and violence) poses risks to the mental health and well-being of lesbian, gay, and bisexual clients.
4. Psychologists strive to understand how inaccurate or prejudicial views of homosexuality or bisexuality may affect the client's presentation in treatment and the therapeutic process.
5. Psychologists strive to be knowledgeable about and respect the importance of lesbian, gay, and bisexual relationships.
6. Psychologists strive to understand the particular circumstances and challenges faced by lesbian, gay, and bisexual clients.
7. Psychologists recognize that the families of lesbian, gay, and bisexual people may include people who are not legally or biologically related.
8. Psychologists strive to understand how a person's homosexual or bisexual orientation may have an impact on their family of origin and the relationship to that family of origin.
9. Psychologists are encouraged to recognize the particular life issues or challenges that are related to multiple and often conflicting cultural norms, values, and beliefs that lesbian, gay, and bisexual members of racial and ethnic minorities face.
10. Psychologists are encouraged to recognize the particular challenges that bisexual individuals experience.
11. Psychologists strive to understand the special problems and risks that exist for lesbian, gay, and bisexual youth.
12. Psychologists consider generational differences within lesbian, gay, and bisexual populations and the particular challenges that lesbian, gay, and bisexual older adults may experience.
13. Psychologists are encouraged to recognize the particular challenges that lesbian, gay, and bisexual individuals experience with physical, sensory, and cognitive-emotional difficulties.
14. Psychologists support the provision of professional education and training on lesbian, gay, and bisexual issues.
15. Psychologists are encouraged to increase their knowledge and understanding of homosexuality and bisexuality through continuing education, training, supervision, and consultation.
16. Psychologists make reasonable efforts to familiarize themselves with relevant mental health, educational, and community resources for lesbian, gay, and bisexual people.

American Psychological Association. (2012b). Guidelines for psychological practice with lesbian, gay, and bisexual clients. *American Psychologist, 67,* 10–42.

treatment of gay, lesbian, and bisexual clients (Table 2); child protection evaluations (Table 3); psychological practice with older adults (Table 4); psychological practice with girls and women (Table 5); and assessment of and intervention with people with disabilities (Table 6). These guidelines are intended to educate practitioners and provide recommendations about professional conduct. They are useful tools for psychologists in practice to develop and maintain competencies and/or learn about new practice areas.

Increasingly, psychologists who specialize in a particular field are seeking board certification with "diplomate status." The American Board of Professional Psychology (ABPP) sets forth criteria for certification of potential diplomates and arranges for their testing by experts in each particular specialty. If you see "ABPP" after a psychologist's signature, this means the individual has received this official certification. Doctoral students in clinical psychology are being advised to track their training so they can qualify for this status early in their careers.

The APA also serves a more general credentialing role in the profession, providing accreditation of clinical training programs, approval of specialty fields (such as neuropsychology or geropsychology), and curriculum standards for programs ranging from high school to postgraduate training in psychology.

Informed Consent

Although you may think only of research when you hear the term *informed consent,* this criterion for ethical behavior applies to other contexts, including psychotherapy. The reason

TABLE 3 Guidelines for Psychological Evaluations in Child Protection Matters

1. The primary purpose of the evaluation is to provide relevant, professionally sound results or opinions in matters where a child's health and welfare may have been and/or may in the future be harmed.
2. When psychologists conduct evaluations in child protection matters to address specific referral questions, they are aware that the interests of the parties in the case may differ from each other.
3. When the referral question in the evaluation addresses concerns about the parent/caretaker and child relationship, psychologists are mindful of: the parent/caretaker's parenting capacities, including circumstances or factors relevant to maltreatment of the child; the child's well-being and psychological needs; and the resulting fit.
4. The role of psychologists who conduct child protection evaluations is that of a professional expert who strives to maintain an unbiased, impartial approach to the evaluation.
5. Psychologists strive to gain competence sufficient to provide effective and ethical forensic services when conducting child protection evaluations and when addressing case-specific issues that may require specialized professional knowledge, training, or skills. I harm.
6. Psychologists strive to be aware of personal biases and societal prejudices and seek to engage in nondiscriminatory practice. The role of the psychologist conducting evaluations is that of a professional expert who strives to maintain an unbiased, objective stance.
7. Psychologists providing child protection evaluations strive to avoid role conflicts and multiple relationships that may compromise their objectivity, competence, or effectiveness, or that may otherwise risk harm or exploitation to the person or identified client (e.g., court, state child protection agency) with whom the professional relationship exists.
8. Based on the nature of referral issues or questions that define the focus and scope of the evaluation, psychologists determine the methods that are appropriate to address the referral issues or questions.
9. In accordance with the Ethics Code, psychologists performing psychological evaluations in child protection matters obtain appropriate informed consent or assent from all adult participants, and as appropriate, inform the child participant.
10. Psychologists use multiple methods of data gathering.
11. Psychologists seek to properly interpret clinical or assessment data that informs or supports their conclusions.
12. Psychologists conducting a psychological evaluation in child protection matters strive to provide opinions only when they have obtained sufficient data to support those opinions.
13. Recommendations, if offered, address the evaluation's specific referral questions, which may encompass various concerns related to the child's welfare and health in a child protection matter.
14. Psychologists create and maintain records in accordance with ethical and legal standards.

Committee on Professional Practice and Standards Board of Professional Affairs (2013). Guidelines for psychological evaluations in child protection matters (published report). American Psychological Association; https://www.apa.org/practice/guidelines/child-protection

is that clinical psychologists are expected to provide their clients with knowledge ahead of time about what they can expect to occur in treatment. At the outset of therapy, clinicians should provide clients with a written statement that outlines the goals of treatment, the process of therapy, the client's rights, the clinician's responsibilities, the treatment risks, the techniques he or she will use, what the client should pay, and the limits of confidentiality. If the treatment includes medication, the clinician should make the client aware of possible short-term and long-term side effects. The clinician has a responsibility to ensure that the client is aware of these issues, receives answers to any questions, and has the opportunity to refuse treatment. The client is then prepared to decide whether to continue in treatment.

There are possible complications. Psychotherapy is an imprecise procedure, and it is not always possible to predict its course, risks, or benefits. The clinician's job, however, is to give a best estimate at the onset of therapy and to provide further information as therapy proceeds. Most people are able to discuss these matters with the clinician and to make an informed choice. There are special cases, however, when prospective clients are unable to understand the issues in order to make informed consent. These cases include children and people who are unable to understand the full nature of the treatment into which they might enter due to cognitive or other psychological disabilities. In these cases, the clinician must work with the individual's family or other legally appointed guardians. Informed consent procedures should also be adapted for non-English-speaking individuals (McMillan, 2020).

TABLE 4 Guidelines for Psychological Practice with Older Adults

Attitudes	
Guideline 1.	Psychologists are encouraged to work with older adults within their scope of competence.
Guideline 2.	Psychologists are encouraged to recognize how their attitudes and beliefs about aging and about older individuals may be relevant to their assessment and treatment of older adults, and to seek consultation or further education about these issues when indicated.
General Knowledge about Adult Development, Aging, and Older Adults	
Guideline 3.	Psychologists strive to gain knowledge about theory and research in aging.
Guideline 4.	Psychologists strive to be aware of the social/psychological dynamics of the aging process.
Guideline 5.	Psychologists strive to understand diversity in the aging process, particularly how sociocultural factors such as gender, ethnicity, socioeconomic status, sexual orientation, disability status, and urban/rural residence may influence the experience and expression of health and of psychological problems in later life.
Guideline 6.	Psychologists strive to be familiar with current information about biological and health-related aspects of aging.
Clinical Issues	
Guideline 7.	Psychologists strive to be familiar with current knowledge about cognitive changes in older adults.
Guideline 8.	Psychologists strive to understand problems in daily living among older adults.
Guideline 9.	Psychologists strive to be knowledgeable about psychopathology within the aging population and cognizant of the prevalence and nature of that psychopathology when providing services to older adults.
Assessment	
Guideline 10.	Psychologists strive to be familiar with the theory, research, and practice of various methods of assessment with older adults, and knowledgeable of assessment instruments that are psychometrically suitable for use with them.
Guideline 11.	Psychologists strive to understand the problems of using assessment instruments created for younger individuals when assessing older adults, and to develop skill in tailoring assessments to accommodate older adults' specific characteristics and contexts.
Guideline 12.	Psychologists strive to develop skill at recognizing cognitive changes in older adults, and in conducting and interpreting cognitive screening and functional ability evaluations.
Intervention, Consultation, and Other Service Provision	
Guideline 13.	Psychologists strive to be familiar with the theory, research, and practice of various methods of intervention with older adults, particularly with current research evidence about their efficacy with this age group.
Guideline 14.	Psychologists strive to be familiar with and develop skill in applying specific psychotherapeutic interventions and environmental modifications with older adults and their families, including adapting interventions for use with this age group.
Guideline 15.	Psychologists strive to understand the issues pertaining to the provision of services in the specific settings in which older adults are typically located or encountered.
Guideline 16.	Psychologists strive to recognize issues related to the provision of prevention and health promotion services with older adults.
Guideline 17.	Psychologists strive to understand issues pertaining to the provision of consultation services in assisting older adults.
Guideline 18.	In working with older adults, psychologists are encouraged to understand the importance of interfacing with other disciplines, and to make referrals to other disciplines and/or to work with them in collaborative teams and across a range of sites, as appropriate.
Guideline 19.	Psychologists strive to understand the special ethical and/or legal issues entailed in providing services to older adults.
Education	
Guideline 20.	Psychologists are encouraged to increase their knowledge, understanding, and skills with respect to working with older adults through continuing education, training, supervision, and consultation.

American Psychological Association. (2018). Guidelines for psychological practice with older adults (published report). Retrieved from http://www.apa.org/practice/guidelines/older-adults.aspx

TABLE 5 Guidelines for Psychological Practice with Girls and Women

Guideline 1.	Psychologists strive to be aware of the effects of socialization, stereotyping, and unique life events on the development of girls and women across diverse cultural groups.
Guideline 2.	Psychologists are encouraged to recognize and utilize information about oppression, privilege, and identity development as they may affect girls and women.
Guideline 3.	Psychologists strive to understand the impact of bias and discrimination upon the physical and mental health of those with whom they work.
Guideline 4.	Psychologists strive to use gender and culturally sensitive, affirming practices in providing services to girls and women.
Guideline 5.	Psychologists are encouraged to recognize how their socialization, attitudes, and knowledge about gender may affect their practice with girls and women.
Guideline 6.	Psychologists are encouraged to employ interventions and approaches that have been found to be effective in the treatment of issues of concern to girls and women.
Guideline 7.	Psychologists strive to foster therapeutic relationships and practices that promote initiative, empowerment, and expanded alternatives and choices for girls and women.
Guideline 8.	Psychologists strive to provide appropriate, unbiased assessments and diagnoses in their work with girls and women.
Guideline 9.	Psychologists strive to consider the problems of girls and women in their sociopolitical context.
Guideline 10.	Psychologists strive to acquaint themselves with and utilize relevant mental health, education, and community resources for girls and women.
Guideline 11.	Psychologists are encouraged to understand and work to change institutional and systemic bias that may impact girls and women.

American Psychological Association. (February 2007). Guidelines for psychological practice with girls and women. Retrieved from https://www.apa.org/practice/guidelines/girls-and-women.aspx

Confidentiality

Several of the standards in the APA Ethics Code cover the issue of confidentiality. This means that the client can expect that what takes place in therapy is private. Confidentiality has long been regarded as a sacred part of the clinician–client relationship and is strictly maintained by licensed psychologists (Fisher & Vacanti-Shova, 2012). Safeguards against the disclosure of confidential information exist within the laws of most states. In order to adhere to the highest standards of professional practice, clinicians should have a clearly articulated protocol regarding the way in which they will inform clients about the nature, extent, and limits of confidentiality.

The content of therapy is privileged communication. In other words, the clinician may not disclose any information about the client in a court of law without the client's express permission. The protection offered by confidentiality allows clients in therapy to freely discuss their symptoms, problems in relationships with others, and early childhood history, all of which may contain extremely personal and delicate information. Confidentiality also protects research subjects from having the information they disclose to an investigator revealed to the public without their express consent.

There are, however, limits to confidentiality. Every state requires some form of mandated reporting by professionals when they learn firsthand of cases of abuse or neglect when victims are children, people with physical or intellectual disabilities, or older adults. Abuse, which can be emotional, verbal, physical or sexual, is an act by a caretaker that causes serious physical or emotional injury. Neglect is the intentional withholding of food, clothing, shelter, or medical care. The purposes of mandated reporting are to protect victims from continued abuse and neglect, to initiate steps toward clinical intervention with the abused individual, and to deter, punish, and rehabilitate abusers. Some states require that psychologists report not only financial, emotional, physical, or sexual abuse but also self-neglect by persons age 60 or older who do not attend to their own needs for food, clothing, safe and secure shelter, personal care, and medical treatment.

TABLE 6 **Guidelines for Assessment of and Intervention with Persons with Disabilities**

Disability Awareness, Training, Accessibility, and Diversity	
Guideline 1.	Psychologists strive to gain awareness of models of disability and an understanding of how these can impact they way they provide services.
Guideline 2.	Psychologists try to examine their own beliefs and reactions toward disabilities and understand how these can affect their work.
Guideline 3.	Psychologists gain education and consultation to improve their knowledge and skills for working with people who have disabilities.
Guideline 4.	Psychologists try to use the language and behavior that will be appropriate and communicate respect for people who have disabilities.
Guideline 5.	To ensure that clients with disabilities can access their services, psychologists work to provide barrier-free environments.
Guideline 6.	Psychologists try to understand both the common and individual experiences that affect their clients with disabilities.
Guideline 7.	Psychologists strive to recognize and learn the diversity of experiences of people with disabilities, including how disability affects the individual's development over the life course.
Guideline 8.	Psychologists gain understanding of the strengths and challenges that face families of people with disabilities.
Guideline 9.	Psychologists strive to recognize the increased risk of abuse that can affect people with disabilities.
Guideline 10.	Psychologists try to learn how assistive technology can be used to benefit individuals with disabilities.
Testing and Assessment	
Guideline 11.	In their assessment of clients with disabilities, psychologists strive to see disability as one among other forms of diversity, and strive to provide appropriate assessment instruments in order to yield valid test scores.
Guideline 12.	Psychologists strive to assess their clients with disabilities through a range of methods in order to understand their strengths and limitations.
Interventions	
Guideline 13.	Psychologists strive to collaborate with their clients, as well as families when appropriate, to plan, develop, and implement psychological interventions.
Guideline 14.	Psychologists strive to be aware of how the environment in which therapy takes place can affect their work with clients who have disabilities.
Guideline 15.	Psychologists strive to provide interventions for clients with disabilities that enhance their well-being as well as reduce distress and help to ameliorate any skill deficits.
Guideline 16.	Maintaining the perspectives of their clients when working with larger treatment or educational systems can allow psychologists to help them achieve self-determination, integration, choice, and availability of the least restrictive alternatives.
Guideline 17.	Psychologists strive to promote the health of individuals with disabilities.

American Psychological Association. (2012a). Guidelines for assessment of and intervention with persons with disabilities. *American Psychologist, 67,* 43–62.

Another exception to the principle of confidentiality occurs when the clinician learns that a client is planning to hurt another person. These cases face the psychologist with a **duty to warn (or otherwise protect)**. The duty-to-warn mandate requires that the clinician inform the intended victim about possible dangers posed by the client's behavior.

duty to warn (or otherwise protect)
The clinician's responsibility to notify a potential victim of a client's harmful intent toward that individual.

In order to provide psychologists with strategies for responding to demands of the legal system for information in the form of subpoenas, the Committee on Legal Issues (COLI) of APA (2016) issued a set of strategies that are consistent with the APA Ethics Code. These include determining whether the request for information carries the force of law, discussing (when appropriate) the request for records with the client, and potentially negotiating with the requestor or even filing a motion to "quash," which would provide relief from the obligation to provide records. A psychologist may also issue a motion to provide a protective order that would protect the client from any negative consequences of disclosing the requested information. Psychologists can also claim privileged information if they are asked to disclose confidential information during testimony. There may be exceptions, however, such as when the client waives the psychotherapist privilege but even then, the release of test results and reports could jeopardize the validity of these tests should their content and scoring be made public. As you can see, then, the ethical standard of confidentiality can have important legal implications.

Duty-to-warn laws have their origins in a famous case, *Tarasoff v. Regents of the University of California* (*Tarasoff v. The Regents of the University of California,* 551 P 2d 334 [California 1976]), in which a community college student named Tatiana Tarasoff was shot and fatally stabbed by Prosenjit Poddar, a graduate student who came from India in 1967 to study electronics and naval architecture at the University of California, Berkeley. Poddar met and began to pursue Tarasoff romantically, but she was not interested in him and in March 1969 rejected his marriage proposal. Poddar became despondent and told his roommate that he wanted to blow up Tarasoff's house. The roommate advised Poddar to seek treatment, and in June 1969 Poddar saw a psychiatrist at the university health services who prescribed antipsychotic medications and referred him to a psychologist for therapy. In August, Poddar repeatedly announced his homicidal thoughts about Tarasoff to the psychologist. After the psychologist warned Poddar that he would restrain him if he continued to express these thoughts, Poddar abruptly discontinued therapy. Although the psychologist and psychiatrist told the police about Poddar's intentions and the police then confronted him, he denied this intention, and the law took no further action. Poddar began to stalk Tarasoff, and in October 1969 he found her home alone and killed her. He then turned himself over to the police. Her parents sued the university and the police for not warning Tarasoff, and finally, in December 1976, the California Supreme Court ruled in favor of the parents. The essential question was "whether a psychotherapist must, on pain of a civil suit for damages, recognize that a patient poses a risk of serious harm or death to an identified third party and then must warn or otherwise protect that third party" (Herbert, 2002, p. 419).

The ramifications of this landmark decision continue to be felt by psychologists, who struggle to differentiate between their clients' serious threats and random fantasies, weighing the client's right of confidentiality against the rights of others. In April 2007, a student at Virginia Polytechnic Institute and State University named Seung-Hui Cho killed 32 people and wounded 25 others. He had received treatment from a mental health facility after having demonstrated threatening and harassing behavior on campus. In Virginia's version of the *Tarasoff* duty-to-warn statute, mental health caregivers must prevent the client from using physical violence or other means of harm to others until the appropriate law enforcement agency can be summoned and take custody of the client.

Duty to warn cases become complicated when clients do not identify specific targets or make threats directly to others. The Nebraska Supreme Court, for example, ruled that psychiatric facilities have a duty to warn in these cases (Burch & Nakic, 2019). The Pennsylvania Supreme Court ruled against healthcare providers who were informed by a client that he wanted to "kill a neighbor" in his 40-unit apartment building, but he did not identify a particular victim. The Court decided that, although not a specific threat, it fell into the duty to warn requirement, and that all the residents should have been informed. Such cases raise the issue of whether informing a large group of people about a potential threat posed by a client could increase the risk of violence. These potentially violent individuals might decide not to confide in a mental health professional and therefore not receive treatment (Ruutiainen & Northrop, 2021).

Even in California, the duty to warn principle continues to evolve as gun law legislation now requires that a clinician must report to the police when a client possesses a gun, but that the potential victim need not be warned (Weinstock et al., 2015). A Michigan survey of police officers found, additionally, that almost all followed up with at least one intervention when informed of a duty to warn. Most of these interventions notifying other police officers, and over half stated they would take action to remove a firearm (Guina, Dornfeld, & Pinals, 2022).

Duty to warn legislation, as in Virginia, may also reflect particular events that occur in a given state. Prior to the Marjorie Stoneman Douglas School (Parkland) shooting, Florida was a "permissive" Tarasoff state until the aftermath of the shooting led to mandatory duty to warn in July 2019 (Hall & Tardif, 2021).

Relationships with Clients, Students, and Research Collaborators

The APA's Ethics Code makes it clear that psychologists must take steps to ensure that they conduct all dealings with other individuals, including other psychologists, with the utmost professionalism. In therapy, clear roles and boundaries are essential in order for the client to feel safe and trusting and for the clinician to maintain objectivity and effectiveness. When a clinician violates boundaries within a therapeutic relationship, clients can experience a variety of nontherapeutic outcomes that only make their symptoms worse.

An extreme form of violation of the therapeutic relationship is sexual intimacy with clients, which is explicitly forbidden in the ethical codes of the mental health professions. In fact, psychologists are prohibited from becoming sexually involved with a client for at least 2 years after treatment ends (or longer in many cases).

Psychologists must also refrain from **multiple relationships**, particularly with their clients in a therapy context. The APA Ethics Code defines multiple relationships as occurring when a psychologist is in a professional role with a person and has another role with that person that could impair the psychologist's "objectivity, competence, or effectiveness in performing their functions as a psychologist" or otherwise risks exploiting or harming the other person. For example, psychologists are forbidden from pursuing professional relationships or friendships with their clients. However, multiple relationships that we would reasonably not believe to cause impairment or risk exploitation or harm are not unethical. For instance, therapists commonly provide individual psychotherapy to their patients while also facilitating a therapy group that the patient participates in.

multiple relationships
Unethical relationships occurring when a psychologist is in a professional role with a person and has another role with that person that could impair the psychologist's "objectivity, competence, or effectiveness in performing their functions as a psychologist" or otherwise risks exploiting or harming the other person.

Other ethical safeguards stipulate that psychologists avoid harming others, refrain from engaging in relationships with any conflict of interest, and not exploit other people with whom they have a professional relationship. When psychologists collaborate on research, for example, they should give or take credit only for work they have actually performed. They must also disclose their source of funding for research they publish in order to report any conflicts of interest.

Record Keeping

With increasing use of electronic health care records (including maintenance of files on cloud-based servers), the need to protect clients becomes even more critical. This need led to passage by the U.S. Congress of a complex series of rules governing patient records in the **Health Insurance Portability and Accountability Act of 1996 (HIPAA)**. HIPAA went into effect in several stages beginning in 2003 and ending in 2008. To enforce the new rules, civil monetary penalties can be levied for failure on the part of the employer, health care provider, or insurance company.

Health Insurance Portability and Accountability Act of 1996 (HIPAA)
U.S. legislation intended to ensure adequate coverage and protect consumers from loss of insurance coverage when they change or lose their jobs.

Title I of HIPAA protects workers and their families from loss of health care insurance when they change or lose their jobs. Prior to HIPAA's passage, people moving from one job to another were vulnerable to losing their health insurance if they had a history of serious illness. For example, someone who was treated for a cancerous condition and took a new job might have encountered the disturbing fact that they could not receive insurance coverage from the new employer because of this "pre-existing" illness.

Title II is intended to regulate the ways in which providers and insurance companies maintain and transmit medical records, called protected health information. Now that organizations send health records, prescriptions, and billing information via the Internet, health care professionals must take special care to protect confidential medical records.

You Be the Judge

Multiple Relationships Between Clients and Psychologists

The APA Ethics Code explicitly prohibits most multiple relationships between psychologists and their clients. However, given the nature of the therapist–client relationship, it is almost inevitable that potential multiple relationships can develop. In evaluating the ethics of a multiple relationship, we should distinguish between sexual and nonsexual. Sexual relationships are prohibited for at least 2 years after the ending of a therapeutic relationship. The boundaries around nonsexual relationships can be much murkier, however. In rural communities or small towns, for example, psychologists may find it almost impossible to avoid such dilemmas in situations ranging from retail sales to education to provision of other professional services. Social interactions between therapists and their clients may also prove difficult, even in larger communities with multiple intersecting social circles. In the chapter "Assessment," you read about the ethical dilemmas facing psychologists in the legal system. Here we will look more generally at multiple relationships as they affect psychologists in their clinical practice.

According to research on multiple relationships (Lamb, Catanzaro, & Moorman, 2004), social interactions are in fact the largest group of situations in which psychologists find themselves facing potential complications from client encounters. Psychologists also reported relationships in the spheres of business, financial dealings, and religious affiliations. These were more likely to occur between psychologists and their former clients than their current clients. In the area of sexual intimacy, the researchers asked psychologists to indicate whether the potential had ever existed for them to have relationships with their clients. However, even though they may have been tempted, these psychologists did not follow through on their interest due to their personal ethics, values, and morals. They also were highly unlikely to pursue a sexual relationship with a former client. At least half the psychologists also indicated that they wished to avoid dual relationships and/or did not want to take advantage of the unequal power dynamics between themselves and clients. Relatively few respondents mentioned that they refrained from these relationships due to possible legal repercussions or to their peers or professional associations sanctioning them.

The results of this survey suggest that psychologists adhere to high ethical standards in their relationships with current and former clients. As the study's authors acknowledge, however, it is possible that the participants who were the guiltiest of multiple relationships were the least likely to respond.

Q: *You be the judge:* Turning back to the ethical issue, consider the pros and cons of multiple relationships. Once a professional relationship is over, is it absolutely necessary for the psychologist not to become involved with a former client, particularly if they had a close connection during the course of treatment? Or is the very nature of the client–therapist relationship such that each party should respect the boundaries, even for years after treatment has ended? Should ethics codes be as stringent as they are in the area of multiple relationships?

The Ethics Code also governs the way in which psychologists charge fees for their services. They must inform clients about their fees prior to beginning any interventions and should reach an agreement with clients about arrangements for billing. Fee practices must also be consistent with the law. Surprisingly, psychologists can barter with their clients for services—that is, accept goods, services, or other nonmonetary remuneration in return for psychological services. They cannot do so, however, if this arrangement is clinically counterindicated or exploits their clients.

15.2 Ethical and Legal Issues in Providing Services

Psychologists and other mental health professionals face a number of issues in ensuring that clients receive the best possible treatment. At the same time, clinicians must balance the rights of clients with those of the community, issues that create ethical and legal dilemmas.

Commitment of Clients

In the best of all possible situations, clients who are in need of psychological treatment seek it themselves; however, clients are not always in a position to judge when they need the care of a psychologist. In these cases, the mental health professional may consider recommending **commitment**, an emergency procedure for involuntary hospitalization. Clinicians begin commitment proceedings in the cases of people who, if not hospitalized, are likely to create harm for self or other people as a result of mental illness.

commitment
An emergency procedure for involuntary psychiatric hospitalization.

The concept of commitment stems from the legal principle that the state has the authority to protect those who are unable to protect themselves. The law refers to this authority as ***parens patriae***, Latin for "the parent of one's country." It is vested in various professionals, such as psychologists, physicians, and nurse specialists, who are authorized to sign an application for a time-limited commitment (usually 10 days). If a health professional is not accessible, a police officer may file commitment papers. In the application, the professional states why failure to hospitalize the individual would result in the likelihood of serious harm due to mental illness.

parens patriae
The state's authority to protect those who are unable to protect themselves.

In some instances, the application for commitment goes to a district court judge, perhaps instigated by the concerns of a family member (though a family member cannot directly apply for commitment). After hearing the reasons for commitment, the judge may issue a warrant to apprehend the person with mental illness in order for that individual to receive a qualified professional assessment. Once the individual has been hospitalized, subsequent applications and hearings may be necessary to extend the period of commitment.

More than two dozen states now give courts, police officers, psychiatrists, mental health professionals, and families the option to coerce individuals with mental illness who have broken the law into treatment rather than to arrest them. Those supporting legislation that permits outpatient commitment assert that the benefits to society, in addition to the therapeutic benefits for the individual, outweigh the risks. In 1999, New York State enacted "Kendra's Law," which provides for the state's court-ordered involuntary outpatient commitment program, termed *assisted outpatient treatment (AOT)*. The law is named after the tragic death of Kendra Webdale, who was pushed in front of a subway train in Manhattan by a stranger who had untreated schizophrenia. The program has resulted in decreased hospitalization and improved service engagement and medication adherence (Swartz et al., 2010).

In California, parole boards may also conduct assessments of prisoners prior to their release to determine whether they should be committed to a state hospital as a condition of parole. A study of nearly 100 cases based on forensic evaluations showed that such evaluations may be unreliable because they depend on who is doing the evaluation, the context of the evaluation, and the length of time elapsing between evaluations (Dahl, DiCiro, Ziegler, & Sterling, 2023).

A case in Massachusetts established a precedent regarding involuntary commitment and the responsibility of colleges and universities to prevent student suicides. In May 2018, the Massachusetts Supreme Judicial Court (SJC) issued a ruling based on a case involving a student's suicide in 2009 at the Massachusetts Institute of Technology (MIT).

The family of graduate student Han Nyugen sued MIT for failure to protect the student despite allegedly having knowledge about his mental health struggles. The lawsuit was originally filed in 2011 and eventually moved up to the SJC, who dismissed all claims against MIT and found that the school was not responsible for Nyugen's death. Part of the ruling stated that a school has the duty to intervene when the school has actual knowledge of either a student's attempted suicide or plan to die by suicide while enrolled or recently prior to enrollment. If this duty is triggered, the SJC ruled that the reasonable measures include either initiating a suicide prevention protocol (if the school has developed such a protocol), or otherwise assisting the student in obtaining clinical care. If the student refuses to seek care, notification of the student's emergency contact is permissible.

It is important to note that the SJC ruling applies to employees and staff who are not licensed mental health clinicians, as clinicians are to abide by their own professional ethical codes when working with students experiencing suicidal ideation. It is likely that this ruling will greatly impact the ways in which colleges and universities manage the care of their students, and although they are not responsible for monitoring all aspects of the lives of their students, the school has a special duty to protect students from harm they may do to themselves.

Right to Treatment

Admission to a psychiatric hospital, whether voluntary or involuntary, is only the beginning of the story. Once admitted, the client enters a world unfamiliar to most people, which can frighten and confuse them. If hospitalized against their will, they may feel outraged. To minimize these reactions, health professionals try to ensure that they give clients appropriate care, including an understanding of their legal rights immediately upon entry to a facility. We have already discussed the importance of obtaining informed consent, when possible, prior to beginning treatment to ensure that clients understand the nature of treatment, the options available, and the client's rights.

right to treatment
Legal right of person entering psychiatric hospital to receive appropriate care.

Perhaps the most important legal right of the person entering a psychiatric hospital is the **right to treatment**. It may seem odd that laws are required to ensure that patients in hospitals receive treatment, but as you read the legal history of these statutes, you will understand why they are necessary. The right to treatment emerged as the outcome of a landmark legal case, *Wyatt v. Stickney* (*Wyatt v. Stickney,* 325 F. Supp. 781 [M.D. Ala. 1971]; 344 F. Supp. [M.D. Ala. 1972]). In this case, a patient named Ricky Wyatt instituted a class-action suit against the commissioner of mental health for the state of Alabama, Dr. Stickney, in response to the horrifying conditions in psychiatric hospitals and facilities devoted to individuals with intellectual developmental disorder. These institutions failed to provide even a minimum of treatment and were so inhumane that they were actually detrimental to the patients' mental health. In ruling against the state of Alabama, the court relied on a principle put forth by a legal scholar invoking the constitutional right to due process. In other words, the court ruled that mental health professionals cannot commit people to an institution that is supposed to help them unless they can guarantee that institutionalization *will* help them. Otherwise, their commitment constitutes the equivalent of imprisonment without a trial. Similarly, people with psychiatric disorders are entitled to treatment in the community rather than relegation to institutions.

Patients also have the right to a humane environment, including privacy, appropriate clothing, opportunities for social interaction, comfortable furnishings, physical exercise, adequate diet, and mail, telephone, and visitation privileges. A related right is that of liberty and safety (*Youngberg v. Romeo,* 457 U.S. 307 [1982]), which includes the right to move about the ward and receive protection from violent patients. Seclusion and mechanical restraints are forbidden unless medically indicated and, when clinicians use them, they can do so only for a limited amount of time and only for appropriate purposes (La Fond, 1994). Clients also have the right to receive treatment that is known to be effective for their disorder (Campbell & Lakeman, 2020).

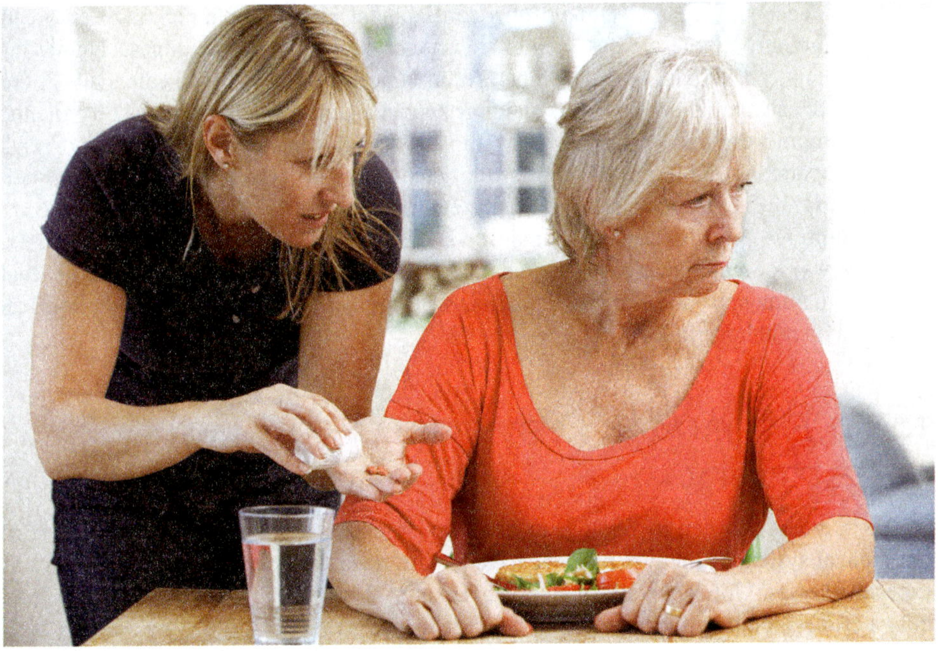

An individual in psychological care has the right to refuse treatment.

Monkey Business Images/Shutterstock

Refusal of Treatment and Least Restrictive Alternative

Medical and psychological treatment are based on the principle that competent adults have the right to either accept or decline medical treatment. In view of the serious side effects of certain psychotherapeutic medications, some U.S. states have enacted laws that give the client the right to refuse unwanted medications. If the client is involuntarily committed, the clinician must obtain a written order from a court of law documenting the need for medication.

Similarly, clients may regard as harsh or even punitive treatments such as the application of aversive noise or unpleasant shock. They may therefore refuse such treatment if they are capable of giving or withholding informed consent. However, cognitively compromised clients incapable of making informed decisions about such interventions may require protection by the law. A court can, in these cases, apply a doctrine called **substituted judgment** for people deemed incompetent of making such treatment decisions themselves. In substituted judgment, health professionals and family members try to make the decision the patient would have made if he or she were able to make decisions (Torke, Alexander, & Lantos, 2008). For example, a judge would attempt to determine whether the client would willingly approve the administration of aversive shock as a treatment designed to stop the client from engaging in life-threatening head-banging behavior.

substituted judgment
A doctrine that allows health professionals and family members to try to make the decision that the patient would have made if he or she were able to make decisions.

Clients also have the right to placement in the **least restrictive alternative** to treatment in an institution, meaning adult protective services provided in a manner no more restrictive of a vulnerable adult's liberty and no more intrusive than necessary to achieve and ensure essential services. This right was established in 1975 by a landmark ruling in the U.S. Supreme Court (*O'Connor v. Donaldson* [1975] 95 S. Ct. 2486). In 1943, Kenneth Donaldson was a 34-year-old father of three working in a General Electric defense plant when he showed what appeared to be symptoms of paranoid schizophrenia. Sent to a state hospital, he was given 23 electroshock treatments and resumed normal life. In the mid-1950s, he developed paranoid delusions that he was being poisoned. At the instigation of his father, Donaldson was committed to Florida's Chattahoochee State Hospital in 1956, where he remained for 15 years. Steadfastly denying he was ill, he refused all treatment and never exhibited signs of threatening behavior. His disorder, which clinicians diagnosed as paranoid schizophrenia, went into remission soon after his commitment. Nevertheless, Donaldson was kept in the hospital for nearly two decades, during which time he was denied many fundamental rights.

least restrictive alternative
A treatment setting that provides the fewest constraints on the client's freedom.

The evidence showed that Donaldson's confinement was a simple regime of enforced custodial care, not a program designed to alleviate or cure his supposed illness. Numerous witnesses had testified that Donaldson had received nothing but custodial care while at the hospital. For substantial periods, he was simply kept in a large room that housed 60 patients, many of whom were under criminal commitment. Donaldson's requests for ground privileges, occupational training, and an opportunity to discuss his case with the hospital superintendent, D. J. B. O'Connor, or other staff members were repeatedly denied.

The Supreme Court's ruling in Donaldson's favor, along with several less-known cases, paved the way for major changes in the mental health system. This case established the legal principle that the presence of mental illness in a person is not sufficient reason for confinement to a mental hospital.

15.3 Forensic Issues in Psychological Treatment

At the interface between psychology and the law, forensic psychologists provide advice to the judicial system in many ways. You have already seen that psychologists may serve as expert witnesses. More generally, they may also help assess whether an individual who commits a crime should be incarcerated or be treated in a mental health facility. Making such determinations requires weighing the complex needs of these offenders and the potential ethical implications of long-term detention (Völlm et al., 2018).

The Insanity Defense

insanity
A legal term that refers to the individual's lack of moral responsibility for committing criminal acts.

insanity defense
The argument, presented by a lawyer acting on behalf of the client, that, because of the existence of a mental disorder, the client should not be held legally responsible for criminal actions.

M'Naghten Rule
The "right-wrong test" used in cases of the insanity defense to determine whether a defendant should be held responsible for a crime.

Insanity is a legal term that describes an individual's lack of moral responsibility for committing criminal acts. The **insanity defense** is the argument a lawyer presents on behalf of a client who, because of the existence of a mental disorder, should not be held legally responsible for criminal actions. Criminal law is based on the principle that people have free choice in their actions and that, if they break the law, they must therefore be held responsible. People determined to be legally insane are judged so on the basis that they to lack the freedom to choose their behavior, as well as the mental competence to distinguish right from wrong. The insanity defense originated as an attempt to protect people with mental disorders from being punished for harmful behavior that resulted from their disturbed psychological state.

The insanity defense emerged from various legal precedents and the legal profession's attempts at clarification. In 1843, the British court handed down the **M'Naghten Rule** in the landmark case of a Scottish woodcutter named Daniel M'Naghten. Under the delusional belief that God was commanding him, M'Naghten killed an English government official. When he went to trial, the defense argued that he should not be held responsible for the murder because his mental disorder prevented him from knowing the difference between right and wrong. He believed he was following the commands of a higher power and, therefore, saw nothing wrong in his behavior. This is why the M'Naghten Rule is referred to as the "right-wrong test."

irresistible impulse
The legal argument that although clients in a forensic setting knew an act was wrong, they were unable to stop themselves from acting on their impulses.

Durham Rule
An expansion of the insanity defense based on determining that the individual was not criminally responsible if the unlawful act was due to the presence of a psychological disorder.

Most jurisdictions in the United States adopted the M'Naghten Rule. U.S. legislatures and courts eventually modified and expanded the definition of insanity, adding the **irresistible impulse** test to take into account the possibility that some disturbed behaviors may result from people's inability to inhibit actions they feel compelled to carry out. Although they may know an act is wrong, they are unable to stop themselves from acting on their impulses.

The **Durham Rule** later expanded the insanity defense after a court decision in 1954 asserted that a person is not criminally responsible if the "unlawful act was the product of mental disease or defect." The intent was to protect individuals with disturbed psychological functioning due to any of a variety of conditions, including personality disorders. This expansion of the insanity defense put the burden on mental health experts to prove a defendant "had a mental disease or defect," even when there was no evidence of overt psychosis.

REAL STORIES

Robert Card

Shortly before 7 P.M. on October 25, 2023, 40-year-old Army Reservist and firearms instructor Robert Card entered a bowling alley in Lewiston Maine, a small town north of Portland, Maine. Using an assault-style rifle, Card opened fire on patrons at random. He then drove 4 miles away to a bar and again shot indiscriminately at patrons before fleeing the scene. In total, he killed 18 people, whose ages ranged from 14 to 76. Thirteen others were critically wounded in this tragic mass shooting (CNN, 2023).

Following the shootings, the local authorities began a manhunt to apprehend Card, who was ultimately found dead in a trailer at a recycling factory from which he was recently fired (CBS News, 2023). Card had shot himself in the head about 12 hours before he was found. During the manhunt, the entire town of Lewiston was put on a shelter-in-place order, stoking intense fear among the small, close-knit community. The ordeal garnered significant national interest as the search for Card went on over an excruciating two-day period. In that time, reports about Card's mental health struggles quickly became the topic of national news, particularly in the context of heated political debates about mental health and gun control. The reports centered around the revelation that Card was placed in an involuntary psychiatric hospitalization just three months prior to the shootings, and after his discharge, he nevertheless was able to legally purchase the assault weapon used in the shootings.

Following the shooting, Card's siblings recounted that he started to show troubling signs of psychosis, including paranoid delusions after a romantic break-up with a girlfriend earlier in the year. Apparently the two had met at the bar which became one of the scenes of his shooting spree. The content of the delusions related to his belief, for which there was no factual basis, that he had been accused online of being a pedophile (New York Times, 2023).

In May 2023, Card's ex-wife and adolescent son because concerned about his mental health enough to the point where they notified the local police that he had become "paranoid and angry," and had recently taken at least 15 guns from his brother's house (New York Times, 2023). Card's family had also been concerned about him due to several episodes of his drinking excessively and talking about shooting people. Law enforcement did not take any formal action related to these concerns.

In July 2023, while at an Army Reserves training camp, Card physically assaulted three fellow soldiers in his unit, stating he believed they were accusing him of being a pedophile. Following the incident, he was taken to a medical facility in the U.S. Military Academy in West Point, New York, and from there was involuntarily committed to a local psychiatric hospital to treat his psychosis. His hospitalization lasted for 14 days, and by all accounts after discharge he did not follow up with outpatient treatment or continue taking medication.

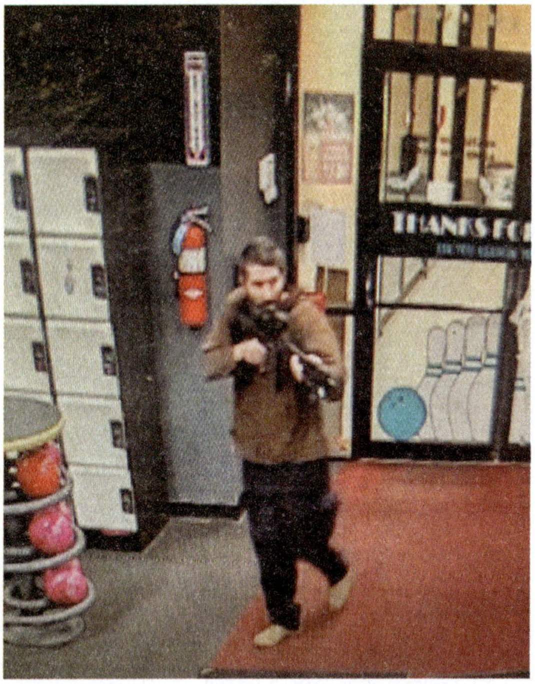

In October 2023, Robert Card opened fire on patrons in a bowling alley and a bar, killing 18 people. Prior to the mass shooting, there were many warning signs that he could be a mass shooter, including concerns that arose during a recent psychiatric hospitalization.

Anadolu/Getty Images

For the next few months, it seems that his mental health continued to deteriorate, and that he repeatedly made violent threats to those around him. The month before the October shooting, he punched another soldier and talked about "shooting up" the army facility where they both trained. The soldier reported his concerns to a superior officer, but the Army did not take steps to follow-up on these concerns. Around that time, the local law enforcement unit had initiated a welfare check to Card's home. He was not home at the time, and there was no further follow-up from that point. Meanwhile, Card had amassed several guns and had even purchased some legally after his hospitalization in July. He had apparently revealed that he had a recent psychiatric hospitalization while completing the background check, but this was not grounds enough to stop him from legally obtaining assault-style weapons, which he went on to use in the October shooting.

Many questions remain as to why the major warning signs about Card's threatening behaviors never turned into direct action to prevent him from committing a mass shooting. The state of Maine has a "yellow flag" warning that law enforcement can initiate if an individual seems like a threat to self or others, which can involve taking away the individual's firearms. That warning was never raised by local law enforcement despite multiple reports of Card's paranoia and threats of violence from many people who knew Card closely. Further, existing laws did not prevent him from legally obtaining assault-style weapons. Little is known about Card's past mental health history apart from what was reported by friends and family following the shooting, and whether he had any form of diagnosis or treatment apart from his known hospitalization. Regardless of his past history though, it seems clear that there were active warning signs of Card's intention to commit a horrific and violent act, linked to his delusional beliefs—that ultimately went ignored by the authorities. The incident added fuel to an already intense national political debate about gun control, and raised major concerns about the law enforcement system, due to the failure of safeguards already in place of preventing such a major, but seemingly predictable, catastrophe.

American Law Institute's (ALI) guidelines
Guidelines proposing that people are not responsible for criminal behavior if their mental disorder prevents them from appreciating the wrongfulness of their behavior or exerting the willpower to control it.

In an attempt to develop uniform standards for the insanity defense, the **American Law Institute's (ALI) guidelines** in 1962 (Sec. 4.01) took a middle position between the pre-Durham Rule codes and the liberal standing the Durham Rule takes. According to ALI, people are not responsible for criminal behavior if their mental disorder prevents them from appreciating the wrongfulness of their behavior or from exerting the necessary willpower to control their acts (the irresistible impulse rule). The important term here is *appreciating.* In other words, knowing what is right and wrong is not equivalent to understanding that your behavior is wrong.

The ALI code allows for the introduction of medical and psychiatric evidence and thus provides a modern test for the insanity defense. Another important feature of the ALI code is the exclusion from the insanity defense of people whose only maladaptive behavior is repeated criminal or otherwise antisocial conduct. The ALI guideline is a more viable standard of insanity than the Durham Rule, because it takes the question of guilt or innocence away from mental health experts and places it in the hands of the jury, who can then make a determination based on the evidence related to the crime itself.

In the years following the publication of the ALI standards, the courts applied the insanity defense much more widely. However, the situation changed once again after John Hinckley Jr. attempted to assassinate President Ronald Reagan in 1981. Hinckley was obsessed with actor Jodie Foster and believed that if he killed the president she would be so impressed that she would fall in love with him and marry him. When the case went to trial, the jury determined that Hinckley's actions justified the insanity defense. He was sent to St. Elizabeth's Hospital in Washington, D.C., where he remained until 2016. This case brought to the nation's attention the rarely used but controversial insanity plea as it had been broadened through the Durham and ALI standards. The public was particularly outraged about the possibility that an assassin could get away with murder on the grounds of having a mental disorder.

In response to the Hinckley case, Congress passed the Insanity Defense Reform Act of 1984, which added the criterion of "severe disturbance" to the insanity defense. This meant that people with personality disorders would no longer be able to plead insanity. The law also moved the burden of proof. Previously, the defense needed to provide reasonable doubt regarding the prosecution's argument that the defendant was sane. The Reform Act meant that the defense must now prove that the defendant fits the legal definition of insanity, which is a more difficult argument to make.

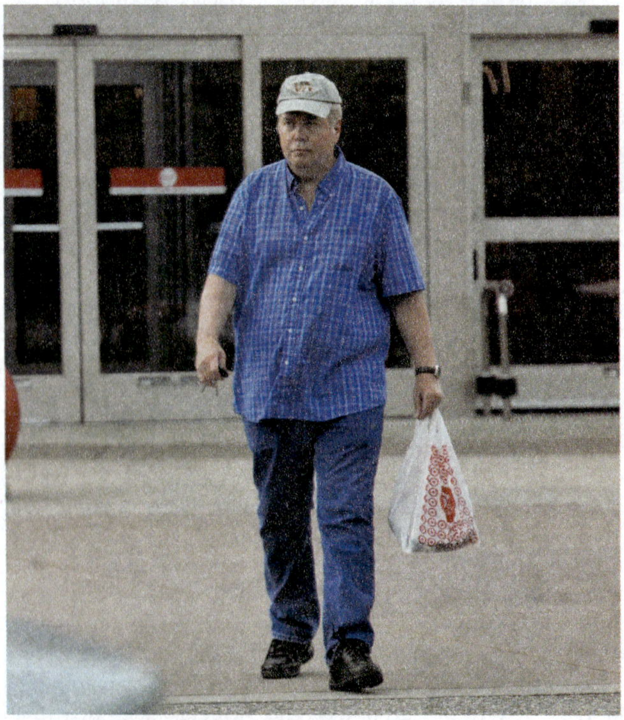

The case of John Hinckley Jr., who in 1981 tried to assassinate President Ronald Reagan, raised public concern over possible misuse of the insanity defense. Hinckley, who was declared insane by the courts, was not imprisoned; instead he was committed for treatment at St. Elizabeth's Hospital in Washington, D.C., until his release in 2016.

Splash News

The nature of the insanity defense varies somewhat by state. Some states separate the matter of guilt from that of mental disorder by allowing the plea of "guilty but mentally ill." The court does not exonerate defendants who use this plea but does give them special consideration in sentencing.

Partly because of the storm of criticism following the Hinckley case, however, the court took a very different route in 1992. This time, a 31-year-old man, Jeffrey Dahmer, had confessed to murdering and dismembering 17 boys and young men in Wisconsin, explaining that he was driven to kill out of a compulsion to have sex with dead bodies. His defense attorney argued that the crimes could have been committed only by someone who fit the legal definition of insanity. The jury rejected the guilty but mentally ill plea because they believed Dahmer to be responsible for his crimes and able to appreciate the wrongfulness of his conduct. Dahmer was sentenced to consecutive life terms for the murders of each of his victims. In 1994, he was killed in prison by another inmate.

Other highly publicized cases since Dahmer's have brought out subtleties in the insanity defense as we currently construe it.

In 1989, California brothers Lyle and Erik Menendez admitted to the premeditated murder of their parents in response, they claimed, to years of abuse. Their defense attorneys presented the argument of "imperfect self-defense," asserting that the brothers, in their twenties at the time, acted in the mistaken belief that their parents were about to kill them, a belief stemming from a lifelong history of physical, emotional, and sexual abuse. The defense argued that on the night of the killings one of the brothers, in an altered mental state, retrieved his shotgun, loaded it, and burst in on his parents. The prosecution, which proved its case, claimed the brothers were instead motivated by the $14 million they stood to inherit.

The irresistible impulse defense came to light in the highly publicized case of Lorena Bobbitt, a Virginia woman who claimed to be temporarily insane as a result of years of physical and psychological abuse by her husband, leading her to cut off his penis. Bobbitt claimed that she had been overcome by what she called "pictures," or mental images, of his abusive actions toward her. The jury concluded that she was temporarily insane and acquitted her of all charges of malicious and unlawful wounding. As mandated by Virginia law, the judge in the case ordered Bobbitt to be evaluated at a state psychiatric hospital to determine whether she posed a danger to herself or others. After the required 45-day period, she was released.

Yet another variant of the insanity defense occurred in the case of Andrea Yates, who in June 2001 drowned her five children in the bathtub of her Texas home. Yates had a history of profound postpartum depression following the births of her fourth and fifth children. Although her case seemed to merit the insanity plea, the court convicted her of capital murder in March 2002. In 2006, however, an appeals court overturned the verdict on the basis that one of the expert witnesses in the trial had presented false testimony relevant to Yates's mental state at the time of the killings. In July 2006, the court moved Yates from a high-security mental health facility to a low-security state mental hospital. The difficulties surrounding this case are reflected in similar cases that have arisen over the past two decades in that the insanity defense in cases of infanticide is inconsistently applied (Nichols, 2023).

The homicide trial of Lee Boyd Malvo and John Allen Muhammad presented the case of two individuals who had committed a crime together, but only one qualified for the insanity defense. The pair were arrested in October 2002 after conducting sniper attacks in which they murdered 10 people in the Washington, D.C., area. The prosecution asserted that Muhammad, a man in his forties, had planned the mass shooting and ordered 17-year-old Malvo to help him. Malvo's defense attorneys pleaded the insanity defense on the grounds that he was indoctrinated and therefore had a form of mental illness. Because he was a teenager under the power of a much older man, they said, Malvo did not know right from wrong. However, the jury rejected this version of the insanity defense. Ultimately, Muhammad was executed by lethal injection in Virginia in 2009, and Malvo was sentenced in 2006 to six consecutive life sentences without the possibility of parole.

The opposite situation occurred in the case of Theodore Kaczynski, known as the Unabomber. From his cabin in Montana, Kaczynski mounted an 18-year campaign against the "industrial-technological system." He admitted that he had killed three people and maimed many others by sending package bombs to government addresses. His history and extensive clinical evaluation offered compelling evidence that he had schizophrenia, paranoid type. However, he refused to use the insanity defense because he did not consider himself to have a psychological disorder. A federal grand jury indicted Kaczynski in April 1996 on 10 counts of illegally transporting, mailing, and using bombs, and three counts of murder; he was held in a maximum security facility in Colorado, and in 2023 he died by suicide in a prison medical center after he was diagnosed with late-stage cancer.

Given the complexity of these key cases, along with the many others that pass through the courts, particularly with the rise of mass shootings, it is essential that psychologists who conduct forensic examinations do so on the basis of standardized training and performance standards (Packer & Kois, 2023). Standardized assessment instruments are

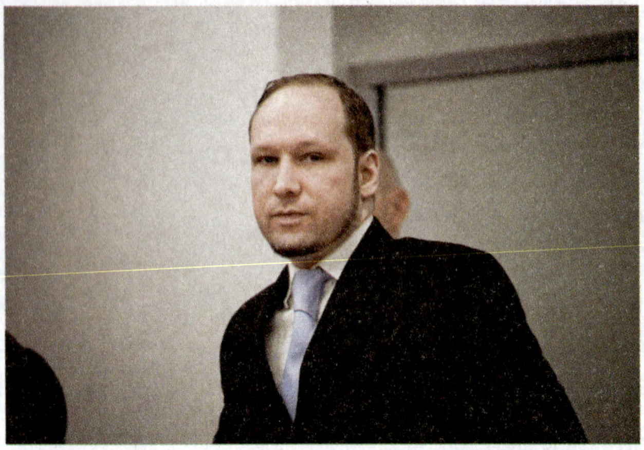

The case of Scott Louis Panetti has been the focus of legal debate and controversy after his death sentence in Texas was overturned by the U.S. Supreme Court on the grounds that Panetti lacked understanding of why he was to be put to death.
Alexander Widding/Alamy Stock Photo

becoming available that can allow such assessments to be made, including those that can detect a criminal's behavior was not linked to a psychological disorder (Parmigiani, Mandarelli, Meynen, & Ferracuti, 2023).

Competency to Stand Trial

Based on the principle that people should be able to participate in their own defense, the finding of **competency to stand trial** asserts that defendants are aware of and able to participate in criminal proceedings against them. To assess competency, a forensic expert evaluates the defendant's cognitive capacity, emotional stamina, and ongoing symptoms at the time of the trial. The court may postpone trial until the defendant's symptoms subside, if necessary, mandating that the individual receive medication. Determination of competency to stand trial can present a challenge, especially when the clinician must simultaneously evaluate the individual's legal sanity (Gardner, Murrie, & Torres, 2022).

competency to stand trial
A prediction by a mental health expert of the defendant's cognitive and emotional stability during the period of the trial.

Understanding the Purpose of Punishment

Separate from the issue of competency to stand trial is the question whether a person with mental illness who is convicted of a capital offense is able to understand the nature and purpose of a death sentence. The case of Scott Louis Panetti, which the U.S. Supreme Court heard in 2007, highlights some of the complexities here.

In 1992, Panetti killed his in-laws while holding hostage his estranged wife and their 3-year-old daughter. Even though Panetti had a lengthy history of mental illness and psychiatric hospitalizations, the Texas court sentenced him to death. In 2003, Panetti petitioned the Texas state appeals court to determine his competency for execution, asserting his belief that satanic forces had sought his execution to prevent him from preaching the Gospel. His defense lawyers claimed that because Panetti could not understand why the jury had sentenced him to death, the death penalty would constitute cruel and unusual punishment and therefore violate the Eighth Amendment of the Constitution. The Texas Department of Criminal Justice objected to this argument, contending that capital punishment in such cases should rest not on whether a convict has rational understanding of the reasons for execution, but on the convict's moral culpability at the time he or she committed the crime.

In 2007, the U.S. Supreme Court blocked Panetti's execution and returned the case to the U.S. District Court in Austin, Texas, returning him to prison in Texas, where he remains on death row. The court based this decision in part on arguments that the American Psychological Association, the American Psychiatric Association, and the National Alliance on Mental Illness put forward. These organizations had jointly submitted a brief stating that individuals with psychotic conditions, such as Panetti, may experience delusions and a disrupted understanding of reality. They may also be unable to connect events or understand cause and effect—namely, the connection between the murder and the punishment.

Concluding Perspectives on Forensic Issues

As you can see from this discussion of forensic issues, there is an entire body of knowledge forming on the border between psychology and the law. Mental health professionals are playing an increasingly important role in the legal system and at the same time finding that they must familiarize themselves with an array of forensic issues. Clearly, the areas of intersection between psychology and the law will continue to grow as society looks for interventions that are humane, ethical, and effective.

Return to the Case: Allison Yang

Allison was hospitalized for 5 days while health care professionals thoroughly assessed her, focusing on her suicidality and depressive symptoms. She attended group therapy and worked with a psychiatrist to change her medication regimen. Once she had stabilized and was no longer suicidal, she was released. Her parents picked her up, and she decided to stay with them for the rest of the semester and return to school the following year.

Before her hospitalization, Allison's parents had not been aware that she was experiencing psychological difficulties. Much to her surprise, they said they understood her need to stay home to recuperate. Since her parents lived several hours away from her school, Allison and her therapist decided to have weekly telephone sessions in order to continue their work together. They focused on the relationship between Allison and her parents, and Allison used the time at home to learn to discuss with her parents how she felt about the pressure they had placed on her and why that been a source of much stress.

Dr. Tobin's reflections: Clinicians are sometimes faced with the difficult decision to hospitalize their therapy clients. Allison's clinician performed the appropriate steps to assess her level of safety and found her in great need of hospitalization because she appeared to be an immediate threat to her own life. Thus, he was ethically bound to break confidentiality and send Allison to the hospital for further evaluation. Luckily, the two had a strong enough alliance that Allison felt she should come in for "one last session" rather than ending her life. This may have been a cry for help because Allison knew her clinician would be able to help her.

Allison's first depressive episode was severe, lasting around 8 months. Usually, the more severe the initial episode, the more persistent and severe subsequent episodes will become. Considering that the current work with her clinician is the first time Allison has received psychological help, part of her treatment will be to help her gain a sense of insight into her psychological struggles. For instance, should she begin to notice the same pattern of symptoms in the future that led to her current depressive episode, she may then recognize that her symptoms could turn more severe if she does not bring them to the attention of her therapist or psychiatrist.

Finally, psychotherapy conducted over the phone or Internet, called teletherapy, is an increasingly common protocol and is covered by the APA's Ethics Code. If both parties agree it is the best way to maintain the therapeutic alliance over a certain period of time, as in Allison's case, it may be a suitable alternative to stopping therapy altogether. Because Allison did plan on returning to school and continuing to work with her therapist in person, it appears that teletherapy was an appropriate way to continue until then and avoid a break in her progress.

SUMMARY

- Ethical guidelines cover the expectations for clinicians to have competence to assess, conceptualize, and treat clients whom they accept into treatment. The American Psychological Association's Ethics Code provides detailed standards that psychologists are required to adhere to.
- Confidentiality is the principle that the therapist must safeguard disclosures in therapy as private. With only a few exceptions, the content of therapy is privileged communication; that is, the clinician may not disclose any information about the client in a court without the client's express permission. Exceptions to confidentiality include instances involving mandated reporting and duty to warn (or otherwise protect). Mental health professionals are mandated by law to report information involving the abuse or neglect of children or other people who are unable to protect themselves. The duty to warn involves the clinician's responsibility to take action to inform a possible victim of a client's intention to do harm to that person.
- In their relationships with clients, clinicians are expected to adhere to the highest standards of ethical and professional conduct. They are to avoid inappropriate relationships, such as sexual intimacy with clients, and must maintain neutrality and distance in their dealings with clients. In overseeing the business aspects of psychotherapy practice, mental health professionals face various challenges, particularly when operating within managed health care delivery systems.
- Clinicians are sometimes involved in the process of commitment, an emergency procedure for the involuntary hospitalization of a person who, if not hospitalized, is likely to create harm for self or others as a result of mental illness. Hospitalized clients have the right to treatment—the right to a humane environment with appropriate amenities, in addition to liberty and safety. Clients also have the right to refuse unwanted treatment, unless a court deems that the client is at risk of harming self or others without needed intervention.

Clients also have the right for placement in the least restrictive alternative to treatment in an institution.

- The major forensic issues that pertain to the field of mental health involve the insanity defense and competency to stand trial. The insanity defense is the legal argument that the lawyer acting on behalf of the client presents, which states that, because of the existence of a mental disorder, the law should not hold the client legally responsible for criminal actions. Various controversies have emerged over the years regarding the insanity defense as courts have struggled with issues of assessing a defendant's responsibility in well-publicized cases involving violent assault and murder. The determination of competency to stand trial pertains to the question of whether defendants are aware of and able to participate in criminal proceedings against them.

KEY TERMS

American Law Institute's (ALI) guidelines
Commitment
Competency to stand trial
Durham Rule
Duty to warn (or otherwise protect)
Emotional competence
Guardian *ad litem*
Health Insurance Portability and Accountability Act of 1996 (HIPAA)
Insanity
Insanity defense
Irresistible impulse
Least restrictive alternative
M'Naghten Rule
Multiple relationships
Parens patriae
Right to treatment
Substituted judgment

GLOSSARY

A

acamprosate An amino acid derivative that appears to moderate glutamate receptors.

acceptance-based perspective A theoretical perspective that is intended to promote psychological flexibility and reduce avoidance of experiences.

acceptance and commitment therapy (ACT) A therapeutic approach that aims to indirectly reduce symptoms by focusing on improving psychological flexibility.

ACT hexaflex In acceptance and commitment therapy (ACT), the six main psychological processes that can become the source of psychological disorders.

active phase A period in the course of schizophrenia in which psychotic symptoms are present.

acute stress disorder An anxiety disorder that develops after a traumatic event, and lasts for up to 1 month with symptoms such as depersonalization, numbing, dissociative amnesia, intense anxiety, hypervigilance, and impairment of everyday functioning.

adaptive testing Testing in which the client's responses to earlier questions determine the subsequent questions presented to them.

affirmative psychotherapy Approach in treating transgender clients in which clinicians help their clients safely explore their gender identity, explore options for gender-affirming medical procedures, and connect with sources of social support.

agoraphobia Intense anxiety triggered by the real or anticipated exposure to situations in which individuals may be unable to get help should they become incapacitated.

akinesia A motor disturbance in which a person's muscles become rigid and movement is difficult to initiate.

alcohol expectancy theory A perspective that emphasizes how expectations about the effects of alcohol use influence actual consumption of alcohol.

alcohol myopia theory Proposes that as individuals consume greater amounts of alcohol, they are more likely to make risky choices because the immediate temptation of the moment overcomes the long-term consequences of the behavior.

allele One of two or more different variations of a gene.

Alternative Model for Personality Disorders (AMPD) A dimensional approach for personality disorders along the dimensions of self and interpersonal functioning.

American Law Institute's (ALI) guidelines Guidelines proposing that people are not responsible for criminal behavior if their mental disorder prevents them from appreciating the wrongfulness of their behavior or exerting the willpower to control it.

amnesia Inability to recall information that was previously learned or to register new memories.

amphetamine A stimulant that affects both the central nervous and the autonomic nervous systems.

amyloid plaques A characteristic of Alzheimer's disease in which clusters of dead or dying neurons become mixed together with fragments of protein molecules.

analog observations Assessments that take place in a setting or context such as a clinician's office or a laboratory specifically designed for observing the target behavior.

anorexia nervosa (AN) An eating disorder characterized by severely restricted eating, an intense fear of gaining weight, and distorted body perception.

anoxia Oxygen deprivation to the brain.

anterograde amnesia Amnesia involving the inability to remember new information.

antisocial behavior The tendency to engage in impulsive and aggressive acts, take risks despite experiencing negative consequences, fail to conform to social or ethical norms, and a history of early behavioral problems or juvenile delinquency.

antisocial personality disorder A personality disorder characterized by a lack of regard for society's moral or legal standards and an impulsive and risky lifestyle.

anxiety A future-oriented and global response, involving both cognitive and emotional components, in which an individual is inordinately apprehensive, tense, and uneasy about the prospect of something terrible happening.

anxiety disorders Disorders characterized by excessive fear and anxiety and related disturbances in behavior.

anxiety sensitivity theory The belief that panic disorder is caused in part by the tendency to interpret cognitive and somatic manifestations of stress and anxiety in a catastrophic manner.

anxiolytic An antianxiety medication.

***APOE* gene** A gene located on chromosome 19 thought to be involved in the late-onset form of Alzheimer's disease.

Applied Behavior Analysis (ABA) Treatment approach within the behavioral perspective that uses principles of reinforcement both to understand and change behavior.

archetypes In Jung's theory, a set of images common to all human experience.

asociality Lack of interest in social relationships.

Asperger's syndrome A term once used to describe individuals with high-functioning autism spectrum disorder.

assertive community treatment (ACT) Treatment modality in which a team of professionals from psychiatry, psychology, nursing, and social work reach out to clients in their homes and workplaces.

assortative mating Entry by a person with a psychological disorder into a long-term relationship with a partner who has the same psychological disorder.

attachment figures Caregivers or adults to whom the individual is attached.

attachment style The way a person relates to a caregiver figure.

attention-deficit/hyperactivity disorder (ADHD) A neurodevelopmental disorder involving a persistent pattern of inattention and/or hyperactivity.

autism spectrum disorder A neurodevelopmental disorder involving impairments in the domains of social communication and the performance of restricted, repetitive behaviors.

automatic thoughts Ideas that are the product of dysfunctional attitudes so deeply entrenched the individual is not even aware they exist.

aversive conditioning Classical conditioning in which the individual associates a maladaptive response with a stimulus that could not itself cause harm.

avoidant/restrictive food intake disorder A disorder in which individuals avoid or restrict food eating to the point that they experience significant threats to their physical health.

avoidant personality disorder A personality disorder in which people have low estimation of their social skills and are fearful of disapproval, rejection, and criticism or being ashamed or embarrassed.

avolition A lack of initiative, either not wanting to take any action or lacking the energy and will to take action.

axis A class of information in previous *DSM*s regarding one dimension of an individual's functioning.

B

behavioral activation Behavioral therapy for depression in which the clinician helps the client identify activities associated with positive mood.

behavioral assessment A form of measurement based on objective recording of the individual's behavior.

behavioral genetics Research area focused on identifying the role of hereditary factors in psychological disorders.

behavioral interviewing Assessment process in which clinicians ask questions about the target behavior's frequency, antecedents, and consequences.

behavioral medicine An interdisciplinary approach to medical conditions affected by psychological factors that is rooted in learning theory.

behavioral perspective A theoretical perspective in which it is assumed that abnormality is caused by faulty learning experiences.

behavioral self-report A method of behavioral assessment in which the individual provides information about the frequency of particular behaviors.

binge alcohol use Drinking four (for women) and five (for men) or more drinks on the same occasion.

binge eating disorder (BED) An eating disorder in which individuals lack control over their eating and engage in binges for at least twice a week for 6 months.

binge eating The ingestion of large amounts of food during a short period of time, even after reaching a point of feeling full, and a lack of control over what or how much is eaten.

biological perspective A theoretical perspective in which it is assumed that disturbances in emotions, behavior, and cognitive processes are caused by abnormalities in the functioning of the body.

biopsychosocial perspective A model in which the interaction of biological, psychological, and sociocultural factors is seen as influencing the development of the individual over time.

bipolar disorder, rapid cycling A form of bipolar disorder involving four or more episodes within the previous year that meet the criteria for manic, hypomanic, or major depressive disorder.

bipolar disorder A mood disorder involving manic episodes—intense and disruptive experiences of heightened mood, possibly alternating with major depressive episodes.

bipolar I disorder A clinical course in which the individual experiences one or more manic episodes with the possibility, although not the necessity, of experiencing one or more major depressive episodes.

bipolar II disorder A clinical course in which the individual has had one or more major depressive episodes and at least one hypomanic episode.

Birth-assigned sex Term that refers to sex assigned to the individual at birth based on either genitalia and/or prenatal sex discernment.

Black-White paradox The fact that the prevalence for depression is lower in Black adults than White adults despite the exposure of Black adults to more life stressors.

Bleuler's "Four A's" According to Swiss psychologist Eugen Bleuler, the four fundamental features of schizophrenia include disorders in association and affect, ambivalence, and autism.

body dysmorphic disorder (BDD) A disorder in which individuals are preoccupied with the idea that a part of their body is ugly or defective.

borderline personality disorder (BPD) A personality disorder characterized by a pervasive pattern of poor impulse control and instability in mood, interpersonal relationships, and sense of self.

Boston Naming Test (BNT) Neuropsychological test intended to assess word retrieval abilities.

bradykinesia A motor disturbance involving a general slowing of motor activity.

brief psychotic disorder A diagnosis clinicians use when an individual develops symptoms of psychosis for more than a day but less than a month.

bulimia nervosa (BN) An eating disorder involving alternation between the extremes of eating large amounts of food in a short time, and then compensating for the added calories either by vomiting or other extreme actions to avoid gaining weight.

buprenorphine A medication used in the treatment of heroin addiction.

caffeine A stimulant found in coffee, tea, chocolate, energy drinks, diet pills, and headache remedies.

Cambridge Neuropsychological Testing Automated Battery (CANTAB) Computerized neuropsychological test battery offering 22 specific tests.

C

case formulation A clinician's analysis of the client's development and the factors that might have influenced his or her current psychological status.

case study An intensive study of a single person described in detail.

catatonia A condition in which the individual shows marked psychomotor disturbances.

childhood-onset fluency disorder (stuttering) A communication disorder that involves a disturbance in the normal fluency and patterning of speech characterized by such verbalizations as sound *repe*titions or prolongations, broken words, the blocking out of sounds, word substitutions to avoid problematic words, or words expressed with an excess of tension.

circadian rhythms Biological clocks that set patterns of sleepfulness and wakefulness on approximately a 24-hour basis.

classical conditioning The process in the behavioral perspective that accounts for the learning of emotional, automatic responses.

client-centered An approach based on the belief held by Rogers that people are innately good and that the potential for self-improvement lies within the individual.

client A person seeking psychological treatment.

climacteric The gradual loss of reproductive potential that occurs in middle and later adulthood.

clinical interview A series of questions that clinicians administer in face-to-face interaction with the client.

clinical psychologist A mental health professional with training in the behavioral sciences who provides direct service to clients.

clinical significance The criterion for a psychological disorder in which the behavior being evaluated includes a measurable degree of impairment that the clinician can observe.

clinician The person providing treatment.

Clock Drawing Test Simple neuropsychological test in which a test-taker draws a picture of an analog clock.

cocaine A highly addictive central nervous system stimulant that an individual snorts, injects, or smokes.

cognitive behavioral perspective An approach that focuses on the role of both maladaptive thoughts and maladaptive behaviors in psychological disorders.

cognitive behavioral therapy (CBT) Treatment method in which clinicians focus on changing both maladaptive thoughts and maladaptive behaviors.

cognitive behavioral therapy for psychosis (CBTp) Method of treating symptoms of psychosis in which clinicians do not try to change clients' delusions or eliminate their hallucinations but instead try to reduce their distress and preoccupation with these symptoms.

cognitive perspective A theoretical perspective in which it is assumed that abnormality is caused by maladaptive thought processes that result in dysfunctional behaviors and emotions.

cognitive restructuring One of the fundamental techniques of cognitive behavioral therapy in which the clinician attempts to change the client's thoughts by questioning and challenging the client's dysfunctional attitudes and irrational beliefs.

cognitive triad According to the cognitive theory of depression, the view that a depressed person's dysphoria results from a negative view of the self, the world, and the future.

commitment An emergency procedure for involuntary psychiatric hospitalization.

communication disorders Neurodevelopmental disorders involving impairment in language, speech, and communication.

community mental health center (CMHC) Outpatient clinic that provides psychological services on a sliding fee scale for individuals who live within a certain geographic area.

comorbidity Co-occurrence of two (or more) disorders within the same individual.

competency to stand trial A prediction by a mental health expert of the defendant's cognitive and emotional stability during the period of the trial.

complex post-traumatic stress disorder Diagnosis in *ICD-11* used to apply to individuals who suffer prolonged exposure to severe stressors or multiple and repeated adverse events from which they cannot escape.

compulsion A repetitive and seemingly purposeful behavior performed in response to uncontrollable urges or according to a ritualistic or stereotyped set of rules.

computed axial tomography (CAT or CT) scan A series of X-rays taken from various angles around the brain that are integrated by computer to produce a composite picture.

concordance rate Agreement ratios between people diagnosed as having a particular disorder and their relatives.

conditioned fear reactions Acquired associations between an internal or external cue and feelings of intense anxiety.

conditions of worth The demands parents place on their children in which they communicate the message that to be loved, they have to meet certain criteria.

conduct disorder An impulse-control disorder that involves repeated violations of the rights of others and society's norms and laws.

contingency management A form of behavioral therapy in which clinicians provide clients with positive reinforcement for performing desired behaviors.

coping The process through which people reduce stress.

correlational design Study in which researchers test the relationships between variables that they cannot experimentally manipulate.

counseling Short-term, problem-focused treatment.

counterconditioning The process of replacing an undesired response to a stimulus with an acceptable response.

couples therapy Treatment provided for both partners in a relationship.

cross-fostering study A type of adoption study in which researchers examine the frequency of the disorder in children whose biological parents had no disorder, but whose adoptive parents do.

cultural concepts of distress Ways that individuals in specific cultural groups experience, understand, and communicate their suffering, behavioral problems, or troubling thoughts and emotions.

cultural formulation A tool that includes the clinician's assessment of the client's degree of identification with the culture of origin, the culture's beliefs about psychological disorders, the ways in which the culture interprets particular events, and the cultural supports available to the client.

Cultural Formulation Interview (CFI) A set of questions that assess the impact of culture on key aspects of the client's clinical presentation and care.

Culturally adapted cognitive behavioral therapy (CA-CBT) Cognitive behavioral approach in which treatment aspects may be modified to take into account culturally relevant material, culturally matched clinicians, language, and session structure.

cyclothymic disorder A mood disorder with symptoms that are more chronic and less severe than those of bipolar disorder.

D

dark triad Personality traits that include psychopathy, extreme self-centeredness, and a tendency to regard other people as objects to be used.

day treatment program A structured program in a community treatment facility that provides activities similar to those provided in a psychiatric hospital.

deep brain stimulation (DBS) Also called neuromodulation, a treatment in which a neurosurgeon implants a microelectrode that delivers a constant flow electrical stimulation to a small region of the brain, powered by an implanted battery.

Default Mode Network Connections of areas within the cortex involved in the processing of internally-generated stimuli.

defense mechanisms Tactics that keep unacceptable thoughts, instincts, and feelings out of conscious awareness and thus protect the ego against anxiety.

deinstitutionalization movement The release of hundreds of thousands of patients from mental hospitals starting in the 1960s.

delayed ejaculation A sexual dysfunction in which a man experiences problems having an orgasm during sexual activity; also known as inhibited male orgasm.

delirium A neurocognitive disorder that is temporary in nature involving disturbances in attention and awareness.

delusional disorder Disorder in which the only symptoms are delusions that have lasted for at least 1 month.

delusion Deeply entrenched false belief not consistent with the client's intelligence or cultural background.

dependent personality disorder A personality disorder whose main characteristic is that the individual is extremely passive and tends to cling to other people, to the point of being unable to make any decisions or to take independent action.

dependent variable The variable whose value is the outcome of the experimenter's manipulation of the independent variable.

depersonalization/derealization disorder A dissociative disorder in which the individual experiences recurrent and persistent episodes of depersonalization, derealization, or both.

depersonalization Condition in which people feel detached from their own body.

depressant A psychoactive substance that causes the depression of central nervous system activity.

depressive disorder A disorder characterized by periods in which, among other symptoms, an individual experiences an unusually intense sad mood.

derealization Condition in which people feel a sense of unreality or detachment from their surroundings.

developmental cascade hypothesis A proposal for the cause of schizophrenia that integrates genetic vulnerabilities, damage occurring in the prenatal and early childhood periods, adversity, and drug abuse as causes of changes in dopamine expressed in psychosis.

developmental coordination disorder A motor disorder characterized by marked impairment in the development of motor coordination.

developmental risk factor model Regards schizophrenia on a continuum, developing in people with a liability to a spectrum of disorders involving psychotic symptoms.

deviation intelligence (IQ) An index of intelligence derived from comparing the individual's score on an intelligence test with the mean score for that individual's reference group.

Diagnostic and Statistical Manual of Mental Disorders, Fifth Edition-Text Revision (DSM-5-TR) A book published by the American Psychiatric Association that contains standard terms and definitions of psychological disorders.

dialectical behavior therapy (DBT) Treatment approach for people with borderline personality disorder that integrates supportive and cognitive behavioral treatments to reduce the frequency of self-destructive acts and to improve the client's ability to handle disturbing emotions, such as anger and dependency.

diathesis-stress model The proposal that people are born with a predisposition (or "diathesis") that places them at risk for developing a psychological disorder if exposed to certain extremely stressful life experiences.

differential diagnosis The process of systematically ruling out alternative diagnoses.

diffusion tensor imaging (DTI) A method to investigate abnormalities in the white matter of the brain.

disinhibited social engagement disorder Diagnosis given to children who engage in culturally inappropriate, overly familiar behavior with people who are relative strangers.

disinhibition An extreme lack of inhibition or control over behavior.

disorganized speech Language that is incomprehensible and incoherent.

disruptive mood dysregulation disorder (DMDD) A depressive disorder in children who exhibit chronic and severe irritability and have frequent temper outbursts.

dissociative amnesia An inability to remember important personal details and experiences; usually associated with traumatic or very stressful events.

dissociative identity disorder (DID) A dissociative disorder in which an individual develops more than one self or personality.

disulfiram Known popularly as Antabuse, a medication used in the treatment of alcoholism that inhibits aldehyde dehydrogenase (ALDH) and causes severe physical reactions when combined with alcohol.

DNA methylation The process that can turn off a gene when a chemical group, methyl, attaches itself to the gene.

double-blind An experimental procedure in which neither the person giving the treatment nor the person receiving the treatment knows whether the participant is in the experimental or control group.

Down syndrome Cause of intellectual developmental disorder in which individuals inherit an extra copy of chromosome 21 and therefore have 47 chromosomes instead of the typical 46.

downward drift A progression observed in people with schizophrenia in which their disorder drives them into poverty, which interferes with their ability to work and earn a living.

dual-process theory A theory regarding alcohol use proposing there are automatic processes that generate an impulse to drink alcohol and controlled, effortful processing that regulates these automatic impulses.

Durham Rule An expansion of the insanity defense based on determining that the individual was not criminally responsible if the unlawful act was due to the presence of a psychological disorder.

duty to warn (or otherwise protect) The clinician's responsibility to notify a potential victim of a client's harmful intent toward that individual.

dyscalculia A pattern of difficulties in number sense, ability to learn arithmetic facts, and calculations.

dysfunctional attitudes Negative beliefs about the self that are deeply ingrained.

dysphoria An unusually elevated sad mood.

E

early-onset familial Alzheimer's disease A form of Alzheimer's disease that begins at the unusually young ages of 40 to 50 years old and is more likely to cluster in families.

eating disorders Diagnosis for people who experience persistent disturbances of eating or eating-related behavior that result in the person's altering the consumption or absorption of food.

echolalia Repetition of the same sounds over and over.

ecstasy (MDMA) A hallucinogenic drug made from a synthetic substance chemically similar to methamphetamine and mescaline.

ego In psychoanalytic theory, the structure of personality that gives the individual the mental powers of judgment, memory, perception, and decision making.

ego psychology Theoretical perspective based on psychodynamic theory emphasizing the ego as the main force in personality.

electroconvulsive therapy (ECT) The application of electric shock to the head for the purpose of inducing therapeutically beneficial seizures.

electroencephalogram (EEG) A measure of changes in the electrical activity of the brain.

elimination disorders Disorders characterized by age-inappropriate incontinence, beginning in childhood.

emotion-focused coping A type of coping in which a person does not change anything about the situation itself but instead tries to improve feelings about the situation.

emotional competence A quality desired in clinicians in which they are free of a diagnosable psychological disorder.

emotional dysregulation Lack of awareness, understanding, or acceptance of emotions; inability to control the intensity or duration of emotions; unwillingness to experience emotional distress as an aspect of pursuing goals; and inability to engage in goal-directed behaviors when experiencing distress.

encopresis An elimination disorder in which the child is incontinent of feces and has bowel movements either in clothes or in another inappropriate place.

endophenotype The expression of a heritable trait that is not outwardly visible.

enuresis An elimination disorder in which the child is incontinent of urine and urinates in clothes or in bed after the age when the child is expected to be continent.

epigenesis The process of inheriting alterations in gene regulation and expression.

erectile disorder Sexual dysfunction in which a man cannot attain or maintain an erection during sexual activity that is sufficient to allow him to initiate or maintain sexual activity.

erotomanic type of delusional disorder Delusional disorder in which individuals falsely believe that another person is in love with them.

euphoria A feeling state that is more cheerful and elated than average, possibly even ecstatic.

evidence-based assessment Assessment that requires the identification of strategies that maximize diagnostic accuracy, informs treatment planning, and makes efficient use of clinician and patient time and resources.

evidence-based practice in psychology Clinical decision making that integrates the best available research evidence and clinical expertise in the context of the cultural background, preferences, and characteristics of clients.

evidence-based treatment Treatment in which clients receive interventions based on the findings of controlled clinical studies.

excoriation (skin-picking) disorder Recurrent picking at one's own skin.

executive functioning The ability to formulate goals, make plans, carry out those plans, and then complete the plans in an effective way.

exhibitionistic disorder A paraphilic disorder in which a person has intense sexual urges and arousing fantasies involving the exposure of genitals to a stranger.

existential psychology The theoretical position that emphasizes the importance of fully appreciating each moment as it occurs.

exorcism A ritual believed to cure psychological disturbance by ritually driving away evil spirits.

expressed emotion (EE) Family interactions with the individual that reflect criticism, hostile feelings, and emotional overinvolvement or overconcern.

extrapyramidal symptoms (EPS) Motor disorders involving rigid muscles, tremors, shuffling movement, restlessness, and muscle spasms affecting posture.

F

factitious disorder imposed on another A condition in which a person induces physical symptoms in another person who is under that person's care.

factitious disorder imposed on self A disorder in which people fake symptoms or disorders not for the purpose of any particular gain but because of an inner need to maintain a sick role.

family inheritance study Research method in genetics that compares disorder rates across relatives with varying degrees of genetic relatedness.

family perspective A theoretical perspective in which it is assumed that abnormality is caused by disturbances in the pattern of interactions and relationships within the family.

family therapy Psychological treatment in which the therapist works with several or all members of the family.

fear The emotional response to real or perceived imminent threat.

female orgasmic disorder A sexual dysfunction in which a woman experiences problems having an orgasm during sexual activity.

female sexual interest/arousal disorder A sexual dysfunction characterized by a persistent or recurrent inability to attain or maintain normal physiological and psychological arousal responses during sexual activity.

fetal alcohol spectrum disorders (FASD) A group of conditions that can occur in a person whose mother drank alcohol during pregnancy.

fetal alcohol syndrome (FAS) A condition associated with intellectual developmental disorder in a child whose mother consumed large amounts of alcohol on a regular basis while pregnant.

fetishistic disorder A paraphilic disorder in which the individual is preoccupied with an object and depends on this object rather than sexual intimacy with a partner for achieving sexual gratification.

first-rank symptom (FRS) Symptom that is truly defining, or key, in the diagnosis of schizophrenia.

Five Factor Model (or "Big Five") Trait theory proposing that there are five basic dispositions in personality, each of which has six facets.

flooding A behavioral technique in which the client is immersed in the sensation of anxiety by being exposed to the feared situation in its entirety.

fragile X syndrome Cause of intellectual disability caused by a change in the gene *FMR1*.

free association A method used in psychoanalysis in which the client speaks freely, saying whatever comes to mind.

frontotemporal neurocognitive disorder (FTD) Neurocognitive disorder that involves the frontotemporal area of the brain.

frotteuristic disorder A paraphilic disorder in which the individual has intense sexual urges and sexually arousing fantasies of rubbing against or fondling an unsuspecting stranger.

fugue An episode of amnesia involving inability to recall some or all of one's past and the loss of identity, with either bewildered wandering or travel that seems focused on a particular purpose.

functional magnetic resonance imaging (fMRI) Provides a picture of how areas of the brain react to stimuli in real time.

functional neurological disorder (conversion disorder) A somatic symptom disorder involving the translation of unacceptable drives or troubling conflicts into physical symptoms.

G

gambling disorder A non-substance-related disorder involving the persistent urge to gamble.

gender-affirming medical procedures Biological treatments including hormone replacement therapy and surgery for people with gender dysphoria.

gender dysphoria Distress that may accompany the incongruence between a person's experienced or expressed gender and that person's birth-assigned sex.

gene mapping The approach used by biological researchers in which they examine genetic variations and connect them to performance on psychological tests or diagnosis of specific disorders.

generalized anxiety disorder An anxiety disorder characterized by anxiety and worry that is not associated with a particular object, situation, or event but seems to be a constant feature of a person's day-to-day existence.

genes The instructions for forming proteins contained within each of the body's cells.

genetic epidemiology Study of the role of genetic factors in disease by studying rates in individuals varying in degree of genetic closeness.

genito-pelvic pain/penetration disorder A sexual dysfunction affecting both males and females that involves recurrent or persistent genital pain before, during, or after sexual intercourse.

genome-wide association studies (GWAS) Genetic method in which researchers scan the entire genome of individuals who are not related to find the associated genetic variations with a particular disease.

genome-wide linkage study Genetic method in which researchers study the families of people with specific psychological traits or disorders.

genotype The genetic makeup of an organism.

Glascow Coma Scale (GCS) Neuropsychological test intended to assess immediate aftermath of brain trauma.

graded *in vivo* A procedure in which clients gradually expose themselves to increasingly challenging anxiety-provoking situations.

grandiose narcissism The form of narcissistic personality disorder in which individuals think of themselves entirely in an inflated and self-aggrandizing way.

grandiose type of delusional disorder An exaggerated view of oneself as possessing special and extremely favorable personal qualities and abilities.

group therapy Psychological treatment in which the therapist facilitates discussion among several clients who talk together about their problems.

guardian *ad litem* A person appointed by the court to represent or make decisions for a minor or an incapacitated adult who is legally incapable of doing so in a civil legal proceeding.

H

halfway house A community treatment facility designed for deinstitutionalized clients leaving a hospital who are not yet ready for independent living.

hallucination A false perception not corresponding to the objective stimuli present in the environment.

hallucinogens Psychoactive substances that cause abnormal perceptual experiences in the form of illusions or hallucinations, usually visual in nature.

hassle A relatively minor event that can cause stress.

health anxiety Undue concern about physical symptoms and illness.

Health Insurance Portability and Accountability Act of 1996 (HIPAA) U.S. legislation intended to ensure adequate coverage and protect consumers from loss of insurance coverage when they change or lose their jobs.

heavy alcohol use Drinking four (for women) and five (for men) drinks on each of five or more days in the past month.

heritability index A decimal ranging from 0 to 1 that shows the extent to which test scores or other measurements are accounted for by genes. Heritability can also be expressed as the percent of variation in a trait accounted for by genetic factors.

heroin A psychoactive substance that is a form of opioid, synthesized from morphine.

HEXACO personality trait model Trait-based approach that proposes personality traits fall into the six categories of honesty: humility, emotional stability, extraversion, agreeableness, and conscientiousness.

histrionic personality disorder A personality disorder characterized by exaggerated emotional reactions, approaching theatricality, in everyday behavior.

hoarding disorder A disorder in which people have persistent difficulties discarding things, even if they have little value.

humanistic perspective A theoretical view of personality and psychological disorder proposing that people are motivated to strive for self-fulfillment and meaning in life.

humanitarian explanations Explanations that regard psychological disorders as the result of cruelty, stress, or poor living conditions.

hypnotic A substance that induces sedation.

hypomanic episode A period of elated mood lasting for up to 4 days.

I

id In psychoanalytic theory, the structure of personality hidden in the unconscious that contains instincts oriented toward fulfilling basic biological drives, including sexual and aggressive needs.

illness anxiety disorder A somatic symptom disorder characterized by the misinterpretation of normal bodily functions as signs of serious illness.

imaginal flooding A behavioral technique in which the client is immersed through imagination into the feared situation.

impulse-control disorder Psychological disorder in which people repeatedly engage in behaviors that are potentially harmful, feeling unable to stop themselves and experiencing a sense of desperation if their attempts to carry out the behaviors are thwarted.

inappropriate affect The extent to which a person's emotional expressiveness fails to correspond either to the social cues present in a situation or to the content of what is being discussed.

incidence The frequency of new cases within a given time period.

independent variable The variable whose level is adjusted or controlled by the experimenter.

individual psychotherapy Psychological treatment in which the therapist works on a one-to-one basis with the client.

inhalants A diverse group of substances that cause psychoactive effects by producing chemical vapors.

inhibitory control The ability to maintain focus rather than attend to irrelevant information.

insanity A legal term that refers to the individual's lack of moral responsibility for committing criminal acts.

insanity defense The argument, presented by a lawyer acting on behalf of the client, that, because of the existence of a mental disorder, the client should not be held legally responsible for criminal actions.

Intellectual developmental disorder (intellectual disability) Diagnosis used to characterize individuals who have intellectual and adaptive deficits that first became evident when they were children.

intermittent explosive disorder An impulse-control disorder involving an inability to hold back urges to express strong angry feelings and associated violent behaviors.

International Classification of Diseases (ICD) The diagnostic system of the World Health Organization (WHO).

interpersonal therapy (IPT) A time-limited form of psychotherapy for treating people with major depressive disorder, based on the assumption that interpersonal stress induces an episode of depression in a person who is genetically vulnerable to this disorder.

***in vivo* flooding** A behavioral technique in which the client is immersed in the actual feared situation.

***in vivo* observation** Process of recording behavior in its natural context, such as the classroom or the home.

irresistible impulse The legal argument that although clients in a forensic setting knew an act was wrong, they were unable to stop themselves from acting on their impulses.

J

jealous type of delusional disorder Delusional disorder in which individuals falsely believe that their romantic partner is unfaithful to them.

K

kleptomania An impulse-control disorder that involves the persistent urge to steal.

Korsakoff's syndrome A permanent form of neurocognitive disorder associated with long-term alcohol use in which the individual develops retrograde and anterograde amnesia, leading to an inability to remember recent events or learn new information.

L

language disorder A communication disorder characterized by having a limited and faulty vocabulary, speaking in short sentences with simplified grammatical structures, omitting critical words or phrases, and putting words together in peculiar order.

late-onset form of Alzheimer's disease The form of Alzheimer's disease that starts at the age of 65 years old or later.

least restrictive alternative A treatment setting that provides the fewest constraints on the client's freedom.

libido An instinctual pressure that strives for gratification of sexual and aggressive desires.

lithium carbonate Naturally occurring salt used to treat bipolar disorder.

loosening of associations Flow of thoughts that is vague, unfocused, and illogical.

lysergic acid diethylamide (LSD) A form of a hallucinogenic drug that users ingest in tablets, capsules, and liquid form.

M

magnetic resonance imaging (MRI) The use of radio waves rather than X-rays to construct a static picture of the living brain based on the water content of various tissues.

mainstreaming A governmental policy to integrate fully into society people with cognitive disabilities.

major depressive disorder A disorder in which the individual experiences acute but time-limited episodes of depressive symptoms.

major depressive episode A period in which the individual experiences intense psychological and physical symptoms accompanying feelings of overwhelming sadness (dysphoria).

major neurocognitive disorder due to another medical condition Cognitive disorders involving the inability to recall previously learned information or to register new memories.

major neurocognitive disorders Disorders involving significant cognitive decline from a previous level of performance.

male hypoactive sexual desire disorder A sexual dysfunction in which the individual has an abnormally low level of interest in sexual activity.

malingering The fabrication of physical or psychological symptoms for some ulterior motive.

maltreated ecophenotype Genetic susceptibility to eating disorders that is strongly influenced by exposure to childhood maltreatment.

manic episode Acute but time-limited period of intense and unusual elation.

marijuana A psychoactive substance derived from the hemp plant whose primary active ingredient is delta-9-tetrahydrocannabinol (THC).

mental hygiene The focus within psychiatry on helping individuals maintain mental health and prevent the development of psychological disorders.

mental status examination A method of objectively assessing a client's behavior and functioning in a number of spheres, with particular attention to the symptoms associated with psychological disturbance.

meta-analysis A statistical approach that evaluates significance of findings across multiple studies and samples.

methadone A synthetic opioid that produces a safer and more controlled reaction than heroin and that is used in treating heroin addiction.

methamphetamine An addictive stimulant drug that is related to amphetamine but provokes more intense central nervous system effects.

Migrants People who move away from their place of usual residence.

mild cognitive impairment A form of neurocognitive disorder referred to as "mild," meaning that the symptoms have not progressed to the level of severity in the more severe form.

mild neurocognitive disorders Disorders involving modest cognitive decline from a previous level of performance.

milieu therapy A treatment approach, used in an inpatient psychiatric facility, in which all facets of the milieu, or environment, are components of the treatment.

mindfulness-based cognitive therapy (MBCT) Treatment that combines cognitive therapy with mindfulness skills.

mindfulness A mental state achieved by intentionally bringing one's awareness to the present moment without judgment of internal or external observations.

Mini-Mental State Examination (MMSE) A structured tool that clinicians use as a brief screening device to assess neurocognitive disorders.

Minnesota Multiphasic Personality Inventory-3 (MMPI-3) Self-report personality inventory containing 335 true/false items, all in the form of statements that describe the individual's thoughts, behaviors, feelings, and attitudes.

minority stress model Approach to psychological disorders that emphasizes the role of discrimination due to minority status.

modality Form in which the clinician offers psychotherapy.

molecular genetics The study of how genes translate hereditary information.

Montreal Cognitive Assessment (MoCA) Brief cognitive screening device used as part of a neuropsychological assessment.

moral treatment The belief that people could develop self-control over their behaviors if they had a quiet and restful environment.

motivational interviewing (MI) A technique that uses empathic understanding as a means of promoting behavioral change in clients.

multi-infarct dementia (MID) A form of neurocognitive disorder caused by transient attacks in which blood flow to the brain is interrupted by a clogged or burst artery.

multiaxial system A multidimensional classification and diagnostic system in previous DSMs summarizing relevant information about an individual's physical and psychological functioning.

multicultural approach Therapy that relies on awareness, knowledge, and skills of the client's sociocultural context.

multicultural assessment Assessment process in which clinicians take into account the person's cultural, ethnic, and racial background.

multiculturally competent care A clinician's ability to demonstrate awareness of and skill in addressing culturally relevant factors when working with individuals from cultural backgrounds that differ from their own.

multiple relationships Unethical relationships occurring when a psychologist is in a professional role with a person and has another role with that person that could impair the psychologist's "objectivity, competence, or effectiveness in performing their functions as a psychologist" or otherwise risks exploiting or harming the other person.

M'Naghten Rule The "right-wrong test" used in cases of the insanity defense to determine whether a defendant should be held responsible for a crime.

N

naltrexone An opioid receptor antagonist that blocks the effects of the body's production of alcohol-induced opioids.

narcissistic personality disorder (NPD) A personality disorder primarily characterized by an unrealistic, inflated sense of self-importance and a lack of sensitivity to the needs of other people.

naturalistic developmental behavioral interventions (NDBI) A behavioral approach for autism spectrum disorders in which teachers or other interventionists can shape the child's behavior in the course of ordinary play or instruction.

negative symptoms The symptoms of schizophrenia that involve functioning below the level of normal behavior.

neologisms Invented ("new") words.

neurocognitive disorder Disorders involving decline acquired in life in one or more domains of cognition associated with alterations in the brain.

neurocognitive disorder due to Alzheimer's disease A neurocognitive disorder associated with progressive, gradual declines in memory, learning, and at least one other cognitive domain.

neurocognitive disorder due to Huntington's disease A hereditary condition causing neurocognitive disorder that involves a widespread deterioration of the subcortical brain structures and parts of the frontal cortex that control motor movements.

neurocognitive disorder due to Parkinson's disease A neurocognitive disorder that involves degeneration of neurons in the subcortical structures that control motor movements.

neurocognitive disorder due to prion disease (Creutzfeldt-Jakob disease) A neurological disease transmitted from animals to humans that leads to neurocognitive disorder and death resulting from abnormal protein accumulations in the brain.

neurocognitive disorder due to traumatic brain injury A disorder in which there is evidence of impact to the head along with cognitive and neurological symptoms that persist past the acute postinjury period.

neurocognitive disorder with Lewy bodies A form of neurocognitive disorder with progressive loss of memory, language, calculation, and reasoning, as well as other higher mental functions resulting from the accumulation of abnormalities called Lewy bodies throughout the brain.

neurodevelopmental disorders Conditions that begin in childhood and have a major impact on social and cognitive functioning.

neurodevelopmental hypothesis Theory proposing that schizophrenia is a disorder of development that arises during adolescence or early adulthood due to alterations in the genetic control of brain maturation.

neurofibrillary tangles A characteristic of Alzheimer's disease in which the material within the cell bodies of neurons becomes filled with densely packed, twisted protein microfibrils, or tiny strands.

neuroimaging Assessment method that provides a picture of the brain's structures or level of activity and therefore is a useful tool for "looking" at the brain.

neuromodulation A treatment in which a neurosurgeon implants a microelectrode that delivers a constant low electrical stimulation to a small region of the brain, powered by an implanted battery.

neuroplasticity Adaptive changes in the brain in response to experience.

neuropsychological assessment A performance-based method assessing cognitive functioning used to examine the cognitive consequences of brain damage, brain disease, and severe mental illness.

neurotransmitter A chemical substance released from a neuron into the synapse, where it can become absorbed by the receiving neuron.

niche-picking The selection by children of environments that match their interests and abilities.

nicotine The psychoactive substance found in cigarettes.

O

object relations A psychodynamically oriented theory that focuses on the relationships people have with the others ("objects") in their lives.

obsession An unwanted thought, word, phrase, or image that persistently and repeatedly comes into a person's mind and causes distress.

obsessive-compulsive disorder (OCD) A disorder characterized by recurrent obsessions or compulsions that are inordinately time consuming or that cause significant distress or impairment.

obsessive-compulsive personality disorder (OCPD) A personality disorder involving intense perfectionism and inflexibility manifested in worrying, indecisiveness, and behavioral rigidity.

Oedipus complex According to Freud, the child's feelings toward the opposite-sex parent peak in early childhood.

one session treatment A treatment for specific phobias in which cognitive behavioral therapy is condensed into one 3-hour session involving exposure and homework.

operant conditioning A learning process in which an individual acquires a response by learning to pair a behavior with its consequences.

opioid A psychoactive substance that relieves pain.

oppositional defiant disorder A disorder characterized by angry or irritable mood, argumentative or defiant behavior, and vindictiveness that results in significant family or school problems.

orthorexia nervosa An unhealthy obsession with staying away from low-quality ingredients or food that may not be properly prepared.

P

Paced Auditory Serial Addition Test (PASAT) Neuropsychological test used to assess processing speed, flexibility, and calculation ability.

panic attack A period of intense fear and physical discomfort accompanied by the feeling that one is being overwhelmed and is about to lose control.

panic disorder An anxiety disorder in which an individual has panic attacks on a recurrent basis or has constant apprehension and worry about the possibility of recurring attacks.

paranoia The irrational belief or perception that others wish to cause you harm.

paranoid personality disorder A personality disorder whose outstanding feature is that the individual is unduly suspicious of others and is always on guard against potential danger or harm.

paraphilias Behaviors in which an individual has recurrent, intense sexually arousing fantasies, sexual urges, or behaviors involving (1) nonhuman objects, (2) children or other nonconsenting persons, or (3) the suffering or humiliation of self or partner.

paraphilic disorder Diagnosis in which a paraphilia causes distress and impairment.

parasuicide Attempted suicide, often a call for help.

parens patriae The state's authority to protect those who are unable to protect themselves.

partialism A paraphilic disorder in which the person is interested solely in sexual gratification from a specific body part, such as feet.

participant modeling A form of therapy in which the therapist first shows the client a desired behavior and then guides the client through the behavioral change.

pathways model Approach to gambling disorder that predicts there are three main developmental paths leading to three distinct subtypes.

patient In health care settings, a person who receives treatment.

pedophilic disorder A paraphilic disorder in which an adult is sexually aroused by children or adolescents.

persecutory type of delusional disorder Delusional disorder in which individuals falsely believe that someone close to them is treating them in a malevolent manner.

persistent depressive disorder Chronic but less severe mood disturbance in which the individual does not experience a major depressive episode.

person-centered theory The humanistic theory that focuses on the uniqueness of each individual, the importance of allowing each individual to achieve maximum fulfillment of potential, and the need for the individual to honestly confront the reality of his or her experiences in the world.

personality disorder A characteristic way of relating to other people, situations, and events involving a rigid and maladaptive pattern of inner experience and behavior, dating back to adolescence or early adulthood.

personality trait An enduring pattern of perceiving, relating to, and thinking about the environment and others.

peyote A form of a hallucinogenic drug whose primary ingredient is mescaline.

pharmacogenetics The use of genetic testing to identify who will and will not improve with a particular medication.

phencyclidine (PCP) A form of a hallucinogenic drug originally developed as an intravenous anesthetic.

phenotype The expression of the genetic program in the individual's physical and psychological attributes.

phenylketonuria (PKU) Condition in which children are born missing an enzyme called phenylalanine hydroxase.

phosphodiesterase (PDE) inhibitors Medications for erectile disorders that increase blood flow to the genital area.

pica A condition in which a person eats inedible substances, such as dirt or feces; commonly associated with intellectual developmental disabilities.

Pick's disease A relatively rare degenerative disease that affects the frontal and temporal lobes of the cerebral cortex and that can cause neurocognitive disorders.

placebo-controlled randomized clinical trial Experimental method in which participants are randomly assigned to a placebo versus treatment group.

placebo condition Condition in an experiment in which participants receive a treatment similar to the experimental treatment, but lacking the key feature of the treatment of interest.

pleasure principle In psychoanalytic theory, a motivating force that seeks the immediate and total gratification of sensual needs and desires.

polygenic A model of inheritance in which more than one gene participates in the process of determining a given characteristic.

polypharmacy The use of multiple prescription medications.

polysomnography A sleep study that records brain waves, blood oxygen levels, heart rate, breathing, eye movements, and leg movements.

positive psychology Perspective that emphasizes the potential for growth and change throughout life.

positive symptoms The symptoms of schizophrenia that represent exaggerations or distortions of normal thoughts, emotions, and behavior.

positron emission tomography (PET) scan A measure of brain activity in which a small amount of radioactive compounds is injected into an individual's bloodstream, following which a computer measures the varying levels of radiation in different parts of the brain and yields a multicolored image.

post-traumatic growth The personal growth that can occur following exposure to a traumatic experience.

post-traumatic stress disorder (PTSD) A disorder in which an individual exposed to a traumatic event continues to experience a range of distressing symptoms for more than a month that include reexperiencing the traumatic event, avoidance of reminders of the trauma, numbing of general responsiveness, and increased arousal.

postconcussion syndrome (PCS) A disorder in which a constellation of physical, emotional, and cognitive symptoms persists from weeks to years.

potentiation The combination of the effects of two or more psychoactive substances such that the total effect is greater than the effect of either substance alone.

prefrontal lobotomy A form of biological treatment in which a neurosurgeon severs the patient's prefrontal lobes from the rest of the brain.

premature (early) ejaculation A sexual dysfunction in which a man reaches orgasm well before he wishes to, perhaps even prior to penetration.

premenstrual dysphoric disorder (PMDD) Changes in mood, irritability, dysphoria, and anxiety that occur during the premenstrual phase of the monthly menstrual cycle and subside after the menstrual period begins for most of the cycles of the preceding year.

prevalence The number of people who have ever had a disorder at a given time or over a specified period.

primary gain The relief from anxiety or responsibility due to the development of physical or psychological symptoms.

principal diagnosis The disorder most closely aligned with the primary reason the individual is seeking professional help.

prion disease A disease caused by an abnormal protein particle that infects brain tissue.

problem-focused coping Coping in which the individual takes action to reduce stress by changing whatever it is about the situation that makes it stressful.

projective test A technique in which the test-taker is presented with an ambiguous item or task and is asked to respond by providing his or her own meaning or perception.

proton magnetic resonance spectroscopy (MRS) A scanning method that measures metabolic activity of neurons and therefore may indicate areas of brain damage.

pseudodementia Literally, false neurocognitive disorder, or a set of symptoms caused by depression that mimic those apparent in the early stages of Alzheimer's disease.

psilocybin A form of a hallucinogenic drug found in certain mushrooms.

psychiatrist Person with a degree in medicine (MD) who receives specialized advanced training in diagnosing and treating people with psychological disorders.

psychodynamic perspective The theoretical orientation in psychology that emphasizes unconscious determinants of behavior.

psychodynamics Interplay among the structures of the mind.

psychological assessment A broad range of measurement techniques, all of which involve having people provide scorable information about their psychological functioning.

psychological disorders Constellations of behavior that receive diagnoses when they are associated with significant impairment and distress.

psychological factors affecting other medical conditions Disorder in which clients have a medical disease or symptom that appears to be exacerbated by psychological or behavioral factors.

psychologist Licensed health care professional offering psychological services.

psychopathology The scientific study of psychological disorders.

psychopathy A cluster of traits that includes lack of empathy, lack of remorse, tendency to manipulate other people, superficial charm, egocentricity, deception, and a grandiosely high sense of self-worth.

psychosexual stages According to psychoanalytic theory, the normal sequence of development through which each individual passes between infancy and adulthood.

psychosurgery A form of brain surgery, the purpose of which is to reduce psychological disturbance.

psychotherapy Treatment modality that focuses on development of a working relationship between clinician and client.

psychotropic medications Medications intended to reduce the symptoms of a psychological disorder by altering the levels of neurotransmitters hypothesized to be involved in the disorder.

purging Eliminating food through unnatural methods, such as vomiting or the excessive use of laxatives.

pyromania An impulse-control disorder involving the persistent and compelling urge to start fires.

Q

qualitative research A method of analyzing data in which researchers use rigorous methods to code the data and summarize information in a way that reflects an objectively applied set of standards.

R

randomized controlled trial (RCT) Experimental method in which participants are randomly assigned to intervention groups.

reactive attachment disorder (RAD) A diagnosis given to children involving a consistent pattern of inhibited, emotionally withdrawn behavior toward adult caregivers along with minimal responsiveness to others and limited positive affect.

reality principle In psychoanalyic theory, the motivational force that leads the individual to confront the constraints of the external world.

reinforcement In operant conditioning, the outcome that makes the individual more likely to repeat the behavior in the future.

relapse prevention A treatment method in which individuals are encouraged not to view lapses from abstinence as signs of certain failure.

relaxation training A behavioral technique used in the treatment of anxiety disorders that involves progressive and systematic patterns of muscle tensing and relaxing.

reliability When used with regard to diagnosis, the degree to which clinicians provide diagnoses consistently across individuals who have a particular set of symptoms.

remission Situation in which the individual's symptoms no longer interfere with his or her behavior and are below those required for a DSM diagnosis.

restricted affect Narrowing of the range of outward expressions of emotions.

retrograde amnesia Amnesia involving loss of memory for past events.

Rett syndrome A rare genetic neurological disorder that develops within the first 18 months of life is more prevalent in girls and is characterized by such symptoms as nearly constant repetitive hand movements, loss of acquired spoken language, gait abnormalities, and partial or complete loss of acquired purposeful hand skills.

right to treatment Legal right of person entering psychiatric hospital to receive appropriate care.

Rorschach Inkblot Test Projective assessment method in which individuals describe their perceptions of each of a set of symmetrical inkblots.

rumination disorder An eating disorder in which the infant or child regurgitates food after it has been swallowed and then either spits it out or reswallows it.

S

schizoaffective disorder A disorder involving the experience of a major depressive episode, a manic episode, or a mixed episode while also meeting the diagnostic criteria for schizophrenia.

schizoid personality disorder A personality disorder primarily characterized by an indifference to social relationships, as well as a limited range of emotional experience and expression.

schizophrenia A disorder with a range of symptoms involving disturbances in content of thought, form of thought, perception, affect, sense of self, motivation, behavior, and interpersonal functioning.

schizophrenia spectrum Range of disorders that reflect a similar underlying disease process as that involved in schizophrenia.

schizophreniform disorder A disorder characterized by psychotic symptoms that are essentially the same as those found in schizophrenia, except for their duration; specifically, symptoms usually last from 1 to 6 months.

schizotypal personality disorder A personality disorder that primarily involves odd beliefs, behavior, appearance, and interpersonal style. People with this disorder may have bizarre ideas or preoccupations, such as magical thinking and beliefs in psychic phenomena.

scientific explanations Explanations that regard psychological disorders as the result of causes that we can objectively measure, such as biological alterations, faulty learning processes, or emotional stressors.

scientific method The process of testing ideas about the nature of psychological phenomena without bias before accepting these ideas as adequate explanations.

secondary gain The sympathy and attention that a sick person receives from other people.

secretases Enzymes that trim part of the APP remaining outside the neuron so that it is flush with the neuron's outer membrane.

sedative A psychoactive substance that has a calming effect on the central nervous system.

selective mutism A disorder originating in childhood in which the individual consciously refuses to talk.

selective serotonin reuptake inhibitor (SSRI) Category of medications that target serotonin pathways in the brain.

self-actualization In humanistic theory, the maximum realization of the individual's potential for psychological growth.

self-efficacy The individual's perception of competence in various life situations.

self-monitoring A self-report technique in which the client keeps a record of the frequency of specified behaviors.

self-report clinical inventory A psychological test with standardized questions having fixed response categories that the test-taker completes independently, self-reporting the extent to which the responses are accurate characterizations.

separation anxiety disorder A childhood disorder characterized by intense and inappropriate anxiety, lasting at least 4 weeks, concerning separation from home or caregivers.

serotonin and norepinephrine reuptake inhibitor (SNRI) Category of medications that target serotonin and norepinephrine pathways in the brain.

sexual dysfunction An abnormality in an individual's sexual responsiveness and reactions.

sexual masochism disorder A paraphilic disorder marked by an attraction to achieving sexual gratification by having painful stimulation applied to one's own body

sexual sadism disorder A paraphilic disorder in which sexual gratification is derived from activities that harm, or from urges to harm, another person.

shared psychotic disorder Delusional disorder in which one or more people develop a delusional system as a result of a close relationship with a psychotic person who is delusional.

single case experimental design (SCED) Design in which the same person serves as the subject in both the experimental and control conditions.

single nucleotide polymorphism (SNP) A small genetic variation that can occur in a person's DNA sequence.

single photon emission computed tomography (SPECT) scan A variant of the PET scan that allows a longer and more detailed imaging analysis to be performed.

social (pragmatic) communication disorder (SPCD) Disorder involving deficits in the ability to use verbal and nonverbal communication in relating to others.

social anxiety disorder An anxiety disorder characterized by marked, or intense, fear or anxiety in social situations in which the individual may be scrutinized by others.

social cognition The ability to read the emotions and thoughts of other people.

social discrimination Prejudicial treatment of a class of individuals, seen in the sociocultural perspective as a cause of psychological problems.

social learning theory Perspective that focuses on understanding how people develop psychological disorders through their relationships with others and through observation of other people.

social support A method of coping in which individuals seek connections with others in order to reduce stress.

sociocultural perspective The theoretical perspective that emphasizes the ways that individuals are influenced by people, social institutions, and social forces in the world around them.

somatic symptom disorder A disorder involving physical symptoms that may or may not be accounted for by a medical condition and accompanied by maladaptive thoughts, feelings, and behaviors.

somatic symptoms Symptoms involving physical problems and/or concerns about medical symptoms.

somatic type of delusional disorder Delusional disorder in which individuals falsely believe that they have a medical condition.

specific learning disorder A delay or deficit in an academic skill that is evident when an individual's achievement and skills are substantially below what would be expected for others of comparable age, education, and level of intelligence.

specific learning disorder with impairment in mathematics A learning disorder in which the individual has difficulty with tasks and concepts involving numbers and numerical reasoning.

specific learning disorder with impairment in reading (dyslexia) A learning disorder in which the individual omits, distorts, or substitutes words when reading and reads in a slow, halting fashion.

specific learning disorder with impairment in written expression A learning disorder in which the individual's writing is characterized by poor spelling, grammatical or punctuation errors, and disorganization of paragraphs.

specific phobia An irrational and unabating fear of a particular object, activity, or situation.

speech sound disorder A communication disorder in which the individual substitutes, omits, or misarticulates speech sounds.

spiritual explanations Explanations that regard psychological disorders as the product of possession by evil or demonic spirits.

splitting A defense, common in people with borderline personality disorder, in which individuals perceive others, or themselves, as being all good or all bad, usually resulting in disturbed interpersonal relationships.

standardization A psychometric criterion that clearly specifies a test's instructions for administration and scoring.

Stanford-Binet 5 (SB5) Individually administered test of intelligence, most commonly used in assessing children.

stereotypic movement disorder A disorder in which the individual engages in repetitive, seemingly driven nonfunctional behaviors.

stigma A negative label that causes certain people to be regarded as different, defective, and set apart from mainstream members of society.

stimulant A psychoactive substance that has an activating effect on the central nervous system.

stressful life event An event that disrupts the individual's life.

stress generation The tendency of people with borderline personality disorder to create stressful situations in their lives as a function of their instability and interpersonal difficulties.

stress The unpleasant emotional reaction that a person has when an event is perceived as threatening.

Structured Clinical Interview for *DSM-5* Disorders (SCID-5) A structured clinical interview developed to assess DSM-5 symptoms.

structured interview A standardized series of assessment questions that follow a predetermined wording and order.

substance-induced disorders Disorders marked by development of a substance-specific syndrome due to recent ingestion of the substance itself.

substance A chemical that alters a person's mood or behavior when it is smoked, injected, drunk, inhaled, snorted, or swallowed.

substance intoxication The temporary maladaptive experience of behavioral or psychological changes that are due to the accumulation of a substance in the body.

substance use disorder A cluster of cognitive, behavioral, and physiological symptoms indicating that the individual uses a substance despite significant substance-related problems.

substituted judgment A doctrine that allows health professionals and family members to try to make the decision that the patient would have made if he or she were able to make decisions.

suicidal ideation Thinking about ending one's life.

suicide A fatal self-inflicted destructive act with explicit or inferred intent to die.

suicide attempt Undertaking nonfatal suicidal behavior.

superego In psychoanalytic theory, the structure of personality that includes the conscience and the ego ideal.

survey A research tool used to gather information from a sample of people considered representative of a particular population, in which participants are asked to answer questions about the topic of concern.

systematic desensitization A variant of counterconditioning that involves presenting the client with progressively more anxiety-provoking images while in a relaxed state.

T

tardive dyskinesia Motor disorder that consists of involuntary movements of the mouth, arms, and trunk of the body.

target behavior A behavior of interest or concern in an assessment.

tau A protein that normally helps maintain the internal support structure of the axons.

Tay-Sachs disease An inherited disease that produces deficits in intellectual functioning due to a lack of hexosaminidase A, an enzyme that helps break down an otherwise toxic chemical in nervous tissue called ganglioside.

telemental health Also referred to as telepsychology, the provision of psychological services using the platform of videoconferencing or telephone.

telepsychology Also referred to as telemental health, the provision of psychological services using the platform of videoconferencing or telephone.

teratogens Environmental hazards mothers experience while pregnant that affect the developing child.

Thematic Apperception Test (TAT) A projective test in which individuals invent a story to explain what is happening in a set of ambiguous pictures.

theoretical perspective An orientation to understanding the causes of human behavior and the treatment of psychological disorders.

tic A rapid, recurring, nonrhythmic, and involuntary movement or vocalization.

token economy A form of contingency management in which a client who performs desired activities earns tokens that can later be exchanged for tangible benefits.

tolerance The extent to which the individual requires larger and larger amounts of a substance in order to achieve its desired effects, or the extent to which the individual feels less of its effects after using the same amount of the substance.

Tourette's disorder A disorder involving a combination of chronic motor and vocal tics.

Trail Making Test (TMT) A simple test of executive functioning involving the ability to trace a path among a set of related stimuli.

transcranial magnetic stimulation The use of repetitive electromagnetic pulses to stimulate nerve cells in the brain associated with mood regulation and depression.

transference-focused psychotherapy A treatment for borderline personality disorder that uses the client–clinician relationship as the framework for helping clients achieve greater understanding of their unconscious feelings and motives.

transference The carrying over of feelings that clients have from their parents to their therapists.

transgender The identity of a person whose assigned gender does not correspond with their gender identity.

transphobia The negative stereotyping and fear of transgender individuals.

transvestic disorder Diagnosis applied to individuals who dress in the clothing of the other sex and have the symptoms of a paraphilic disorder.

trauma-informed care An approach to treatment that acknowledges the role that trauma can have on the mental health of individuals.

trauma Response experienced by an individual to an event that is harmful or life threatening that can have lasting adverse effects on the individual's functioning and mental health.

traumatic brain injury (TBI) Damage to the brain caused by exposure to trauma.

treatment plan The outline for how therapy should take place.

trephining The process of cutting a hole in the skull to allow so-called, "evil spirits" to escape.

trichotillomania (hair-pulling disorder) An impulse-control disorder involving the compulsive, persistent urge to pull out one's own hair.

type A behavior pattern Set of behaviors that purportedly include being hard-driving, competitive, impatient, cynical, suspicious of and hostile toward others, and easily irritated.

type D personality A personality type seen in those who experience emotions that include anxiety, irritation, and depressed mood.

U

unconditional positive regard A method in client-centered therapy in which the clinician gives total acceptance of what the client says, does, and feels.

unstructured interview A series of open-ended questions aimed at determining the client's reasons for being in treatment, symptoms, health status, family background, and life history.

uplifts Events that boost your feelings of well-being.

V

validity The extent to which a test, diagnosis, or rating accurately and distinctly characterizes a person's psychological status.

vascular neurocognitive disorder A form of neurocognitive disorder resulting from a vascular disease that causes deprivation of the blood supply to the brain.

vicarious reinforcement A form of learning in which a new behavior is acquired through the process of watching someone else receive reinforcement for the same behavior.

virtual reality exposure therapy (VRET) A method of exposure therapy that uses virtual reality, in which clients become immersed in computer-generated environments that resemble the situations they fear.

voyeuristic disorder A paraphilic disorder in which the individual has a compulsion to derive sexual gratification from observing the nudity or sexual activity of others.

vulnerability The idea that individuals have a biologically determined predisposition to developing schizophrenia but that the disorder develops only when certain environmental conditions are in place.

vulnerable narcissism The form of narcissistic personality disorder in which individuals have an internally weak sense of self and so become despondent when they feel that someone who is important to them is humiliating or betraying them.

W

Wechsler Adult Intelligence Scale (WAIS) The first comprehensive individual test that researchers specifically designed to measure adult intelligence.

Wernicke's disease A reversible form of neurocognitive disorder associated with long-term alcohol use.

Wisconsin Card Sorting Test (WCST) Test used in neuropsychological assessment involving the ability to form higher-order abstract concepts.

withdrawal Physiological and psychological changes that occur when an individual stops taking a substance.

REFERENCES

A

Abé, C., Ekman, C., Sellgren, C., Petrovic, P., Ingvar, M., & Landén, M. (2015). Manic episodes are related to changes in frontal cortex: A longitudinal neuroimaging study of bipolar disorder *Brain: A Journal of Neurology, 138* (11), 3440–3448. https://doi.org/10.1093/brain/awv266

Abecassis, S., Magen, H., & Weintraub, N. (2023). Typing performance and technique of higher education students with specific learning disorders. *Learning Disabilities Research & Practice, 38* (2), 119–128. https://doi.org/10.1111/ldrp.12305

Aboujaoude, E., Gamel, N., & Koran, L. M. (2004). Overview of kleptomania and phenomenological description of 40 patients. *Primary Care Companion Journal of Clinical Psychiatry, 6,* 244–247.

Abraham, K. (1911/1968). Notes on the psychoanalytic investigation and treatment of manic-depressive insanity and allied conditions. In K. Abraham (Ed.), *Selected papers of Karl Abraham.* Basic Books.

Abram, S. V., Wisner, K. M., Fox, J. M., Barch, D. M., Wang, L., Csernansky, J. G., . . . Smith, M. J. (2017). Fronto-temporal connectivity predicts cognitive empathy deficits and experiential negative symptoms in schizophrenia. *Human Brain Mapping, 38* (3), 1111–1124. https://doi.org/10.1002/hbm.23439

Achenbach, T. M. (2020). Bottom-up and top-down paradigms for psychopathology: A half-century odyssey. *Annual Review of Clinical Psychology, 16,* 1–24. https://doi.org/10.1146/annurev-clinpsy-071119-115831

Achterhof, R., Dorahy, M. J., Rowlands, A., Renouf, C., Britt, E., & Carter, J. D. (2018). Predictors of posttraumatic growth 10–11 months after a fatal earthquake. *Psychological Trauma: Theory, Research, Practice, and Policy, 10* (2), 208–215. https://doi.org/10.1037/tra0000286

Adam, Y., Meinlschmidt, G., Gloster, A. T., & Lieb, R. (2012). Obsessive-compulsive disorder in the community: 12-Month prevalence, comorbidity and impairment. *Social Psychiatry and Psychiatric Epidemiology, 47* (3), 339–349. https://doi.org/10.1007/s00127-010-0337-5

Aerts, J. E. M., Rijckmans, M. J. N., Bogaerts, S., & van Dam, A. (2023). Establishing an optimal working relationship with patients with an antisocial personality disorder Aspects and processes in the therapeutic alliance. *Psychology and Psychotherapy: Theory, Research and Practice.* https://doi.org/10.1111/papt.12492

Agarwal, P., Leurgans, S. E., Agrawal, S., Aggarwal, N. T., Cherian, L. J., James, B. D., . . . Schneider, J. A. (2023). Association of Mediterranean-DASH Intervention for neurodegenerative delay and Mediterranean diets with Alzheimer Disease pathology. *Neurology, 100* (22), e2259–e2268. https://doi.org/10.1212/wnl.0000000000207176

Ahlberg, R., Du Rietz, E., Ahnemark, E., Andersson, L. M., Werner-Kiechle, T., Lichtenstein, P., Larsson, H., & Garcia-Argibay, M. (2023). Real-life instability in ADHD from young to middle adulthood: A nationwide register-based study of social and occupational problems. *BMC Psychiatry, 23* (1). https://doi.org/10.1186/s12888-023-04713-z

Aiello, E. N., Fiabane, E., Manera, M. R., Radici, A., Grossi, F., Ottonello, M., Pain, D., & Pistarini, C. (2022). Screening for cognitive sequelae of SARS-CoV-2 infection: A comparison between the Mini-Mental State Examination (MMSE) and the Montreal Cognitive Assessment (MoCA). *Neurological Sciences, 43* (1), 81–84. https://doi.org/10.1007/s10072-021-05630-3

Ainsworth, M. D. S., Blehar, M. C., Waters, E., & Wall, S. (1978). *Patterns of attachment: A psychological study of the strange situation.* Lawrence Erlbaum.

Aji, M., Glozier, N., Bartlett, D. J., Grunstein, R. R., Calvo, R. A., Marshall, N. S., White, D. P., & Gordon, C. (2022). The dffectiveness of digital insomnia treatment with adjunctive wearable technology: A pilot randomized dontrolled trial. *Behavioral Sleep Medicine, 20* (5), 570–583. https://doi.org/10.1080/15402002.2021.1967157

Alavi, S. M., Kia-Keating, M., & Nerenberg, C. (2023). Secondary traumatic stress and burnout in health care providers: A post-disaster study. *Traumatology, 29* (3), 389–401 https://doi.org/10.1037/trm0000418 10.1037/trm0000418.supp (Supplemental)

Aldridge, R. W., Story, A., Hwang, S. W., Nordentoft, M., Luchenski, S. A., Hartwell, G., . . . Hayward, A. C. (2018). Morbidity and mortality in homeless individuals, prisoners, sex workers, and individuals with substance use disorders in high-income countries: A systematic review and meta-analysis. *The Lancet, 391* (10117), 241–250 https://doi.org/10.1016/S0140-6736(17)31869-X

Aliane, V., Pérez, S., Bohren, Y., Deniau, J.-M., & Kemel, M.-L. (2011). Key role of striatal cholinergic interneurons in processes leading to arrest of motor stereotypes. *Brain: A Journal of Neurology, 134,* 110–118.

Allami, Y., Williams, R. J., Hodgins, D. C., Stevens, R., Shaw, C. A., el-Guebaly, N., . . . Belanger, Y. D. (2023). Predictors of problem gambling remission in adults: A Canadian longitudinal study. *Psychology of Addictive Behaviors.* https://doi.org/10.1037/adb0000964 10.1037/adb0000964.supp (Supplemental)

Allen, M. S., & Walter, E. E. (2019). Erectile dysfunction: An umbrella review of meta-analyses of risk-factors, treatment, and prevalence outcomes. *Journal of Sexual Medicine, 16* (4), 531–541. https://doi.org/10.1016/j.jsxm.2019.01.314

Allen, T. A., Dombrovski, A. Y., Soloff, P. H., & Hallquist, M. N. (2020). Borderline personality disorder: Stress reactivity or stress generation? A prospective dimensional study. *Psychological Medicine.* https://doi.org/10.1017/S003329172000255X

Almalki, S. (2021). A qualitative study of supported employment practices in Project SEARCH. *International Journal of Developmental Disabilities, 67* (2), 140–150. https://doi.org/10.1080/20473869.2019.1627793

Alosco, M. L., Tripodis, Y., Rowland, B., Chua, A. S., Liao, H., Martin, B., . . . Lin, A. (2020). A magnetic resonance spectroscopy investigation in symptomatic former NFL players. *Brain Imaging and Behavior, 14* (5), 1419–1429. https://doi.org/10.1007/s11682-019-00060-4

Altunoz, U., Kokurcan, A., Kirici, S., Bastug, G., & Ozel-Kizil, E. T. (2018). Clinical characteristics of generalized anxiety disorder: Older vs. young adults. *Nordic Journal of Psychiatry, 72* (2), 97–102. https://doi.org/10.1080/08039488.2017.1390607

Alzheimer, A. (1907/1987). About a peculiar disease of the cerebral cortex. *Alzheimer's Disease and Associated Disorders, 1,* 7–8.

Alzheimer's Association. (2023). 2023 Alzheimer's Disease Facts and Figures. https://www.alz.org/media/Documents/alzheimers-facts-and-figures.pdf

American Psychiatric Association. (2022). *DSM-5: Diagnostic and statistical manual of mental disorders.* American Psychiatric Association.

American Psychological Association Presidential Task Force on Evidence-Based Practice. (2006). Evidence-based practice in psychology. *American Psychologist, 61,* 271–285.

American Psychological Association. (2010). *Ethical principles of psychologists and code of conduct.* http://www.apa.org/ethics/code/index.aspx

American Psychological Association. (2013). Guidelines for psychological evaluations in child protection matters. https://www.apa.org/practice/guidelines/child-protection

American Psychological Association. (2014). What are telehealth and telepsychology? https://www.apa.org/pi/disability/resources/publications/telepsychology

American Psychological Association. (2015a). Guidelines for psychological practice with transgender and gender nonconforming people. *American Psychologist, 70* (9), 832–864. https://doi.org/10.1037/a0039906

American Psychological Association. (2017). Ethical principles of psychologists and code of conduct. https://www.apa.org/ethics/code. Accessed 3/18/21.

American Psychological Association. (2017). Multicultural guidelines: An ecological approach to context, identity, and intersectionality. http://www.apa.org/about/policy/multicultural-guidelines.pdf

American Psychological Association. (2018). APA RESOLUTION for the use of the term patient in American Psychological Association policies, rules, and public relations activities when referring to the health-related and scientific activities of health service psychologists. https://www.apa.org/about/policy/resolution-term-patient.pdf

American Psychological Association. (2020). *Gender.* https://apastyle.apa.org/style-grammar-guidelines/bias-free-language/gender. Accessed 3/1/21.

American Psychological Association. (2021). Inclusive language guidelines. https://www.apa.org/about/apa/equitydiversity-inclusion/language-guidelines.pdf

Amiri, S., & Khan, M. A. B. (2023). Prevalence of non-suicidal self-injury, suicidal ideation, suicide attempts, suicide mortality in eating disorders: A systematic review and meta-analysis. *Eating Disorders: The Journal of Treatment & Prevention, 31* (5), 487–525. https://doi.org/10.1080/10640266.2023.2196492

Andreasen, N. C. (2010). The lifetime trajectory of schizophrenia and the concept of neurodevelopment. *Dialogues in Clinical Neuroscience, 12,* 409–415.

Anestis, J. C., Rodriguez, T. R., O'Dell, C., Preston, O. C., Harrop, T. M., & Charles, N. E. (2023). Psychometric properties of the MMPI-3 in a sample of black and white American undergraduate students: Examining group differences and convergent/discriminant validity with the ASEBA adult self-report. *Journal of Personality Assessment.* https://doi.org/10.1080/00223891.2023.2214817

Angelakis, I., Gooding, P. A., & Panagioti, M. (2016). Suicidality in body dysmorphic disorder (BDD): A systematic review with meta-analysis. *Clinical Psychology Review, 49,* 55–66. https://doi.org/10.1016/j.cpr.2016.08.002

Applied Behavior Analysis. (2020). How is Greta Thunberg affected by autism? https://www.appliedbehavioranalysisprograms.com/faq/autism-affects-greta-thunberg/

Arán Filippetti, V., Krumm, G. L., & Raimondi, W. (2020). Computerized versus manual versions of the Wisconsin Card Sorting Test: Implications with typically developing and ADHD children. *Applied Neuropsychology: Child, 9* (3), 230–245. https://doi.org/10.1080/21622965.2019.1570198

Arbona, C., Fan, W., & Olvera, N. (2018). College stress, minority status stress, depression, grades, and persistence intentions among Hispanic female students: A mediation model. *Hispanic Journal of Behavioral Sciences, 40* (4), 414–420. https://doi.org/10.1177/0739986318799077

Arch, J. J., Eifert, G. H., Davies, C., Vilardaga, J. C. P., Rose, R. D., & Craske, M. G. (2012). Randomized clinical trial of cognitive behavioral therapy (CBT) versus acceptance and commitment therapy (ACT) for mixed anxiety disorders. *Journal of Consulting and Clinical Psychology, 80* (5), 750.

Archibald, T., & Bryant-Waugh, R. (2023). Current evidence for avoidant restrictive food intake disorder: Implications for clinical practice and future directions. *JCPP Advances, 3* (2). https://doi.org/10.1002/jcv2.12160

Arias, V. B., Ponce, F. P., & Martínez-Molina, A. (2022). How a few inconsistent respondents can confound the structure of personality survey data: An example with the Core-Self Evaluations Scale. *European Journal of Psychological Assessment.* https://doi.org/10.1027/1015-5759/a000719

Ariza, M., Cano, N., Segura, B., Adan, A., Bargalló, N., Caldú, X., . . . Garolera, M. (2022). Neuropsychological impairment in post-COVID condition individuals with and without cognitive complaints. *Frontiers in Aging Neuroscience, 14.* https://doi.org/10.3389/fnagi.2022.1029842

Arnatkeviciute, A., Lemire, M., Morrison, C., Mooney, M., Ryabinin, P., Roslin, N. M., . . . Bellgrove, M. A. (2023). Trans-ancestry meta-analysis of genome wide association studies of inhibitory control. *Molecular Psychiatry.* https://doi.org/10.1038/s41380-023-02187-9

Arnoldussen, I. A. C., Sundh, V., Backman, K., Kern, S., Ostling, S., Blennow, K., Gustafson, D. R. (2018). A 10-year follow-up of adiposity and dementia in Swedish adults aged 70 years and older. *Journal of Alzheimer's DIsease, 63* (4), 1325–1335. https://doi.org/10.3233/jad-180099

Arria, A. M., Caldeira, K. M., Bugbee, B. A., Vincent, K. B., & O'Grady, K. E. (2017). Trajectories of energy drink consumption and subsequent drug use during young adulthood. *Drug and Alcohol Dependence, 179,* 424–432. https://doi.org/0.1016/j.drugalcdep.2017.06.008

Arts, L. P. J., Oerlemans, S., Schoormans, D., Sanders, A. L. T. M., Stevens, W. B. C., Posthuma, E. F. M., Tick, L. W., & van de Poll-Franse, L. V. (2021). Psychological distress among patients with lymphoma: The association with personality and coping strategies. *Journal of Psychosocial Oncology Research & Practice, 3* (1), 1–6. https://doi.org/10.1097/OR9.0000000000000041

Asami, Y., Nomura, K., Shimada, H., Nakagawa, K., Sugano, M., Koshiba, A., . . . Ohishi, M. (2022). Cognitive behavioural group therapy with mindfulness for kleptomania: An open trial. *The Cognitive Behaviour Therapist, 15.* https://doi.org/10.1017/S1754470X22000290

Asaoka, Y., Won, M., Morita, T., Ishikawa, E., & Goto, Y. (2023). Distinct situational cue processing in individuals with kleptomania: A preliminary study. *International Journal of Neuropsychopharmacology, 26* (5), 340–349. https://doi.org/10.1093/ijnp/pyad005

Asselmann, E., & Specht, J. (2020). Taking the ups and downs at the rollercoaster of love: Associations between major life events in the domain of romantic relationships and the Big Five personality traits. *Developmental Psychology, 56* (9), 1803–1816. https://doi.org/10.1037/dev0001047

Associated Press. (2007). False-imprisonment charge dropped against Broncos' Marshall. *ESPN.* Retrieved 3/16/21 from https://www.espn.com/nfl/news/story?id=2882758

Associated Press. (2020). Brandon Marshall tries to break the stigma of mental illness. *USA Today.* https://www.usatoday.com/story/sports/nfl/2020/11/27/brandon-marshall-tries-to-break-the-stigma-of-mental-illness/43199299/

Assumpção, A. A., Garcia, F. D., Garcia, H. D., Bradford, J. W., & Thibaut, F. (2014). Pharmacologic treatment of paraphilias. *Psychiatric Clinics of North America, 37,* 173–181. https://doi.org/10.1016/j.psc.2014.03.002

Austin, A., & Craig, S. L. (2015). Transgender affirmative cognitive behavioral therapy: Clinical considerations and applications. *Professional Psychology: Research and Practice, 46* (1), 21.

Axelsson, E., & Hedman-Lagerlöf, E. (2022). Validity and clinical utility of distinguishing between DSM-5 somatic symptom disorder and illness anxiety disorder in pathological health anxiety: Should we close the chapter? *Journal of Psychosomatic Research.* https://doi.org/10.1016/j.jpsychores.2022.111133

Axt, J. R., Conway, M. A., Westgate, E. C., & Buttrick, N. R. (2021). Implicit transgender attitudes independently predict beliefs about gender and transgender people. *Personality and Social Psychology Bulletin, 47* (2), 257–157. https://doi.org/10.1177/0146167220921065

Ayers, C. R., Najmi, S., Mayes, T. L., & Dozier, M. E. (2015). Hoarding disorder in older adulthood. *The American Journal of Geriatric Psychiatry, 23,* 416–422. https://doi.org/10.1016/j.jagp.2014.05.009

B

Bader, S. M., Schoeneman-Morris, K. A., Scalora, M. J., & Casady, T. K. (2008). Exhibitionism: Findings from a Midwestern police contact sample. *International Journal of Offender Therapy and Comparative Criminology, 52,* 270–279.

Badji, S., Black, N., & Johnston, D. W. (2020). Association between density of gaming venues in a geographical area and prevalence of insolvency: Longitudinal evidence from Australia. *Addiction, 115* (12), 2349–2356. https://doi.org/10.1111/add.15090

Bagby, R. M., & Widiger, T. A. (2020). Assessment of the *ICD-11* dimensional trait model: An introduction to the special section. *Psychological Assessment, 32* (1), 1-7. https://doi.org/10.1037/pas0000785

Bahji, A., Mazhar, M. N., Hudson, C. C., Nadkarni, P., MacNeil, B. A., & Hawken, E. (2019). Prevalence of substance use disorder comorbidity among individuals with eating disorders: A systematic review and meta-analysis. *Psychiatry Research, 273,* 58-66. https://doi.org/10.1016/j.psychres.2019.01.007

Bahji, A., Vazquez, G. H., & Zarate, C. A., Jr (2021). Comparative efficacy of racemic ketamine and esketamine for depression: A systematic review and meta-analysis. *Journal of affective disorders, 278,* 542-555. https://doi.org/10.1016/j.jad.2020.09.071

Balaratnasingam, S., & Janca, A. (2015). Normal personality, personality disorder and psychosis: Current views and future perspectives. *Current Opinion in Psychiatry, 28,* 30-34. https://doi.org/10.1097/YCO.0000000000000124

Banaj, N., Vecchio, D., Piras, F., De Rossi, P., Bustillo, J., Ciufolini, S., . . . Piras, F. (2023). Cortical morphology in patients with the deficit and non-deficit syndrome of schizophrenia: A worldwide meta- and mega-analyses. *Molecular Psychiatry*. https://doi.org/10.1038/s41380-023-02221-w

Band-Winterstein, T., Goldblatt, H., Lev, S., & Harel, D. (2021). Forms of sexual assault against older women in the context of acquaintance relationships: An intersectional perspective. *Health & Social Care in the Community*. https://doi.org/10.1111/hsc.13672

Bandura, A. (1971). Psychotherapy based upon modeling principles. In A. E. Bergin & S. L. Garfield (Eds.), *Handbook of psychotherapy and behavior change* (pp. 653-708). Wiley.

Barbaree, H. E., & Blanchard, R. (2008). Sexual deviance over the lifespan: Reductions in deviant sexual behavior in the aging sex offender. In D. R. Laws & W. T. O'Donohue (Eds.), *Sexual deviance: Theory, assessment, and treatment* (2nd ed., pp. 37-60). New York: Guilford Press.

Barber, K. E., Capel, L. K., Merl, N., Twohig, M. P., Saunders, S. M., Compton, S. N., Franklin, M. E., & Woods, D. W. (2023). Pulling sites in trichotillomania: Exploring differences in characteristics, phenomenology, and contextual variables. *Cognitive Therapy and Research*. https://doi.org/10.1007/s10608-023-10419-z

Barbonetti, A., D'Andrea, S., Cavallo, F., Martorella, A., Francavilla, S., & Francavilla, F. (2019). Erectile dysfunction and premature ejaculation in homosexual and heterosexual men: A systematic review and meta-analysis of comparative studies. *Journal of Sexual Medicine, 16* (5), 624-632. https://doi.org/10.1016/j.jsxm.2019.02.014

Barbour, S. (2019). Lamar Odom admits to sleeping with more than 2,000 women and having a sex addiction. *Cosmopolitan*. https://www.cosmopolitan.com/entertainment/celebs/a27483678/lamar-odom-sex-2000-women-drug-addiction. Accessed 2/27/21.

Barbour, S. (2020). Lady Gaga's "911" lyrics are about taking antipsychotic medication. *Cosmopolitan*. Retrieved 2/23/21 from https://www.cosmopolitan.com/entertainment/music/a34075153/lady-gaga-911-lyrics-meaning-antipsychotic-medication

Barker, T. H., Pollock, D., Stone, J. C., Klugar, M., Scott, A. M., Stern, C., . . . Munn, Z. (2023). How should we handle predatory journals in evidence synthesis? A descriptive survey-based cross-sectional study of evidence synthesis experts. *Research Synthesis Methods, 14* (3), 370-381. https://doi.org/10.1002/jrsm.1613

Barkley, R. A., & Benton, C. M. (2021). Taking charge of adult ADHD (Second edition): Proven strategies to succeed at work, at home, and in relationships. Guilford Press.

Barnes, D. M., & Bates, L. M. (2017). Do racial patterns in psychological distress shed light on the Black-White depression paradox? A systematic review. *Social Psychiatry and Psychiatric Epidemiology: The International Journal for Research in Social and Genetic Epidemiology and Mental Health Services, 52* (8), 913-928. https://doi.org/10.1007/s00127-017-1394-9

Barr, S. M., Snyder, K. E., Adelson, J. L., & Budge, S. L. (2022). Posttraumatic stress in the trans community: The roles of anti-transgender bias, non-affirmation, and internalized transphobia. *Psychology of Sexual Orientation and Gender Diversity, 9* (4), 410-421. https://doi.org/10.1037/sgd0000500 10.1037/sgd0000500.supp (Supplemental)

Barrett, J., Gonsalvez, C. J., & Shires, A. (2019). Evidence-based practice within supervision during psychology practitioner training: A systematic review. *Clinical Psychologist*. https://doi.org/10.1111/cp.12196

Barrett, J., Gonsalvez, C. J., & Shires, A. (2020). Evidence-based practice within supervision during psychology practitioner training: A systematic review. *Clinical Psychologist, 24* (1), 3-17. https://doi.org/10.1111/cp.12196

Bartels, J. M., & Peters, D. (2017). Coverage of Rosenhan's "On being sane in insane places" in Abnormal Psychology Textbooks. *Teaching of Psychology, 44* (2), 169-173. https://doi.org/10.1177/0098628317692634

Bártová, K., Androvičová, R., Krejčová, L., Weiss, P., & Klapilová, K. (2020). The prevalence of paraphilic interests in the Czech population: Preference, arousal, the use of pornography, fantasy, and behavior. *Journal of Sex Research*. https://doi.org/10.1080/00224499.2019.1707468

Basavarajappa, B. S., & Subbanna, S. (2023). Synaptic plasticity abnormalities in fetal alcohol spectrum disorders. *Cells, 12* (3). https://doi.org/10.3390/cells12030442

Bayless, S. J., & Harvey, A. J. (2017). Testing Alcohol Myopia Theory: Examining the effects of alcohol intoxication on simultaneous central and peripheral attention. *Perception, 46* (1), 90-99. https://doi.org/10.1177/0301006616672221

BBC News. (2020). Greta Thunberg: Who is she and what does she want? https://www.bbc.com/news/world-europe-49918719

Beck, A. T. (1967). *Depression: Clinical, experimental, and theoretical aspects.* Harper & Row.

Beck, A. T., & Weishaar, M. (1989). Cognitive therapy. In A. Freeman, K. M. Simon, L. E. Beutler, & H. Arkowitz (Eds.), *Comprehensive handbook of cognitive therapy* (pp. 21-36). Plenum Press.

Beck, A. T., Freeman, A., & Davis, D. D. (2004). *Cognitive therapy of personality disorders* (2nd ed.). Guilford Press.

Beck, A. T., Rush, A. J., Shaw, B. F., & Emery, G. (1979). *Cognitive therapy of depression: A treatment manual.* Guilford Press.

Beck, F., Léger, D., Fressard, L., Peretti-Watel, P., & Verger, P. (2021). COVID-19 health crisis and lockdown associated with high level of sleep complaints and hypnotic uptake at the population level. *Journal of Sleep Research, 30* (1). https://doi.org/10.1111/jsr.13119

Bedics, J. D., Atkins, D. C., Harned, M. S., & Linehan, M. M. (2015). The therapeutic alliance as a predictor of outcome in dialectical behavior therapy versus nonbehavioral psychotherapy by experts for borderline personality disorder. *Psychotherapy, 52,* 67-77. https://doi.org/10.1037/a0038457

Begley, R., Farrell, L., Lyttle, N., Alty, J., Curran, D., Williams, S., & Graham, C. D. (2023). Clinicians' implicit and explicit attitudes about the legitimacy of functional neurological disorders correlate with referral decisions. *British Journal of Health Psychology, 28* (2), 604-618. https://doi.org/10.1111/bjhp.12643

Behary, W. T., & Dieckmann, E. (2013). Schema therapy for pathological narcissism: The art of adaptive reparenting. In J. S. Ogrodniczuk (Ed.), *Understanding and treating pathological narcissism* (pp. 285-300). Washington, DC: American Psychological Association. https://doi.org/10.1037/14041-017

Bekk, M., Meland, K. J., Moen, E., Nøstvik, L. I., Gausdal, A. L., & Hummelen, B. (2023). Group-based comprehensive behavioral intervention for tics (CBIT) for adults with Tourette syndrome or chronic tic disorders: A pilot study. *Scandinavian Journal of Psychology*. https://doi.org/10.1111/sjop.12942

Bemporad, J. R. (1985). Long-term analytic treatment of depression. In E. E. Beckham & W. R. Leber (Eds.), *Handbook of depression: Treatment, assessment, and research* (pp. 82-89). Dorsey Press.

Ben-Porath, Y. S., & Tellegen, A. (2020). *Minnesota Multiphasic Personality Inventory-3 (MMPI-3): Manual for administration, scoring, and interpretation.* Pearson.

Benarous, X., Renaud, J., Breton, J. J., Cohen, D., Labelle, R., & Guilé, J.-M. (2020). Are youths with disruptive mood dysregulation disorder different from youths with major depressive disorder or persistent depressive disorder? *Journal of Affective Disorders, 265,* 207–215. https://doi.org/10.1016/j.jad.2020.01.020

Berezowski, L., Ludwig, L., Martin, A., Löwe, B., & Shedden-Mora, M. C. (2022). Early psychological interventions for somatic symptom disorder and functional somatic syndromes: A systematic review and meta-analysis. *Psychosomatic Medicine, 84* (3), 325–338. https://doi.org/10.1097/PSY.0000000000001011

Beringer, R., de Vries, B., Gill, P., & Gutman, G. (2023). Beyond mortality: The social and health impacts of COVID-19 among older (55+) BIPOC and LGBT respondents in a Canada-wide survey. *Healthcare (Basel), 11* (14). https://doi.org/10.3390/healthcare11142044

Berlin, F. S. (2014). Pedophilia and *DSM-5*: The importance of clearly defining the nature of a pedophilic disorder. *Journal of the American Academy of Psychiatry and the Law, 42,* 404–407.

Berrettini, W., & Lohoff, F. W. (2017). Genetics of bipolar and unipolar disorders. In R. J. DeRubeis & D. R. Strunk (Eds.), *The Oxford handbook of mood disorders* (pp. 111–119). Oxford University Press.

Besser, A., & Priel, B. (2010). Grandiose narcissism versus vulnerable narcissism in threatening situations: Emotional reactions to achievement failure and interpersonal rejection. *Journal of Social and Clinical Psychology, 29,* 874–902.

Beutel, M., Krakau, L., Kaufhold, J., Bahrke, U., Grabhorn, A., Hautzinger, M., . . . Leuzinger-Bohleber, M. (2022). Recovery from chronic depression and structural change: 5-year outcomes after psychoanalytic and cognitive-behavioural long-term treatments (lac depression study). *Clinical Psychology & Psychotherapy*. https://doi.org/10.1002/cpp.2793

Beyer, K. M., Szabo, A., Hoormann, K., & Stolley, M. (2018). Time spent outdoors, activity levels, and chronic disease among American adults. *Journal of Behavioral Medicine, 1* (4), 494–503. https://doi.org/10.1007/s10865-018-9911-1

Biasutti, W. R., Leffers, K. S. H., & Callaghan, R. C. (2020). Systematic review of cannabis use and risk of occupational injury. *Substance Use & Misuse, 55* (11), 1733–1745. https://doi.org/10.1080/10826084.2020.1759643

Bierer, L. M., Bader, H. N., Daskalakis, N. P., Lehrner, A., Provençal, N., Wiechmann, T., . . . Yehuda, R. (2020). Intergenerational effects of maternal holocaust exposure on FKBP5 methylation. *The American Journal of Psychiatry, 177* (8), 744–753. https://doi.org/10.1176/appi.ajp.2019.19060618

Bigdeli, T. B., Genovese, G., Georgakopoulos, P., Meyers, J. L., Peterson, R. E., Iyegbe, C. O., . . . Pato, C. N. (2020). Contributions of common genetic variants to risk of schizophrenia among individuals of African and Latino ancestry. *Molecular Psychiatry, 25* (10), 2455–2467. https://doi.org/10.1038/s41380-019-0517-y

Bighelli, I., Wallis, S., Reitmeir, C., Schwermann, F., Salahuddin, N. H., & Leucht, S. (2023). Effects of psychological treatments on functioning in people with schizophrenia: A systematic review and meta-analysis of randomized controlled trials. *European Archives of Psychiatry and Clinical Neuroscience, 273* (4), 779–810. https://doi.org/10.1007/s00406-022-01526-1

Bilder, R. M., Widaman, K. F., Bauer, R. M., Drane, D., Loring, D. W., Umfleet, L. G., . . . Shih, S. (2023). Construct identification in the neuropsychological battery: What are we measuring? *Neuropsychology, 37* (4), 351–372. https://doi.org/10.1037/neu0000832 10.1037

Bilet, T., Olsen, T., Andersen, J. R., & Martinsen, E. W. (2020). Cognitive behavioral group therapy for panic disorder in a general clinical setting: A prospective cohort study with 12 to 31-years follow-up. *BMC Psychiatry, 20*. https://doi.org/10.1186/s12888-020-02679-w

Binaco, R., Calzaretto, N., Epifano, J., McGuire, S., Umer, M., Emrani, S., . . . Polikar, R. (2020). Machine learning analysis of digital clock drawing test performance for differential classification of mild cognitive impairment subtypes versus Alzheimer's disease. *Journal of the International Neuropsychological Society, 26* (7), 690–700. https://doi.org/10.1017/S1355617720000144

Biography. (2021). Lady Gaga Biography 2016. https://www.biography.com/musician/lady-gaga

Bitsko, R. H., Claussen, A. H., Lichstein, J., Black, L. I., Jones, S. E., Danielson, M., . . . Ghandour, R. M. (2022). Mental health surveillance among children — United States, 2013–2019. *Morbidity and Mortality Weekly Report (MMWR), 71* (Suppl-2), 1–42. https://doi.org/http://dx.doi.org/10.15585/mmwr.su7102a1

Bjornsson, A. S., Didie, E. R., & Phillips, K. A. (2010). Body dysmorphic disorder. *Dialogues in Clinical Neuroscience, 12* (2), 221–232. https://doi.org/10.31887/DCNS.2010.12.2/abjornsson

Blanchard, R. (2010). The *DSM* diagnostic criteria for transvestic fetishism. *Archives of Sexual Behavior, 39,* 363–372.

Blashfield, R. K., Reynolds, S. M., & Stennett, B. (2012). The death of histrionic personality disorder. In T. A. Widiger (Ed.), *The Oxford handbook of personality disorders* (pp. 603–627). New York: Oxford University Press. https://doi.org/10.1093/oxfordhb/9780199735013.013.0028

Bockting, C. L. H., Klein, N. S., Elgersma, H. J., van Rijsbergen, G. D., Slofstra, C., Ormel, J., . . . Burger, H. (2018). Effectiveness of preventive cognitive therapy while tapering antidepressants versus maintenance antidepressant treatment versus their combination in prevention of depressive relapse or recurrence (DRD study): A three-group, multicentre, randomised controlled trial. *The Lancet Psychiatry, 5* (5), 401 doi:10.1016/S2215-0366(18)30100-7

Boe, H. J., Holgersen, K. H., & Holen, A. (2011). Mental health outcomes and predictors of chronic disorders after the North Sea oil rig disaster: 27-year longitudinal follow-up study. *Journal of Nervous and Mental Disease, 199,* 49–54.

Boer, E. M. J. d., Orie, V. K., Williams, T., Baker, M. R., Oliveira, H. M. D., Polvikoski, T., . . . Vucic, S. (2021). TDP-43 proteinopathies: A new wave of neurodegenerative diseases. *Journal of Neurology, Neurosurgery & Psychiatry, 92* (1), 86–95. https://doi.org/10.1136/jnnp-2020-322983

Boerwinkle, A. H., Gordon, B. A., Wisch, J., Flores, S., Henson, R. L., Butt, O. H., . . . Ances, B. M. (2023). Comparison of amyloid burden in individuals with Down syndrome versus autosomal dominant Alzheimer's disease: A cross-sectional study. *The Lancet Neurology, 22* (1), 55–65. https://doi.org/10.1016/S1474-4422(22)00408-2

Bohus, M., Kleindienst, N., Hahn, C., Müller-Engelmann, M., Ludäscher, P., Steil, R., . . . Priebe, K. (2020). Dialectical Behavior Therapy for Posttraumatic Stress Disorder (DBT-PTSD) compared with cognitive processing therapy (CPT) in complex presentations of PTSD in women survivors of childhood abuse: A randomized clinical trial. *JAMA Psychiatry, 77* (12), 1235–1245. https://doi.org/10.1001/jamapsychiatry.2020.2148

Bomyea, J., Ramsawh, H., Ball, T. M., Taylor, C. T., Paulus, M. P., Lang, A. J., & Stein, M. B. (2015). Intolerance of uncertainty as a mediator of reductions in worry in a cognitive behavioral treatment program for generalized anxiety disorder. *Journal of Anxiety Disorders,* 3390–3394. https://doi.org/10.1016/j.janxdis.2015.05.004

Bond, K., & Anderson, I. M. (2015). Psychoeducation for relapse prevention in bipolar disorder: A systematic review of efficacy in randomized controlled trials. *Bipolar Disorders, 17,* 349–362. https://doi.org/10.1111/bdi.12287

Bouchard, K., Gareau, A., Greenman, P. S., Lalande, K., Sztajerowska, K., & Tulloch, H. (2023). What's love got to do with it? Relationship quality appraisals and quality of life in couples facing cardiovascular disease. *Health Psychology and Behavioral Medicine, 11* (1). https://doi.org/10.1080/21642850.2023.2237564

Bowlby, J. (1980). *Attachment and loss: Vol. III. Loss: Sadness and depression.* Basic Books.

Brady, W. (Author). (2017). Our Dr. Freda Lewis-Hall talks depression with actor and comedian, Wayne Brady. https://www.youtube.com/watch?v=8NthKtEK3wY 2/22/21

Brænden, A., Coldevin, M., Zeiner, P., Stubberud, J., & Melinder, A. (2023). Executive function in children with disruptive mood dysregulation disorder compared to attention-deficit/hyperactivity disorder and oppositional defiant disorder, and in children with different irritability levels. *European Child & Adolescent Psychiatry.* https://doi.org/10.1007/s00787-023-02143-6

Brauer, L., & Reinecke, M. A. (2015). Dependent personality disorder. In A. T. Beck, D. D. Davis, & A. Freeman (Eds.), *Cognitive therapy of personality disorders* (3rd ed., pp. 155–173). Guilford Press.

Breiner, C. E., Miller, M. L., Hamilton, A. L., Cruz Garcia, S., Sanzari, C. M., & Hormes, J. M. (2023). Exploring the relationship between food disgust and avoidant/restrictive food intake disorder (ARFID) presentations in a non-clinical collegiate sample. *International Journal of Eating Disorders, 56* (7), 1444–1448. https://doi.org/10.1002/eat.23955

Bretherton, I., Thrower, E., Zwickl, S., Wong, A., Chetcuti, D., Grossmann, M., . . . Cheung, A. S. (2020). The health and well-being of transgender Australians: A national community survey. *LGBT Health.* https://doi.org/10.1089/lgbt.2020.0178

Britton, T. C., Wilkinson, E. H., & Hall, S. S. (2020). Examining the specificity of forms and functions of aggressive behavior in boys with fragile X syndrome. *American Journal on Intellectual and Developmental Disabilities, 125* (4), 247–259. https://doi.org/10.1352/1944-7558-125.4.247

Brown, L. A., Fernandez, C. A., Kohn, R., Saldivia, S., & Vicente, B. (2018). Pre-disaster PTSD as a moderator of the relationship between natural disaster and suicidal ideation over time. *Journal of Affective Disorders, 230,* 7–14. https://doi.org/10.1016/j.jad.2017.12.096

Bruijniks, S. J. E., Meeter, M., Lemmens, L. H. J. M., Peeters, F., Cuijpers, P., & Huibers, M. J. H. (2022). Temporal and specific pathways of change in cognitive behavioral therapy (CBT) and interpersonal psychotherapy (IPT) for depression. *Behaviour Research and Therapy, 151,* 1–13. https://doi.org/10.1016/j.brat.2021.104010

Bryant-Waugh, R., Markham, L., Kreipe, R. E., & Walsh, B. T. (2010). Feeding and eating disorders in childhood. *International Journal of Eating Disorders, 43,* 98–111.

Budman, E., Deeb, W., Martinez-Ramirez, D., Pilitsis, J. G., Peng-Chen, Z., Okun, M. S., & Ramirez-Zamora, A. (2018). Potential indications for deep brain stimulation in neurological disorders: An evolving field. *European Journal of Neurology, 25* (3), 434–e30. https://doi.org/10.1111/ene.13548

Bueno, A. (Producer). (2014). Wayne Brady opens up about his depression: "I had a complete breakdown." https://www.etonline.com/news/153335_wayne_brady_opens_up_about_his_depression 2/22/21

Burch, E., & Nakic, M. (2019). A duty to protect without a clearly communicated threat? *Journal of the American Academy of Psychiatry and the Law, 47* (1), 117–119.

Bursch, B., Emerson, N. D., & Sanders, M. J. (2021). Evaluation and management of factitious disorder imposed on another. *Journal of Clinical Psychology in Medical Settings, 28* (1), 67–77. https://doi.org/10.1007/s10880-019-09668-6

Burton, P. R. S., McNiel, D. E., & Binder, R. L. (2012). Firesetting, arson, pyromania, and the forensic mental health expert. *Journal of the American Academy of Psychiatry and the Law, 40* (3), 355–365.

C

Cabé, N., Lanièpce, A., & Pitel, A. L. (2021). Physical activity: A promising adjunctive treatment for severe alcohol use disorder. *Addictive Behaviors, 113.* https://doi.org/10.1016/j.addbeh.2020.106667

Cai, W., Mizuno, Y., Tomoda, A., & Menon, V. (2023). Bayesian dynamical system analysis of the effects of methylphenidate in children with attention-deficit/hyperactivity disorder: A randomized trial. *Neuropsychopharmacology.* https://doi.org/10.1038/s41386-023-01668-3

Calabrese, W. R., Martin Lopez, M., Koenigsberg, H. W., New, A. S., Rosell, D. R., Hazlett, E. A., McClure, M. M., & Perez-Rodriguez, M. M. (2023). The structure of antagonism: A hierarchical model of self- and interview-rated psychopathology. *Personality Disorders: Theory, Research, and Treatment, 14* (4), 441–451. https://doi.org/10.1037/per0000603 10.1037/per0000603.supp (Supplemental)

Caligor, E., Levy, K. N., & Yeomans, F. E. (2015). Narcissistic personality disorder: Diagnostic and clinical challenges. American Journal of Psychiatry, 172(5), 415–422. https://doi.org/10.1176/appi.ajp.2014.14060723

Campbell, K., & Lakeman, R. (2020). Borderline personality disorder: A case for the right treatment, at the right dose, at the right time. *Issues in Mental Health Nursing.* https://doi.org/10.1080/01612840.2020.1833119

Campbell, W. G. (2003). Addiction: A disease of volition caused by a cognitive impairment. *Canadian Journal of Psychiatry, 48,* 669–674.

Campos-Magdaleno, M., Leiva, D., Pereiro, A. X., Lojo-Seoane, C., Mallo, S. C., Facal, D., & Juncos-Rabadán, O. (2020). Changes in visual memory in mild cognitive impairment: A longitudinal study with CANTAB. *Psychological Medicine.* https://doi.org/10.1017/S0033291720001142

Cañedo-Ayala, M., Rice, D. B., Levis, A. W., Chiovitti, M., & Thombs, B. D. (2020). Balance of group sizes in randomized controlled trials published in American Psychological Association journals. *Health Psychology: Official Journal of the Division of Health Psychology, American Psychological Association, 39* (11)(1930-7810 (Electronic)), 956–965. https://doi.org/10.1037/hea0001020

Canty, A. L., Cao, Y., Neumann, D., & Shum, D. H. K. (2021). The functional significance of cognitive empathy and theory of mind in early and chronic schizophrenia. *Psychiatry Research, 299.* https://doi.org/10.1016/j.psychres.2021.113852

Carl, J. R., Miller, C. B., Henry, A. L., Davis, M. L., Stott, R., Smits, J. A. J., . . . Espie, C. A. (2020). Efficacy of digital cognitive behavioral therapy for moderate-to-severe symptoms of generalized anxiety disorder: A randomized controlled trial. *Depression and Anxiety, 37* (12), 1168–1178. https://doi.org/10.1002/da.23079

Carpenter, J. K., Andrews, L. A., Witcraft, S. M., Powers, M. B., Smits, J. J., & Hofmann, S. G. (2018). Cognitive behavioral therapy for anxiety and related disorders: A meta-analysis of randomized placebo-controlled trials. *Depression and Anxiety, 35* (6), 502–514. https://doi.org/10.1002/da.22728

Carpenter, K. M., Vickerman, K. A., Salmon, E. E., Javitz, H. S., Epel, E. S., & Lovejoy, J. C. (2019). A randomized pilot study of a phone-based mindfulness and weight loss program. *Behavioral Medicine, 45* (4), 271–281. https://doi.org/10.1080/08964289.2017.1384359

Carrollo, K. (2011). NFL star Brandon Marshall has borderline personality disorder. *ABC News.* https://abcnews.go.com/Health/miami-dolphins-wide-receiver-brandon-marshall-reveals-borderline/story?id=Accessed 3/18/21.

Cash, T. F., & Smolak, L. (2011). *Body image: A handbook of science, practice, and prevention,* 2nd ed. The Guilford Press.

Castellini, G., Rellini, A. H., Appignanesi, C., Pinucci, I., Fattorini, M., Grano, E., . . . Ricca, V. (2018). Deviance or normalcy? The relationship among paraphilic thoughts and behaviors, hypersexuality, and psychopathology in a sample of university students. *Journal of Sexual Medicine, 15* (9), 1322–1335. https://doi.org/10.1016/j.jsxm.2018.07.015

CBS News. (2014). Wayne Brady opens up about his depression: "I had a complete breakdown." https://www.cbsnews.com/news/wayne-brady-opens-up-about-his-depression-i-had-a-complete-breakdown/

Centers for Disease Control and Prevention. (2023). Facts about suicide. https://www.cdc.gov/suicide/facts/index.html

Centers for Disease Control and Prevention. (2023). Fetal alcohol spectrum disorders (FASDs). https://www.cdc.gov/ncbddd/fasd/data.html

Centers for Disease Control and Prevention. (2023). TBI Data. https://www.cdc.gov/traumaticbraininjury/data/index.html

Cerea, S., Ghisi, M., Bottesi, G., Manoli, T., Carraro, E., & Doron, G. (2021). Cognitive behavioral training using a mobile application reduces body image-related symptoms in high-risk female university students: A randomized controlled study. *Behavior Therapy, 52* (1), 170–182. https://doi.org/10.1016/j.beth.2020.04.002

Cervin, M., Miguel, E. C., Güler, A. S., Ferrão, Y. A., Erdoğdu, A. B., Lazaro, L., . . . Mataix-Cols, D. (2021). Towards a definitive symptom structure of obsessive–compulsive disorder: A factor and network analysis of 87 distinct symptoms in 1366 individuals. *Psychological Medicine*. https://doi.org/10.1017/S0033291720005437

Cesar, K. G., Yassuda, M. S., Porto, F. H. G., Brucki, S. M. D., & Nitrini, R. (2019). MoCA Test: Normative and diagnostic accuracy data for seniors with heterogeneous educational levels in Brazil. *Arquivos de Neuro-Psiquiatria, 77* (11), 775–781. https://doi.org/10.1590/0004-282x20190130

Chang, H., Cai, X., Li, H.-J., Liu, W.-P., Zhao, L.-J., Zhang, C.-Y., . . . Xiao, X. (2020). Functional genomics identify a regulatory risk variation rs4420550 in the 16p112 schizophrenia-associated locus. *Biological Psychiatry*. https://doi.org/10.1016/j.biopsych.2020.09.016

Chapman, A. L. (2019). Borderline personality disorder and emotion dysregulation. *Development and Psychopathology*. https://doi.org/10.1017/S0954579419000658

Chatwin, H., Holde, K., Yilmaz, Z., Larsen, J. T., Albiñana, C., Vilhjálmsson, B. J., . . . Petersen, L. V. (2023). Risk factors for anorexia nervosa: A population-based investigation of sex differences in polygenic risk and early life exposures [Article]. *International Journal of Eating Disorders, 56* (9), 1703–1716. https://doi.org/10.1002/eat.23997

Chen, L., Lu, X., Yuan, J., Luo, J., Luo, J., Xie, Z., & Li, D. (2020). A social media study on the associations of flavored electronic cigarettes with health symptoms: Observational study. *Journal of Medical Internet Research, 22* (6). https://doi.org/10.2196/17496

Cheng, Z. H., Perko, V. L., Fuller-Marashi, L., Gau, J. M., & Stice, E. (2019). Ethnic differences in eating disorder prevalence, risk factors, and predictive effects of risk factors among young women. *Eating Behaviors, 32*, 23–30. https://doi.org/10.1016/j.eatbeh.2018.11.004

Chia, K., Pasalich, D. S., Fassnacht, D. B., Ali, K., Kyrios, M., Maclean, B., & Grisham, J. R. (2021). Interpersonal attachment, early family environment, and trauma in hoarding: A systematic review. *Clinical Psychology Review, 90*,102096. https://doi.org/10.1016/j.cpr.2021.102096

Child Mind Institute. (2017). Wayne Brady has depression. https://childmind.org/blog/wayne-brady-myyoungerself/ 2/22/21

Cho, Y., Choi, Y., & Kim, S. (2021). Role of panic appraisal in predicting the severity of panic and agoraphobic symptoms. *Journal of Clinical Psychology, 77* (1), 298–311. doi:10.1002/jclp.23028

Chodosh, J., Thorpe, L. E., & Trinh-Shevrin, C. (2018). Changing faces of cognitive impairment in the US: Detection strategies for underserved communities. *American Journal of Preventive Medicine, 54* (6), 842–844. https://doi.org/10.1016/j.amepre.2018.02.016

Chóliz, M., Marcos, M., & Lázaro-Mateo, J. (2019). The risk of online gambling: A study of gambling disorder prevalence rates in Spain. *International Journal of Mental Health and Addiction*. https://doi.org/10.1007/s11469-019-00067-4

Chou, C. Y., Tsoh, J. Y., Shumway, M., Smith, L. C., Chan, J., Delucchi, K., . . . Mathews, C. A. (2020). Treating hoarding disorder with compassion-focused therapy: A pilot study examining treatment feasibility, acceptability, and exploring treatment effects. *British Journal of Clinical Psychology, 59* (1), 1–21. https://doi.org/10.1111/bjc.12228

Choy, Y., Fyer, A. J., & Lipsitz, J. D. (2007). Treatment of specific phobia in adults. *Clinical Psychology Review, 27*, 266–286.

Ciafrè, S., Ferraguti, G., Greco, A., Polimeni, A., Ralli, M., Ceci, F. M., . . . Fiore, M. (2020). Alcohol as an early life stressor: Epigenetics, metabolic, neuroendocrine and neurobehavioral implications. *Neuroscience and Biobehavioral Reviews, 118*, 654–668. https://doi.org/10.1016/j.neubiorev.2020.08.018

Ciao, A. C., Accurso, E. C., Fitzsimmons-Craft, E. E., & Le Grange, D. (2015). Predictors and moderators of psychological changes during the treatment of adolescent bulimia nervosa. *Behaviour Research and Therapy, 69*, 48–53. https://doi.org/10.1016/j.brat.2015.04.002

Citrome, L., & Volavka, J. (2021). Specific anti-hostility effects of atypical antipsychotics in persons with schizophrenia: From clozapine to cariprazine. *Harvard Review of Psychiatry, 29* (1), 20–34. https://doi.org/10.1097/HRP.0000000000000275 (Violence and Mental Illness)

Clark, S. K., Jeglic, E. L., Calkins, C., & Tatar, J. R. (2016). More than a nuisance: The prevalence and consequences of frotteurism and exhibitionism. *Sexual Abuse: Journal of Research and Treatment, 28* (1), 3–19. https://doi.org/10.1177/1079063214525643

Clauss-Ehlers, C. S., Hunter, S. J., Morse, G. S., & Tummala-Narra, P. (2024). Conducting culturally informed work in psychology: Multicultural guideline In *Applying multiculturalism: An ecological approach to the APA guidelines* (pp. 201–217). American Psychological Association. https://doi.org/10.1037/0000348-011

Clayton, A. H., & Valladares Juarez, E. M. (2017). Female sexual dysfunction. *Psychiatric Clinics of North America, 40* (2), 267–284. https://doi.org/10.1016/j.psc.2017.01.004

Clinch, D & Levitan, C. (September, 2014). A Lesson in Humility from Adam Duriz. Men's Health. https://www.menshealth.com/trending-news/a19518814/adam-duritz-interview/

Coccaro, E. F., & McCloskey, M. S. (2019). Chapter Three–Phenomenology of impulsive aggression and intermittent explosive disorder. In E. F. Coccaro & M. S. McCloskey (Eds.), *Intermittent explosive disorder* (pp. 37–65). Academic Press. https://doi.org/10.1016/B978-0-12-813858-8.00003-6

Coelho, C. M., Goncalves, D. C., Purkis, H., Pocinho, M., Pachana, N. A., & Byrne, G. J. (2010). Specific phobias in older adults: Characteristics and differential diagnosis. *International Psychogeriatrics, 22*, 702–711.

Coffino, J. A., Grilo, C. M., & Udo, T. (2020). Childhood food neglect and adverse experiences associated with *DSM-5* eating disorders in US national sample. *Journal of Psychiatric Research, 127*, 75–79. https://doi.org/10.1016/j.jpsychires.2020.05.011

Cohen, A. S., Auster, T. L., MacAulay, R. K., & McGovern, J. E. (2014). Illusory superiority and schizotypal personality: Explaining the discrepancy between subjective/objective psychopathology. *Personality Disorders: Theory, Research, and Treatment, 5*, 413–418. https://doi.org/10.1037/per0000080

Cohen, B. M., Öngür, D., Babb, S. M., & Harris, P. Q. (2022). Diagnostic terms psychiatrists prefer to use for common psychotic and personality disorders. *Journal of Psychiatric Research, 155*, 226–231. https://doi.org/10.1016/j.jpsychires.2022.08.026

Cole, C. S. (2011). Sleep and primary care of adults and older adults. In N. S. Redeker & G. McEnany (Eds.), *Sleep disorders and sleep promotion in nursing practice* (pp. 291–308). Springer Publishing Co.

Coleman, E., Bockting, W., Botzer, M., Cohen-Kettenis, P., DeCuypere, G., Feldman, J., . . . Monstrey, S. (2012). Standards of care for the health of transsexual, transgender, and gender-nonconforming people, version 7. *International Journal of Transgenderism, 13* (4), 165–232.

Coleman, J. R. I., Peyrot, W. J., Purves, K. L., Davis, K. A. S., Rayner, C., Choi, S. W., . . . Breen, G. (2020). Genome-wide gene-environment analyses of major depressive disorder and reported lifetime traumatic experiences in UK Biobank. *Molecular Psychiatry, 25* (7), 1430–1446. https://doi.org/10.1038/s41380-019-0546-6

Colle, L., Gabbatore, I., Riberi, E., Borroz, E., Bosco, F. M., & Keller, R. (2019). Mindreading abilities and borderline personality disorder: A comprehensive assessment using the Theory of Mind Assessment Scale. *Psychiatry Research, 272,* 609–617. https://doi.org/10.1016/j.psychres.2018.12.102

Collins, L. (2017). *Unfiltered: No shame, no regrets, just me.* HarperCollins.

Committee on Legal Issues American Psychological Association. (2016). Strategies for private practitioners coping with subpoenas or compelled testimony for client/patient records or test data or test materials. *Professional Psychology: Research and Practice, 47* (1), 1–11. https://doi.org/10.1037/pro0000063

Connolly, D., & Gilchrist, G. (2020). Prevalence and correlates of substance use among transgender adults: A systematic review. *Addictive Behaviors, 111.* https://doi.org/10.1016/j.addbeh.2020.106544

Connors, M. H., Teixeira-Pinto, A., Ames, D., Woodward, M., & Brodaty, H. (2023). Distinguishing apathy and depression in dementia: A longitudinal study. *Australian and New Zealand Journal of Psychiatry, 57* (6), 884–894. https://doi.org/10.1177/00048674221114597

Conroy, D. E., Ram, N., Pincus, A. L., Coffman, D. L., Lorek, A. E., Rebar, A. L., & Roche, M. J. (2015). Daily physical activity and alcohol use across the adult lifespan. *Health Psychology, 34,* 653–660. https://doi.org/10.1037/hea0000157

Conroy, D. E., Wu, J., Lee, A. M., Brunke-Reese, D., & Lagoa, C. M. (2023). Dose-response relations between the frequency of two types of momentary feedback prompts and daily physical activity. *Health Psychology, 42* (3), 151–160. https://doi.org/10.1037/hea0001271 10.1037/hea0001271.supp (Supplemental)

Cook, R., Pan, P., Silverman, R., & Soltys, S. M. (2010). Do-not-resuscitate orders in suicidal patients: Clinical, ethical, and legal dilemmas. *Psychosomatics: Journal of Consultation Liaison Psychiatry, 51,* 277–282.

Coon, J. C., & Rapp, J. T. (2018). Application of multiple baseline designs in behavior analytic research: Evidence for the influence of new guidelines. *Behavioral Interventions, 33* (2), 160–172. https://doi.org/10.1002/bin.1510

Correll, C. U., Agid, O., Crespo-Facorro, B., de Bartolomeis, A., Fagiolini, A., Seppälä, N., & Howes, O. D. (2022). A guideline and checklist for initiating and managing clozapine treatment in patients with treatment-resistant schizophrenia. *CNS Drugs, 36* (7), 659–679. https://doi.org/10.1007/s40263-022-00932-2

Corrigall, K. A., & Schellenberg, G. (2015). Predicting who takes music lessons: Parent and child characteristics. *Frontiers in Psychology, 6.* https://doi.org/10.3389/fpsyg.2015.00282

Cosh, S. M., Olson, J., & Tully, P. J. (2023). Exploration of orthorexia nervosa and diagnostic overlap with eating disorders, anorexia nervosa and obsessive-compulsive disorder. *International Journal of Eating Disorders.* https://doi.org/10.1002/eat.24051

Costa, D. S. J., Mercieca-Bebber, R., Tesson, S., Seidler, Z., & Lopez, A. L. (2019). Patient, client, consumer, survivor or other alternatives? A scoping review of preferred terms for labelling individuals who access healthcare across settings. *BMJ Open, 9* (3), e025166. https://doi.org/10.1136/bmjopen-2018-025166

Costa, P. T., Jr., & McCrae, R. R. (1992). *NEO-PI-R manual.* Psychological Assessment Resources.

Covey, T. J., Shucard, J. L., Wang, X., Gregory, M. A., & Shucard, D. W. (2023). Cognitive skill learning in multiple sclerosis: A meaningful component of the neuropsychological profile. *Brain and Cognition, 166,* 1–11. https://doi.org/10.1016/j.bandc.2023.105959

Craske, M. G., Kircanski, K., Epstein, A., Wittchen, H. U., Pine, D. S., Lewis-Fernandez, R., . . . Posttraumatic and Dissociative Disorder Work Group (2010). Panic disorder: A review of *DSM-IV* panic disorder and proposals for *DSM-V. Depression and Anxiety, 27,* 93–112.

Crump, F. M., Arndt, L., Grivel, M., Horga, G., Corcoran, C. M., Brucato, G., & Girgis, R. R. (2017). Attenuated first-rank symptoms and conversion to psychosis in a clinical high-risk cohort. *Early Intervention in Psychiatry.* https://doi.org/10.1111/eip.12529

Currie, C. J., Katz, B. A., & Yovel, I. (2017). Explicit and implicit shame aversion predict symptoms of avoidant and borderline personality disorders. *Journal of Research in Personality, 71,* 13–16. https://doi.org/10.1016/j.jrp.2017.08.006

Cyranowski, J. M., Andersen, B. L., Glowacka, M., Vannier, S. A., Rosen, N. O., O'Sullivan, L. F., . . . Zimmer-Gembeck, M. J. (2020). Self-concept and self-esteem. In R. R. Milhausen, J. K. Sakaluk, T. D. Fisher, C. M. Davis, & W. L. Yarber (Eds.), *Handbook of sexuality-related measures* (4th ed., pp. 532–565). New York, NY: Routledge/Taylor & Francis Group.

D

D'Agostino, A., Ferrara, P., Terzoni, S., Ostinelli, E. G., Carrara, C., Prunas, C., . . . Destrebecq, A. (2020). Efficacy of Triple Chronotherapy in unipolar and bipolar depression: A systematic review of the available evidence. *Journal of Affective Disorders, 276,* 297–304. https://doi.org/10.1016/j.jad.2020.07.026

D'Agostino, A., Pepi, R., & Starcevic, V. (2022). Borderline personality disorder and ageing: Myths and realities. *Current Opinion in Psychiatry, 35* (1), 68–72. https://doi.org/10.1097/YCO.0000000000000764

Dahl, T. A., DiCiro, M., Ziegler, E., & Sterling, S. (2023). Field reliability of forensic mental health evaluations of offenders for post-prison civil commitment. *Journal of Forensic Psychology Research and Practice.* https://doi.org/10.1080/24732850.2023.2249451

Dall' Aglio, L., Rijlaarsdam, J., Mulder, R. H., Neumann, A., Felix, J. F., Kok, R., . . . Cecil, C. A. M. (2020). Epigenome-wide associations between observed maternal sensitivity and offspring DNA methylation: A population-based prospective study in children. *Psychological Medicine.* https://doi.org/10.1017/S0033291720004353

Daubney, M., & Bateman, A. (2015). Mentalization-based therapy (MBT): An overview. *Australasian Psychiatry, 23,* 132–135. https://doi.org/10.1177/1039856214566830

Davis, E. B., McElroy-Heltzel, S. E., Lemke, A. W., Cowden, R. G., VanderWeele, T. J., Worthington, E. L., Jr., . . . Aten, J. D. (2021). Psychological and spiritual outcomes during the COVID-19 pandemic: A prospective longitudinal study of adults with chronic disease. *Health Psychology, 40* (6), 347–356. https://doi.org/10.1037/hea0001079

Davis, H. L. (Writer). (2017). *Demi Lovato: Simply complicated.* In P. Productions (Producer).

Davis, L. W., Luedtke, B. L., Monson, C., Siegel, A., Daggy, J. K., Yang, Z., . . . Ertl, M. (2021). Testing adaptations of cognitive-behavioral conjoint therapy for PTSD: A randomized controlled pilot study with veterans. *Couple and Family Psychology: Research and Practice, 10* (2), 71–86. https://doi.org/10.1037/cfp0000148 10.1037/cfp0000148

Davis, T. E., III, & Ollendick, T. H. (2011). Specific phobias. In D. McKay & E. A. Storch (Eds.), *Handbook of child and adolescent anxiety disorders* (pp. 231–244). New York: Springer Science + Business Media.

Dawson, S. J., Bannerman, B. A., & Lalumière, M. L. (2016). Paraphilic interests: An examination of sex differences in a nonclinical sample. *Sexual Abuse: Journal of Research and Treatment, 28* (1), 20– https://doi.org/10.1177/1079063214525645

Day, N. J. S., Townsend, M. L., & Grenyer, B. F. S. (2022). Living with pathological narcissism: Core conflictual relational themes within intimate relationships. *BMC Psychiatry, 22.* https://doi.org/10.1186/s12888-021-03660-x

de Andrade Teles, R. B., Diniz, T. C., Costa Pinto, T. C., de Oliveira Júnior, R. G., Gama E Silva, M., de Lavor, É. M., . . . da Silva Almeida, J. R. G. (2018). Flavonoids as therapeutic agents in Alzheimer's and Parkinson's Diseases: A systematic review of preclinical evidences. *Oxidative Medicine and Cellular Longevity, 2018,* 7043213–7043213. https://doi.org/10.1155/2018/7043213

de Jong, P. J., & Merckelbach, H. (2000). Phobia-relevant illusory correlations: The role of phobic responsivity. Journal of Abnormal Psychology, 109, 597–601.

de Jong, P. J., & Peters, M. L. (2007). Blood-injection-injury fears: Harm- vs.

disgust-relevant selective outcome associations. *Journal of Behavior Therapy and Experimental Psychiatry, 38,* 263–274.

De Leon, A. N., Woerner, J., Dvorak, R. D., Cox, J., Magri, T. D., Hayden, E. R., Ahuja, M., & Haeny, A. M. (2023). An examination of discrimination on stress, depression, and oppression-based trauma during the COVID-19 pandemic and the racial awakening of *Chronic Stress, 7.* https://doi.org/10.1177/24705470231152953

de Lijster, J. M., Dierckx, B., Utens, E. J., Verhulst, F. C., Zieldorff, C., Dieleman, G. C., & Legerstee, J. S. (2017). The age of onset of anxiety disorders: A meta-analysis. *The Canadian Journal of Psychiatry / La Revue Canadienne De Psychiatrie, 62* (4), 237–246. https://doi.org/10.1177/070674371 6640757org/10.1177/0706743716640757

de Vries, A. L. C., Beek, T. F., Dhondt, K., de Vet, H. C. W., Cohen-Kettenis, P. T., Steensma, T. D., & Kreukels, B. P. C. (2021). Reliability and clinical utility of gender identity-related diagnoses: Comparisons between the *ICD-11, ICD-10, DSM-IV,* and *DSM-5. LGBT Health.* https://doi.org/10.1089/lgbt.2020.0272

Dechsling, A., Orm, S., Kalandadze, T., Sütterlin, S., Øien, R. A., Shic, F., & Nordahl-Hansen, A. (2022). Virtual and augmented reality in social skills interventions for individuals with autism spectrum disorder: A scoping review. *Journal of Autism and Developmental Disorders, 52* (11), 4692–4707. https://doi .org/10.1007/s10803-021-05338-5

degli Espinosa, F., Metko, A., Raimondi, M., Impenna, M., & Scognamiglio, E. (2020). A model of support for families of children with autism living in the COVID-19 lockdown: Lessons from Italy. *Behavior Analysis in Practice, 13* (3), 550–558. https://doi.org/10.1007/s40617-020-00438-7

Dela Cruz, G. A., Johnstone, S., Kim, H. S., & Castle, D. J. (2023). Review of third-wave therapies for substance use disorders in people of color and collectivist cultures: Current evidence and future directions. Psychology of Addictive Behaviors, 37(5), 681–694. https://doi.org/10.1037/adb0000883

delCacho-Tena, A., Merced, K., Perrin, P. B., Arango-Lasprilla, J. C., Olabarrieta-Landa, L., & Rivera, D. (2023). 15-item version of the Boston Naming Test: Normative data for the Latin American Spanish-speaking adult population. *Neuropsychology, 37* (5), 607–614. https://doi.org/10.1037/neu0000889

Delgadillo, J., Branson, A., Kellett, S., Myles-Hooton, P., Hardy, G. E., & Shafran, R. (2020). Therapist personality traits as predictors of psychological treatment outcomes. *Psychotherapy Research.* https://doi.org/10.1080/10503307.2020.1731927

Delpino, F. M., da Silva, C. N., Jerônimo, J. S., Mulling, E. S., da Cunha, L. L., Weymar, M. K., Alt, R., Caputo, E. L., & Feter, N. (2022). Prevalence of anxiety during the COVID-19 pandemic: A systematic review and meta-analysis of over 2 million people. *Journal of Affective Disorders, 318,* 272–282. https://doi.org/10.1016/j.jad.2022.09.003

Deng, Z.-D., Robins, P. L., Regenold, W., Rohde, P., Dannhauer, M., & Lisanby, S. H. (2023). How electroconvulsive therapy works in the treatment of depression: Is it the seizure, the electricity, or both? *Neuropsychopharmacology.* https://doi.org/10.1038/s41386-023-01677-2

Derogatis, L. R. (1994). *Manual for the symptom check list-90 revised (SCL-90-R).* Pearson Publishers.

DeTure, M. A., & Dickson, D. W. (2019). The neuropathological diagnosis of Alzheimer's disease. *Molecular Neurodegeneration, 14* (1), 32. https://doi.org/10.1186/s13024 -019-0333 5

Devi, G. (2023). A how-to guide for a precision medicine approach to the diagnosis and treatment of Alzheimer's disease. *Frontiers in Aging Neuroscience, 15.* https://doi.org/10.3389/fnagi.2023.1213968

Dhejne, C., Van Vlerken, R., Heylens, G., & Arcelus, J. (2016). Mental health and gender dysphoria: A review of the literature. *International Review of Psychiatry, 28* (1), 44–57. https://doi.org/10.3109/09540261.201 5.1115753

Diamond, D., Yeomans, F., & Keefe, J. R. (2021). Transference-focused psychotherapy for pathological narcissism and narcissistic personality disorder (TFP-N). *Psychodynamic Psychiatry, 49* (2), 244–272. https://doi.org/10.1521/pdps.2021.49.2.244

Díaz-Blancat, G., García-Prieto, J., Maestú, F., & Barceló, F. (2018). Fast neural dynamics of proactive cognitive control in a task-switching analogue of the Wisconsin Card Sorting Test. *Brain Topography, 31* (3), 407–418. https://doi.org/10.1007/s10548 -017-0607-6

Dickerson, F. B., Tenhula, W. N., & Green-Paden, L. D. (2005). The token economy for schizophrenia: Review of the literature and recommendations for future research. *Schizophrenia Research, 75,* 405–416.

Dimidjian, S., Gallop, R., Levy, J., Beck, A., & Segal, Z. V. (2023). Mediators of change in online mindfulness-based cognitive therapy: A secondary analysis of a randomized trial of mindful mood balance. *Journal of Consulting and Clinical Psychology, 91* (8), 496–502. https://doi.org/10.1037/ccp0000825

Dimitrova, L. I., Dean, S. L., Schlumpf, Y. R., Vissia, E. M., Nijenhuis, E. R. S., Chatzi, V., . . . Reinders, A. A. T. S. (2023). A neurostructural biomarker of dissociative amnesia: A hippocampal study in dissociative identity disorder. *Psychological Medicine, 53* (3), 805–813. https://doi.org/10.1017/S0033291721002154

Disney, K. L., Weinstein, Y., & Oltmanns, T. F. (2012). Personality disorder symptoms are differentially related to divorce frequency. *Journal of Family Psychology, 26,* 959–965. https://doi.org/10.1037/a0030446

Disney, K. L., Weinstein, Y., & Oltmanns, T. F. (2012). Personality disorder symptoms are differentially related to divorce frequency. *Journal of Family Psychology, 26,* 959–965. https://doi.org/10.1037/a0030446

Dittrich, L. (2016). *Patient H.M.: A story of memory, madness, and family secrets.* Random House.

Doherty, A., Bracken, M., & Gormley, L. (2018). Teaching children with autism to initiate and respond to peer mands using picture exchange communication system (PECS). *Behavior Analysis in Practice, 11* (4), 279–288. https://doi.org/10.1007/s40617-018-00311-8

Donaldson, K. R., Jonas, K. G., Tian, Y., Larsen, E. M., Klein, D. N., Mohanty, A., Bromet, E. J., & Kotov, R. (2022). Dynamic interplay between life events and course of psychotic disorders: 10-year longitudinal study following first admission. *Psychological Medicine, 52* (11), 2116–2123. https://doi.org/10.1017/S0033291720003992

Donoghue, K., Elzerbi, C., Saunders, R., Whittington, C., Pilling, S., & Drummond, C. (2015). The efficacy of acamprosate and naltrexone in the treatment of alcohol dependence, Europe versus the rest of the world: A meta-analysis. *Addiction, 110* (6), 920–930. https://doi.org/10.1111/add.12875

Doroszkiewicz, C., Gold, D., Green, R., Tartaglia, M. C., Ma, J., & Tator, C. H. (2021). Anxiety, depression, and quality of life: A long-term follow-up study of patients with persisting concussion symptoms. *Journal of Neurotrauma, 38* (4), 493–505. https://doi.org/10.1089/neu.2020.7313

Doyle, J. N., Smith, M. M., Watt, M. C., Cohen, J. N., & Couture, M.-E. (2023). Higher baseline emotion dysregulation predicts treatment dropout in outpatients with borderline personality disorder. *Personality Disorders: Theory, Research, and Treatment, 14* (5), 579–583. https://doi.org/10.1037/per0000627 10.1037/per0000627

Dreher, D. E. (2013). Abnormal psychology in the Renaissance. In T. G. Plante (Ed.), *Abnormal psychology across the ages, Vol. 1: History and conceptualizations, Vol. 2: Disorders and treatments, Vol. 3: Trends and future directions* (pp. 33–50). Praeger/ABC-CLIO.

Driessen, E., & Hollon, S. D. (2010). Cognitive behavioral therapy for mood disorders: Efficacy, moderators and mediators. *Psychiatric Clinics of North America, 33,* 537–555.

Driessen, E., Van, H. L., Don, F. J., Peen, J., Kool, S., Westra, D., . . . Dekker, J. J. (2013). The efficacy of cognitive-behavioral therapy and psychodynamic therapy in the outpatient treatment of major depression: A randomized clinical trial. *American Journal of Psychiatry, 170* (9), 1041–1050. https://doi.org/10.1176/appi.ajp.2013.12070899

Drill, R., Malone, J., Flouton-Barnes, M., Cotton, L., Keyes, S., Wasserman, R., . . . Beinashowitz, J. (2019). Inclusive language regarding gender, sexual orientation, and relationship status: The ongoing process and outcome of revising psychiatric materials. *The Journal of Mental Health Training, Education and Practice, 14* (6), 385–398. https://doi.org/10.1108/JMHTEP-02-2018-0009

Druker, K. C., Mazzucchelli, T. G., & Beilby, J. M. (2019). An evaluation of an integrated fluency and resilience program for early developmental stuttering disorders. *Journal of Communication Disorders, 78,* 69–83. https://doi.org/10.1016/j.jcomdis.2019.02.002

Dubey, M. J., Ghosh, R., Chatterjee, S., Biswas, P., Chatterjee, S., & Dubey, S. (2020). COVID-19 and addiction. *Diabetes and Metabolic Syndrome, 14* (5), 817–823. https://doi.org/10.1016/j.dsx.2020.06.008

Ducharme, E. L. (2017). Best practices in working with complex trauma and dissociative identity disorder. *Practice Innovations, 2* (3), 150–161. https://doi.org/10.1037/pri0000050

Dudley, M. D., Barker-Collo, S. L., Wilson, D. L., & Garrett, N. K. (2019). Factors associated with Māori performance on the WAIS-IV. *Archives of Clinical Neuropsychology, 34* (7), 1203–1216. https://doi.org/10.1093/arclin/acy110

Dudley, M., Goldney, R., & Hadzi-Pavlovic, D. (2010). Are adolescents dying by suicide taking SSRI antidepressants? A review of observational studies. *Australasian Psychiatry, 18,* 242–245.

Duke, D. C., Bodzin, D. K., Tavares, P., Geffken, G. R., & Storch, E. A. (2009). The phenomenology of hairpulling in a community sample. *Journal of Anxiety Disorders, 23,* 1118–1125.

Dumarkaite, A., Truskauskaite-Kuneviciene, I., Andersson, G., Mingaudaite, J., & Kazlauskas, E. (2021). Effects of mindfulness-based internet intervention on ICD-11 posttraumatic stress disorder and complex posttraumatic stress disorder symptoms: A pilot randomized controlled trial. *Mindfulness, 12* (11), 2754–2766. https://doi.org/10.1007/s12671-021-01739-w

Dunbar, N. (2023). Dead dinosaurs and creative beginnings: A case study of a 3-year-old boy who started nursery shortly after the loss of his mother. *British Journal of Psychotherapy.* https://doi.org/10.1111/bjp.12858

Durazzo, T. C., Meyerhoff, D. J., & Yoder, K. K. (2018). Cigarette smoking is associated with cortical thinning in anterior frontal regions, insula and regions showing atrophy in early Alzheimer's disease. *Drug and Alcohol Dependence, 192,* 277–284. https://doi.org/10.1016/j.drugalcdep.2018.08.009

Duritz, A. (2008). The lonely disease: Mens Health. Retrieved 05/20/2024 from https://www.menshealth.com/health/a19542157/mental-illness/

E

Earlywine, J. J., Bagley, S. M., Rodean, J., Zima, B. T., Chadi, N., Leslie, D. L., & Hadland, S. E. (2023). Medications for alcohol use disorder and retention in care in medicaid-enrolled youth, 2014–2019. *Journal of Adolescent Health.* https://doi.org/10.1016/j.jadohealth.2023.03.005

Eckes, T., Buhlmann, U., Holling, H.-D., & Möllmann, A. (2023). Comprehensive ABA-based interventions in the treatment of children with autism spectrum disorder—a meta-analysis. *BMC Psychiatry, 23* (1). https://doi.org/10.1186/s12888-022-04412-1

Eddy, K. T., Thomas, J. J., Hastings, E., Edkins, K., Lamont, E., Nevins, C. M., . . . Becker, A. E. (2015). Prevalence of *DSM-5* avoidant/restrictive food intake disorder in a pediatric gastroenterology healthcare network. *International Journal of Eating Disorders, 48* (5), 464–470. https://doi.org/10.1002/eat.22350

Edwards, L. M., Burkard, A. W., Adams, H. A., & Newcomb, S. A. (2017). A mixed-method study of psychologists' use of multicultural assessment. *Professional Psychology: Research and Practice, 48* (2), 131–138. https://doi.org/10.1037/pro0000095

Ehlers, A., Wild, J., Warnock-Parkes, E., Grey, N., Murray, H., Kerr, A., . . . Clark, D. M. (2023). Therapist-assisted online psychological therapies differing in trauma focus for post-traumatic stress disorder (STOP-PTSD): A UK-based, single-blind, randomised controlled trial. *The Lancet Psychiatry, 10* (8), 608–622. https://doi.org/10.1016/S2215-0366(23)00181-5

Eilenberg, T., Fink, P., Jensen, J. S., Rief, W., & Frostholm, L. (2016). Acceptance and commitment group therapy (ACT-G) for health anxiety: A randomized controlled trial. *Psychological Medicine, 46* (1), 103–115. https://doi.org/10.1017/S0033291715001579

Eisendrath, S. J., Gillung, E., Delucchi, K., Mathalon, D. H., Yang, T. T., Satre, D. D., . . . Wolkowitz, O. M. (2015). A preliminary study: Efficacy of mindfulness-based cognitive therapy versus sertraline as first-line treatments for major depressive disorder. *Mindfulness, 6,* 475–482. https://doi.org/10.1007/s12671-014-0280-8

Eisma, M. C., Janshen, A., Huber, L. F. T., & Schroevers, M. J. (2023). Cognitive reappraisal, emotional expression and mindfulness in adaptation to bereavement: A longitudinal study. *Anxiety, Stress & Coping: An International Journal.* https://doi.org/10.1080/10615806.2023.2165647

Eley, T. C., McAdams, T. A., Rijsdijk, F. V., Lichtenstein, P., Narusyte, J., Reiss, D., . . . Neiderhiser, J. M. (2015). The intergenerational transmission of anxiety: A children-of-twins study. *The American Journal of Psychiatry, 172,* 630–637. https://doi.org/10.1176/appi.ajp.2015.14070818

Elharake, J. A., Akbar, F., Malik, A. A., Gilliam, W., & Omer, S. B. (2023). Mental health impact of COVID-19 among children and college students: A systematic review. *Child Psychiatry and Human Development, 54* (3), 913–925. https://doi.org/10.1007/s10578-021-01297-1

Ellen, B. P., III, Alexander, K. C., Mackey, J. D., McAllister, C. P., & Carson, J. E. (2021). Portrait of a workplace deviant: A clearer picture of the Big Five and Dark Triad as predictors of workplace deviance. *Journal of Applied Psychology.* https://doi.org/10.1037/apl0000880

Elliott, M. L., Knodt, A. R., Ireland, D., Morris, M. L., Poulton, R., Ramrakha, S., . . . Hariri, A. R. (2020). What is the test-retest reliability of common task-functional MRI measures? New empirical evidence and a meta-analysis. *Psychological Science, 31* (7), 792–806. https://doi.org/10.1177/0956797620916786

Ellis, A. (2005). *The myth of self-esteem.* Prometheus.

Ellison, W. D., Acuff, M. C., Kealy, D., Joyce, A. S., & Ogrodniczuk, J. S. (2020). Narcissism and quality of life: The mediating role of relationship patterns. *Journal of Nervous and Mental Disease, 208* (8), 613–618. https://doi.org/10.1097/NMD.0000000000001170

ElSayed, M., & Gupta, R. (2020). Does degarelix hold potential for the treatment of pedophilic disorder? *JAMA Psychiatry, 77* (10), 1084–1085. https://doi.org/10.1001/jamapsychiatry.2020.2594

Enserink, M. (1998). First Alzheimer's disease confirmed. *Science, 279,* 2037.

Epstein, E. E., McCrady, B. S., Hallgren, K. A., Cook, S., Jensen, N. K., & Hildebrandt, T. (2018). A randomized trial of female-specific cognitive behavior therapy for alcohol dependent women. *Psychology of Addictive Behaviors, 32* (1), 1–15. https://doi.org/10.1037/adb0000330

Eschweiler, G. W., Czornik, M., Herrmann, M. L., Knauer, Y. P., Forkavets, O., von Arnim, C. A. F., . . . Rapp, M. A. (2021). Presurgical screening improves risk prediction for delirium in elective surgery of older patients: The PAWEL RISK study. *Frontiers in Aging Neuroscience, 13.* https://doi.org/10.3389/fnagi.2021.679933

Esposito, R., Cieri, F., di Giannantonio, M., & Tartaro, A. (2018). The role of body image and self-perception in anorexia nervosa: The neuroimaging perspective. *Journal of Neuropsychology, 12* (1), 41–52. https://doi.org/10.1111/jnp.12106

Estévez, A., Jauregui, P., Lopez-Gonzalez, H., Macia, L., López, N., Zamora, L., . . . Jiménez-Murcia, S. (2021). Exploring the predictive value of gambling motives, cognitive distortions, and materialism on problem gambling severity in adolescents and young adults. *Journal of Gambling Studies, 37* (2), 643–661. https://doi.org/10.1007/s10899-020-09972-z

Eysenck, H. J. (2021). "Prediction of cancer and coronary heart disease mortality by means of a personality inventory: Results of a 15-year follow-up study": Retraction. *Psychological Reports, 124* (2), 920–921. http://silk.library.umass.edu/login?url=https://search.ebscohost.com/login.aspx?direct=true&db=psyh&AN=2021-19859-031&site=ehost-live&scope=site

F

Falkenburg, J., & Tracy, D. K. (2014). Sex and schizophrenia: A review of gender differences. *Psychosis: Psychological, Social and Integrative Approaches, 6,* 61–69. https://doi.org/10.1080/17522439.2012.733405

Fancy, F., Rodrigues, N. B., Di Vincenzo, J. D., Chau, E. H., Sethi, R., Husain, M. I., . . . Rosenblat, J. D. (2023). Real-world effectiveness of repeated ketamine infusions for treatment-resistant bipolar depression. *Bipolar Disorders, 25* (2), 99–109. https://doi.org/10.1111/bdi.13284

Fang, A., & Hofmann, S. G. (2010). Relationship between social anxiety disorder and body dysmorphic disorder. *Clinical Psychology Review, 30,* 1040–1048.

Fang, A., & Wilhelm, S. (2015). Clinical features, cognitive biases, and treatment of body dysmorphic disorder. *Annual Review of Clinical Psychology, 11,* 187–212. https://doi.org/10.1146/annurev-clinpsy-032814-112849

Farabaugh, A., Nyer, M. B., Holt, D. J., Fisher, L. B., Cheung, J. C., Anton, J., . . . Mischoulon, D. (2019). CBT delivered in a specialized depression clinic for college students with depressive symptoms. *Journal of Rational-Emotive & Cognitive-Behavior Therapy, 37* (1), 52–61. https:10.1007/s10942-018-0300-z

Farrell, H. M. (2010). Dissociative identity disorder: No excuse for criminal activity. *Current Psychiatry, 10,* 33–40.

Farrell, H. M. (2011). Dissociative identity disorder: Medicolegal challenges. *Journal of the American Academy of Psychiatry and the Law, 39,* 402–406.

Farros, J. N., Legaspi, D., & Wallace, M. (2023). Functional analyses conducted via telehealth with caregivers as primary therapists. *Behavioral Interventions.* https://doi.org/10.1002/bin.1965

Faustino, B., Oliveira, J., & Lopes, P. (2022). Normative scores of the Wisconsin Card Sorting Test in a sample of the adult Portuguese population. *Applied Neuropsychology: Adult, 29* (4), 767–774. https://doi.org/10.1080/23279095.2020.1810040

Fazel, S., Yoon, I. A., & Hayes, A. J. (2017). Substance use disorders in prisoners: An updated systematic review and meta-regression analysis in recently incarcerated men and women. *Addiction, 112* (10), 1725–1739. https://doi.org/10.1111/add.13877

Feinstein, B. A., Christophe, N. K., Chang, C. J., Silvia, P. J., Starr, L. R., Stein, G. L., & Vrshek-Schallhorn, S. (2022). Measurement invariance of the Interpersonal Needs Questionnaire (INQ-15) across sexual orientation, gender identity, and race/ethnicity in a sample of sexual minority young adults. *Psychological Assessment, 34* (10), 978–984. https://doi.org/10.1037/pas0001159 10.1037

Fernández-Modamio, M., Gil-Sanz, D., Arrieta-Rodríguez, M., Santacoloma-Cabero, I., Bengochea-Seco, R., González-Fraile, E., & Muñiz, J. (2020). A randomized study on the efficacy of the Social Cognition Training Program-brief version in a sample of patients with schizophrenia. *Psychiatric Rehabilitation Journal.* https://doi.org/10.1037/prj0000410

Fernández, R. S., Crivelli, L., Guimet, N. M., Allegri, R. F., & Pedreira, M. E. (2020). Psychological distress associated with COVID-19 quarantine: Latent profile analysis, outcome prediction and mediation analysis. *Journal of Affective Disorders, 277,* 75–84. https://doi.org/10.1016/j.jad.2020.07.133

Ferrari, C., Lombardi, G., Polito, C., Lucidi, G., Bagnoli, S., Piaceri, I., . . . Sorbi, S. (2018). Alzheimer's disease progression: Factors influencing cognitive decline. *Journal of Alzheimer's Disease, 61* (2), 785–791. https://doi.org/10.3233/JAD-170665

Filipčíková, M., & McDonald, S. (2023). Inhibitory control impairment in social disinhibition following severe traumatic brain injury: An experimental study using social and nonsocial go/no-go task. *Neuropsychology.* https://doi.org/10.1037/neu0000923

Fiquer, J. T., Moreno, R. A., Brunoni, A. R., Barros, V. B., Fernandes, F., & Gorenstein, C. (2018). What is the nonverbal communication of depression? Assessing expressive differences between depressive patients and healthy volunteers during clinical interviews. *Journal of Affective Disorders, 238,* 636–644. https://doi.org/10.1016/j.jad.2018.05.071

First, M. B., Williams, J. B. W., Karg, R. S., & Spitzer, R. L. (2016). *Structured Clinical Interview for DSM-5 Disorders (SCID-5-CV): Clinician Version.* American Psychiatric Association.

Fišar, Z. (2023). Biological hypotheses, risk factors, and biomarkers of schizophrenia. *Progress in Neuro-Psychopharmacology & Biological Psychiatry, 120,* 1–18. https://doi.org/10.1016/j.pnpbp.2022.110626

Fisher, C. B., & Vacanti-Shova, K. (2012). The responsible conduct of psychological research: An overview of ethical principles, APA Ethics Code standards, and federal regulations. In S. J. Knapp, M. C. Gottlieb, M. M. Handelsman, & L. D. VandeCreek (Eds.), *APA handbook of ethics in psychology* (Vol. 2, pp. 335–369). American Psychological Association.

Fisher, C., & Ravetch, J. (2008). *Wishful drinking.* Simon and Schuster.

Fiske, A., Henningsen, P., & Buyx, A. (2019). Your robot therapist will see you now: Ethical implications of embodied artificial intelligence in psychiatry, psychology, and psychotherapy. *Journal of Medical Internet Research, 21* (5), e13216. https://doi.org/10.2196/13216

Fiske, K. E., Isenhower, R. W., Bamond, M. J., & Lauderdale-Littin, S. (2020). An analysis of the value of token reinforcement using a multiple-schedule assessment. *Journal of Applied Behavior Analysis, 53* (1), 563–571. https://doi.org/10.1002/jaba.613

Fiske, K. E., Isenhower, R. W., Bamond, M. J., Delmolino, L., Sloman, K. N., & LaRue, R. H. (2015). Assessing the value of token reinforcement for individuals with autism. *Journal of Applied Behavior Analysis, 48,* 448–453. https://doi.org/10.1002/jaba.207

Flannigan, K., Coons-Harding, K. D., Anderson, T., Wolfson, L., Campbell, A., Mela, M., & Pei, J. (2020). A systematic review of interventions to improve mental health and substance use outcomes for individuals with prenatal alcohol exposure and Fetal Alcohol Spectrum Disorder [Report]. *Alcoholism: Clinical and Experimental Research, 44* (12),2401. https://doi.org/10.1111/acer.14490

Florence, C., Luo, F., & Rice, K. (2021). The economic burden of opioid use disorder and fatal opioid overdose in the United States, *Drug and Alcohol Dependence, 218,* 108350. https://doi.org/10.1016/j.drugalcdep.2020.108350

Folstein, M. F., Folstein, S. E., & McHugh, P. R. (1975). Mini-Mental State: A practical method for grading the cognitive state of patients for the clinician. *Journal of Psychiatric Research, 12,* 189–198.

Food and Drug Administration. (2023). MedWatch: The FDA Safety Information and Adverse Event Reporting Program. https://www.fda.gov/safety/medwatch-fda-safety-information-and-adverse-event-reporting-program

Forcen, F. E. (2017). The Edinburgh medical garden, Benjamin Rush, and the seeds of pharmacology. *The American Journal of Psychiatry, 174* (3), 215–215. https://doi.org/10.1176/appi.ajp.2016.16080877

Ford-Paz, R. E., Gouze, K. R., Kerns, C. E., Ballard, R., Parkhurst, J. T., Jha, P., & Lavigne, J. (2020). Evidence-based assessment in clinical settings: Reducing assessment burden for a structured measure of child and adolescent anxiety. *Psychological Services, 17* (3), 343–354. https://doi.org/10.1037/ser0000367

Forejtová, Z., Serranová, T., Sieger, T., Slovák, M., Nováková, L., Věchetová, G., Růžička, E., & Edwards, M. J. (2023). The complex syndrome of functional neurological disorder. *Psychological Medicine, 53* (7), 3157–3167. https://doi.org/10.1017/S0033291721005225

Forrest, L. N., Grilo, C. M., & Udo, T. (2020). Suicide attempts among people with eating disorders and adverse childhood experiences: Results from a nationally representative sample of adults. *International Journal of Eating Disorders*. https://doi.org/10.1002/eat.23457

Forsyth, K., Maciver, D., Howden, S., Owen, C., & Shepherd, C. (2008). Developmental coordination disorder: A synthesis of evidence to underpin an allied health professions' framework. *International Journal of Disability, Development and Education, 55,* 153–172.

Fortuna, L. R., Falgas-Bague, I., Ramos, Z., Porche, M. V., & Alegría, M. (2020). Development of a cognitive behavioral therapy with integrated mindfulness for Latinx immigrants with co-occurring disorders: Analysis of intermediary outcomes. *Psychological Trauma: Theory, Research, Practice, and Policy, 12* (8), 825–835. https://doi.org/10.1037/tra0000949 (Complementary Medicine and Integrative Approaches to Trauma Therapy and Recovery)

Foubert-Samier, A., Helmer, C., Le Goff, M., Guillet, F., Proust-Lima, C., Jacqmin-Gadda, H., . . . Tison, F. (2020). Cognitive and functional changes in prediagnostic phase of Parkinson disease: A population-based study. *Parkinsonism & Related Disorders, 79,* 40–46. https://doi.org/10.1016/j.parkreldis.2020.08.022

Fox, M. J. (2002). *Lucky man: A memoir.* Hyperion.

Fox, M. J. (2009). *Always looking up: The adventures of an incurable optimist.* Hyperion.

Fox, M. J. (2020). *No time like the future: An optimist considers mortality.* Flatiron Books.

Frank, E. (2007). Interpersonal and social rhythm therapy: A means of improving depression and preventing relapse in bipolar disorder. *Journal of Clinical Psychology, 63,* 463–473.

Frankl, V. (1963). *Man's search for meaning.* Simon & Schuster.

Franko, D. L., Keshaviah, A., Eddy, K. T., Krishna, M., Davis, M. C., Keel, P. K., & Herzog, D. B. (2013). A longitudinal investigation of mortality in anorexia nervosa and bulimia nervosa. *The American Journal of Psychiatry, 170,* 917–925. https://doi.org/10.1176/appi.ajp.2013.12070868

Frattaroli, J. (2006). Experimental disclosure and its moderators: A meta-analysis. *Psychological Bulletin, 132,* 823–865.

Freeman, A., & Fox, S. (2013). Cognitive behavioral perspectives on the theory and treatment of the narcissistic character. In J. S. Ogrodniczuk (Ed.), *Understanding and treating pathological narcissism* (pp. 301–320). Washington, DC: American Psychological Association. https://doi.org/10.1037/14041-018

Freud, S. (1911). *Formulations of the two principles of mental functioning* (J. Strachey, Trans.). In J. Strachey (Ed.), *The standard edition of the complete psychological works of Sigmund Freud* (Vol. 12). Hogarth.

Freud, S. (1923). *The ego and the id* (J. Strachey, Trans.). In J. Strachey (Ed.), *The standard edition of the complete psychological works of Sigmund Freud* (Vol. 19). Hogarth.

Friedrich, A., & Schlarb, A. A. (2018). Let's talk about sleep: A systematic review of psychological interventions to improve sleep in college students. *Journal of Sleep Research, 27* (1), 4–22. https://doi.org/10.1111/jsr.12568

Fuller, E. K., Gatner, D. T., & Douglas, K. S. (2023). Concurrent, convergent, and discriminant validity of the DSM-5 section III psychopathy specifier. *Assessment, 30* (6), 1790–1810. https://doi.org/10.1177/10731911221124344

Furness, D. (July, 2015). Counting Crows' Adam Duritz Discusses Mental Health and Metaphors. Miami New Times. https://www.miaminewtimes.com/music/counting-crows-adam-duritz-discusses-mental-health-and-metaphors-7781223

Furnham, A. (2014). A bright side, facet analysis of histrionic personality disorder: The relationship between the HDS colourful factor and the NEO-PI-R facets in a large adult sample. *The Journal of Social Psychology, 154,* 527–536. https://doi.org/10.1080/00224545.2014.953026

G

Gál, É., Ştefan, S., & Cristea, I. A. (2021). The efficacy of mindfulness meditation apps in enhancing users' well-being and mental health related outcomes: A meta-analysis of randomized controlled trials. *Journal of Affective Disorders, 279,* 131–142. https://doi.org/10.1016/j.jad.2020.09.134

Gallagher, B. J., III. (2018). Social class and schizophrenia: A review of early and recent findings in the United States. *Current Psychiatry Reviews, 14* (3), 187–194. https://doi.org/10.2174/157340051466618101511544 2

Gallinat, C., Moessner, M., Haenssle, H. A., Winkler, J. K., Backenstrass, M., & Bauer, S. (2019). Help-seeking attitudes and experiences in individuals affected by skin picking. *Journal of Obsessive-Compulsive and Related Disorders, 23.* https://doi.org/10.1016/j.jocrd.2019.100483

Gao, P., Gao, J., Wang, Y., Peng, D., Zhang, Y., Li, H., . . . Zhang, X. (2021). Temperament-character traits and attitudes toward premature ejaculation in 4 types of premature ejaculation. *Journal of Sexual Medicine, 18* (1), 72–82. https://doi.org/10.1016/j.jsxm.2020.11.001

Garcia, R. (2017). Neurobiology of fear and specific phobias. *Learning and Memory, 24* (9), 462–471. https://doi.org/10.1101/lm.044115.116

Gardner, B. O., Murrie, D. C., & Torres, A. N. (2022). To proceed or not proceed: Conducting sanity evaluations of incompetent defendants. *Psychology, Public Policy, and Law, 28* (1), 67–77. https://doi.org/10.1037/law0000304

Garnett, C., Oldham, M., Angus, C., Beard, E., Burton, R., Field, M., . . . Brown, J. (2021). Evaluating the effectiveness of the smartphone app, Drink Less, compared with the NHS alcohol advice webpage, for the reduction of alcohol consumption among hazardous and harmful adult drinkers in the UK at 6-month follow-up: Protocol for a randomised controlled trial. *Addiction, 116* (2), 412–425. https://doi.org/10.1111/add.15287

Gatov, E., Rosella, L., Chiu, M., & Kurdyak, P. A. (2017). Trends in standardized mortality among individuals with schizophrenia, 1993–2012: A population-based, repeated cross-sectional study. *Canadian Medical Association Journal, 189* (37), E1177–E1187. https://doi.org/10.1503/cmaj.161351

Gatzunis, K. S., Weiss, M. J., Ala'i-Rosales, S., Fahmie, T. A., & Syed, N. Y. (2023). Using behavioral skills training to teach functional assessment interviewing, cultural responsiveness, and empathic and compassionate care to students of applied behavior analysis. *Behavior Analysis in Practice*. https://doi.org/10.1007/s40617-023-00794-0

GBD 2016 Alcohol Collaborators. (2018). Alcohol use and burden for 195 countries and territories, 1990–2016: A systematic analysis for the Global Burden of Disease Study 2016. *Lancet, 392* (10152), 1015–1035. https://doi.org/10.1016/s0140-6736(18)31310-2

GBD 2016 Disease and Injury Incidence and Prevalence Collaborators. (2017). Global, regional, and national incidence, prevalence, and years lived with disability for 328 diseases and injuries for 195 countries, 1990-2016: A systematic analysis for the Global Burden of Disease Study 2016. *Lancet, 390* (10100), 1211–1259. https://doi.org/10.1016/s0140-6736(17)32154-2

Gbiri, C. A. O., & Akumabor, J. C. (2023). Effectiveness of physiotherapy interventions in the management male sexual dysfunction: A systematic review. *International Journal of Sexual Health, 35* (1), 52–66. https://doi.org/10.1080/19317611.2022.2155288

Gebauer, J. E., Nehrlich, A. D., Stahlberg, D., Sedikides, C., Hackenschmidt, A., Schick, D., . . . Mander, J. (2018). Mind-body practices and the self: Yoga and meditation do not quiet the ego but instead boost self-enhancement. *Psychological Science, 29* (8), 1299–1308. https://doi.org/10.1177/0956797618764621

George, W. H. (2019). Alcohol and sexual health behavior: "What we know and how we know it." *Journal of Sex Research, 56* (4–5), 409–424. https://doi.org/10.1080/00224499.2019.1588213

Gesualdo, C., & Pinquart, M. (2023). Influences on change in expected and actual health behaviors among first-year university students. *Health Psychology and Behavioral Medicine, 11* (1). https://doi.org/10.1080/21642850.2023.2174697

Ghamkhar Fard, Z., Pourshahbaz, A., Anderson, J. L., Boland, J. K., Shakiba, S., & Mirabzadeh, A. (2021). The continuity between DSM-5 criterion-based and trait-based models for personality disorders in an iranian community sample. *Current Psychology: A Journal for Diverse Perspectives on Diverse Psychological Issues*. https://doi.org/10.1007/s12144-021-01751-2

Giami, A. (2015). Between *DSM* and ICD: Paraphilias and the transformation of sexual norms. *Archives of Sexual Behavior, 44,* 1127–1138. https://doi.org/10.1007/s10508-015-0549-6

Gibbons, A., & Warne, R. T. (2019). First publication of subtests in the Stanford-Binet 5, WAIS-IV, WISC-V, and WPPSI-IV. *Intelligence, 75,* 9–18. https://doi.org/10.1016/j.intell.2019.02.005

Gigante, A. D., Barenboim, I. Y., Dias, R. da S., Toniolo, R. A., Mendonça, T., Miranda-Scippa, Â., ... Lafer, B. (2016). Psychiatric and clinical correlates of rapid cycling bipolar disorder: A cross-sectional study. *Revista Brasileira de Psiquiatria, 38* (4), 270–274. https://doi-org.silk.library.umass.edu/10.1590/1516-4446-2015-1789

Gilbert, K., Codd, R. T., III, Hoyniak, C., Tillman, R., Baudinet, J., Pires, P. P., . . . Lynch, T. R. (2023). Processes of change in a randomized clinical trial of radically open dialectical behavior therapy (RO DBT) for adults with treatment-refractory depression. *Journal of Consulting and Clinical Psychology, 91* (2), 71–81. https://doi.org/10.1037/ccp0000795

Gillespie, C., Murphy, M., Kells, M., & Flynn, D. (2022). Individuals who report having benefitted from dialectical behaviour therapy (DBT): A qualitative exploration of processes and experiences at long-term follow-up. *Borderline Personality Disorder and Emotion Dysregulation, 9*. https://doi.org/10.1186/s40479-022-00179-9

Gillett, G. (2011). The gold-plated leucotomy standard and deep brain stimulation. *Journal of Bioethical Inquiry, 8,* 35–44.

Girard, T. D., Exline, M. C., Carson, S. S., Hough, C. L., Rock, P., Gong, M. N., . . . Ely, E. W. (2018). Haloperidol and ziprasidone for treatment of delirium in critical illness. *New England Journal of Medicine, 379* (26), 2506–2516. https://doi.org/10.1056/NEJMoa1808217

Gisslen, M., Hagberg, L., Brew, B. J., Cinque, P., Price, R. W., & Rosengren, L. (2007). Elevated cerebrospinal fluid neurofilament light protein concentrations predict the development of AIDS dementia complex. *Journal of Infectious Diseases, 195,* 1774–1778.

Glazer, K. B., Sonneville, K. R., Micali, N., Swanson, S. A., Crosby, R., Horton, N. J., . . . Field, A. E. (2019). The course of eating disorders involving bingeing and purging among adolescent girls: Prevalence, stability, and transitions. *Journal of Adolescent Health, 64* (2), 165–171. https://doi.org/10.1016/j.jadohealth.2018.09.023

Gleason, M. M., Fox, N. A., Drury, S., Smyke, A., Egger, H. L., Nelson, C. A., III, ... Zeanah, C. H. (2011). Validity of evidence-derived criteria for reactive attachment disorder: Indiscriminately social/disinhibited and emotionally withdrawn/inhibited types. *Journal of the American Academy of Child & Adolescent Psychiatry,* 50(3), 216–231. https://doi.org/10.1016/j.jaac.2010.12.012

GMA Team. (2020). Demi Lovato gives 1st major public performance since 2018 overdose at the Grammy Awards. https://www.goodmorningamerica.com/culture/story/demi-lovato-perform-song-grammys-wrote-shortly-2018-68505121

Goetter, E. M., Frumkin, M. R., Palitz, S. A., Swee, M. B., Baker, A. W., Bui, E., & Simon, N. M. (2020). Barriers to mental health treatment among individuals with social anxiety disorder and generalized anxiety disorder. *Psychological Services, 17* (1), 5–12. https://doi.org/10.1037/ser0000254

Goldsmith, S. K., Pellmar, T. C., Kleinman, A. M., & Bunney, W. E. (Eds.). (2002). *Reducing suicide: A national imperative*. The National Academies Press.

Gomathi, M., Padmapriya, S., & Balachandar, V. (2020). Drug studies on Rett syndrome: From bench to bedside. *Journal of Autism and Developmental Disorders, 50* (8), 2740–2764. https://doi.org/10.1007/s10803-020-04381-y

Gonidakis, F., Kravvariti, V., & Varsou, E. (2015). Sexual function of women suffering from anorexia nervosa and bulimia nervosa. *Journal of Sex & Marital Therapy, 41,* 368–378. https://doi.org/10.1080/0092623X.2014.915904

Gonzalez Aguilar, M. J., & Alba Ferrara, L. (2020). CSIS: Proposal for a new combined screening interpretation score for patients with mild cognitive impairment. *Experimental Aging Research*. https://doi.org/10.1080/0361073X.2020.1861839

Goodman, W. K., Storch, E. A., & Sheth, S. A. (2021). Harmonizing the neurobiology and treatment of obsessive-compulsive disorder. *The American Journal of Psychiatry, 178* (1), 17–29. https://doi.org/10.1176/appi.ajp.2020.20111601

Goodwin, R. D., Dierker, L. C., Wu, M., Galea, S., Hoven, C. W., & Weinberger, A. H. (2022). Trends in U.S. depression prevalence from 2015 to 2020: The widening treatment gap. *American Journal of Preventive Medicine, 63* (5), 726–733. https://doi.org/10.1016/j.amepre.2022.05.014

Gordon-King, K., Schweitzer, R. D., & Dimaggio, G. (2019). Metacognitive interpersonal therapy for personality disorders: The case of a man with obsessive-compulsive personality disorder and avoidant personality disorder. *Journal of Contemporary Psychotherapy: On the Cutting Edge of Modern Developments in Psychotherapy, 49* (1), 39–47. https://doi.org/10.1007/s10879-018-9404-0

Gordovez, F. J. A., & McMahon, F. J. (2020). The genetics of bipolar disorder. *Molecular Psychiatry, 25* (3), 544–559. https:10.1038/s41380-019-0634-7

Gosdin, L. K., Deputy, N. P., Kim, S. Y., Dang, E. P., & Denny, C. H. (2022). Alcohol consumption and binge drinking during pregnancy among adults aged 18-49 years of age: United States 2018–2020. *Morbidity and Mortality Weekly Report (MMWR), 2022* (71), 10–13. https://doi.org/ http://dx.doi.org/10.15585/mmwr.mm7101a2external

Grady, M. D., Levenson, J. S., Mesias, G., Kavanagh, S., & Charles, J. (2019). "I can't talk about that": Stigma and fear as barriers to preventive services for minor-attracted persons. *Stigma and Health, 4* (4), 400–410. https://doi.org/10.1037/sah0000154

Graham Holmes, L., Zampella, C. J., Clements, C., McCleery, J. P., Maddox, B. B., Parish-Morris, J., . . . Miller, J. S. (2020). A lifespan approach to patient-reported outcomes and quality of life for people on the autism spectrum. *Autism Research, 13* (6), 970–987. https://doi.org/10.1002/aur.2275

Graham, C. A., Štulhofer, A., Lange, T., Hald, G. M., Carvalheira, A. A., Enzlin, P., & Træen, B. (2020). Prevalence and predictors of sexual difficulties and associated distress among partnered, sexually active older women in Norway, Denmark, Belgium, and Portugal. Archives of Sexual Behavior, 49(8), 2951–2961. https://doi.org/10.1007/s10508-020-01742-7

Granero, R., Jiménez-Murcia, S., Fernández-Aranda, F., del Pino-Gutiérrez, A., Mena-Moreno, T., Mestre-Bach, G., Gómez-Peña, M., Moragas, L., Aymamí, N., Giroux, I., Grall-Bronnec, M., Sauvaget, A., Codina, E., Vintró-Alcaraz, C., Lozano-Madrid, M., Camozzi, M., Agüera, Z., Sánchez-González, J., Casalé-Salayet, G., . . . Menchón, J. M. (2022). Contribution of stressful life events to gambling activity in older age. Ageing & Society, 42(7), 1513–1537. https://doi.org/10.1017/S0144686X20001592

Grant, J. E. (2005). Clinical characteristics and psychiatric comorbidity in males with exhibitionism. *Journal of Clinical Psychiatry, 66,* 1367–1371.

Grant, J. E. (2006). Kleptomania. In E. Hollander & D. J. Stein (Eds.), *Clinical manual of impulse-control disorders* (pp. 175–201). American Psychiatric Publishing, Inc.

Grant, J. E., & Kim, S. W. (2007). Clinical characteristics and psychiatric comorbidity of pyromania. *Journal of Clinical Psychiatry, 68,* 1717–1722.

Grant, J. E., & Odlaug, B. L. (2010). Impulse control disorders. In D. McKay, J. S. Abramowitz & S. Taylor (Eds.), *Cognitive-behavioral therapy for refractory cases: Turning failure into success* (pp. 231–254). American Psychological Association. https://doi.org/10.1037/12070-011

Grant, J. E., Collins, M., Chesivoir, E., & Chamberlain, S. R. (2023). Hazardous alcohol use in trichotillomania. *Psychiatric Quarterly, 94* (3), 361–369. https://doi.org/10.1007/s11126-023-10042-x

Grant, J. E., Dougherty, D. D., & Chamberlain, S. R. (2020). Prevalence, gender correlates, and co-morbidity of trichotillomania. *Psychiatry Research, 288,* 112948. https://doi.org/10.1016/j.psychres.2020.112948

Grant, J. E., Levine, L., Kim, D., & Potenza, M. N. (2005). Impulse control disorders in adult psychiatric inpatients. *American Journal of Psychiatry, 162,* 2184–2188.

Grant, J. E., Odlaug, B. L., & Kim, S. W. (2010). Kleptomania: Clinical characteristics and relationship to substance use disorders. *The American Journal of Drug and Alcohol Abuse, 36,* 291–295.

Grant, J. E., Odlaug, B. L., Davis, A., & Kim, S. W. (2009). Legal consequences of kleptomania. *Psychiatric Quarterly, 80,* 251–259.

Grant, J. E., Odlaug, B. L., Medeiros, G., Christianine, A. R., & Tavares, H. (2015). Cross-cultural comparison of compulsive stealing (kleptomania). *Annals of Clinical Psychiatry, 27,* 150–151.

Grant, J. E., Peris, T. S., Ricketts, E. J., Lochner, C., Stein, D. J., Stochl, J., . . . Keuthen, N. J. (2021). Identifying subtypes of trichotillomania (hair pulling disorder) and excoriation (skin picking) disorder using mixture modeling in a multicenter sample. *Journal of Psychiatric Research, 137,* 603–612. https://doi.org/10.1016/j.jpsychires.2020.11.001

Grant, J. E., Peris, T. S., Ricketts, E. J., Lochner, C., Stein, D. J., Stochl, J., . . . Keuthen, N. J. (2020). Identifying subtypes of trichotillomania (hair pulling disorder) and excoriation (skin picking) disorder using mixture modeling in a multicenter sample. *Journal of Psychiatric Research.* https://doi.org/10.1016/j.jpsychires.2020.11.001

Greene, D. J., Koller, J. M., Hampton, J. M., Wesevich, V., Van, A. N., Nguyen, A. L., . . . Dosenbach, N. U. F. (2018). Behavioral interventions for reducing head motion during MRI scans in children. *NeuroImage, 171,* 234–245. https://doi.org/10.1016/j.neuroimage.2018.01.023

Grenier, S., Payette, M. C., Gunther, B., Askari, S., Desjardins, F. F., Raymond, B., & Berbiche, D. (2019). Association of age and gender with anxiety disorders in older adults: A systematic review and meta-analysis. *International Journal of Geriatric Psychiatry, 34* (3), 397–407. https://doi.org/10.1002/gps.5035

Grenyer, B. F. S., & Marceau, E. M. (2022). Helping patients master core conflictual relationship themes in psychotherapy. *Journal of Clinical Psychology, 78* (3), 386–395. https://doi.org/10.1002/jclp.23314

Gritti, E. S., Meyer, G. J., Bornstein, R. F., Marino, D. P., & Marco, J. d. (2020). Narcissism and reactions to a self-esteem insult: An experiment using predictions from self-report and the Rorschach task. *Journal of Personality Assessment.* https://doi.org/10.1080/00223891.2020.1848854

Gross, A. L., Tommet, D., D'Aquila, M., Schmitt, E., Marcantonio, E. R., Helfand, B., . . . for the B. S. G. (2018). Harmonization of delirium severity instruments: A comparison of the DRS-R-98, MDAS, and CAM-S using item response theory. *BMC Medical Research Methodology, 18* (1), 92. https://doi.org/10.1186/s12874-018-0552-4

Guay, D. R. P. (2009). Drug treatment of paraphilic and nonparaphilic sexual disorders. *Clinical Therapeutics: The International Peer-Reviewed Journal of Drug Therapy, 31,* 1–31.

Gueorguieva, R., Wu, R., Tsai, W., O'Connor, P. G., Fucito, L., Zhang, H., & O'Malley, S. S. (2015). An analysis of moderators in the COMBINE study: Identifying subgroups of patients who benefit from acamprosate. *European Neuropsychopharmacology, 25,* 1586–1599. https://doi.org/10.1016/j.euroneuro.2015.06.006

Guina, J., Dornfeld, B., & Pinals, D. A. (2022). A 20-year follow-up survey of police officers' experience with tarasoff warnings: How law enforcement reacts to clinicians' duty to protect. *Behavioral Sciences & the Law.* https://doi.org/10.1002/bsl.2564

Gunst, A., Ventus, D., Arver, S., Dhejne, C., Görts-Öberg, K., Zamore-Söderström, E., & Jern, P. (2019). A randomized, waiting-list-controlled study shows that brief, mindfulness-based psychological interventions are effective for treatment of women's low sexual desire. *Journal of Sex Research, 56* (7), 913–929. https://doi.org/10.1080/00224499.2018.1539463

Guo, W., Liu, F., Xiao, C., Zhang, Z., Liu, J., Yu, M., . . . Zhao, J. (2015). Decreased insular connectivity in drug-naive major depressive disorder at rest. *Journal of Affective Disorders, 179,* 31–37. https://doi.org/10.1016/j.jad.2015.03.028

Güzel, Â., Mutlu, N. L., & Molendijk, M. (2023). COVID-19-related changes in eating disorder pathology, emotional and binge eating and need for care: A systematic review with frequentist and Bayesian meta-analyses. *Eating & Weight Disorders, 28* (1), 1–11. https://doi.org/10.1007/s40519-023-01547-2

Gyereh, J., & Shukla, M. (2023). Risk factors of and interventions for mental health problems in learning disabilities: A systematic review of psychological therapies for parents and children. *Current Psychology: A Journal for Diverse Perspectives on Diverse Psychological Issues.* https://doi.org/10.1007/s12144-023-04527-y

H

Haaland, Å. T., Eskeland, S. O., Moen, E. M., Vogel, P. A., Haseth, S., Mellingen, K., . . . Hummelen, B. (2017). ACT-enhanced behavior therapy in group format for trichotillomania: An effectiveness study. *Journal of Obsessive-Compulsive and Related Disorders, 12,* 109–116. https://doi.org/10.1016/j.jocrd.2017.01.005

Hackett, R. A., Ronaldson, A., Bhui, K., Steptoe, A., & Jackson, S. E. (2020). Racial discrimination and health: A prospective study of ethnic minorities in the United Kingdom. *BMC Public Health, 20* (1), 1652. https://doi.org/10.1186/s12889-020-09792-1

Haderlein, T. P., Wong, M. S., Yuan, A., Llorente, M. D., & Washington, D. L. (2020). Association of PTSD with COVID-19 testing and infection in the veterans health administration. *Journal of Psychiatric Research.* https://doi.org/10.1016/j.jpsychires.2020.11.033

Hagger, M. S., Hankonen, N., Kangro, E. M., Lintunen, T., Polet, J., Pagaduan, J., Ries, F., & Hamilton, K. (2019). Trait self-control, social cognition constructs, and intentions: Correlational evidence for mediation and moderation effects in diverse health behaviours. *Applied Psychology: Health and Well-Being, 11* (3), 407–437. https://doi.org/10.1111/aphw.12153

Haji, I. (2010). Psychopathy, ethical perception, and moral culpability. *Neuroethics, 3,* 135–150.

Hall, B. J., Tolin, D. F., Frost, R. O., & Steketee, G. (2013). An exploration of comorbid symptoms and clinical correlates of clinically significant hoarding symptoms. *Depression and Anxiety, 30,* 67–76. https://doi.org/10.1002/da.22015

Hall, R. C. W., & Tardif, I. (2021). Florida law enforcement policies for and experience with Tarasoff-like reporting. *Journal of the American Academy of Psychiatry and the Law, 49* (1), 77–86.

Hallberg, J., Kaldo, V., Arver, S., Dhejne, C., Piwowar, M., Jokinen, J., & Öberg, K. G. (2020). Internet-administered cognitive behavioral therapy for hypersexual disorder, with or without paraphilia(s) or paraphilic disorder(s) in men: A pilot study. *Journal of Sexual Medicine, 17* (10), 2039–2054. https://doi.org/10.1016/j.jsxm.2020.07.018

Hamdi, N. R., Krueger, R. F., & South, S. C. (2015). Socioeconomic status moderates genetic and environmental effects on the amount of alcohol use. *Alcoholism: Clinical and Experimental Research, 39,* 603–610. https://doi.org/10.1111/acer.12673

Hamilton, K., Gibbs, I., Keech, J. J., & Hagger, M. S. (2020). Reasoned and implicit processes in heavy episodic drinking: An integrated dual-process model. *British Journal of Health Psychology, 25* (1), 189–209. https://doi.org/10.1111/bjhp.12401

Han, J., Zhou, F., Zhang, L., Su, Y., & Mao, L. (2020). Psychological symptoms of cancer survivors during the COVID-19 outbreak: A longitudinal study. *Psycho-Oncology.* https://doi.org/10.1002/pon.5588

Hang, Y., Zhong, Y., Zhang, G., Wu, Z., Kong, J., Wang, Q., . . . Zhang, N. (2022). Altered spontaneous neural activity in frontal and visual regions in patients with acrophobia. *Journal of Affective Disorders, 303*, 340–345. https://doi.org/10.1016/j.jad.2022.02.022

Hannaford, S., Shaw, R., & Walker, R. (2019). Older adults' perceptions of psychotherapy: What is it and who is responsible? *Australian Psychologist, 54* (1), 37–45. https://doi.org/10.1111/ap.12360

Hantsoo, L., & Payne, J. L. (2023). Towards understanding the biology of premenstrual dysphoric disorder: From genes to GABA. *Neuroscience and Biobehavioral Reviews, 149*. https://doi.org/10.1016/j.neubiorev.2023.105168

Hare, R. D. (1997). *Hare psychopathy checklist–Revised (PCL-R).* Personality Assessment Resources.

Harkness, G. V. (2023). *Rain king: The life and music of Adam Duritz and Counting Crows*. Carol Press.

Harnois-Leblanc, S., Van Hulst, A., Sabiston, C. M., Maximova, K., Béland, M., Doré, I., . . . Henderson, M. (2021). Self-reported weight loss attempts and weight-related stress in childhood: Heightening the risk of obesity in early adolescence. *International Journal of Eating Disorders*. https://doi.org/10.1002/eat.23474

Harstad, E., Sideridis, G., Sherritt, L., Shrier, L. A., Ziemnik, R., & Levy, S. (2016). Concurrent validity of caffeine problems and diagnostic criteria for substance use disorders. *Journal of Caffeine Research, 6* (4), 141–147. https://doi.org/10.1089/jcr.2016.0006

Hartman, C. A., Larsson, H., Vos, M., Bellato, A., Libutzki, B., Solberg, B. S., . . . Reif, A. (2023). Anxiety, mood, and substance use disorders in adult men and women with and without attention-deficit/hyperactivity disorder: A substantive and methodological overview. *Neuroscience and Biobehavioral Reviews, 151*. https://doi.org/10.1016/j.neubiorev.2023.105209

Hartmann, E., & Opaas, M. (2023). Convergence in a multi-method study between Rorschach and self-report data of traumatized refugees assessed before and after psychotherapy. *Journal of Clinical Psychology, 79* (5), 1357–1370. https://doi.org/10.1002/jclp.23484

Hasan, S. S., Pearson, J. S., Morris, J., & Whorwell, P. J. (2019). Skype hypnotherapy for irritable bowel syndrome: Effectiveness and comparison with face-to-face treatment. *International Journal of Clinical and Experimental Hypnosis, 67* (1), 69–80. https://doi.org/10.1080/00207144.2019.1553766

Hasin, D. S., Sarvet, A. L., Meyers, J. L., Saha, T. D., Ruan, W. J., Stohl, M., & Grant, B. F. (2018). Epidemiology of adult DSM-5 major depressive disorder and its specifiers in the United States. *JAMA Psychiatry, 75* (4), 336–346. https://doi.org/10.1001/jamapsychiatry.2017.4602

Hatchett, G. T. (2015). Treatment guidelines for clients with antisocial personality disorder. *Journal of Mental Health Counseling, 37*, 15–27.

Hawkins, M., Sockalingam, S., Bonato, S., Rajaratnam, T., Ravindran, M., Gosse, P., & Sheehan, K. A. (2021). A rapid review of the pathoetiology, presentation, and management of delirium in adults with COVID-19. *Journal of Psychosomatic Research, 141*, 110350–110350. https://doi.org/10.1016/j.jpsychores.2020.110350

Hay, P. (2021). Is orthorexia nervosa a healthy way of being or a mental health disorder? Commentary on He et al. (2020). *International Journal of Eating Disorders*. https://doi.org/10.1002/eat.23465

Hayes, J. F., Miles, J., Walters, K., King, M., & Osborn, D. J. (2015). A systematic review and meta-analysis of premature mortality in bipolar affective disorder. *Acta Psychiatrica Scandinavica, 131*, 417–425. https://doi.org/10.1111/acps.12408

Hayes, S. C., Luoma, J. B., Bond, F. W., Masuda, A., & Lillis, J. (2006). Acceptance and commitment therapy: Model, processes and outcomes. *Behavior Research and Therapy, 44* (1), 1–125. https://doi.org/10.1016/j.brat.2005.06.006

Hebert, E. A., & Dugas, M. J. (2019). Behavioral experiments for intolerance of uncertainty: Challenging the unknown in the treatment of generalized anxiety disorder. *Cognitive and Behavioral Practice, 26* (2), 421–436. https://doi.org/10.1016/j.cbpra.2018.07.007

Heeren, A., & McNally, R. J. (2018). Social anxiety disorder as a densely interconnected network of fear and avoidance for social situations. *Cognitive Therapy and Research, 42* (1), 103–113. https://doi.org/10.1007/s10608-017-9876-3

Hein, C., Forgues, A., Piau, A., Sommet, A., Vellas, B., & Nourhashémi, F. (2014). Impact of polypharmacy on occurrence of delirium in elderly emergency patients. *Journal of the American Medical Directors Association, 15* (11), 850.e811–855. https://doi.org/10.1016/j.jamda.2014.08.012

Hendershot, C. S., Wardell, J. D., Samokhvalov, A. V., & Rehm, J. (2017). Effects of naltrexone on alcohol self-administration and craving: Meta-analysis of human laboratory studies. *Addiction Biology, 22* (6), 1515–1527. https://doi.org/10.1111/adb.12425

Henssler, J., Brandt, L., Müller, M., Liu, S., Montag, C., Sterzer, P., & Heinz, A. (2020). Migration and schizophrenia: Meta-analysis and explanatory framework. *European Archives of Psychiatry and Clinical Neuroscience, 270* (3), 325–335. https://doi.org/10.1007/s00406-019-01028-7

Herbert, P. B. (2002). The duty to warn: A reconsideration and critique. *Journal of the American Academy of Psychiatry and the Law, 30*, 417–424.

Hettema, J. M., van den Oord, E. J. C. G., Zhao, M., Xie, L. Y., Copeland, W. E., Penninx, B. W. J. H., Aberg, K. A., & Clark, S. L. (2023). Methylome-wide association study of anxiety disorders. *Molecular Psychiatry*. https://doi.org/10.1038/s41380-023-02205-w

Hill, C. E., Knox, S., & Duan, C. (2023). Psychotherapist advice, suggestions, recommendations: A research review. *Psychotherapy, 60* (3), 295–305. https://doi.org/10.1037/pst0000476 (Evidence-Based Psychotherapy Skills and Methods)

Hilleary, M. (May, 2021). Counting Crows' Adam Duritz on Nostalgia, Dissociative Disorder and His Band's New EP. Inside Hook. https://www.insidehook.com/article/music/counting-crows-adam-duritz-interview

Hillemacher, T., Heberlein, A., Muschler, M. A., Bleich, S., & Frieling, H. (2011). Opioid modulators for alcohol dependence. *Expert Opinion on Investigational Drugs, 20*, 1073–1086.

Hipolito, G., Pagnamenta, E., Stacey, H., Wright, E., Joffe, V., Murayama, K., & Creswell, C. (2023). A systematic review and meta-analysis of nonpharmacological interventions for children and adolescents with selective mutism. *JCPP Advances*. https://doi.org/10.1002/jcv2.12166

Hobbs, K. A., Mann, F. D., Latzman, R. D., Zimmermann, J., Jaeger, U., Markon, K., & Krueger, R. F. (2023). Pathological personality in relation to multiple domains of quality of life and impairment: Evidence for the specific relevance of the maladaptive poles of major trait domains. *Journal of Psychopathology and Clinical Science, 132* (2), 135–144. https://doi.org/10.1037/abn0000810 10.103

Hoffman, S. J., Vukovich, M. M., Fulkerson, J., Gewirtz, A., Robertson, C. L., Fredkove, W. M., & Gaugler, J. (2023). The impact of parent torture and family functioning on youth adjustment in war-affected families: A path analysis describing intergenerational trauma and the family system. *Journal of Family Nursing, 29* (3), 288–300. https://doi.org/ https://doi.org/10.1177/10748407231164747

Hoge, C. W., Castro, C. A., Messer, S. C., McGurk, D., Cotting, D. I., & Koffman, R. L. (2004). Combat duty in Iraq and Afghanistan, mental health problems, and barriers to care. *New England Journal of Medicine, 351*, 13–22.

Hoge, C. W., Terhakopian, A., Castro, C. A., Messer, S. C., & Engel, C. C. (2007). Association of posttraumatic stress disorder with somatic symptoms, health care visits, and absenteeism among Iraq war veterans. *American Journal of Psychiatry, 164*, 150–153.

Hollingshead, A. B., & Redlich, F. C. (1958). *Social class and mental illness: A community study.* Wiley.

Hollon, S. D., & Ponniah, K. (2010). A review of empirically supported psychological therapies for mood disorders in adults. *Depression and Anxiety, 27*, 891–932.

Holmes, T. H., & Rahe, R. H. (1967). The social readjustment rating scale. *Journal of Psychosomatic Research, 11,* 213–218.

Holvoet, L., Huys, W., Coppens, V., Seeuws, J., Goethals, K., & Morrens, M. (2017). Fifty shades of Belgian gray: The prevalence of BDSM-related fantasies and activities in the general population. *Journal of Sexual Medicine, 14* (9), 1152–1159. https://doi.org/10.1016/j.jsxm.2017.07.003

Horn, M., Wathelet, M., Amad, A., Martignène, N., Lathiere, T., Khelfaoui, K., . . . D'Hondt, F. (2023). Persistent physical symptoms after COVID-19 infection and the risk of somatic symptom disorder. *Journal of Psychosomatic Research, 166,* 1–7. https://doi.org/10.1016/j.jpsychores.2023.111172

Howe, E. (2008). Ethical considerations when treating patients with schizophrenia. *Psychiatry (Edgmont), 5,* 59–64.

Huang, H., Botao, Z., Jiang, Y., Tang, Y., Zhang, T., Tang, X., . . . Wang, J. (2020). Aberrant resting-state functional connectivity of salience network in first-episode schizophrenia. *Brain Imaging and Behavior, 14* (5), 1350–1360. https://doi.org/10.1007/s11682-019-00040-8

Hubers, N., Hagenbeek, F. A., Pool, R., Déjean, S., Harms, A. C., Roetman, P. J., . . . Boomsma, D. I. (2023). Integrative multi-omics analysis of genomic, epigenomic, and metabolomics data leads to new insights for attention-deficit/hyperactivity disorder. *American Journal of Medical Genetics Part B: Neuropsychiatric Genetics.* https://doi.org/10.1002/ajmg.b.32955

Hudson, C. G. (2012). Patterns of residential mobility of people with schizophrenia: Multi-level tests of downward geographic drift. *Journal of Sociology and Social Welfare, 39* (3), 149–179.

Hughes, S. D., & Hammack, P. L. (2020). Narratives of the origins of kinky sexual desire held by users of a kink-oriented social networking website. *Journal of Sex Research.* https://doi.org/10.1080/00224499.2020.1840495

Hummelen, B., Pedersen, G., Wilberg, T., & Karterud, S. (2015). Poor validity of the *DSM-IV* schizoid personality disorder construct as a diagnostic category. *Journal of Personality Disorders, 29,* 334–346. https://doi.org/10.1521/pedi_2014_28_159

Humphreys, K. L., Nelson, C. A., Fox, N. A., & Zeanah, C. H. (2017). Signs of reactive attachment disorder and disinhibited social engagement disorder at age 12 years: Effects of institutional care history and high-quality foster care. *Development and Psychopathology, 29* (2), 675–684. https://doi.org/10.1017/S0954579417000256

Huppert, J. D., Foa, E. B., McNally, R. J., & Cahill, S. P. (2009). Role of cognition in stress-induced and fear circuitry disorders. In G. Andrews, D. S. Charney, P. J. Sirovatka, & D. A. Regier (Eds.), *Stress-induced and fear circuitry disorders: Advancing the research agenda for DSM-V* (pp. 175–193). Arlington, VA: American Psychiatric Publishing, Inc.

I

Ilchena, C., Slayen, C., Rennie, S., Cheung, K., Gaulke, T., & Theule, J. (2023). Parenting stress and FASD: A scoping review [Report]. *Research in Developmental Disabilities, 137.* https://doi.org/10.1016/j.ridd.2023.104498

Imbimbo, B. P., Ippati, S., Watling, M., & Balducci, C. (2022). A critical appraisal of tau-targeting therapies for primary and secondary tauopathies. *Alzheimer's & Dementia, 18* (5), 1008–1037. https://doi.org/10.1002/alz.12453

Iwase, S., Bérubé, N. G., Zhou, Z., Kasri, N. N., Battaglioli, E., Scandaglia, M., & Barco, A. (2017). Epigenetic etiology of intellectual disability. *The Journal of Neuroscience, 37* (45), 10773–10782.

J

Jackson, C. E., Ciarleglio, M. M., Aslan, M., Marx, B. P., Ko, J., Concato, J., . . . Vasterling, J. J. (2021). Associations among increases in posttraumatic stress symptoms, neurocognitive performance, and long-term functional outcomes in US Iraq war veterans. *Journal of Traumatic Stress.* https://doi.org/10.1002/jts.22663

Jackson, S. E., Hackett, R. A., Grabovac, I., Smith, L., & Steptoe, A. (2019). Perceived discrimination, health and wellbeing among middle-aged and older lesbian, gay and bisexual people: A prospective study. *PLoS ONE, 14* (5), e0216497. https://doi.org/10.1371/journal.pone.0216497

Jahnke, S., Philipp, K., & Hoyer, J. (2015). Stigmatizing attitudes towards people with pedophilia and their malleability among psychotherapists in training. *Child Abuse & Neglect, 40,* 93–102. https://doi.org/10.1016/j.chiabu.2014.07.008

Jain, A., & Davis, A. M. (2021). Initiating pharmacologic treatment in tobacco-dependent adults. *Journal of the American Medical Association, 325* (3), 301–302. https://doi.org/10.1001/jama.2020.24790

James, S. L., Abate, D., Abate, K. H., Abay, S. M., Abbafati, C., Abbasi, N., . . . Murray, C. J. L. (2018). Global, regional, and national incidence, prevalence, and years lived with disability for 354 diseases and injuries for 195 countries and territories, 1990–2017: A systematic analysis for the Global Burden of Disease Study 2017. *The Lancet, 392* (10159), 1789–1858. https://doi.org/10.1016/S0140-6736(18)32279-7

Jauk, E., Ulbrich, L., Jorschick, P., Höfler, M., Kaufman, S. B., & Kanske, P. (2022). The nonlinear association between grandiose and vulnerable narcissism: An individual data meta-analysis. *Journal of Personality, 90* (5), 703–726. https://doi.org/10.1111/jopy.12692

Jelsma, L. D., Cavalcante Neto, J. L., Smits-Engelsman, B., Targino Gomes Draghi, T., Araújo Rohr, L., & Tudella, E. (2023). Type of active video-games training does not impact the effect on balance and agility in children with and without developmental coordination disorder: A randomized comparator-controlled trial. *Applied Neuropsychology: Child, 12* (1), 64–73. https://doi.org/10.1080/21622965.2022.2030740

Jenkins, S. R. (2017). Not your same old story: New rules for thematic apperceptive techniques (TATs). *Journal of Personality Assessment, 99* (3), 238–253. https://doi.org/10.1080/00223891.2016.1248972

Ji, Y., Du, Z., Zheng, K., Jiang, Y., Ren, C., Zhu, H., Xiao, M., & Wang, T. (2023). Bidirectional causal association between ischemic stroke and five mental disorders. *Acta Psychiatrica Scandinavica.* https://doi.org/10.1111/acps.13606

Ji, Y., Zhang, X., Wang, Z., Qin, W., Liu, H., Xue, K., . . . Yu, C. (2021). Genes associated with gray matter volume alterations in schizophrenia. *NeuroImage, 225.* https://doi.org/10.1016/j.neuroimage.2020.117526

Jiang, H., Xiang, X., Room, R., & Hao, W. (2016). Alcohol and the sustainable development goals. *The Lancet, 388* (10051), 1279–1280. https://doi.org/10.1016/S0140-6736(16)31673-7

Jiang, M. Y. W., Upton, E., & Newby, J. M. (2020). A randomised wait-list controlled pilot trial of one-session virtual reality exposure therapy for blood-injection-injury phobias. *Journal of Affective Disorders, 276,* 636–645. doi:10.1016/j.jad.2020.07.076

John, E. (2012). *Love is the cure: On life, loss and the end of AIDS.* Little, Brown, and Company.

John, E. (2013). Elton John: My life in 20 songs. *Rolling Stone.* https://www.rollingstone.com/music/music-lists/elton-john-my-life-in-20-songs-10473/empty-sky-226400/

John, E. (2019a). *Me.* St. Martin's Griffin.

John, E. (2019b). Elton John recalls performing: "I Was Terrified". https://variety.com/2019/music/uncategorized/elton-john-sober-addiction-recovery-1203392566/

John, E. (2019b). Elton John recalls performing for the first time since getting sober: "I Was Terrified". *Variety.* https://variety.com/2019/music/uncategorized/elton-john-sober-addiction-recovery-1203392566. Accessed 4/14/21.

Johnson-Munguia, S., Negi, S., Chen, Y., Thomeczek, M. L., & Forbush, K. T. (2023). Eating disorder psychopathology, psychiatric impairment, and symptom frequency of atypical anorexia nervosa versus anorexia nervosa: A systematic review and meta-analysis. *International Journal of Eating Disorders.* https://doi.org/10.1002/eat.23989

Johnson, E. C., Kapoor, M., Hatoum, A. S., Zhou, H., Polimanti, R., Wendt, F. R., . . . Agrawal, A. (2023). Investigation of convergent and divergent genetic influences underlying schizophrenia and alcohol use disorder. *Psychological Medicine, 53* (4), 1196–1204. https://doi.org/10.1017/S003329172100266X

Johnson, E. C., Paul, S. E., Baranger, D. A. A., Hatoum, A. S., Colbert, S. M. C., Lin, S., . . . Agrawal, A. (2023). Characterizing alcohol expectancies in the ABCD study: Associations with sociodemographic factors, the immediate social environment, and genetic propensities. *Behavior Genetics, 53* (3), 265–278. https://doi.org/10.1007/s10519-023-10133-2

Johnston, L. D., Miech, R. A., Patrick, M. E., O'Malley, P. M., Schulenberg, J. E., & Bachman, J. G. (2023). Monitoring the Future national survey results on drug use 1975–2022: Overview, key findings on adolescent drug use. https://monitoringthefuture.org/wp-content/uploads/2023/01/mtfoverview2022.pdf

Jolley, S., & Grice, S. (2023). State of the art in psychological therapies for psychosis: Family interventions for psychosis. *Psychology and Psychotherapy: Theory, Research and Practice.* https://doi.org/10.1111/papt.12487

Jonason, P. K., Strosser, G. L., Kroll, C. H., Duineveld, J. J., & Baruffi, S. A. (2015). Valuing myself over others: The dark triad traits and moral and social values. *Personality and Individual Differences, 81,* 102–106. https://doi.org/10.1016/j.paid.2014.10.045

Jongenelis, M. I., Morley, B., Worrall, C., & Talati, Z. (2021). Grandparents' perceptions of the barriers and strategies to providing their grandchildren with a healthy diet: A qualitative study. *Appetite, 159.* https://doi.org/10.1016/j.appet.2020.105061

Jonsson, U., Linton, S. J., Ybrandt, H., Ringborg, A., Leander, L., Moberg, K., Hultcrantz, M., & Arnberg, F. K. (2023). Internet-delivered psychological treatment as an add-on to treatment as usual for common mental disorders: A systematic review with meta-analysis of randomized trials. *Journal of Affective Disorders, 322,* 221–234. https://doi.org/10.1016/j.jad.2022.11.036

Joo, M., & Park, S. W. (2019). Depression is associated with negativity in TAT narratives: The mediating role of agency. *Current Psychology: A Journal for Diverse Perspectives on Diverse Psychological Issues.* https://doi.org/10.1007/s12144-019-00245-6

Jorstad-Stein, E. C., & Heimberg, R. G. (2009). Social phobia: An update on treatment. *Psychiatric Clinics of North America, 32,* 641–663.

Jumaili, W. A., Trivedi, C., Chao, T., Kubosumi, A., & Jain, S. (2022). The safety and efficacy of ketamine NMDA receptor blocker as a therapeutic intervention for PTSD review of a randomized clinical trial. *Behavioural Brain Research, 424,* 1–5. https://doi.org/10.1016/j.bbr.2022.113804

Jung, C. G. (1961). *Memories, dreams, reflections.* Pantheon.

K

Kabat-Zinn, J. (2003). Mindfulness-based interventions in context: Past, present, and future. *Clinical Psychology: Science and Practice, 10* (2), 144–156.

Kaehne, A. (2016). Project SEARCH UK—Evaluating its employment outcomes. *Journal of Applied Research in Intellectual Disabilities, 29* (6), 519–530. https://doi.org/10.1111/jar.12207

Kaiser, R. H., Andrews-Hanna, J. R., Wager, T. D., & Pizzagalli, D. A. (2015). Large-scale network dysfunction in major depressive disorder: A meta-analysis of resting-state functional connectivity. *JAMA Psychiatry, 72,* 603–611. https:10.1001/jamapsychiatry.2015.0071

Kalk, N. J., Nutt, D. J., & Lingford-Hughes, A. R. (2011). The role of central noradrenergic dysregulation in anxiety disorders: Evidence from clinical studies. *Journal of Psychopharmacology, 25,* 3–16.

Kamody, R. C., Grilo, C. M., & Udo, T. (2020). Disparities in *DSM-5* defined eating disorders by sexual orientation among US adults. *International Journal of Eating Disorders, 53* (2), 278–287. https://doi.org/10.1002/eat.23193

Kananian, S., Soltani, Y., Hinton, D., & Stangier, U. (2020). Culturally adapted cognitive behavioral therapy plus problem management (ca-cbt+) with Afghan refugees: A randomized controlled pilot study. *Journal of Traumatic Stress.* https://doi.org/10.1002/jts.22615

Kao, S. Y. S., Li, A. C. M., Mak, W. W. S., & Cheung, R. Y. M. (2023). The efficacy of acceptance and commitment therapy on self-stigma reduction among people with mental illness: A quasi-experimental design. *Stigma and Health.* https://doi.org/10.1037/sah0000474

Karlsson, A., & Håkansson, A. (2018). Gambling disorder, increased mortality, suicidality, and associated comorbidity: A longitudinal nationwide register study. *Journal of Behavioral Addictions, 7* (4), 1091–1099. https://doi.org/10.1556/2006.7.2018.112

Kaur, M., Floyd, A., & Balta, A.-M. (2022). Oppositional defiant disorder: Evidence-based review of behavioral treatment programs. *Annals of Clinical Psychiatry, 34* (1), 44–58.

Kealy, D., Goodman, G., Rasmussen, B., Weideman, R., & Ogrodniczuk, J. S. (2017). Therapists' perspectives on optimal treatment for pathological narcissism. *Personality Disorders: Theory, Research, and Treatment, 8* (1), 35–45. https://doi.org/10.1037/per0000164

Kearney, C. A., & Vecchio, J. L. (2007). When a child won't speak. *The Journal of Family Practice, 56,* 917–921.

Keefe, J. R., Levy, K. N., Sowislo, J. F., Diamond, D., Doering, S., Hörz-Sagstetter, . . . Clarkin, J. F. (2023). Reflective functioning and its potential to moderate the efficacy of manualized psychodynamic therapies versus other treatments for borderline personality disorder. *Journal of Consulting and Clinical Psychology, 91* (1), 50–56. https://doi.org/10.1037/ccp0000760

Keefe, J. R., McMain, S. F., McCarthy, K. S., Zilcha-Mano, S., Dinger, U., Sahin, Z., . . . Barber, J. P. (2020). A meta-analysis of psychodynamic treatments for borderline and cluster C personality disorders. *Personality Disorders: Theory, Research, and Treatment, 11* (3), 157–169. https://doi.org/10.1037/per0000382

Kellas, J. K., Horstman, H. K., Willer, E. K., & Carr, K. (2015). The benefits and risks of telling and listening to stories of difficulty over time: Experimentally testing the expressive writing paradigm in the context of interpersonal communication between friends. *Health Communication, 30,* 843–858. https://doi.org/10.1080/10410236.2013.850017

Kennedy, J. H. (2021). For Michael J. Fox, nothing easy about looking on the bright side. https://vineyardgazette.com/news/2021/02/18/mj-fox

Kenton, J. A., Ontiveros, T., Bird, C. W., Valenzuela, C. F., & Brigman, J. L. (2020). Moderate prenatal alcohol exposure alters the number and function of GABAergic interneurons in the murine orbitofrontal cortex. *Alcohol, 88,* 33–41. doi:10.1016/j.alcohol.2020.06.001

Kerckhof, M. E., Kreukels, B. P. C., Nieder, T. O., Becker-Hébly, I., van de Grift, T. C., Staphorsius, A. S., . . . Elaut, E. (2019). Prevalence of sexual dysfunctions in transgender persons: Results from the ENIGI Follow-Up Study. *Journal of Sexual Medicine, 16* (12), 2018–2029. https://doi.org/10.1016/j.jsxm.2019.09.003

Kerekes, N., Zouini, B., Karlsson, E., Cederholm, E., Lichtenstein, P., Anckarsäter, H., & Råstam, M. (2020). Conduct disorder and somatic health in children: A nationwide genetically sensitive study. *BMC Psychiatry, 20.* https://doi.org/10.1186/s12888-020-03003-2

Kerkemeyer, L., Wasem, J., Neumann, A., Brannath, W., Mester, B., Timm, J., . . . Biermann, J. (2018). Effectiveness and cost-effectiveness of an integrated care program for schizophrenia: An analysis of routine data. *European Archives of Psychiatry and Clinical Neuroscience, 268* (6), 611–619. https://doi.org/10.1007/s00406-017-0830-x

Kessing, L. V., Vradi, E., McIntyre, R. S., & Andersen, P. K. (2015). Causes of decreased life expectancy over the life span in bipolar disorder. *Journal of Affective Disorders, 180,* 142–147. https://doi.org/10.1016/j.jad.2015.03.027

Kessler, R. C., Berglund, P., Demler, O., Jin, R., Merikangas, K. R., & Walters, E. E. (2005). Lifetime prevalence and age-of-onset distributions of *DSM-IV* disorders in the National Comorbidity Survey Replication. *Archives of General Psychiatry, 62,* 593–602.

Kessler, R. C., Chiu, W. T., Demler, O., Merikangas, K. R., & Walters, E. E. (2005). Prevalence, severity, and comorbidity of 12-month *DSM-IV* disorders in the National Comorbidity Survey Replication. *Archives of General Psychiatry, 62* (6), 617–627.

Kessler, R. C., Petukhova, M., Sampson, N. A., Zaslavsky, A. M., & Wittchen, H. U. (2012). Twelve-month and lifetime prevalence and lifetime morbid risk of anxiety and mood disorders in the United States. *International Journal of Methods in Psychiatric Research, 21* (3), 169–184. https://doi.org/10.1002/mpr.1359

Khubchandani, J., Price, J. H., Sharma, S., Wiblishauser, M. J., & Webb, F. J. (2022). COVID-19 pandemic and weight gain in American adults: A nationwide population-based study. *Diabetes and Metabolic Syndrome, 16* (1), 102392. https://doi.org/10.1016/j.dsx.2022.102392

Kilpela, L. S., Marshall, V. B., Hooper, S. C., Becker, C. B., Keel, P. K., LaCroix, A. Z., Musi, N., & Espinoza, S. E. (2023). Binge eating age of onset, frequency, and associated emotional distress among women aged 60 years and over. *Eating Disorders: The Journal of Treatment & Prevention, 31* (5), 479–486. https://doi.org/10.1080/10640266.2023.2192600

Kiluk, B. D. (2019). Computerized cognitive behavioral therapy for substance use disorders: A summary of the evidence and potential mechanisms of behavior change. *Perspectives on Behavior Science, 42* (3), 465–478. https://doi.org/10.1007/s40614-019-00205-2

Kim, B.-H., Nho, K., & Lee, J.-M. (2021). Genome-wide association study identifies susceptibility loci of brain atrophy to nfia and st18 in Alzheimer's disease. *Neurobiology of Aging.* https://doi.org/10.1016/j.neurobiolaging.2021.01.021

Kim, B.-N. (2020). Behavioral activation system (BAS) dysregulation and bipolar spectrum psychopathology in daily life: An online-diary study. *Psychiatry Research, 291.* https://doi.org/10.1016/j.psychres.2020.113180

Kim, H. S., Hodgins, D. C., Torres, A. R., Fontenelle, L. F., do Rosário, M. C., de Mathis, M. A., . . . Tavares, H. (2018). Dual diagnosis of obsessive compulsive and compulsive buying disorders: Demographic, clinical, and psychiatric correlates. *Comprehensive Psychiatry, 86,* 67–73. https://doi.org/10.1016/j.comppsych.2018.07.013

Kimhi, S., Eshel, Y., Marciano, H., Adini, B., & Bonanno, G. A. (2021). Trajectories of depression and anxiety during COVID-19 associations with religion, income, and economic difficulties. *Journal of Psychiatric Research, 144,* 389–396. https://doi.org/10.1016/j.jpsychires.2021.10.043

Kimmel, R. J., Roy-Byrne, P. P., & Cowley, D. S. (2015). Pharmacological treatments for panic disorder, generalized anxiety disorder, specific phobia, and social anxiety disorder. In P. E. Nathan & J. M. Gorman (Eds.), *A guide to treatments that work* (pp. 463–505). New York: Oxford University Press.

King, J. D., McQuaid, A., Leeson, V. C., Samuel, O., Grant, J., Imran Azeem, M. S., Barnicot, K., & Crawford, M. J. (2023). The association of severe COVID anxiety with poor social functioning, quality of life, and protective behaviours among adults in United Kingdom: A cross-sectional study. *BMC Psychiatry, 23.* https://doi.org/10.1186/s12888-023-04595-1

Kings College London. (2019). King's College London enquiry into publications authored by Professor Hans Eysenck with Professor Ronald Grossarth Maticek. https://retractionwatch.com/wp-content/uploads/2019/10/HE-Enquiry.pdf

Kinsey, A. C., Pomeroy, W. B., & Martin, C. E. (1948). *Sexual behavior in the human male.* Philadelphia, PA: Saunders.

Kinsey, A. C., Pomeroy, W. B., Martin, C. E., & Gebhard, P. H. (1953). *Sexual behavior in the human female.* Philadelphia, PA: Saunders.

Kiosses, D. N., & Marino, P. (2019). Assessment of depression and anxiety in older adults. In L. D. Ravdin & H. L. Katzen (Eds.), *Handbook on the neuropsychology of aging and dementia* (2nd ed., pp. 49–59). Springer Nature Switzerland AG.

Klippel, A., Myin-Germeys, I., Chavez-Baldini, U., Preacher, K. J., Kempton, M., Valmaggia, L., . . . Reininghaus, U. (2017). Modeling the interplay between psychological processes and sdverse, stressful contexts and experiences in pathways to psychosis: An experience sampling study. *Schizophrenia Bulletin, 43* (2), 302–315. https://doi.org/10.1093/schbul/sbw185

Knapp, S., & VandeCreek, L. (2001). Ethical issues in personality assessment in forensic psychology. *Journal of Personality Assessment, 77,* 242–254.

Knopman, D. S. (2020). The enigma of decreasing dementia incidence. *JAMA Network Open, 3* (7), e2011199–e2011199. https://doi.org/10.1001/jamanetworkopen.2020.11199

Knutson, D., & Koch, J. M. (2019). Performance involvement, identity, and emotion among cisgender male drag queens. *Journal of Creativity in Mental Health, 14* (1), 54–69. https://doi.org/10.1080/15401383.2018.1549517

Ko, H.-C., & Kuo, F.-Y. (2009). Can blogging enhance subjective well-being through self-disclosure? *CyberPsychology & Behavior, 12,* 75–79.

Ko, K. Y., Ridley, N., Bryce, S. D., Allott, K., Smith, A., & Kamminga, J. (2022). Screening tools for cognitive impairment in adults with substance use disorders: A systematic review. *Journal of the International Neuropsychological Society, 28* (7), 756–779. https://doi.org/10.1017/S135561772100103X

Kocovski, N. L., Fleming, J. E., Hawley, L. L., Ho, M. R., & Antony, M. M. (2015). Mindfulness and acceptance-based group therapy and traditional cognitive behavioral group therapy for social anxiety disorder: Mechanisms of change. *Behaviour Research and Therapy,* 7011–7022. https://doi.org/10.1016/j.brat.2015.04.005

Kogan, S. M., Bae, D., Lei, M.-K., & Brody, G. H. (2019). Family-centered alcohol use prevention for African American adolescents: A randomized clinical trial. *Journal of Consulting and Clinical Psychology, 87* (12), 1085–1092. https://doi.org/10.1037/ccp0000448

Kohut, H. (1966). Forms and transformations of narcissism. *Journal of the American Psychoanalytic Association, 14,* 243–272.

Kohut, H. (1971). *The analysis of the self.* New York: International Universities Press.

Krick, L. C., Berman, M. E., McCloskey, M. S., Coccaro, E. F., & Fanning, J. R. (2022). Gender moderates the association between exposure to interpersonal violence and intermittent explosive disorder diagnosis. *Journal of Interpersonal Violence, 37* (15–16), NP14746–NP14771. https://doi.org/10.1177/08862605211013951

Krist, L., Keller, T., Sebald, L., Yesil-Jürgens, R., Ellert, U., Reich, A., . . . Liman, T. G. (2019). The Montreal Cognitive Assessment (MoCA) in a population-based sample of Turkish migrants living in Germany. *Aging & Mental Health, 23* (1), 30–https://doi.org/10.1080/13607863.2017.1396577

Kristjansson, A. L., Mann, M. J., Smith, M. L., Kogan, S. M., Lilly, C. L., & James, J. E. (2022). Caffeine consumption and onset of alcohol use among early adolescents. *Preventive Medicine: An International Journal Devoted to Practice and Theory, 163,* 1–4. https://doi.org/10.1016/j.ypmed.2022.107208

Krizan, Z., & Herlache, A. D. (2018). The narcissism spectrum model: A synthetic view of narcissistic personality. *Personality and Social Psychology Review, 22* (1), 3–31. https://doi.org/10.1177/1088868316685018

Kroon, E., Kuhns, L., & Cousijn, J. (2021). The short-term and long-term effects of cannabis on cognition: Recent advances in the field. *Current Opinion in Psychology, 38,* 49–55. https://doi.org/10.1016/j.copsyc.2020.07.005

Krueger, R. B., Reed, G. M., First, M. B., Marais, A., Kismodi, E., & Briken, P. (2017). Proposals for paraphilic disorders in the International Classification of Diseases and Related Health Problems, eleventh revision (ICD-11). *Archives of Sexual Behavior, 46* (5), 1529–1545. https://doi.org/10.1007/s10508-017-0944-2

Kuhl, E. S., Hoodin, F., Rice, J., Felt, B. T., Rausch, J. R., & Patton, S. R. (2010). Increasing daily water intake and fluid adherence in children receiving treatment for retentive encopresis. *Journal of Pediatric Psychology, 35,* 1144–1151.

Kuhn, J. (2015). Developmental dyscalculia: Causes, characteristics, and interventions. *Zeitschrift Für Psychologie, 223* (2), 67–68. https://doi.org/10.1027/2151-2604/a000204

Kuppalli, S., Seth, R., Orhurhu, V., Urits, I., Kaye, A. D., Hunter, C., . . . Jones, M. R. (2021). Recent advances in the treatment of opioid use disorder. *Current Pain and Headache Reports, 25* (4), 23. https://doi.org/10.1007/s11916-021-00941-8

Kvarstein, E. H., Antonsen, B. T., Klungsøyr, O., Pedersen, G., & Wilberg, T. (2021). Avoidant personality disorder and social functioning: A longitudinal, observational study investigating predictors of change in a clinical sample. *Personality Disorders: Theory, Research, and Treatment.* https://doi.org/10.1037/per0000471

Kysow, K., Bratiotis, C., Lauster, N., & Woody, S. R. (2020). How can cities tackle hoarding? Examining an intervention program bringing together fire and health authorities in Vancouver. *Health & Social Care in the Community, 28* (4), 1160–1169. https://doi.org/10.1111/hsc.12948

L

La Fond, J. Q. (1994). Law and the delivery of involuntary mental health services. *American Journal of Orthopsychiatry, 64,* 209–222.

Lady Gaga. (2016). "Head Stuck in a Cycle I Look Off and I Stare" A personal letter from Gaga. Retrieved 2/23/21 from https://bornthisway.foundation/personal-letter-gaga

Lady Gaga. (2020) *Lady Gaga tells Oprah she was " repeatedly " raped at 19 and developed PTSD/ Interviewer: C. Gillespie.* https://www.health.com/condition/ptsd/lady-gaga-rape-ptsd

Ladygaga [@ladygaga]. (2020). Video 911. Retrieved 2/23/21

Lahaie, M., Amsel, R., Khalifé, S., Boyer, S., Faaborg-Andersen, M., & Binik, Y. M. (2015). Can fear, pain, and muscle tension discriminate vaginismus from dyspareunia/provoked vestibulodynia? Implications for the new *DSM-5* diagnosis of genito-pelvic pain/penetration disorder. *Archives of Sexual Behavior, 44,* 1537–1550. https://doi.org/10.1007/s10508-014-0430-z

Laing, R. D. (1959). *The divided self.* Penguin.

Lam, C., & Chung, M.-H. (2021). A meta-analysis of the effect of interpersonal and social rhythm therapy on symptom and functioning improvement in patients with bipolar disorders. *Applied Research in Quality of Life, 16* (1), 153–165. https://doi.org/10.1007/s11482-019-09740-1

Lamb, D. H., Catanzaro, S. J., & Moorman, A. S. (2004). A preliminary look at how psychologists identify, evaluate, and proceed when faced with possible multiple relationship dilemmas. *Professional Psychology: Research and Practice, 35,* 248–254.

Lambert, H. K., & McLaughlin, K. A. (2019). Impaired hippocampus-dependent associative learning as a mechanism underlying PTSD: A meta-analysis. *Neuroscience and Biobehavioral Reviews, 107,* 729–749. https://doi.org/10.1016/j.neubiorev.2019.09.024

Lampe, L. (2016). Avoidant personality disorder as a social anxiety phenotype: Risk factors, associations and treatment. *Current Opinion in Psychiatry, 29* (1), 64–69. https://doi.org/10.1097/YCO.0000000000000211

Landgren, V., Malki, K., Bottai, M., Arver, S., & Rahm, C. (2020). Effect of gonadotropin-releasing hormone antagonist on risk of committing child sexual abuse in men with pedophilic disorder: A randomized clinical trial. *JAMA Psychiatry, 77* (9), 897–905. https://doi.org/10.1001/jamapsychiatry.2020.0440

Langevin, S., Mascheretti, S., Côté, S. M., Vitaro, F., Boivin, M., Turecki, G., Tremblay, R. E., & Ouellet-Morin, I. (2019). Cumulative risk and protection effect of serotonergic genes on male antisocial behaviour: Results from a prospective cohort assessed in adolescence and early adulthood. *The British Journal of Psychiatry, 214* (3), 137–145. https://doi.org/10.1192/bjp.2018.251

Långström, N. (2010). The *DSM* diagnostic criteria for exhibitionism, voyeurism, and frotteurism. *Archives of Sexual Behavior, 39,* 317–324.

Långström, N., & Seto, M. C. (2006). Exhibitionistic and voyeuristic behavior in a Swedish national population survey. *Archives of Sexual Behavior, 35,* 427–435.

Lantto, R., & Lundberg, T. (2022). (Un) desirable approaches in therapy with Swedish individuals practicing BDSM: Client's perspectives and recommendations for affirmative clinical practices. *Psychology & Sexuality, 13* (3), 742–755. https://doi.org/10.1080/19419899.2021.1918230

Laumann, E. O., & Waite, L. J. (2008). Sexual dysfunction among older adults: Prevalence and risk factors from a nationally representative U.S. probability sample of men and women 57–85 years of age. *Journal of Sexual Medicine, 5,* 2300–2311.

Lawrance, E. L., Thompson, R., Newberry Le Vay, J., Page, L., & Jennings, N. (2022). The impact of climate change on mental health and emotional wellbeing: A narrative review of current evidence, and its implications. *International Review of Psychiatry, 34* (5), 443–498. https://doi.org/10.1080/09540261.2022.2128725

Lawson, K. M., Kellerman, J. K., Kleiman, E. M., Bleidorn, W., Hopwood, C. J., & Robins, R. W. (2021). The role of temperament in the onset of suicidal ideation and behaviors across adolescence: Findings from a 10-year longitudinal study of Mexican-origin youth. *Journal of Personality and Social Psychology.* https://doi.org/10.1037/pspp0000382

Lazarus, A. A. (1968). Learning theory and the treatment of depression. *Behaviour Research and Therapy, 6,* 83–89.

Lazarus, R. S., & Folkman, S. (1984). *Stress, appraisal, and coping.* Springer.

LeBeau, R. T., Glenn, D., Liao, B., Wittchen, H. U., Beesdo-Baum, K., Ollendick, T., Craske, M. G. (2010). Specific phobia: A review of *DSM-IV* specific phobia and preliminary recommendations for *DSM-V. Depression and Anxiety, 27,* 148–167.

Lee, E. J., & Zwicker, J. G. (2021). Early identification of children with/at risk of developmental coordination disorder: A scoping review. *Developmental Medicine & Child Neurology.* https://doi.org/10.1111/dmcn.14803

Lee, K., & Ashton, M. C. (2004). Psychometric properties of the HEXACO personality inventory. *Multivariate Behavioral Research, 39* (2), 329–358. https://doi.org/10.1207/s15327906mbr3902_8

Lehmann, S., Breivik, K., Heiervang, E. R., Havik, T., & Havik, O. E. (2015). Reactive attachment disorder and disinhibited social engagement disorder in school-aged foster children—a confirmatory approach to dimensional measures. *Journal of Abnormal Child Psychology, 44* (3), 445–457. https://doi.org/10.1007/s10802-015-0045-4

Lei, D., Pinaya, W. H. L., van Amelsvoort, T., Marcelis, M., Donohoe, G., Mothersill, D. O., . . . Mechelli, A. (2020). Detecting schizophrenia at the level of the individual: Relative diagnostic value of whole-brain images, connectome-wide functional connectivity and graph-based metrics. *Psychological Medicine, 50* (11), 1852–1861. https://doi.org/10.1017/S0033291719001934

Leichsenring, F., & Steinert, C. (2017). Short-term psychodynamic therapy for obsessive-compulsive disorder: A manual-guided approach to treating the "inhibited rebel." *Bulletin of the Menninger Clinic, 81* (4), 341–389. https://doi.org/10.1521/bumc_2017_81_07

Lemer, J. L., Salafia, E. B., & Benson, K. E. (2013). The relationship between college women's sexual attitudes and sexual activity: The mediating role of body image. *International Journal of Sexual Health, 25,* 104–114. https://doi.org/10.1080/19317611.2012.722593

Lemieux, J. (2019). Mary J. Blige on recovery, healing, and taking care of herself. *Self.com.* https://www.self.com/story/mary-j-blige. Accessed 3/12/21.

Leonard, M.-J., Vasiliadis, H.-M., Leclerc, M.-È., & Brunet, A. (2023). Traumatic stress in Canadian lawyers: A longitudinal study. *Psychological Trauma: Theory, Research, Practice, and Policy, 15* (Suppl 2),

S259–S267. https://doi.org/10.1037/tra0001177 (Secondary Trauma)

Leong, F. T. L., Lui, P. P., & Kalibatseva, Z. (2020). Multicultural issues in clinical psychological assessment. In M. Sellbom & J. A. Suhr (Eds.), *The Cambridge handbook of clinical assessment and diagnosis* (pp. 25–37). Cambridge University Press.

Levaque, E., Dawson, S. J., Wan, C., & Lalumière, M. L. (2021). Sex drive as a possible mediator of the gender difference in the prevalence of paraphilic interests in a nonclinical sample. *Archives of Sexual Behavior*. https://doi.org/10.1007/s10508-021-02074-w

Levy, K. N., Johnson, B. N., Clouthier, T. L., Scala, J. W., & Temes, C. M. (2015). An attachment theoretical framework for personality disorders. *Canadian Psychology/Psychologie Canadienne, 56,* 197–207. https://doi.org/10.1037/cap0000025

Lewinsohn, P. M. (1974). A behavioral approach to depression. In R. J. Friedman & M. M. Katz (Eds.), *The psychology of depression: Contemporary theory and research* (pp. 157–174). John Wiley & Sons.

Lewis, R. W., Fugl-Meyer, K. S., Corona, G., Hayes, R. D., Laumann, E. O., Moreira, E. D., Jr., . . . Segraves, T. (2010). Definitions/epidemiology/risk factors for sexual dysfunction. *Journal of Sexual Medicine, 7,* 1598–1607.

Li, X., Li, S., Xiang, M., Fang, Y., Qian, K., Xu, J., . . . Wang, B. (2020). The prevalence and risk factors of PTSD symptoms among medical assistance workers during the COVID-19 pandemic. *Journal of Psychosomatic Research, 139.* https://doi.org/10.1016/j.jpsychores.2020.110270

Li, X., Tang, Y., Wang, C., & de Leon, J. (2015). Clozapine for treatment-resistant bipolar disorder: A systematic review. *Bipolar Disorders, 17,* 235–247. https://doi.org/10.1111/bdi.12272

Li, Z., Guo, Z., Wang, N., Xu, Z., Qu, Y., Wang, X., . . . Kingdon, D. (2015). Cognitive-behavioural therapy for patients with schizophrenia: A multicentre randomized controlled trial in Beijing, China. *Psychological Medicine, 45,* 1893–1905. https://doi.org/10.1017/S0033291714002992

Lim, J., Greenspoon, D., Hunt, A., & McAdam, L. (2020). Rehabilitation interventions in Rett syndrome: A scoping review. *Developmental Medicine & Child Neurology, 62* (8), 906–916. https://doi.org/10.1111/dmcn.14565

Lima Pereira, V., Freitas, S., Simões, M. R., & Gerardo, B. (2023). Montreal cognitive assessment (MoCA): A validation study among prisoners. *Criminal Behaviour and Mental Health.* https://doi.org/10.1002/cbm.2306

Lin, N., Bacala, L., Martin, S., Bratiotis, C., & Muroff, J. (2023). Hoarding disorder: The current evidence in conceptualization, intervention, and evaluation. *Psychiatric Clinics of North America, 46* (1), 181–196. https://doi.org/10.1016/j.psc.2022.10.007

Lin, P., Li, L., Wang, Y., Zhao, Z., Liu, G., Chen, W., . . . Gao, X. (2018). Type D personality, but not Type A behavior pattern, is associated with coronary plaque vulnerability. *Psychology, Health & Medicine, 23* (2), 216–223. https://doi.org/10.1080/13548506.2017.1344254

Linardon, J., Fairburn, C. G., Fitzsimmons-Craft, E. E., Wilfley, D. E., & Brennan, L. (2017). The empirical status of the third-wave behaviour therapies for the treatment of eating disorders: A systematic review. *Clinical Psychology Review, 58,* 125–140. https://doi.org/10.1016/j.cpr.2017.10.005

Lindberg, N., Holi, M. M., Tani, P., & Virkkunen, M. (2005). Looking for pyromania: Characteristics of a consecutive sample of Finnish male criminals with histories of recidivist fire-setting between 1973 and 1993. *BMC Psychiatry, 5,* 47.

Linde, J., Luoma, J. B., Rück, C., Ramnerö, J., & Lundgren, T. (2023). Acceptance and compassion-based therapy targeting shame in body dysmorphic disorder: A multiple baseline study. *Behavior Modification, 47* (3), 693–718. https://doi.org/10.1177/01454455221129989

Linden-Carmichael, A. N., & Lau-Barraco, C. (2017). A daily diary examination of caffeine mixed with alcohol among college students. *Health Psychology, 36* (9), 881–889. https://doi.org/10.1037/hea0000506

Lindley, L., & Galupo, M. P. (2020). Gender dysphoria and minority stress: Support for inclusion of gender dysphoria as a proximal stressor. *Psychology of Sexual Orientation and Gender Diversity, 7* (3), 265–275. https://doi.org/10.1037/sgd0000439

Linehan, M. (1993). *Cognitive-behavioral treatment of borderline personality disorder.* Guilford Press.

Linehan, M. (2014). *DBT® skills training manual.* Guilford Publications.

Linehan, M. M., Cochran, B. N., & Kehrer, C. A. (2001). Dialectical behavior therapy for borderline personality disorder. In D. H. Barlow (Ed.), *Clinical handbook of psychological disorders: A step-by-step treatment manual* (3rd ed., pp. 470–522). New York: Guilford Press.

Lino, F., & Chieffo, D. P. R. (2022). Developmental coordination disorder and most prevalent comorbidities: A narrative review. *Children (Basel), 9* (7). https://doi.org/10.3390/children9071095

Lintunen, J., Lähteenvuo, M., Tanskanen, A., Tiihonen, J., & Taipale, H. (2023). Non-adherence to mood stabilizers and antipsychotics among persons with bipolar disorder: A nationwide cohort study. *Journal of Affective Disorders, 333,* 403–408. https://doi.org/10.1016/j.jad.2023.04.030

Lisanby, S. H. (2007). Electroconvulsive therapy for depression. *New England Journal of Medicine, 357,* 1939–1945.

Lisko, J. G., Lee, G. E., Kimbrell, J. B., Rybak, M. E., Valentin-Blasini, L., & Watson, C. H. (2017). Caffeine concentrations in coffee, tea, chocolate, and energy drink flavored e-liquids. *Nicotine & Tobacco Research, 19* (4), 484–492.

Liu, C. I., Hua, M. H., Lu, M. L., & Goh, K. K. (2023). Effectiveness of cognitive behavioural-based interventions for adults with attention-deficit/hyperactivity disorder extends beyond core symptoms: A meta-analysis of randomized controlled trials. *Psychology and Psychotherapy: Theory, Research and Practice.* https://doi.org/10.1111/papt.12455

Liu, J., Teh, W. L., Tan, R. H. S., Tan, Y. B., Tang, C., Chandwani, N., & Subramaniam, M. (2023). Sleep disturbance as transdiagnostic mediator between adverse childhood experiences and psychopathology in children and adolescents: A structural equation modeling meta-analysis. *JCPP Advances.* https://doi.org/10.1002/jcv2.12156

Liu, M., Wang, N., Wang, P., Wu, H., Ding, X., & Zhao, F. (2021). Negative emotions and job burnout in news media workers: A moderated mediation model of rumination and empathy. *Journal of Affective Disorders, 279,* 75–82. https://doi.org/10.1016/j.jad.2020.09.123

Liu, W., Hua, M., Qin, J., Tang, Q., Han, Y., Tian, H., . . . Zhuo, C. (2020). Disrupted pathways from frontal-parietal cortex to basal ganglia and cerebellum in patients with unmedicated obsessive compulsive disorder as observed by whole-brain resting-state effective connectivity analysis—A small sample pilot study. *Brain Imaging and Behavior.* https://doi.org/10.1007/s11682-020-00333-3

Liu, W., Williams, K., Batchelor, M., Perkhounkova, Y., & Hein, M. (2021). Mealtime verbal interactions among nursing home staff and residents with dementia: A secondary behavioural analysis of videotaped observations. *Journal of Advanced Nursing, 77* (3), 1244–1257. https://doi.org/10.1111/jan.14647

Livingston, N. A., Farmer, S. L., Mahoney, C. T., Marx, B. P., & Keane, T. M. (2022). Longitudinal course of mental health symptoms among veterans with and without cannabis use disorder. *Psychology of Addictive Behaviors, 36* (2), 131–143. https://doi.org/10.1037/adb0000736

Lochner, C., Grant, J. E., Odlaug, B. L., & Stein, D. J. (2012). *DSM-5* field survey: Skin picking disorder. *Annals of Clinical Psychiatry, 24,* 300–304.

Lochner, C., Roos, A., & Stein, D. J. (2017). Excoriation (skin-picking) disorder: A systematic review of treatment options. *Neuropsychiatric Disease and Treatment, 13,* 1867–1872. https://doi.org/10.2147/NDT.S121138.

Lovato, D. (2013). *Staying strong: 365 days a year.* Feiwel & Friends.

Lui, P. P., & Zamboanga, B. L. (2018). A critical review and meta-analysis of the associations between acculturation and alcohol use outcomes among Hispanic Americans. *Alcoholism: Clinical and Experimental Research, 42* (10), 1841–1862. https://doi.org/10.1111/acer.13845

Lunsky, Y., Langdon, P. E., Redquest, B., & Summers, J. (2021). Intellectual and developmental disabilities and mental health. In L. M. Glidden, L. Abbeduto, L. L. McIntyre, & M. J. Tassé (Eds.), *APA handbook of intellectual and developmental disabilities: Foundations., Vol. 1.* (pp. 451–472). Washington, DC: American Psychological Association.

Luo, X., Law, S. F., Wang, X., Shi, J., Zeng, W., Ma, X., . . . Phillips, M. R. (2019). Effectiveness of an Assertive Community Treatment program for people with severe schizophrenia in mainland China–A 12-month randomized controlled trial. *Psychological Medicine, 49* (6), 969–979. https://doi.org/10.1017/S0033291718001629

Luoni, C., Scorza, M., Stefanelli, S., Fagiolini, B., & Termine, C. (2023). A neuropsychological profile of developmental dyscalculia: The role of comorbidity. *Journal of Learning Disabilities, 56* (4), 310–323. https://doi.org/10.1177/00222194221102925

Lynch, M. E., Kable, J. A., & Coles, C. D. (2015). Prenatal alcohol exposure, adaptive function, and entry into adult roles in a prospective study of young adults. *Neurotoxicology and Teratology, 51,* 52–60. https://doi.org/10.1016/j.ntt.2015.07.008

M

Mackenzie, K. (2018). Stereotypic movement disorders. *Seminars in Pediatric Neurology, 25,* 19–https://doi.org/https://doi.org/10.1016/j.spen.2017.12.004

Maggio, J. B., Ospina, J. P., Callahan, J., Hunt, A. L., Stephen, C. D., & Perez, D. L. (2020). Outpatient physical therapy for functional neurological disorder: A preliminary feasibility and naturalistic outcome study in a US cohort. *The Journal of Neuropsychiatry and Clinical Neurosciences, 32* (1), 85–89. https://doi.org/10.1176/appi.neuropsych.19030068

Magill, M., Apodaca, T. R., Borsari, B., Gaume, J., Hoadley, A., Gordon, R. F., . . . Moyers, T. (2018). A meta-analysis of motivational interviewing process: Technical, relational, and conditional process models of change. *Journal of Consulting and Clinical Psychology, 86* (2), 140–157. https://doi.org/10.1037/ccp0000250

Mahfoud, D., Hallit, S., Haddad, C., Fekih-Romdhane, F., & Haddad, G. (2023). The moderating effect of cognitive impairment on the relationship between inner speech and auditory verbal hallucinations among chronic patients with schizophrenia. *BMC Psychiatry, 23* (1). https://doi.org/10.1186/s12888-023-04940-4

Mai, C. T., Isenburg, J. L., Canfield, M. A., Meyer, R. E., Correa, A., Alverson, C. J., . . . Kirby, R. S. (2019). National population-based estimates for major birth defects, 2010–2014. *Birth Defects Res, 111* (18), 1420–1435. https://doi.org/10.1002/bdr2.1589

Maier, C. A., Riger, D., & Morgan-Sowada, H. (2021). "It's splendid once you grow into it": Client experiences of relational teletherapy in the era of COVID-19. *Journal of Marital and Family Therapy, 47* (2), 304–319. https://doi.org/10.1111/jmft.12508

Maniglio, R. (2014). Prevalence of sexual abuse among children with conduct disorder: A systematic review. *Clinical Child and Family Psychology Review, 17* (3), 268–282. https://doi.org/10.1007/s10567-013-0161-z

Mao, A. R., Babcock, T., & Brams, M. (2011). ADHD in adults: Current treatment trends with consideration of abuse potential of medications. *Journal of Psychiatric Practice, 17,* 241–250.

Marceau, K., McMaster, M. T. B., Smith, T. F., Daams, J. G., van Beijsterveldt, C. E. M., Boomsma, D. I., & Knopik, V. S. (2016). The prenatal environment in twin studies: A review on chorionicity. *Behavior Genetics, 46* (3), 286–303. https://doi.org/10.1007/s10519-016-9782-6

Maric, M., & Kok, S. I. (2023). How did the treatment work for Robin? And for Dylan? Studying individual youth treatment mediators using single-case experimental designs. *Clinical Child and Family Psychology Review.* https://doi.org/10.1007/s10567-023-00442-7

Marra, D. E., Hamlet, K. M., Bauer, R. M., & Bowers, D. (2020). Validity of teleneuropsychology for older adults in response to COVID-19: A systematic and critical review. *The Clinical Neuropsychologist, 34* (7–8), 1411–1452. https://doi.org/10.1080/13854046.2020.1769192

Marshall, V. B., Hooper, S. C., Gomez, F., Middlemass, K. M., Kilpela, L. S., & Becker, C. B. (2023). Posttraumatic stress disorder and other mental health correlates in a predominantly Latino/Hispanic sample living with food insecurity. *Psychological Trauma: Theory, Research, Practice, and Policy, 15* (7), 1094–1101. https://doi.org/10.1037/tra0001503

Martin-Vivar, M., Villena-Moya, A., Mestre-Bach, G., Hurtado-Murillo, F., & Chiclana-Actis, C. (2022). Treatments for persistent genital arousal disorder in women: A scoping review. *Journal of Sexual Medicine, 19* (6), 961–974. https://doi.org/10.1016/j.jsxm.2022.03.220

Martin, C. S., Steinley, D. L., Vergés, A., & Sher, K. J. (2011). The proposed 2/11 symptom algorithm for *DSM-5* substance use disorders is too lenient. *Psychological Medicine: A Journal of Research in Psychiatry and the Allied Sciences, 41,* 2008–2010.

Martino, D., & Pringsheim, T. M. (2018). Tourette syndrome and other chronic tic disorders: An update on clinical management. *Expert Review of Neurotherapeutics, 18* (2), 125–137. https://doi.org/10.1080/14737175.2018.1413938

Maslow, A. H. (1962). *Toward a psychology of being.* Van Nostrand.

Masters, W. H., & Johnson, V. E. (1966). *Human sexual response*. Boston, MA: Little Brown.

Masters, W. H., & Johnson, V. E. (1970). *Human sexual inadequacy.* Boston, MA: Little Brown.

Masterson, J. F. (1981). *The narcissistic and borderline disorders: An integrated developmental approach.* New York: Brunner/Mazel.

May, P. A., Marais, A.-S., Kalberg, W. O., de Vries, M. M., Buckley, D., Hasken, J. M., . . . Parry, C. D. H. (2023). Multifaceted case management during pregnancy is associated with better child outcomes and less fetal alcohol syndrome. *Annals of Medicine, 55* (1), 926–945. https://doi.org/10.1080/07853890.2023.2185808

May, R. (1983). *The discovery of being: Writings in existential psychology.* Norton.

Maye, M., Sanchez, V. E., Stone-MacDonald, A., & Carter, A. S. (2020). Early interventionists' appraisals of intervention strategies for toddlers with autism spectrum disorder and their peers in inclusive childcare classrooms. *Journal of Autism and Developmental Disorders, 50* (11), 4199–4208. https://doi.org/10.1007/s10803-020-04456-w

Mayne, S., Bowden, A., Sundvall, P.-D., & Gunnarsson, R. (2019). The scientific evidence for a potential link between confusion and urinary tract infection in the elderly is still confusing–A systematic literature review. *BMC Geriatrics, 19* (1), 32–32. https://doi.org/10.1186/s12877-019-1049-7

McAshan, B. (2017). NFL receiver Brandon Marshall speaks on borderline personality disorder at Menninger luncheon. https://www.tmc.edu/news/2019/05/nfl-receiver-brandon-marshall-speaks-on-borderline-personality-disorder-at-menninger-luncheon. Accessed 3/18/21.

McCabe, G. A., Smith, M. M., & Widiger, T. A. (2023). Psychopathy and antisocial personality disorder in the fifth edition of the American Psychiatric Association's Diagnostic and Statistical Manual of Mental Disorders: An attempted replication of Wygant et al. (2016). *Personality Disorders: Theory, Research, and Treatment.* https://doi.org/10.1037/per0000626 10.1037

McCabe, M. P., & Connaughton, C. (2014). How the prevalence rates of male sexual dysfunction vary using different criteria. *International Journal of Sexual Health, 26,* 229–237. https://doi.org/10.1080/19317611.2013.873104

McClintock, A. S., & Anderson, T. (2015). The application of mindfulness for interpersonal dependency: Effects of a brief intervention.

Mindfulness, 6, 243–252. https://doi.org/10.1007/s12671-013-0253-3

McClintock, A. S., & McCarrick, S. M. (2017). An examination of dependent personality disorder in the alternative *DSM-5* model for personality disorders. *Journal of Psychopathology and Behavioral Assessment, 39* (4), 635–641. https://doi.org/10.1007/s10862-017-9621-y

McCloskey, M. S., Chen, E. Y., Olino, T. M., & Coccaro, E. F. (2022). Cognitive-behavioral versus supportive psychotherapy for intermittent explosive disorder: A randomized controlled trial. *Behavior Therapy, 53* (6), 1133–1146. https://doi.org/10.1016/j.beth.2022.05.001

McCloskey, M. S., Kleabir, K., Berman, M. E., Chen, E. Y., & Coccaro, E. F. (2010). Unhealthy aggression: Intermittent explosive disorder and adverse physical health outcomes. *Health Psychology, 29,* 324–332.

McCrae, R. R., & Costa, P. T., Jr. (1987). Validation of the five-factor model of personality across instruments and observers. *Journal of Personality and Social Psychology, 52,* 81–90.

McDonald, S., Melkonian, M., Karin, E., Dear, B. F., Titov, N., & Wootton, B. M. (2023). Predictors of response to cognitive behavioural therapy (CBT) for individuals with obsessive-compulsive disorder (OCD): A systematic review. *Behavioural and Cognitive Psychotherapy, 51* (4), 302–319. https://doi.org/10.1017/S1352465823000103

McGuire, A., Steele, R. G., & Singh, M. N. (2021). Systematic review on the application of trauma-focused cognitive behavioral therapy (tf-cbt) for preschool-aged children. *Clinical Child and Family Psychology Review.* doi:10.1007/s10567-020-00334-0

McGuire, J. F., Myers, N. S., Lewin, A. B., Storch, E. A., & Rahman, O. (2020). The influence of hair pulling styles in the treatment of trichotillomania. *Behavior Therapy, 51* (6), 895–904. https://doi.org/10.1016/j.beth.2019.12.003

McHugh, R. K., Peckham, A. D., Björgvinsson, T., Korte, F. M., & Beard, C. (2020). Benzodiazepine misuse among adults receiving psychiatric treatment. *Journal of Psychiatric Research, 128,* 33–37. https://doi.org/10.1016/j.jpsychires.2020.05.020

McHugh, R. K., Whitton, S. W., Peckham, A. D., Welge, J. A., & Otto, M. W. (2013). Patient preference for psychological vs. pharmacological treatment of psychiatric disorders: A meta-analytic review. *Journal of Clinical Psychiatry, 74,* 595–602. https://doi.org/10.4088/JCP.12r07757

McKenna, K., Bray, M. A., Fitzmaurice, B., Choi, D., DeMaio, E., Bray, C. R., & Bernstein, C. (2023). Self-monitoring with goal-setting: Decreasing disruptive behavior in children with attention-deficit/hyperactivity disorder. *Psychology in the Schools.* https://doi.org/10.1002/pits.23026

McMillan, G. (2020). IRB policies for obtaining informed consent from non-English-speaking people. *Ethics & Human Research, 42* (3), 21–29. doi:10.1002/eahr.500050

McNamara, K. (2023). Lowering the age of consent: Legal, ethical, and clinical implications of adolescent-directed therapy. *Family Court Review, 61* (3), 472–477. https://doi.org/10.1111/fcre.12722

McQuillan, V. A., Swanwick, R. A., Chambers, M. E., Schlüter, D. K., & Sugden, D. A. (2021). A comparison of characteristics, developmental disorders and motor progression between children with and without developmental coordination disorder. *Human Movement Science, 78.* https://doi.org/10.1016/j.humov.2021.102823

Melikyan, Z. A., Agranovich, A. V., & Puente, A. E. (2019). Fairness in psychological testing. In G. Goldstein, D. N. Allen, & J. DeLuca (Eds.), *Handbook of psychological assessment* (4th ed., pp. 551–572). Elsevier Academic Press.

Melikyan, Z. A., Puente, A. E., & Agranovich, A. V. (2021). Cross-cultural comparison of rural healthy adults: Russian and American groups. *Archives of Clinical Neuropsychology, 36* (3), 359–370. https://doi.org/10.1093/arclin/acz071

Mennigen, E., & Bearden, C. E. (2020). Psychosis risk and development: What do we know from population-based studies? *Biological Psychiatry, 88* (4), 315–325. https://doi.org/10.1016/j.biopsych.2019.12.014

Menzel, J. (2018). Avoidant/restrictive food intake disorder: Assessment and treatment. In L. K. Anderson, S. B. Murray, & W. H. Kaye (Eds.), *Clinical handbook of complex and atypical eating disorders* (pp. 149–168). Oxford University Press.

Merced, K., Pugh, M., Jr., Klyce, D. W., Ohayagha, C., & Perrin, P. B. (2022). Exploring racial performance disparities with the Modified Mini-Mental State Exam (3MS) in an acute brain injury rehabilitation setting. *Rehabilitation Psychology, 67* (4), 597–601. https://doi.org/10.1037/rep0000465

Merikangas, K. R., Jin, R., He, J.-P., Kessler, R. C., Lee, S., Sampson, N. A., . . . Zarkov, Z. (2011). Prevalence and correlates of bipolar spectrum disorder in the World Mental Health Survey Initiative. *Archives of General Psychiatry, 68* (3), 241–251. https://doi.org/10.1001/archgenpsychiatry.2011.12

Mersha, A. G., Eftekhari, P., Bovill, M., Tollosa, D. N., & Gould, G. S. (2021). Evaluating level of adherence to nicotine replacement therapy and its impact on smoking cessation: A systematic review and meta-analysis. *Archives of Public Health, 79* (1), 26. https://doi.org/10.1186/s13690-021-00550-2

Metz, M. E., Epstein, N. B., & McCarthy, B. (2018). *Cognitive-behavioral therapy for sexual dysfunction.* Routledge/Taylor & Francis Group.

Meyer, G. J., & Eblin, J. J. (2012). An overview of the Rorschach Performance Assessment System (R-PAS). *Psychological Injury and Law, 5* (2), 107–121. https://doi.org/10.1007/s12207-012-9130-y

Michalski, S. C., Ellison, C., Szpak, A., & Loetscher, T. (2021). Vocational training in virtual environments for people with neurodevelopmental disorders: A systematic review. *Frontiers in Psychology, 12.* https://doi.org/10.3389/fpsyg.2021.627301

Michel, E., Molitor, S., & Schneider, W. (2018). Differential changes in the development of motor coordination and executive functions in children with motor coordination impairments. *Child Neuropsychology, 24* (1), 20–45. https://doi.org/10.1080/09297049.2016.1223282

Milinkovic, M. S., & Tiliopoulos, N. (2020). A systematic review of the clinical utility of the *DSM-5* section III alternative model of personality disorder. *Personality Disorders: Theory, Research, and Treatment, 11* (6), 377–397. https://doi.org/10.1037/per0000408

Mills, L., Lee, J. C., Boakes, R., & Colagiuri, B. (2023). Reduction in caffeine withdrawal after open-label decaffeinated coffee. *Journal of Psychopharmacology, 37* (2), 181–191. https://doi.org/10.1177/02698811221147152

Miranda, A. R., Franchetto Sierra, J., Martínez Roulet, A., Rivadero, L., Serra, S. V., & Soria, E. A. (2020). Age, education and gender effects on Wisconsin card sorting test: Standardization, reliability and validity in healthy Argentinean adults. *Aging, Neuropsychology, and Cognition, 27* (6), 807–825. https://doi.org/10.1080/13825585.2019.1693491

Mitchell, D., Tafrate, R. C., & Freeman, A. (2015). Antisocial personality disorder. In A. T. Beck, D. D. Davis, & A. Freeman (Eds.), *Cognitive therapy of personality disorders* (3rd ed., pp. 346–365). Guilford Press.

Modlin, N. L., Miller, T. M., Rucker, J. J., Kirlic, N., Lennard-Jones, M., Schlosser, D., & Aaronson, S. T. (2023). Optimizing outcomes in psilocybin therapy: Considerations in participant evaluation and preparation. *Journal of Affective Disorders, 326,* 18–https://doi.org/10.1016/j.jad.2023.01.077

Mohajerin, B., Lynn, S. J., Bakhtiyari, M., & Dolatshah, B. (2019). Evaluating the unified protocol in the treatment of dissociative identify disorder. *Cognitive and Behavioral Practice.* https://doi.org/10.1016/j.cbpra.2019.07.012

Mohd Hasim, M. J., Hashim, N. H., & Mustafa, H. (2023). Married life: Measuring adult romantic attachment and satisfaction. *Couple and Family Psychology: Research and Practice, 12* (3), 119–131. https://doi.org/10.1037/cfp0000188

Molitor, S. J., & LeNoble, J. (2023). Integrating parent mental health assessment into pediatric psychology: Applying an ethics-based model. *Clinical Practice in*

Pediatric Psychology, 11 (3), 350–356. https://doi.org/10.1037/cpp0000457

Mond, J., Mitchison, D., Latner, J., Hay, P., Owen, C., & Rodgers, B. (2013). Quality of life impairment associated with body dissatisfaction in a general population sample of women. *BMC Public Health, 13,* https://doi.org/10.1186/1471-2458-13-920

Monroe, S. M., Anderson, S. F., & Harkness, K. L. (2019). Life stress and major depression: The mysteries of recurrences. *Psychological Review, 126* (6), 791–816. https://doi.org/10.1037/rev0000157

Montalvo-Ortiz, J. L., Zhang, H., Chen, C., Liu, C., & Coccaro, E. F. (2018). Genome-wide DNA methylation changes associated with intermittent explosive disorder: A gene-based functional enrichment analysis. *International Journal of Neuropsychopharmacology, 21* (1), 12–20. https://doi.org/10.1093/ijnp/pyx087

Monteleone, A. M., Cascino, G., Ruzzi, V., Pellegrino, F., Patriciello, G., Barone, E., . . . Maj, M. (2020). Emotional traumatic experiences significantly contribute to identify a maltreated ecophenotype sub-group in eating disorders: Experimental evidence. *European Eating Disorders Review.* https://doi.org/10.1002/erv.2818

Moore, A. A., Silberg, J. L., Roberson-Nay, R., & Mezuk, B. (2017). Life course persistent and adolescence limited conduct disorder in a nationally representative US sample: Prevalence, predictors, and outcomes. *Social Psychiatry and Psychiatric Epidemiology: The International Journal for Research in Social and Genetic Epidemiology and Mental Health Services, 52* (4), 435–443. https://doi.org/10.1007/s00127-017-1337-5

Morin, J. W., & Levenson, J. S. (2008). Exhibitionism: Assessment and treatment. In D. R. Laws & W. T. O'Donohue (Eds.), *Sexual deviance: Theory, assessment, and treatment* (2nd ed., pp. 76–107). New York: Guilford Press.

Morina, N., Ijntema, H., Meyerbröker, K., & Emmelkamp, P. M. (2015). Can virtual reality exposure therapy gains be generalized to real-life? A meta-analysis of studies applying behavioral assessments. *Behaviour Research and Therapy,* 7418–7424. https://doi.org/10.1016/j.brat.2015.08.010

Morishita, C., Inoue, T., Honyashiki, M., Ono, M., Iwata, Y., Tanabe, H., Kusumi, I., & Masuya, J. (2022). Roles of childhood maltreatment, personality traits, and life stress in the prediction of severe premenstrual symptoms. *BioPsychoSocial Medicine, 16.* https://doi.org/10.1186/s13030-022-00240-7

Moritz, S., Penney, D., Bruhns, A., Weidinger, S., & Schmotz, S. (2023). Habit reversal training and variants of decoupling for use in body-focused repetitive behaviors A randomized controlled trial. *Cognitive Therapy and Research, 47* (1), 109–122. https://doi.org/10.1007/s10608-022-10334-9.

Morland, L. A., Knopp, K. C., Khalifian, C. E., Macdonald, A., Grubbs, K. M., Mackintosh, . . . Monson, C. M. (2022). A randomized trial of brief couple therapy for PTSD and relationship satisfaction. *Journal of Consulting and Clinical Psychology, 90* (5), 392–404. https://doi.org/10.1037/ccp0000731

Morreale, M., Holingue, C., Samuels, J., & Nestadt, G. (2021). Long-term physical health outcomes of obsessive-compulsive personality disorder traits. *Journal of Clinical Psychology, 77* (11), 2626–2637. https://doi.org/10.1002/jclp.23207

Morris, E. R., Lindley, L., & Galupo, M. P. (2020). "Better issues to focus on": Transgender microaggressions as ethical violations in therapy. *The Counseling Psychologist, 48* (6), 883–915. https://doi.org/10.1177/0011000020924391

Mufson, E. J., Perez, S. E., Nadeem, M., Mahady, L., Kanaan, N. M., Abrahamson, E. E., . . . McKee, A. C. (2016). Progression of tau pathology within cholinergic nucleus basalis neurons in chronic traumatic encephalopathy: A chronic effects of neurotrauma consortium study. *Brain Injury, 30* (12), 1399–1413. https://doi.org/10.1080/02699052.2016.1219058

Müller, C. P., Schumann, G., Rehm, J., Kornhuber, J., & Lenz, B. (2023). Self-management with alcohol over lifespan: Psychological mechanisms, neurobiological underpinnings, and risk assessment. *Molecular Psychiatry.* https://doi.org/10.1038/s41380-023-02074-3

Müller, E., & VanGilder, R. (2014). The relationship between participation in Project SEARCH and job readiness and employment for young adults with disabilities. *Journal of Vocational Rehabilitation, 40* (1), 15–26.

Müller, K. W., Wölfling, K., Dickenhorst, U., Beutel, M. E., Medenwaldt, J., & Koch, A. (2017). Recovery, relapse, or else? Treatment outcomes in gambling disorder from a multicenter follow-up study. *European Psychiatry, 43,* 28–34. https://doi.org/10.1016/j.eurpsy.2017.01.326

Muris, P., & Ollendick, T. H. (2021). Selective mutism and its relations to social anxiety disorder and autism spectrum disorder. *Clinical Child and Family Psychology Review.* https://doi.org/10.1007/s10567-020-00342-0

Murnen, S. K., & Smolak, L. (2019). The CASH effect: Shaping the research conversation on body image and eating disorders. *Body Image, 31,* 288–293. https://doi.org/10.1016/j.bodyim.2019.01.001

Murphy, R., Calugi, S., Cooper, Z., & Dalle Grave, R. (2020). Challenges and opportunities for enhanced cognitive behaviour therapy (CBT-E) in light of COVID- *The Cognitive Behaviour Therapist, 13.* https://doi.org/10.1017/S1754470X20000161

Murphy, W. D., & Page, I. J. (2008). Exhibitionism: Psychopathology and theory. In D. R. Laws & W. T. O'Donohue (Eds.), *Sexual deviance: Theory, assessment, and treatment* (2nd ed., pp. 61–75). New York: Guilford Press.

Murray, R. M., Bhavsar, V., Tripoli, G., & Howes, O. (2017). 30 years on: How the neurodevelopmental hypothesis of schizophrenia morphed into the developmental risk factor model of psychosis. *Schizophrenia Bulletin, 43* (6), 1190–1196. https://doi.org/10.1093/schbul/sbx121

Musetti, A., Eboli, G., Cavallini, F., & Corsano, P. (2019). Social relationships, self-esteem, and loneliness in adolescents with learning disabilities. *Clinical Neuropsychiatry: Journal of Treatment Evaluation, 16* (4), 165–172.

Mushtaq, A., & Khan, M. A. (2023). Social isolation, loneliness, and mental health among older adults during COVID-19: A scoping review. *Journal of Gerontological Social Work.* https://doi.org/10.1080/01634372.2023.2237076

N

Na, S., & King, T. Z. (2019). Performance discrepancies on the Boston Naming Test in African-American and non-Hispanic White American young adults. *Applied Neuropsychology: Adult, 26* (3), 236–246. https://doi.org/10.1080/23279095.2017.1393427

Nadeau, M. M., Rochlen, A. B., & Tyminski, R. (2019). The psychology of shoplifting: Development of a new typology for repeated shoplifting. *International Journal of Offender Therapy and Comparative Criminology, 63* (13), 2338–2355. https://doi.org/10.1177/0306624X19845979

Nagata, J. M., Ganson, K. T., & Austin, S. B. (2020). Emerging trends in eating disorders among sexual and gender minorities. *Current Opinion in Psychiatry, 33* (6), 562–567. https://doi.org/10.1097/YCO.0000000000000645

Nagoshi, J. L., & Brzuzy, S. I. (2010). Transgender theory: Embodying research and practice. *Affilia: Journal of Women & Social Work, 25,* 431–443.

Nahas, A. (2019). Lamar Odom feels deep regret about cheating on and lying to Ex Khloé Kardashian. *People.* Retrieved 3/3/21 from https://people.com/tv/lamar-odom-feels-deep-regret-about-cheating-on-lying-to-khloe-kardashian

Nakama, N., Usui, N., Doi, M., & Shimada, S. (2023). Early life stress impairs brain and mental development during childhood increasing the risk of developing psychiatric disorders. *Progress in Neuro-Psychopharmacology & Biological Psychiatry, 126,* 1–8. https://doi.org/10.1016/j.pnpbp.2023.110783

Naoi, M., Maruyama, W., & Shamoto-Nagai, M. (2018). Type A monoamine oxidase and serotonin are coordinately involved in depressive disorders: From neurotransmitter imbalance to impaired neurogenesis. *Journal*

of Neural Transmission, 125 (1), 53–66. https://doi.org/10.1007/s00702-017-1709-8

Naragon-Gainey, K., & Watson, D. (2018). What lies beyond neuroticism? An examination of the unique contributions of social-cognitive vulnerabilities to internalizing disorders. *Assessment, 25* (2), 143–158. https://doi.org/10.1177/1073191116659741

Nasreddine, Z. S., & Patel, B. B. (2016). Validation of Montreal cognitive assessment, MoCA, alternate French versions. *The Canadian Journal of Neurological Sciences / Le Journal Canadien Des Sciences Neurologiques, 43* (5), 665–671. https://doi.org/10.1017/cjn.2016.273

Nasreddine, Z. S., Phillips, N. A., Bédirian, V., Charbonneau, S., Whitehead, V., Collin, I., . . . Chertkow, H. (2005). The Montreal Cognitive Assessment, MoCA: A brief screening tool for mild cognitive impairment. *Journal of the American Geriatrics Society, 53* (4), 695–699. https://doi.org/10.1111/j.1532-5415.2005.53221.x

National Institute of Drug Abuse. (2019). *Substance use and military life.* https://www.drugabuse.gov/publications/drugfacts/substance-use-military-life. Accessed 3/8/21.

National Institute of Mental Health. (2020). Questions and answers about the National Comorbidity Survey Replication (NCSR) study. https://www.nimh.nih.gov/health/topics/ncsr-study/questions-and-answers-about-the-national-comorbidity-survey-replication-ncsr-study.shtml

National Institute of Mental Health. (2023). Major depression. Retrieved 9/13/23 from https://www.nimh.nih.gov/health/statistics/major-depression

National Institute of Mental Health. (2023). Schizophrenia. Retrieved 9/8/23 from https://www.nimh.nih.gov/health/statistics/schizophrenia

National Institute on Aging. (2023a). Stages of Alzheimer's disease. https://www.nia.nih.gov/health/alzheimers-disease-fact-sheet#stages

National Institute on Aging. (2023b). Age-related forgetfulness or signs of dementia? https://www.nia.nih.gov/health/infographics/age-related-forgetfulness-or-signs-dementia

National Institute on Alcohol Abuse and Alcoholism. (2007). Helping patients who drink too much: A clinician's guide. https://pubs.niaaa.nih.gov/publications/practitioner/cliniciansguide2005/guide.pdf. Accessed 6/5/2018.

National Institute on Drug Abuse. (2020a). Common comorbidities with substance use disorders research report. https://www.drugabuse.gov/download/1155/common-comorbidities-substance-use-disorders-research-report.pdf?v=5d6a5983e0e9353d46d01767fb20354b. Accessed 3/5/21.

Nelson, J. (2021). Lady Gaga talks show-stopping inauguration performance: "It was the honor of my lifetime". *People.* Retrieved 2/23/21 from https://people.com/music/lady-gaga-calls-inauguration-performance-honor-of-lifetime

Nelson, P. T., Dickson, D. W., Trojanowski, J. Q., Jack, C. R., Boyle, P. A., Arfanakis, K., . . . Schneider, J. A. (2019). Limbic-predominant age-related TDP-43 encephalopathy (LATE): Consensus working group report. *Brain, 142* (6), 1503–1527. https://doi.org/10.1093/brain/awz099

Neumann, N., Dubischar-Krivec, A. M., Braun, C., Löw, A., Poustka, F., Bölte, S., & Birbaumer, N. (2010). The mind of the mnemonists: An MEG and neuropsychological study of autistic memory savants. *Behavioural Brain Research, 215,* 114–121.

Newbury-Helps, J., Feigenbaum, J., & Fonagy, P. (2017). Offenders with antisocial personality disorder display more impairments in mentalizing. *Journal of Personality Disorders, 31* (2), 232–255. https://doi.org/10.1521/pedi_2016_30_246

Newcomb, M. E., Hill, R., Buehler, K., Ryan, D. T., Whitton, S. W., & Mustanski, B. (2020). High burden of mental health problems, substance use, violence, and related psychosocial factors in transgender, non-binary, and gender diverse youth and young adults. *Archives of Sexual Behavior, 49* (2), 645–659. https://doi.org/10.1007/s10508-019-01533-9

Newcorn, J. H., Krone, B., & Dittmann, R. W. (2022). Nonstimulant treatments for ADHD. *Child and Adolescent Psychiatric Clinics of North America, 31* (3), 417–435. https://doi.org/10.1016/j.chc.2022.03.005

News release. (2018). NIH launches HEAL initiative, doubles funding to accelerate scientific solutions to stem national opioid epidemic. National Institute of Health. https://www.nih.gov/news-events/news-releases/nih-launches-heal-initiative-doubles-funding-accelerate-scientific-solutions-stem-national-opioid-epidemic. Accessed 4/12/2018.

Nguyen, H. (2014). Buddhism-based exorcism and spirit-calling as a form of healing for mental problems: Stories from Vietnam. *Journal of Religion & Spirituality in Social Work: Social Thought, 33* (1), 33–48. https://doi.org/10.1080/15426432.2014.873648

Nichols, A. (2023). Twenty years after Andrea: Postpartum psychosis and the insanity defense. *Family Court Review, 61* (2), 443–457. https://doi.org/10.1111/fcre.12702

Nielsen, J. D., Mennies, R. J., & Olino, T. M. (2020). Application of a diathesis-stress model to the interplay of cortical structural development and emerging depression in youth. *Clinical Psychology Review, 82.* https://doi.org/10.1016/j.cpr.2020.101922

Niemyjska, A., & Parzuchowski, M. (2020). You make all things special: Developing a scale to measure sympathetic magic in romantic relationships. *Current Psychology: A Journal for Diverse Perspectives on Diverse Psychological Issues, 39* (5), 1635–1647. https://doi.org/10.1007/s12144-018-9861-3

Nikstat, A., Beam, C. R., & Riemann, R. (2023). Gene-environment interplay in internalizing problem behavior. *Developmental Psychology, 59* (8), 1470–1483. https://doi.org/10.1037/dev0001567 10.1037/dev0001567.supp (Supplemental)

Njoroge, W. F. M., Forkpa, M., & Bath, E. (2021). Impact of racial discrimination on the mental health of minoritized youth. *Current Psychiatry Reports, 23* (12), 81. https://doi.org/10.1007/s11920-021-01297-x

Nobakht, H. N., Steinsbekk, S., & Wichstrøm, L. (2023). Development of symptoms of oppositional defiant disorder from preschool to adolescence: The role of bullying victimization and emotion regulation. *Journal of Child Psychology and Psychiatry.* https://doi.org/10.1111/jcpp.13845

Nøhr, A. K., Eriksson, H., Hobart, M., Moltke, I., Buller, R., Albrechtsen, A., & Lindgreen, S. (2021). Predictors and trajectories of treatment response to SSRIs in patients suffering from PTSD. *Psychiatry Research, 301.* https://doi.org/10.1016/j.psychres.2021.113964

Nolte, K., Romo, E., Stopka, T. J., Drew, A., Dowd, P., Del Toro-Mejias, L., Bianchet, E., & Friedmann, P. D. (2023). "I've been to more of my friends' funerals than I've been to my friends' weddings": Witnessing and responding to overdose in rural Northern New England. *The Journal of Rural Health, 39* (1), 197–211. https://doi.org/10.1111/jrh.12660

Nota, L., Ginevra, M. C., & Soresi, S. (2019). School inclusion of children with intellectual disability: An intervention program. *Journal of Intellectual and Developmental Disability, 44* (4), 439–446. https://doi.org/10.3109/13668250.2018.1428785

Novak, C. E., Keuthen, N. J., Stewart, S. E., & Pauls, D. L. (2009). A twin concordance study of trichotillomania. *American Journal of Medical Genetics Series B: Neuropsychiatry of Genetics, 150B,* 944–949.

Nower, L., Blaszczynski, A., & Anthony, W. L. (2022). Clarifying gambling subtypes: The revised pathways model of problem gambling. *Addiction, 117* (7), 2000–2008. https://doi.org/10.1111/add.15745

Nübel, J., Guhn, A., Müllender, S., Le, H. D., Cohrdes, C., & Köhler, S. (2020). Persistent depressive disorder across the adult lifespan: Results from clinical and population-based surveys in Germany. *BMC Psychiatry, 20.* https://doi.org/10.1186/s12888-020-2460-5

O

Ó Ciardha, C., Ildeniz, G., & Karoğlu, N. (2022). The prevalence of sexual interest in children and sexually harmful behavior self-reported by men recruited through an online crowdsourcing platform. *Sexual Abuse: Journal of Research and Treatment, 34* (2), 207–226. https://doi.org/10.1177/10790632211013811

O'Connor v. Donaldson. (1975). 95 S. Ct. 2486.

O'Connor, L. K., Yanos, P. T., & Firmin, R. L. (2018). Correlates and moderators of stigma resistance among people with severe mental illness. *Psychiatry Research, 270,* 198–204. https://doi.org/10.1016/j.psychres.2018.09.040

Oakley, S. H., Vaccaro, C. M., Crisp, C. C., Estanol, M. V., Fellner, A. N., Kleeman, S. D., & Pauls, R. N. (2014). Clitoral size and location in relation to sexual function using pelvic MRI. *Journal of Sexual Medicine, 11,* 1013–1022. https://doi.org/10.1111/jsm.12450

Oberai, T., Laver, K., Crotty, M., Killington, M., & Jaarsma, R. (2018). Effectiveness of multicomponent interventions on incidence of delirium in hospitalized older patients with hip fracture: A systematic review. *International Psychogeriatrics, 30* (4), 481–492. https://doi.org/10.1017/S1041610217002782

Oberheim, S. T., Swank, J. M., & DePue, M. K. (2017). Building culturally sensitive assessments for transgender clients: Best practices for instrument development and the adaptation process. *Journal of LGBT Issues in Counseling, 11* (4), 259–270. https://doi.org/10.1080/15538605.2017.1380554

Odom, L. (2019). *Darkness to light: A memoir.* Dallas TX: BenBella Books, Inc.

Oh, E. S., Fong, T. G., Hshieh, T. T., & Inouye, S. K. (2017). Delirium in older persons: Advances in diagnosis and treatment. *Journal of the American Medical Association, 318* (12), 1161–1174. https://doi.org/10.1001/jama.2017.12067

Oh, S., & Shillingford-Butler, A. (2020). The client assessment of multicultural competent behavior (CAMCB): Development and validation. *Measurement and Evaluation in Counseling and Development.* https://doi.org/10.1080/07481756.2020.1745651

Olbrich, S., Jahn, I., & Stengler, K. (2019). Exposure and response prevention therapy augmented with naltrexone in kleptomania: A controlled case study using galvanic skin response for monitoring. *Behavioural and Cognitive Psychotherapy, 47* (5), 622–627. https://doi.org/10.1017/S1352465819000213

Olfson, M., Gerhard, T., Huang, C., Crystal, S., & Stroup, T. S. (2015). Premature mortality among adults with schizophrenia in the United States. *JAMA Psychiatry, 72* (12), 1172–1181. https://doi.org/10.1001/jamapsychiatry.2015.1737

Olivari, C., Di Cugno, M., & Caselli, G. (2023). Sexual dysfunctions and metacognitive beliefs: A prisma-compliant systematic review. *Sexual and Relationship Therapy.* https://doi.org/10.1080/14681994.2023.2253742

Ollendick, T. H., Öst, L., Ryan, S. M., Capriola, N. N., & Reuterskiöld, L. (2017). Harm beliefs and coping expectancies in youth with specific phobias. *Behaviour Research and Therapy, 91,* 51–57. https://doi.org/10.1016/j.brat.2017.01.007

Ollikainen, M., Smith, K. R., Joo, E. J., Ng, H. K., Andronikos, R., Novakovic, B., . . . Craig, J. M. (2010). DNA methylation analysis of multiple tissues from newborn twins reveals both genetic and intrauterine components to variation in the human neonatal epigenome. *Human Molecular Genetics, 19,* 4176–4188.

Olusanya, B. O., Smythe, T., Ogbo, F. A., Nair, M. K. C., Scher, M., & Davis, A. C. (2023). Global prevalence of developmental disabilities in children and adolescents: A systematic umbrella review. *Frontiers in Public Health, 11,* 1122009. https://doi.org/10.3389/fpubh.2023.1122009

Omer, J., Mohammed, S. H., Salih, R. Q., Kakamad, F. H., Mikael, T. M., Mohammed, K. K., . . . Salih, A. M. (2019). Predatory journals in psychiatry. *The Lancet Psychiatry, 6* (7), 564–565. https://doi.org/10.1016/S2215-0366(19)30185-3

Orjiakor, C. T., Sellbom, M., Keeley, J. W., & Bagby, R. M. (2023). Measurement invariance of the Personality Inventory for the DSM-5 (PID-5) for Nigerian and White American university students. *Psychological Assessment, 35* (8), 715–720. https://doi.org/10.1037/pas0001251

Osa, N., Penelo, E., Navarro, J. B., Trepat, E., & Ezpeleta, L. (2019). Prevalence, comorbidity, functioning and long-term effects of subthreshold oppositional defiant disorder in a community sample of preschoolers. *European Child & Adolescent Psychiatry.* https://doi.org/10.1007/s00787-019-01300-0

Oshana, A., Klimek, P., & Blashill, A. J. (2020). Minority stress and body dysmorphic disorder symptoms among sexual minority adolescents and adult men. *Body Image, 34,* 167–174. https://doi.org/10.1016/j.bodyim.2020.06.001

Osório, F. L., Loureiro, S. R., Hallak, J. E. C., Machado-de-Sousa, J. P., Ushirohira, J. M., Baes, C. V. W., . . . Crippa, J. A. S. (2019). Clinical validity and intrarater and test-retest reliability of the Structured Clinical Interview for DSM-5—Clinician Version (SCID-5-CV). *Psychiatry and Clinical Neurosciences, 73* (12), 754–760. https://doi.org/10.1111/pcn.12931

Ottisova, L., Smith, P., & Oram, S. (2018). Psychological consequences of human trafficking: Complex posttraumatic stress disorder in trafficked children. *Behavioral Medicine, 44* (3), 234–241. https://doi.org/10.1080/08964289.2018.1432555

Overk, C. R., & Masliah, E. (2014). Pathogenesis of synaptic degeneration in Alzheimer's disease and Lewy body disease. *Biochemical Pharmacology, 88* (4), 508–516. https://doi.org/10.1016/j.bcp.2014.01.015

Oxman, T. E., Barrett, J. E., Sengupta, A., & Williams, J. W., Jr. (2000). The relationship of aging and dysthymia in primary care. *The American Journal of Geriatric Psychiatry, 8,* 318–326.

P

Packard, G., Molloy, A., & Anderson, P. L. (2022). Trait mindfulness is related to attention bias toward threat and attention bias variability in social anxiety disorder. *Current Psychology: A Journal for Diverse Perspectives on Diverse Psychological Issues.* https://doi.org/10.1007/s12144-022-02817-5

Packer, I. K., & Kois, L. E. (2023). Criminal responsibility evaluations. In D. DeMatteo & K. C. Scherr (Eds.), *The Oxford handbook of psychology and law* (pp. 170–185). Oxford University Press. https://doi.org/10.1093/oxfordhb/9780197649138.013.10

Padmanabhan, A., Lynch, C. J., Schaer, M., & Menon, V. (2017). The Default Mode Network in autism. *Biological Psychiatry: Cognitive Neuroscience and Neuroimaging, 2* (6), 476–486. https://doi.org/10.1016/j.bpsc.2017.04.004

Palermo, G. B. (2015). A look at firesetting, arson, and pyromania. *International Journal of Offender Therapy and Comparative Criminology, 59* (7), 683–684. https://doi.org/10.1177/0306624X15586217

Palma-Gudiel, H., Córdova-Palomera, A., Navarro, V., & Fañanás, L. (2020). Twin study designs as a tool to identify new candidate genes for depression: A systematic review of DNA methylation studies. *Neuroscience and Biobehavioral Reviews, 112,* 345–https://doi.org/10.1016/j.neubiorev.2020.02.017

Panayotis, N., Ehinger, Y., Felix, M. S., & Roux, J. C. (2023). State-of-the-art therapies for Rett syndrome. *Developmental Medicine & Child Neurology, 65* (2), 162–170. https://doi.org/10.1111/dmcn.15383

Papola, D., Ostuzzi, G., Tedeschi, F., Gastaldon, C., Purgato, M., Del Giovane, . . . Barbui, C. (2022). Comparative efficacy and acceptability of psychotherapies for panic disorder with or without agoraphobia: Systematic review and network meta-analysis of randomised controlled trials. *The British Journal of Psychiatry, 221* (3), 507–519. https://doi.org/10.1192/bjp.2021.148

Park, R.H., Liu, Y.T., Samuel, A., Gurganus, M., Gampper, T.J., Corbett, S.T., Shahane, A., & Stranix, J.T. (2022). Long-term outcomes after gender-affirming surgery: 40-Year follow-up study. *Annals of Plastic Surgery, 89* (4), 431–436. https://doi.org/10.1097/SAP.0000000000003233. PMID: 36149983.

Parker, D. A., Cubells, J. F., Imes, S. L., Ruban, G. A., Henshey, B. T., Massa, N. M., . . . Ousley, O. Y. (2023). Deep psychophysiological phenotyping of adolescents and adults with 22q112 deletion syndrome: A multilevel approach to defining core disease processes. *BMC Psychiatry, 23* (1). https://doi.org/10.1186/s12888-023-04888-5

Parmigiani, G., Mandarelli, G., Meynen, G., & Ferracuti, S. (2023). Structured instruments for insanity defense evaluations: Opportunities and limitations. *Behavioral Sciences & the Law*. https://doi.org/10.1002/bsl.2618

Patel, T. A., Summers, B. J., Wilver, N. L., & Cougle, J. R. (2023). Reliability and validity of the self-report version of the Yale-Brown Obsessive-Compulsive Scale modified for body dysmorphic disorder. *Assessment, 30* (6), 1935–1946. https://doi.org/10.1177/10731911221124341

Peixoto, M. M., & Nobre, P. (2015). Prevalence of sexual problems and associated distress among lesbian and heterosexual women. *Journal of Sex & Marital Therapy, 41* (4), 427–439. https://doi.org/10.1080/0092623X.2014.918066

Pellecchia, M., Dickson, K. S., Vejnoska, S. F., & Stahmer, A. C. (2021). The autism spectrum: Diagnosis and epidemiology. In L. M. Glidden, L. Abbeduto, L. L. McIntyre, & M. J. Tassé (Eds.), *APA handbook of intellectual and developmental disabilities: Foundations., Vol. 1.* (pp. 207–237). Washington, DC: American Psychological Association.

Pellicano, G. R., Carola, V., Bussone, S., Cecchini, M., Tambelli, R., & Lai, C. (2020). Beyond the dyad: The role of mother and father in newborns' global DNA methylation during the first month of life—A pilot study. *Developmental Psychobiology*. https://doi.org/10.1002/dev.22072

Penberthy, J. K., Konig, A., Gioia, C. J., Rodríguez, V. M., Starr, J. A., Meese, W., . . . Natanya, E. (2015). Mindfulness-based relapse prevention: History, mechanisms of action, and effects. *Mindfulness, 6,* 151–158. https://doi.org/10.1007/s12671-013-0239-1

Pennebaker, J. W., Colder, M., & Sharp, L. K. (1990). Accelerating the coping process. *Journal of Personality and Social Psychology, 58,* 528–537.

Peralta, V., & Cuesta, M. J. (2020). Schneider's first-rank symptoms have neither diagnostic value for schizophrenia nor higher clinical validity than other delusions and hallucinations in psychotic disorders. *Psychological Medicine*. https://doi.org/10.1017/S0033291720003293

Pereira, D. C. S., Coutinho, E. S. F., Corassa, R. B., Andrade, L. H., & Viana, M. C. (2020). Prevalence and psychiatric comorbidities of intermittent explosive disorders in metropolitan São Paulo, Brazil. *Social Psychiatry and Psychiatric Epidemiology: The International Journal for Research in Social and Genetic Epidemiology and Mental Health Services*. https://doi.org/10.1007/s00127-020-01869-x

Perez, M., Perko, V., Yu, K. Y., Hernández, J. C., Ohrt, T. K., & Stadheim, J. (2021). Identifying central symptoms of eating disorders among ethnic and racial minority women. *Journal of Abnormal Psychology, 130* (7), 748–760. https://doi.org/10.1037/abn0000695

Perlstein, S., Fair, M., Hong, E., & Waller, R. (2023). Treatment of childhood disruptive behavior disorders and callous-unemotional traits: A systematic review and two multilevel meta-analyses. *Journal of Child Psychology and Psychiatry, 64* (9), 1372–1387. https://doi.org/10.1111/jcpp.13774

Pfaffenseller, B., Kapczinski, F., Gallitano, A. L., & Klamt, F. (2018). EGR3 immediate early gene and the brain-derived neurotrophic factor in bipolar disorder. *Frontiers in Behavioral Neuroscience, 12.* https://doi.org/10.3389/fnbeh.2018.00015

Phillips, K. A., Menard, W., Fay, C., & Pagano, M. E. (2005). Psychosocial functioning and quality of life in body dysmorphic disorder. *Comprehensive Psychiatry*, 46, 254–260.

Piantella, S., Dragano, N., Marques, M., McDonald, S. J., & Wright, B. J. (2021). Prospective increases in depression symptoms and markers of inflammation increase coronary heart disease risk—The Whitehall II cohort study. *Journal of Psychosomatic Research, 151*. https://doi.org/10.1016/j.jpsychores.2021.110657

Pietkiewicz, I. J., Kłosińska, U., Tomalski, R., & van der Hart, O. (2021). Beyond dissociative disorders: A qualitative study of Polish Catholic women reporting demonic possession. *European Journal of Trauma & Dissociation, 5* (4). https://doi.org/10.1016/j.ejtd.2021.100204

Pijnenborg, G. H. M., Withaar, F. K., Evans, J. J., Van Den Bosch, R. J., Timmerman, M. E., & Brouwer, W. H. (2009). The predictive value of measures of social cognition for community functioning in schizophrenia: Implications for neuropsychological assessment. *Journal of the International Neuropsychological Society, 15* (2), 239–247. https://doi.org/10.1017/S1355617709090341

Ploutarchou, G., Savva, C., Karagiannis, C., Pavlou, K., O'Sullivan, K., & Korakakis, V. (2023). The effectiveness of cognitive behavioural therapy in chronic neck pain: A systematic review with meta-analysis. *Cognitive Behaviour Therapy, 52* (5), 523–563. https://doi.org/10.1080/16506073.2023.2236296

Pocnet, C., Popp, J., & Jopp, D. (2020). The power of personality in successful ageing: A comprehensive review of larger quantitative studies. *European Journal of Ageing*. https://doi.org/10.1007/s10433-020-00575-6

Pollack, M. H., & Simon, N. M. (2009). Pharmacotherapy for panic disorder and agoraphobia. In M. M. Antony & M. B. Stein (Eds.), *Oxford handbook of anxiety and related disorders* (pp. 295–307). New York: Oxford University Press.

Post, R. M., Altshuler, L. L., Kupka, R., McElroy, S. L., Frye, M. A., Rowe, M., . . . Nolen, W. A. (2020). More assortative mating in US compared to European parents and spouses of patients with bipolar disorder: Implications for psychiatric illness in the offspring. *European Archives of Psychiatry and Clinical Neuroscience, 270* (2), 237–245. https://doi.org/10.1007/s00406-018-0934-y

Prescott, D. S., & Levenson, J. S. (2010). Sex offender treatment is not punishment. *Journal of Sexual Aggression, 16,* 275–285.

Prom-Wormley, E. C., Ebejer, J., Dick, D. M., & Bowers, M. S. (2017). The genetic epidemiology of substance use disorder: A review. *Drug and Alcohol Dependence, 180,* 241–259. https://doi.org/10.1016/j.drugalcdep.2017.06.040

Q

Qiao, Y., Chi, Y., Zhang, Q., & Ma, Y. (2023). Safety and efficacy of lecanemab for Alzheimer's disease: A systematic review and meta-analysis of randomized clinical trials. *Frontiers in Aging Neuroscience, 15*. https://doi.org/10.3389/fnagi.2023.1169499

Quang, H., Nguyen, A. L., Do, C., McDonald, S., & Nguyen, C. (2023). Examining the Vietnamese Montreal Cognitive Assessment in healthy and moderate-to-severe traumatic brain injury populations. *The Clinical Neuropsychologist, 37* (5), 1062–1077. https://doi.org/10.1080/13854046.2023.2170281

Quimby, A. E., & Shamy, M. C. F. (2015). The Canadian management of bovine spongiform encephalopathy in historical and scientific perspective, 1990–2014. *The Canadian Journal of Neurological Sciences / Le Journal Canadien Des Sciences Neurologiques, 42* (6), 472–481. https://doi.org/10.1017/cjn.2015.286

R

Radević, L., & Dinić, B. M. (2022). The effects of dark tetrad and hexaco traits on laboratory-induced malice behaviors. *Current Psychology: A Journal for Diverse Perspectives on Diverse Psychological Issues*. https://doi.org/10.1007/s12144-022-03720-9

Radonjić, N. V., Bellato, A., Khoury, N. M., Cortese, S., & Faraone, S. V. (2023). Nonstimulant medications for Attention-Deficit/Hyperactivity Disorder (ADHD) in adults: Systematic review and meta-analysis. *CNS Drugs, 37* (5), 381–397. https://doi.org/10.1007/s40263-023-01005-8

Raison, A., & Andrea, S. (2023). Childhood trauma in patients with Dissociative Identity Disorder: A systematic review of data from 1990 to 2022. *European Journal of Trauma & Dissociation, 7* (1). https://doi.org/10.1016/j.ejtd.2022.100310

Rajan, K. B., Weuve, J., Barnes, L. L., McAninch, E. A., Wilson, R. S., & Evans, D. A. (2021). Population estimate of people with clinical Alzheimer's disease and mild cognitive impairment in the United States (2020–2060). *Alzheimer's & Dementia, 17* (12), 1966–1975. https://doi.org/10.1002/alz.12362

Rambau, S., Forstner, A. J., Wegener, I., Mücke, M., Wissussek, C. S., Staufenbiel, S. M., . . . Conrad, R. (2018). Childhood adversities, bonding, and personality in social anxiety disorder with alcohol use disorder. *Psychiatry Research, 262,* 295–302. https://doi.org/10.1016/j.psychres.2018.02.006

Rammal, S., Abi Chahine, J., Rammal, M., Fares, Y., & Abou Abbas, L. (2019). Modified Wisconsin Card Sorting Test (M-WCST): Normative data for the Lebanese adult population. *Developmental Neuropsychology, 44* (5), 397–408. https://doi.org/10.1080/87565641.2019.1652828

Rape Abuse & Incest National Network (RAINN). (2021). Children and teens: Statistics. https://www.rainn.org/statistics/children-and-teens 2/26/21

Raspa, M., Wheeler, A., Okoniewski, K. C., Edwards, A., & Scott, S. (2023). Research gaps in Fragile X syndrome: An updated literature review to inform clinical and public health practice. *Journal of Developmental and Behavioral Pediatrics, 44* (1), e56–e65. https://doi.org/10.1097/DBP.0000000000001134

Rauch, S. A. M., Kim, H. M., Acierno, R., Ragin, C., Wangelin, B., Blitch, K., . . . Zivin, K. (2023). Improving function through primary care treatment of posttraumatic stress disorder study outcomes: A randomized controlled trial of prolonged exposure for primary care in veterans. *Families, Systems, & Health*. https://doi.org/10.1037/fsh0000823 10.1037/fsh0000823.supp (Supplemental)

Reas, D. L., Kjelsas, E., Heggestad, T., Eriksen, L., Nielsen, S., Gjertsen, F., & Gotestam, K. G. (2005). Characteristics of anorexia nervosa-related deaths in Norway (1992–2000): Data from the National Patient Register and the Causes of Death Register. *International Journal of Eating Disorders, 37,* 181–187.

Rector, N. A., Richter, M. A., Katz, D., & Leybman, M. (2019). Does the addition of cognitive therapy to exposure and response prevention for obsessive compulsive disorder enhance clinical efficacy? A randomized controlled trial in a community setting. *British Journal of Clinical Psychology, 58* (1), 1–18. https://doi.org/10.1111/bjc.12188

Reed, G. M., First, M. B., Kogan, C. S., Hyman, S. E., Gureje, O., Gaebel, W., . . . Saxena, S. (2019). Innovations and changes in the ICD-11 classification of mental, behavioural and neurodevelopmental disorders. *World Psychiatry: Official Journal of the World Psychiatric Association (WPA), 18* (1), 3–19. https://doi.org/10.1002/wps.20611

Rees, G., & Garcia, J. R. (2017a). An investigation into the solitary and interpersonal aspects of sexual object fetishism: A mixed-methods approach. *Psychology & Sexuality, 8* (4), 252–267.

Rees, G., & Garcia, J. R. (2017b). All I need is shoe: An investigation into the obligatory aspect of sexual object fetishism. *International Journal of Sexual Health, 29* (4), 303–312. https://doi.org/10.1080/19317611.2017.1309483

Reid, H., & Bahar, R. J. (2006). Treatment of encopresis and chronic constipation in young children: Clinical results from interactive parent-child guidance. *Clinical Pediatrics, 45,* 157–164.

Reinders, A. A. T. S., & Veltman, D. J. (2020). Dissociative identity disorder: Out of the shadows at last? *The British Journal of Psychiatry*. doi:10.1192/bjp.2020.168

Rentmeesters, N., & Hermans, D. (2023). Posttraumatic stress disorder in Belgian police officers: Prevalence and the effects of exposure to traumatic events. *European Journal of Psychotraumatology, 14* (1). https://doi.org/10.1080/20008066.2022.2156558

Results from the 2019 National Survey on Drug Use and Health: Detailed tables. Rockville, MD: Center for Behavioral Health Statistics and Quality, Substance Abuse and Mental Health Services. Retrieved from https://www.samhsa.gov/data/report/2019-nsduh -detailed-tables.

Rezayat, A. A., Sahebdel, S., Jafari, S., Kabirian, A., Rahnejat, A. M., Farahani, R. H., Mosaed, R., & Nour, M. G. (2020). Evaluating the prevalence of PTSD among children and adolescents after earthquakes and floods: A systematic review and meta-analysis. *Psychiatric Quarterly, 91* (4), 1265–1290. https://doi.org/10.1007/s11126-020-09840-4

Ribeiro, W. S., Romeo, R., King, D., Owens, S., Gronholm, P. C., Fisher, H. L., Laurens, K. R., & Evans-Lacko, S. (2023). Influence of stigma, sociodemographic and clinical characteristics on mental health-related service use and associated costs among young people in the United Kingdom. *European Child & Adolescent Psychiatry, 32* (8), 1363–1373. https://doi.org/10.1007/s00787-022-01947-2

Ricketts, E. J., Woods, D. W., Espil, F. M., McGuire, J. F., Stiede, J. T., Schild, J., . . . Piacentini, J. (2022). Childhood predictors of long-term tic severity and tic impairment in Tourette's disorder. *Behavior Therapy, 53* (6), 1250–1264. https://doi.org/10.1016/j.beth.2022.07.002

Riederer, P., & ter Meulen, V. (2020). Coronaviruses: A challenge of today and a call for extended human postmortem brain analyses. *Journal of Neural Transmission, 127* (9), 1217–1228. https://doi.org/10.1007/s00702-020-02230-x

Riggs, S. E., & Creed, T. A. (2017). A model to transform psychosis milieu treatment using CBT-informed interventions. *Cognitive and Behavioral Practice, 24* (3), 353–362. https://doi.org/10.1016/j.cbpra.2016.08.001

Rincón-Hernández, A. I., Parra-Carrillo, W. C., Álvarez-Muelas, A., Peñuela-Trujillo, C., Rosero, F., Espitia de la Hoz, F., . . . Vallejo-Medina, P. (2021). Temporal stability and clinical validation of the Spanish version of the female sexual function inventory (FSFI). *Women & Health, 61* (2), 189–198. https://doi.org/10.1080/03630242.2020.1819940

Ringen, P. A., Engh, J. A., Birkenaes, A. B., Dieset, I., & Andreassen, O. A. (2014). Increased mortality in schizophrenia due to cardiovascular disease—A non-systematic review of epidemiology, possible causes, and interventions. *Frontiers in Psychiatry, 5,* 137.

Ritterband, L. M., Thorndike, F. P., Lord, H. R., Borowitz, S. M., Walker, L. S., Ingersoll, K. S., Sutphen, J. L., & Cox, D. J. (2013). An RCT of an internet intervention for pediatric encopresis with one-year follow-up. *Clinical Practice in Pediatric Psychology, 1* (1), 68–80. https://doi.org/10.1037/cpp0000007

Roberts, C. A., Quednow, B. B., Montgomery, C., & Parrott, A. C. (2018). MDMA and brain activity during neurocognitive performance: An overview of neuroimaging studies with abstinent "Ecstasy" users. *Neuroscience and Biobehavioral Reviews, 84,* 470–482. https://doi.org/10.1016/j.neubiorev.2017.07.015

Rodriguez-Monguio, R., Brand, E., & Volberg, R. (2018). The economic burden of pathological gambling and co-occurring mental health and substance use disorders. *Journal of Addiction Medicine, 12* (1), 53–60.

Rody, T., De Amorim, J. A., & De Felice, F. G. (2022). The emerging neuroprotective roles of exerkines in Alzheimer's disease. *Frontiers in Aging Neuroscience, 14*. https://doi.org/10.3389/fnagi.2022.965190

Rogers, C. R. (1951). *Client-centered therapy: Its current practice implications, and theory.* Houghton Mifflin.

Roivainen, E. (2019). European and American WAIS IV norms: Cross-national differences in perceptual reasoning, processing speed and working memory subtest scores. *Scandinavian Journal of Psychology, 60* (6), 513–519. https://doi.org/10.1111/sjop.12581

Romano, M., Moscovitch, D. A., Saini, P., & Huppert, J. D. (2020). The effects of positive interpretation bias on cognitive reappraisal and social performance: Implications for social anxiety disorder. *Behaviour Research and Therapy, 131*. https://doi.org/10.1016/j.brat.2020.103651

Roos, H., Fälth, L., Karlsson, L., Nilvius, C., Selenius, H., & Svensson, I. (2023). Promoting basic arithmetic competence in early school years–using a response to intervention model. *Journal of Research in Special Educational Needs, 23* (4), 313–322. https://doi.org/10.1111/1471-3802.12602

Rose, E., Schreiber-Agus, N., Bajaj, K., Klugman, S., & Goldwaser, T. (2016). Challenges of pre- and post-test counseling for Orthodox Jewish individuals in the premarital phase. *Journal of Genetic Counseling, 25* (1), 18–24. https://doi.org/10.1007/s10897-015-9880-2

Roselló, B., Berenguer, C., Baixauli, I., Mira, Á., Martinez-Raga, J., & Miranda, A. (2020). Empirical examination of executive functioning, ADHD associated behaviors, and functional impairments in adults with persistent ADHD, remittent ADHD, and without ADHD. *BMC Psychiatry, 20*. https://doi.org/10.1186/s12888-020-02542-y

Rosen, R., Brown, C., Heiman, J., Leiblum, S., Meston, C., Shabsigh, R., . . . D'Agostino, R., Jr. (2000). The Female Sexual Function Index (FSFI): A multidimensional self-report instrument for the assessment of female sexual function. *Journal of Sex & Marital Therapy, 26,* 191–208.

Roth, Y., Barnea-Ygael, N., Carmi, L., Storch, E. A., Tendler, A., & Zangen, A. (2020). Deep transcranial magnetic stimulation for obsessive-compulsive disorder is efficacious even in patients who failed multiple medications and CBT. *Psychiatry Research, 290.* https://doi.org/10.1016/j.psychres.2020.113179

Rowa, K., Cameron, D., Soreni, N., LeMoult, J., & McCabe, R. E. (2020). Outcome of CBT for problematic hoarding in a naturalistic setting: Impact on symptoms and distress tolerance. *Behaviour Change, 37* (1), 13–21. https://doi.org/10.1017/bec.2019.17

Rowland, D. L., & Kolba, T. N. (2016). Understanding orgasmic difficulty in women. *Journal of Sexual Medicine, 13* (8), 1246–1254. https://doi.org/10.1016/j.jsxm.2016.05.014

Ruckle, M. M., Bednar, M. K., Suen, K., & Falligant, J. M. (2023). Brief assessment and treatment of pica using differential reinforcement, response interruption and redirection, and competing stimuli. *Behavioral Interventions, 38* (1), 255–267. https://doi.org/10.1002/bin.1881

Rudd, M. D., Bryan, C. J., Wertenberger, E. G., Peterson, A. L., Young-McCaughan, S., Mintz, J., . . . Bruce, T. O. (2015). Brief cognitive-behavioral therapy effects on post-treatment suicide attempts in a military sample: Results of a randomized clinical trial with 2-year follow-up. *The American Journal of Psychiatry, 172,* 441–449. https://doi.org/10.1176/appi.ajp.2014.14070843

Russo, D. (Writer). (2012). *Demi Lovato: Stay strong.* In S. Storr, D. Sirulnik, J. Wilkes, & J. Mussman (Producer): MTV.

Rutherford, B. R., Choi, C. J., Chrisanthopolous, M., Salzman, C., Zhu, C., Montes-Garcia, C., . . . Roose, S. P. (2020). The COVID-19 pandemic as a traumatic stressor: Mental health responses of older adults with chronic PTSD. *The American Journal of Geriatric Psychiatry.* https://doi.org/10.1016/j.jagp.2020.10.010

Ruutiainen, T., & Northrop, J. (2021). Defining the scope of duty to warn readily identifiable individuals. *Journal of the American Academy of Psychiatry and the Law, 49* (2), 265–267.

Ryding, F. C., & Kuss, D. J. (2020). The use of social networking sites, body image dissatisfaction, and body dysmorphic disorder: A systematic review of psychological research. *Psychology of Popular Media, 9* (4), 412–435. https://doi.org/10.1037/ppm0000264

S

Saez, C. M., Davies, M. S., Kazemi, E., & Fields, A. (2023). Factors affecting parent treatment decisions for children with autism spectrum disorders: A brief review. *Behavior Analysis in Practice, 16* (1), 93–101. https://doi.org/10.1007/s40617-022-00716-6

Sajjadi, S. F., Gross, J., Sellbom, M., & Hayne, H. (2021, January 7). Narrative Identity in Borderline Personality Disorder. *Personality Disorders: Theory, Research, and Treatment.* Advance online publication. http://dx.doi.org/10.1037/per0000476

Saks, E. (2007). *The center cannot hold: My journey through madness.* Hachette Books.

Sala, G., Inagaki, H., Ishioka, Y., Masui, Y., Nakagawa, T., Ishizaki, T., . . . Gondo, Y. (2020). The psychometric properties of the Montreal Cognitive Assessment (MoCA): A comprehensive investigation. *Swiss Journal of Psychology, 79* (3–4), 155–161. https://doi.org/10.1024/1421-0185/a000242

Salekin, R. T., Worley, C., & Grimes, R. D. (2010). Treatment of psychopathy: A review and brief introduction to the mental model approach for psychopathy. *Behavioral Sciences & the Law, 28,* 235–266.

Salvatore, J. E., Han, S., Farris, S. P., Mignogna, K. M., Miles, M. F., & Agrawal, A. (2018). Beyond genome-wide significance: Integrative approaches to the interpretation and extension of GWAS findings for alcohol use disorder. *Addiction Biology.* https://doi.org/10.1111/adb.12591

Samalin, L., & Belzeaux, R. (2023). Why does non-adherence to treatment remain a leading cause of relapse in patients with bipolar disorder? *European Neuropsychopharmacology, 73,* 16–18. https://doi.org/10.1016/j.euroneuro.2023.04.012

Samuel, D. B., & Gore, W. L. (2012). Maladaptive variants of conscientiousness and agreeableness. *Journal of Personality, 80,* 1669–1696. https://doi.org/10.1111/j.1467-6494.2012.00770.x

Samuel, D. B., Balling, C. E., & Bucher, M. A. (2022). The alternative model of personality disorder is inadequate for capturing obsessive-compulsive personality disorder. *Personality Disorders: Theory, Research, and Treatment, 13* (4), 418–421. https://doi.org/10.1037/per0000544 (The DSM-5 Alternative Model of Personality Disorders: A Ten-Year Retrospective)

Sanders, N., Smeets, P. M., van Elburg, A. A., Danner, U. N., van Meer, F., Hoek, H. W., & Adan, R. H. (2015). Altered food-cue processing in chronically ill and recovered women with anorexia nervosa. *Frontiers in Behavioral Neuroscience, 9,* 46.

Sansone, R. A., Dittoe, N., Hahn, H. S., & Wiederman, M. W. (2011). The prevalence of borderline personality disorder in a consecutive sample of cardiac stress test patients. *The Primary Care Companion for CNS Disorders, 13* (3), PCC.10l01087. https://doi.org/10.4088/PCC.10l01087

Saraçaydın, G., Ruisch, I. H., van Rooij, D., Sprooten, E., Franke, B., Buitelaar, J. K., Dietrich, A., & Hoekstra, P. J. (2023). Shared genetic etiology between ADHD, task-related behavioral measures and brain activation during response inhibition in a youth ADHD case-control study. *European Archives of Psychiatry and Clinical Neuroscience.* https://doi.org/10.1007/s00406-023-01632-8

Sassenrath, C., Keller, J., Stöckle, D., Kesberg, R., Nielsen, Y. A., & Pfattheicher, S. (2023). I like it because it hurts you: On the association of everyday sadism, sadistic pleasure, and victim blaming. *Journal of Personality and Social Psychology.* https://doi.org/10.1037/pspp0000464

Sauer-Zavala, S., Southward, M. W., Fruhbauerova, M., Semcho, S. A., Stumpp, N. E., Hood, C. O., . . . Cravens, L. (2023). BPD compass: A randomized controlled trial of a short-term, personality-based treatment for borderline personality disorder. *Personality Disorders: Theory, Research, and Treatment, 14* (5), 534–544. https://doi.org/10.1037/per0000612 10.1037

Saul, J., Griffiths, S., & Norbury, C. F. (2023). Prevalence and functional impact of social (pragmatic) communication disorders. *Journal of Child Psychology and Psychiatry, 64* (3), 376–387. https://doi.org/10.1111/jcpp.13705

Savoie, J., Root, K., Villers, J., Goldsmith, K. M., & Short, M. (2019). Boston naming test performance in French-speaking Acadians. *Aphasiology, 33* (5), 561–578. https://doi.org/10.1080/02687038.2018.1490387

Schaakxs, R., Comijs, H. C., Lamers, F., Beekman, A. F., & Penninx, B. H. (2017). Age-related variability in the presentation of symptoms of major depressive disorder. *Psychological Medicine, 47* (3), 543–552. https://doi.org/10.1017/S0033291716002579

Scherf-Clavel, M., Weber, H., Wurst, C., Stonawski, S., Hommers, L., Unterecker, S., . . . Deckert, J. (2022). Effects of pharmacokinetic gene variation on therapeutic drug levels and antidepressant treatment response. *Pharmacopsychiatry, 55* (5), 246–254. https://doi.org/10.1055/a-1872-0613

Scheveneels, S., De Witte, N., & Van Daele, T. (2023). The first steps in facing your fears: The acceptability of virtual reality and in vivo exposure treatment for specific fears. *Journal of Anxiety Disorders, 95,* 102695. https://doi.org/https://doi.org/10.1016/j.janxdis.2023.102695

Schick, M. R., Spillane, N. S., & Hostetler, K. L. (2020). A call to action: A systematic review examining the failure to include females and members of minoritized racial/ethnic groups in clinical trials of pharmacological treatments for alcohol use disorder. *Alcoholism: Clinical and Experimental Research, 44* (10), 1933–1951. https://doi.org/10.1111/acer.14440

Schieber, K., Kollei, I., de Zwaan, M., & Martin, A. (2015). Classification of body dysmorphic disorder—What is the advantage of the new *DSM-5* criteria? *Journal of Psychosomatic Research, 78,* 223–227. https://doi.org/10.1016/j.jpsychores.2015.01.002

Schienle, A., Hettema, J. M., Cáceda, R., & Nemeroff, C. B. (2011). Neurobiology and genetics of generalized anxiety disorder. *Psychiatric Annals, 41* (2), 113–123.

Schippers, E. E., Smid, W. J., Huckelba, A. L., Hoogsteder, L. M., Beekman, A. T. F., & Smit, J. H. (2021). Exploratory factor analysis of unusual sexual interests. *Journal of Sexual Medicine, 18* (9), 1615–1631. https://doi.org/10.1016/j.jsxm.2021.07.002

Schmitt, A., Bendig, E., Baumeister, H., Hermanns, N., & Kulzer, B. (2021). Associations of depression and diabetes distress with self-management behavior and glycemic control. *Health Psychology, 40* (2), 113–124. https://doi.org/10.1037/hea0001037

Schröder, J., Werkle, N., Cludius, B., Jelinek, L., Moritz, S., & Westermann, S. (2020). Unguided Internet-based cognitive-behavioral therapy for obsessive-compulsive disorder: A randomized controlled trial. *Depression and Anxiety, 37* (12), 1208–1220. https://doi.org/10.1002/da.23105

Schulz, A., Rost, S., Flasinski, T., Dierolf, A. M., Lutz, A. P. C., Münch, E. E., . . . Vögele, C. (2020). Distinctive body perception mechanisms in high versus low symptom reporters: A neurophysiological model for medically-unexplained symptoms. *Journal of Psychosomatic Research, 137*. https://doi.org/10.1016/j.jpsychores.2020.110223

Schwarzmeier, H., Kleint, N. I., Wittchen, H. U., Ströhle, A., Hamm, A. O., & Lueken, U. (2019). Characterizing the nature of emotional-associative learning deficits in panic disorder: An fMRI study on fear conditioning, extinction training and recall. *European Neuropsychopharmacology, 29* (2), 306–318. https://doi.org/10.1016/j.euroneuro.2018.11.1108

Segal, Z. V., Williams, J. M. G., & Teasdale, J. D. (2002). *Mindfulness-based cognitive therapy for depression: A new approach to preventing relapse.* Guilford Press.

Seim, A. R., Jozefiak, T., Wichstrøm, L., Lydersen, S., & Kayed, N. S. (2020). Reactive attachment disorder and disinhibited social engagement disorder in adolescence: Co-occurring psychopathology and psychosocial problems. *European Child & Adolescent Psychiatry*. https://doi.org/10.1007/s00787-020-01673-7

Seretis, D., Hart, C. M., & Maguire, T. (2023). Validity of a Revised Obsessive-Compulsive Personality Disorder (OCPD) trait profile and its relationship with social interaction anxiety and coping. *Journal of Personality Assessment, 105* (5), 647–656. https://doi.org/10.1080/00223891.2022.2145963

Seto, M. C., Curry, S., Dawson, S. J., Bradford, J. M. W., & Chivers, M. L. (2021). Concordance of paraphilic interests and behaviors. *Journal of Sex Research, 58* (4), 424–437. https://doi.org/10.1080/00224499.2020.1830018

Shakya, I., Bergen, G., Haddad, Y. K., Kakara, R., & Moreland, B. L. (2020). Fall-related emergency department visits involving alcohol among older adults. *Journal of Safety Research, 74*, 125–131. https://doi.org/10.1016/j.jsr.2020.06.001

Shanok, N. A., Rodriguez, S., Muzac, S., Del Pino, C. H., Brown, L., & Rodriguez, R. (2023). Deep transcranial magnetic stimulation alters resting-state neurophysiological traits in major depressive disorder. *Journal of Affective Disorders, 337*, 104–111. https://doi.org/10.1016/j.jad.2023.05.066

Sharrock, M. J., Mahoney, A. E. J., Haskelberg, H., Millard, M., & Newby, J. M. (2021). The uptake and outcomes of Internet-based cognitive behavioural therapy for health anxiety symptoms during the COVID-19 pandemic. *Journal of Anxiety Disorders, 84*. https://doi.org/10.1016/j.janxdis.2021.102494

Shedler, J. (2010). The efficacy of psychodynamic psychotherapy. *American Psychologist, 65*, 98–109.

Shepard, J. A., Poler, J. E., Jr., & Grabman, J. H. (2017). Evidence-based psychosocial treatments for pediatric elimination disorders. *Journal of Clinical Child and Adolescent Psychology, 46* (6), 767–797. https://doi.org/10.1080/15374416.2016.1247356

Shepard, J. A., Poler, J. J., & Grabman, J. H. (2017). Evidence-based psychosocial treatments for pediatric elimination disorders. *Journal of Clinical Child and Adolescent Psychology, 46* (6), 767–797. https://doi.org/10.1080/15374416.2016.1247356

Shepler, D. K., Smendik, J. M., Cusick, K. M., & Tucker, D. R. (2018). Predictors of sexual satisfaction for partnered lesbian, gay, and bisexual adults. *Psychology of Sexual Orientation and Gender Diversity, 5* (1), 25–35. https://doi.org/10.1037/sgd0000252

Sher, L. (2019). Resilience as a focus of suicide research and prevention. *Acta Psychiatrica Scandinavica, 140* (2), 169–180. https://doi.org/10.1111/acps.13059

Sherzai, D., Sherzai, A., Lui, K., Pan, D., Chiou, D., Bazargan, M., & Shaheen, M. (2016). The association between diabetes and dementia among elderly individuals: A nationwide inpatient sample analysis. *Journal of Geriatric Psychiatry Neurology, 29* (3), 120–125. https://doi.org/10.1177/0891988715627016

Shipherd, J. C., Lynch, K., Gatsby, E., Hinds, Z., DuVall, S. L., & Livingston, N. A. (2021). Estimating prevalence of PTSD among veterans with minoritized sexual orientations using electronic health record data. *Journal of Consulting and Clinical Psychology, 89* (10), 856–868. https://doi.org/10.1037/ccp0000691

Shir, R., & Tishby, O. (2023). Therapy matchmaking: Patient-therapist match in personality traits and attachment style. *Psychotherapy Research*. https://doi.org/10.1080/10503307.2023.2195054

Shusterman, A., Feld, L., Baer, L., & Keuthen, N. (2009). Affective regulation in trichotillomania: Evidence from a large-scale Internet survey. *Behaviour Research and Therapy*, 47, 637–644.

Shuttleworth-Edwards, A. B. (2016). Generally representative is representative of none: Commentary on the pitfalls of IQ test standardization in multicultural settings. *Clinical Neuropsychology, 30* (7), 975–998. https://doi.org/10.1080/13854046.2016.1204011

Siegmann, P., Teismann, T., Fritsch, N., Forkmann, T., Glaesmer, H., Zhang, X. C., . . . Margraf, J. (2018). Resilience to suicide ideation: A cross-cultural test of the buffering hypothesis. *Clinical Psychology & Psychotherapy, 25* (1), e1– e9. https://doi.org/10.1002/cpp.211

Siev, J., Rasmussen, J., Sullivan, A. D. W., & Wilhelm, S. (2021). Clinical features of scrupulosity: Associated symptoms and comorbidity. *Journal of Clinical Psychology, 77* (1), 173–188. https://doi.org/10.1002/jclp.23019

Silarova, B., Giltay, E. J., Van Reedt Dortland, A., Van Rossum, E. C., Hoencamp, E., Penninx, B. H., & Spijker, A. T. (2015). Metabolic syndrome in patients with bipolar disorder: Comparison with major depressive disorder and non-psychiatric controls. *Journal of Psychosomatic Research, 78*, 391–398. https://doi.org/10.1016/j.jpsychores.2015.02.010

Silén, Y., & Keski-Rahkonen, A. (2022). Worldwide prevalence of DSM-5 eating disorders among young people. *Current Opinion in Psychiatry, 35* (6), 362–371. https://doi.org/10.1097/YCO.0000000000000818

Sillon, G., Allard, P., Drury, S., Rivière, J. B., & Bie, I. (2020). The incidence and carrier frequency of Tay-Sachs disease in the French-Canadian population of Quebec based on retrospective data from 24 years, 1992–2015. *Journal of Genetic Counseling, 29* (6), 1173–1185. https://doi.org/10.1002/jgc4.1284

Silove, D., Alonso, J., Bromet, E., Gruber, M., Sampson, N., Scott, K., . . . Kessler, R. C. (2015). Pediatric-onset and adult-onset separation anxiety disorder across countries in the World Mental Health Survey. *The American Journal of Psychiatry, 172*, 647–656. https://doi.org/10.1176/appi.ajp.2015.14091185

Silove, D., Alonso, J., Bromet, E., Gruber, M., Sampson, N., Scott, K., . . . Kessler, R. C. (2015). Pediatric-onset and adult-onset separation anxiety disorder across countries in the World Mental Health Survey. *The American Journal of Psychiatry, 172* (7), 647–656. https://doi.org/10.1176/appi.ajp.2015.14091185

Silva, M. A., Jaramillo, Y., Paris, M., Jr., Añez-Nava, L., Frankforter, T. L., & Kiluk, B. D. (2020). Changes in *DSM* criteria following a culturally-adapted computerized CBT for Spanish-speaking individuals with substance use disorders. *Journal of Substance Abuse Treatment, 110*, 42–48. https://doi.org/10.1016/j.jsat.2019.12.006

Silva, R. d. M. F. d., Brunoni, A. R., Goerigk, S., Batistuzzo, M. C., Costa, D. L. d. C.,

Diniz, J. B., . . . Shavitt, R. G. (2021). Efficacy and safety of transcranial direct current stimulation as an add-on treatment for obsessive-compulsive disorder: A randomized, sham-controlled trial. *Neuropsychopharmacology*. https://doi.org/10.1038/s41386-020-00928-w

Silver, Z., Coger, M., Barr, S., & Drill, R. (2020). Psychotherapy at a public hospital in the time of COVID-19: Telehealth and implications for practice. *Counselling Psychology Quarterly*. https://doi.org/10.1080/09515070.2020.1777390

Silvestre, G., Iglesias, R. M., & Silvestre, E. (2018). Boston Naming Test norms for the Dominican population. *Aphasiology, 32* (3), 340–365. https://doi.org/10.1080/02687038.2017.1338662

Silveus, S. A., Schmit, M. K., Oliveira, J. T., & Hughes, L. E. (2023). Meta-analysis of culturally adapted cognitive behavioral therapy for anxiety and depression. *Journal of Counseling & Development, 101* (2), 129–142. https://doi.org/10.1002/jcad.12463

Simon, J. A., Thorp, J., & Millheiser, L. (2019). Flibanserin for premenopausal hypoactive sexual desire disorder: Pooled analysis of clinical trials. *Journal of Women's Health, 28* (6), 769–777. https://doi.org/10.1089/jwh.2018.7516

Siskind, D., Dark, F., Carney, K., Gore-Jones, V., Kar Ray, M., Steginga, A., Suetani, S., & Kisely, S. (2021). Placing rehabilitation at the core of assertive community treatment. *Australasian Psychiatry, 29* (1), 47–51. https://doi.org/10.1177/1039856220928876

Sitnikova, K., Leone, S. S., van Marwijk, H. W. J., Twisk, J., van der Horst, H. E., & van der Wouden, J. C. (2019). Effectiveness of a cognitive behavioural intervention for patients with undifferentiated somatoform disorder: Results from the CIPRUS cluster randomized controlled trial in primary care. *Journal of Psychosomatic Research, 127*. https://doi.org/10.1016/j.jpsychores.2019.109745

Sivaratnam, L., Selimin, D. S., Abd Ghani, S. R., Nawi, H. M., & Nawi, A. M. (2021). Behavior-related erectile dysfunction: A systematic review and meta-analysis. *Journal of Sexual Medicine, 18* (1), 121–143. https://doi.org/10.1016/j.jsxm.2020.09.009

Skinner, B. F. (1953). *Science and human behavior.* Free Press.

Smart, D., Youssef, G. J., Sanson, A., Prior, M., Toumbourou, J. W., & Olsson, C. A. (2017). Consequences of childhood reading difficulties and behaviour problems for educational achievement and employment in early adulthood. *British Journal of Educational Psychology, 87* (2), 288–308. https://doi.org/10.1111/bjep.12150

Smith, M., & South, S. (2020). Romantic attachment style and borderline personality pathology: A meta-analysis. *Clinical Psychology Review, 75*. https://doi.org/10.1016/j.cpr.2019.101781

Snorrason, I., Belleau, E. L., & Woods, D. W. (2012). How related are hair pulling disorder (trichotillomania) and skin picking disorder? A review of evidence for comorbidity, similarities and shared etiology. *Clinical Psychology Review, 32,* 618–629. https://doi.org/10.1016/j.cpr.2012.05.008

Snorrason, I., Berlin, G. S., & Lee, H. (2015). Optimizing psychological interventions for trichotillomania (hair-pulling disorder): An update on current empirical status. *Psychology Research and Behavior Management, 8,* 105–113.

Solé, B., Verdolini, N., Amoretti, S., Montejo, L., Rosa, A. R., Hogg, B., . . . Torrent, C. (2021). Effects of the COVID-19 pandemic and lockdown in Spain: Comparison between community controls and patients with a psychiatric disorder preliminary results from the BRIS-MHC STUDY. *Journal of Affective Disorders, 281,* 13–23. https://doi.org/10.1016/j.jad.2020.11.099

Solem, S., Håland, Å. T., Vogel, P. A., Hansen, B., & Wells, A. (2009). Change in metacognitions predicts outcome in obsessive-compulsive disorder patients undergoing treatment with exposure and response prevention. *Behaviour Research and Therapy, 47,* 301–307.

Song, P., Zha, M., Yang, Q., Zhang, Y., Li, X., & Rudan, I. (2021). The prevalence of adult attention-deficit hyperactivity disorder: A global systematic review and meta-analysis. *Journal of Global Health, 11, 04009.* https://doi.org/10.7189/jogh.11.04009

Soose, R. J., Araujo, M., Faber, K., Roy, A., Lee, K., Ni, Q., Srivastava, J., & Strollo, P. J. (2022). Cluster analysis of upper airway stimulation adherence patterns and implications on clinical care. *Sleep: Journal of Sleep and Sleep Disorders Research, 45* (11), 1–7. https://doi.org/10.1093/sleep/zsac049

Sørensen, K. D., Råbu, M., Wilberg, T., & Berthelsen, E. (2019). Struggling to be a person: Lived experience of avoidant personality disorder. *Journal of Clinical Psychology, 75* (4), 664–680. https://doi.org/10.1002/jclp.22740

Sørensen, K. D., Wilberg, T., Berthelsen, E., & Råbu, M. (2020). Subjective experience of the origin and development of avoidant personality disorder. *Journal of Clinical Psychology, 76* (12), 2232–2248. https://doi.org/10.1002/jclp.23013

Specht, M. W., Mahone, E. M., Kline, T., Waranch, R., Brabson, L., Thompson, C. B., & Singer, H. S. (2017). Efficacy of parent-delivered behavioral therapy for primary complex motor stereotypies. *Developmental Medicine & Child Neurology, 59* (2), 168–173. https://doi.org/10.1111/dmcn.13164

Spence, S. H., Prosser, S. J., March, S., & Donovan, C. L. (2020). Internet-delivered cognitive behavior therapy with minimal therapist support for anxious children and adolescents: Predictors of response. *Journal of Child Psychology and Psychiatry, 61* (8), 914–927. https://doi.org/10.1111/jcpp.13257

Sperling, R. A., Donohue, M. C., Raman, R., Rafii, M. S., Johnson, K., Masters, C. L., . . . Aisen, P. S. (2023). Trial of Solanezumab in preclinical Alzheimer's Disease. *New England Journal of Medicine, 389* (12), 1096–1107. https://doi.org/10.1056/NEJMoa2305032

Sperry, L., & Casteleiro, G. (2022). Avoidant personality disorder. In R. E. Feinstein (Ed.), *Personality disorders* (pp. 545–564). Oxford University Press. http://silk.library.umass.edu/login?url=https://search.ebscohost.com/login.aspx?direct=true&db=psyh&AN=2023-22399-022&site=ehost-live&scope=site

Spetie, L., & Arnold, L. E. (2007). Ethical issues in child psychopharmacology research and practice: Emphasis on preschoolers. *Psychopharmacology, 191,* 15–26.

Spinhoven, P., van Hemert, A. M., & Penninx, B. H. (2017). Experiential avoidance and bordering psychological constructs as predictors of the onset, relapse and maintenance of anxiety disorders: One or many? *Cognitive Therapy and Research, 41* (6), 867–880. https://doi.org/10.1007/s10608-017-9856-7

Stahl, E. A., Breen, G., Forstner, A. J., McQuillin, A., Ripke, S., Trubetskoy, V., . . . Sklar, P. (2019). Genome-wide association study identifies 30 loci associated with bipolar disorder. *Nature Genetics, 51* (5), 793–803. https://doi.org/10.1038/s41588-019-0397-8

Stamates, A. L., Preonas, P. D., Linden-Carmichael, A. N., Junkin, E., Roberts, R., & Lau-Barraco, C. (2023). Daily positive alcohol expectancies and alcohol use outcomes among college students. *Addiction Research & Theory*. https://doi.org/10.1080/16066359.2023.2241358

State v. Darnall. (1980). 161, 614 P. 2d 120 (Or. Ct. App.)

State v. Greene. (1998). 960 P.2d 980 (Wash. Ct. App.)

State v. Jones. (1998). 743 P. 2d 276 P 2d 1183, 1185 (Washington Court Appellate 1987. Affiliated 759.)

State v. Lockhart. (2000). 542 S.E.2d 443 (W. Va.)

State v. Milligan, **No. 77-CR-11-2908 (Franklin County, Ohio. Dec. 4, 1978).**

Stea, J. N., Hodgins, D. C., & Fung, T. (2015). Abstinence versus moderation goals in brief motivational treatment for pathological gambling. *Journal of Gambling Studies, 31,* 1029–1045. https://doi.org/10.1007/s10899-014-9461-6

Stech, E. P., Lim, J., Upton, E. L., & Newby, J. M. (2020). Internet-delivered cognitive behavioral therapy for panic disorder with or without agoraphobia: A systematic review and meta-analysis. *Cognitive Behaviour Therapy, 49* (4), 270–293. https://doi.org/10.1080/16506073.2019.1628808

Stein, D. J., Palk, A. C., & Kendler, K. S. (2021). What is a mental disorder? An exemplar-focused approach. *Psychological Medicine, 51* (6), 894–901. https://doi.org/10.1017/S0033291721001185

Stein, M. B., & Gelernter, J. (2014). Genetic factors in social anxiety disorder. In J. W. Weeks (Ed.), *The Wiley Blackwell handbook of social anxiety disorder* (pp. 53–66). Hoboken, NJ: Wiley-Blackwell. https://doi.org/10.1002/9781118653920.ch3

Stephenson, K. R., Zippan, N., & Brotto, L. A. (2021). Feasibility of a cognitive behavioral online intervention for women with Sexual Interest/Arousal Disorder. *Journal of Clinical Psychology, 77* (9), 1877–1893. https://doi.org/10.1002/jclp.23137

Stevenson, A. (1989). *Bitter fame: A life of Sylvia Plath*. Houghton Mifflin.

Stewart, K. E., Sumantry, D., & Malivoire, B. L. (2020). Family and couple integrated cognitive-behavioural therapy for adults with OCD: A meta-analysis. *Journal of Affective Disorders, 277,* 159–168. https://doi.org/10.1016/j.jad.2020.07.140

Stilo, S. A., & Murray, R. M. (2010). The epidemiology of schizophrenia: Replacing dogma with knowledge. *Dialogues in Clinical Neuroscience, 12,* 305–315.

Stone, L. E., Segal, D. L., & Krus, G. C. (2021). Relationships between pathological narcissism and maladaptive personality traits among older adults. *Aging & Mental Health, 25* (5), 930–935. https://doi.org/10.1080/13607863.2020.1725802

Straub, K. T., & Kerns, J. G. (2021). Positive schizotypy, maladaptive openness, and openness facets. *Personality Disorders: Theory, Research, and Treatment, 12* (1), 51–58. https://doi.org/10.1037/per0000407

Studart-Neto, A., Moraes, N. C., Spera, R. R., Merlin, S. S., Parmera, J. B., Jaluul, O., . . . Nitrini, R. (2022). Translation, cross-cultural adaptation, and validity of the Brazilian version of the Cognitive Function Instrument. *Dementia & Neuropsychologia, 16* (1), 79–88. https://doi.org/10.1590/1980-5764-dn-2021-0057

Sturgeon, M. (2023). The impact of mindfulness interventions for staff on the care, treatment, and experiences of people with intellectual disabilities: A systematic review [Article]. *Journal of Applied Research in Intellectual Disabilities, 36* (5), 978–999. https://doi.org/10.1111/jar.13140

Sturmey, P. (2009). Behavioral activation is an evidence-based treatment for depression. *Behavior Modification, 33,* 818–829.

Suárez Santiago, J. E., Roldán, G. R., & Picazo, O. (2023). Ketamine as a pharmacological tool for the preclinical study of memory deficit in schizophrenia. *Behavioural Pharmacology, 34* (2-3), 80–91. https://doi.org/10.1097/FBP.0000000000000689

Substance Abuse and Mental Health Services Administration. (2014). SAMHSA's concept of trauma and guidance for a trauma-informed approach. (HHS Publication No. SMA 14-4884). Rockville, MD: Substance Abuse and Mental Health Services Administration.

Substance Abuse and Mental Health Services Administration. (2022). Key substance use and mental health indicators in the United States: Results from the 2021 National Survey on Drug Use and Health (HHS Publication No. PEP22-07-01-005, NSDUH Series H-57), Rockville, MD: Center for Behavioral Health Statistics and Quality, Substance Abuse and Mental Health Services Administration. https://www.samhsa.gov/data/report/2021-nsduh-annual-national-report

Suchy, Y. (2023). Disorders of executive functioning. In G. G. Brown, T. Z. King, K. Y. Haaland, & B. Crosson (Eds.), *APA handbook of neuropsychology, Volume 1: Neurobehavioral disorders and conditions: Accepted science and open questions* (Vol. 1, pp. 185–203). American Psychological Association. https://doi.org/10.1037/0000307-009

Summers, K. (2020). For the greater good? Ethical reflections on interviewing the "rich" and "poor" in qualitative research. *International Journal of Social Research Methodology: Theory & Practice, 23* (5), 593–602. https://doi.org/10.1080/13645579.2020.1766772

Sun, H., Caporaso, A., Cantor, D., Davis, T., & Blake, K. (2023). The effects of prompt interventions on web survey response rate and data quality measures. *Field Methods, 35* (2), 100–116. https://doi.org/10.1177/1525822X211072358

Sunderland, T., Hill, J. L., Mellow, A. M., Lawlor, B. A., Gundersheimer, J., Newhouse, P. A., & Grafman, J. H. (1989). Clock drawing in Alzheimer's disease: A novel measure of dementia severity. *Journal of the American Geriatrics Society, 37,* 725–729.

Sutherland, K., & Cistulli, P. A. (2015). Recent advances in obstructive sleep apnea pathophysiology and treatment. *Sleep and Biological Rhythms, 13,* 26–40. https://doi.org/10.1111/sbr.12098

Swartz, M. S., Wilder, C. M., Swanson, J. W., Van Dorn, R. A., Robbins, P. C., Steadman, H. J., . . . Monahan, J. (2010). Assessing outcomes for consumers in New York's assisted outpatient treatment program. *Psychiatric Services, 61,* 976–981.

Sweeney, M. M., Weaver, D. C., Vincent, K. B., Arria, A. M., & Griffiths, R. R. (2020). Prevalence and correlates of caffeine use disorder symptoms among a United States sample. *Journal of Caffeine and Adenosine Research, 10* (1), 4–11. https://doi.org/10.1089/caff.2019.0020

Syriopoulou-Delli, C. K., & Sarri, K. (2023). Vocational rehabilitation of adolescents and young adults with autism spectrum disorder: A review. *International Journal of Developmental Disabilities,* 1–20. https://doi.org/10.1080/20473869.2023.2208898

Szuhany, K. L., & Simon, N. M. (2022). Anxiety disorders: A review. JAMA: *Journal of the American Medical Association, 328* (24), 2431–2445. https://doi.org/10.1001/jama.2022.22744

T

Tan, S. (2023). "Just put it in perspective": The perception of sexual voyeurism and violence in Singapore evaluated through Facebook comments. *Journal of Gender Studies, 32* (1), 59–73. https://doi.org/10.1080/09589236.2021.1979483

Tanck, J. A., Hartmann, A. S., Svaldi, J., Hagena, S., Osen, B., Stierle, C., & Vocks, S. (2022). What happens in the course of positive mirror exposure? Effects on eating pathology, body satisfaction, affect, and subjective physiological arousal in patients with anorexia and bulimia nervosa. *European Eating Disorders Review, 30* (6), 797–814. https://doi.org/10.1002/erv.2929

Tang, Y. (2020). The MoCA as a cognitive screening tool for Mild Cognitive Impairment (MCI) in elderly adults in China. *Psychiatry Research, 291.* https://doi.org/10.1016/j.psychres.2020.113210

Tarasoff v. The Regents of the University of California. (1976). 551 P 2d334 (California).

Tariq, S. H., Tumosa, N., Chibnall, J. T., Perry, M. H., 3rd, & Morley, J. E. (2006). Comparison of the Saint Louis University mental status examination and the mini-mental state examination for detecting dementia and mild neurocognitive disorder—A pilot study. *American Journal of Geriatric Psychiatry, 14* (11), 900–910. https://doi.org/10.1097/01.Jgp.0000221510.33817.86

Taylor, M. J., Martin, J., Butwicka, A., Lichtenstein, P., D'Onofrio, B., Lundström, S., Larsson, H., & Rosenqvist, M. A. (2023). A twin study of genetic and environmental contributions to attention-deficit/hyperactivity disorder over time. *Journal of Child Psychology and Psychiatry.* https://doi.org/10.1111/jcpp.13854

Teasdale, G., Maas, A., Lecky, F., Manley, G., Stocchetti, N., & Murray, G. (2014). The Glasgow Coma Scale at 40 years: Standing the test of time. *The Lancet Neurology, 13* (8), 844–854. https://doi.org/10.1016/S1474-4422(14)70120-6

Ter Kuile, M. M., Melles, R. J., Tuijnman-Raasveld, C. C., de Groot, H. E., & van Lankveld, J. J. D. M. (2015). Therapist-aided exposure for women with lifelong vaginismus: Mediators of treatment outcome: A randomized waiting list control trial. *Journal of Sexual Medicine, 12* (8), 1807–1819. https://doi.org/10.1111/jsm.12935

Thibaut, F., Cosyns, P., Fedoroff, J. P., Briken, P., Goethals, K., & Bradford, J. M. W. (2020). The World Federation of Societies of Biological Psychiatry (WFSBP) 2020 guidelines for the pharmacological treatment of paraphilic disorders. *The World Journal of Biological Psychiatry, 21* (6), 412–490. https://doi.org/10.1080/15622975.2020.1744723

Thomasius, R., Zapletalova, P., Petersen, K., Buchert, R., Andresen, B., Wartberg, L., . . . Schmoldt, A. (2006). Mood, cognition and serotonin transporter availability in current and former ecstasy (MDMA) users: The longitudinal perspective. *Journal of Psychopharmacology, 20,* 211–225.

Thompson-Hollands, J., Lunney, C. A., Sloan, D. M., Wiltsey Stirman, S., & Schnurr, P. P. (2023). Treatment length and symptom improvement in prolonged exposure and present-centered therapy for posttraumatic stress disorder: Comparing dose–response and good-enough level models in two manualized interventions. *Journal of Consulting and Clinical Psychology, 91* (10), 596–605. https://doi.org/10.1037/ccp0000834

Thompson, A. (2013). Blige opens up about drugs and depression. *USA Today*. https://www.usatoday.com/story/life/people/2013/01/09/blige-opens-up-about-drugs-and-depression/1820431. Accessed 3/12/21.

Thompson, A., Petrie, T., Balcom, K., Tackett, B., & Edward Watkins, C. (2020). Psychosocial predictors of eating classification in female athletes: From collegiate sport to retirement. *International Journal of Eating Disorders*. https://doi.org/10.1002/eat.23456

Thunberg, G. (2019). School strike for climate–Save the world by changing the rules. *TedX Stockholm*. https://www.ted.com/talks/greta_thunberg_school_strike_for_climate_save_the_world_by_changing_the_rules/transcript?language=en

Thunberg, G. (2020). *I am Greta*. Hulu Films.

Thunberg, G. [@GretaThunberg]. (2020). They are starting to get more and more desperate...This shows that we're winning. [Twitter]. Retrieved 4/14/21.

Thurber, S. (2017). Childhood enuresis: Current diagnostic formulations, salient findings, and effective treatment modalities. *Archives of Psychiatric Nursing, 31* (3), 319–323. https://doi.org/10.1016/j.apnu.2016.11.005

Tick, B., Bolton, P., Happé, F., Rutter, M., & Rijsdijk, F. (2016). Heritability of autism spectrum disorders: A meta-analysis of twin studies. *Journal of Child Psychology and Psychiatry, 57* (5), 585–595. https://doi.org/10.1111/jcpp.12499

Tieges, Z., Evans, J. J., Neufeld, K. J., & MacLullich, A. M. J. (2018). The neuropsychology of delirium: Advancing the science of delirium assessment. *International Journal of Geriatric Psychiatry, 33* (11), 1501–1511. https://doi.org/10.1002/gps.4711

Tielbeek, J. J., Uffelmann, E., Williams, B. S., Colodro-Conde, L., Gagnon, É., Mallard, T. T., . . . Posthuma, D. (2022). Uncovering the genetic architecture of broad antisocial behavior through a genome-wide association study meta-analysis. *Molecular Psychiatry, 27* (11), 4453–4463. https://doi.org/10.1038/s41380-022-01793-3

Toms, J. (2010). Mind the gap: MIND, the mental hygiene movement and the trapdoor in measurements of intellect. *Journal of Intellectual Disability Research : JIDR, 54 Suppl 1* (0 1), 16–27. https://doi.org/10.1111/j.1365-2788.2009.01234.x

Torales, J., González, I., Castaldelli-Maia, J. M., & Ventriglio, A. (2020). Kleptomania as a neglected disorder in psychiatry. *International Review of Psychiatry*. https://doi.org/10.1080/09540261.2020.1756635

Torke, A. M., Alexander, G. C., & Lantos, J. (2008). Substituted judgment: The limitations of autonomy in surrogate decision making. *Journal of General Internal Medicine, 23,* 1514–1517. https://doi.org/http://doi.org/10.1007/s11606-008-0688-8

Traeen, B., Fischer, N., & Grøndahl, P. (2022). Norwegian data on prevalence, sexual risk behaviors, sexual problems, and sexual satisfaction in men who have sex exclusively with women, men who have sex exclusively with men, and men who have sex with men and women. *International Journal of Sexual Health*. https://doi.org/10.1080/19317611.2022.2126056

Traish, A. M., Feeley, R. J., & Guay, A. T. (2009). Testosterone therapy in women with gynecological and sexual disorders: A triumph of clinical endocrinology from 1938 to 2008. *Journal of Sexual Medicine, 6,* 334–351.

Tran, A., Smallidge, M., Cadavos, B., Tran, V., & Mattie, H. (2020). Unhealthy weight control behaviors among a sample of US journalists. *International Journal of Eating Disorders, 53* (12), 2067–2072. https://doi.org/0.1002/eat.23388

Trethewey, E., Evans, S., McIver, S., O'Brien, J., Lowndes, J., Pepin, G., & O'Shea, M. (2023). One size may not fit all: A mapping review of yoga-based interventions for the treatment of eating disorders. *Complementary Therapies in Clinical Practice, 53,* 101779. https://doi.org/10.1016/j.ctcp.2023.101779

Tripathi, S., Messias, E., Spollen, J., & Salomon, R. M. (2019). Modern-day relics of psychiatry. *Journal of Nervous and Mental Disease, 207* (9), 701–704. https://doi.org/10.1097/NMD.0000000000001059

Trombello, J. M., South, C., Sánchez, A., Kahalnik, F., Kennard, B. D., & Trivedi, M. H. (2020). Two trajectories of depressive symptom reduction throughout behavioral activation teletherapy among underserved, ethnically diverse, primary care patients: A VitalSign[6] report. *Behavior Therapy, 51* (6), 958–971. https://doi.org/10.1016/j.beth.2020.01.002

Trzepacz, P. T., Mittal, D., Torres, R., Kanary, K., Norton, J., & Jimerson, N. (2001). Validation of the Delirium Rating Scale-Revised-98: Comparison with the Delirium Rating Scale and the Cognitive Test for Delirium. *The Journal of Neuropsychiatry and Clinical Neurosciences, 13,* 229–242.

Tung, I., Li, J. J., Meza, J. I., Jezior, K. L., Kianmahd, J. S. V., Hentschel, P. G., . . . Lee, S. S. (2016). Patterns of comorbidity among girls with ADHD: A meta-analysis. *Pediatrics, 138* (4), 1–13.

Turner, D., & Briken, P. (2018). Treatment of paraphilic disorders in sexual offenders or men with a risk of sexual offending with luteinizing hormone-releasing hormone agonists: An updated systematic review. *Journal of Sexual Medicine, 15* (1), 77–93. https://doi.org/10.1016/j.jsxm.2017.11.013

Turner, D., Wolf, A. J., Barra, S., Müller, M., Gregório Hertz, P., Huss, M., . . . Retz, W. (2021). The association between adverse childhood experiences and mental health problems in young offenders. *European Child & Adolescent Psychiatry*. https://doi.org/10.1007/s00787-020-01608-2

Tzeng, N.-S., Yeh, H.-W., Chung, C.-H., Chang, H.-A., Kao, Y.-C., Chiang, W.-S., & Chien, W.-C. (2019). Risk of psychiatric morbidity in psychosexual disorders in male patients: A nationwide, cohort study in Taiwan. *American Journal of Men's Health, 13* (2). https://doi.org/10.1177/1557988319842985

U

Uhlmann, A., Dias, A., Taljaard, L., Stein, D. J., Brooks, S. J., & Lochner, C. (2020). White matter volume alterations in hair-pulling disorder (trichotillomania). *Brain Imaging and Behavior, 14* (6), 2202–2209. https://doi.org/10.1007/s11682-019-00170-z

UK ECT Review Group. (2003). Efficacy and safety of electroconvulsive therapy in depressive disorders: A systematic review and meta-analysis. *The Lancet, 361,* 799–808.

Unity Behavioral Health. (2021). Lamar Odom on the addiction recovery path. https://unityrehab.com/recovery-in-the-news/addiction-recovery-lamar-odom. Accessed 2/27/21.

Ussher, J. M., Hawkey, A., Perz, J., Liamputtong, P., Sekar, J., Marjadi, B., . . . Brook, E. (2020). Crossing boundaries and fetishization: Experiences of sexual violence for trans women of color. *Journal of Interpersonal Violence*. https://doi.org/10.1177/0886260520949149

V

Valdés-Florido, M. J., López-Díaz, Á., Palermo-Zeballos, F. J., Garrido-Torres, N., Álvarez-Gil, P., Martínez-Molina, I., . . . Ruiz-Veguilla, M. (2022). Clinical characterization of brief psychotic disorders triggered by the COVID-19 pandemic: A multicenter observational study. *European Archives of Psychiatry and Clinical Neuroscience, 272* (1), 5–15. https://doi.org/10.1007/s00406-021-01256-w

Valenzuela, F., Lock, J., Le Grange, D., & Bohon, C. (2018). Comorbid depressive symptoms and self-esteem improve after either cognitive-behavioural therapy or family-based treatment for adolescent bulimia nervosa. *European Eating Disorders Review, 26* (3), 253–258. https://doi.org/10.1002/erv.2582

Valle, S., & Grant, J. E. (2022). Quality of life in trichotillomania: An assessment of specific life domains. *Annals of Clinical Psychiatry, 34* (1), 27–32. https://doi.org/10.12788/acp.0052

Valleur, M., Codina, I., Venisse, J., Romo, L., Magalon, D., Fatseas, M., . . . Challet-Bouju, G. (2016). Towards a validation of the three pathways model of pathological gambling. *Journal of Gambling Studies, 32* (2), 757–771. https://doi.org/10.1007/s10899-015-9545-y

van Dis, E. A. M., van Veen, S. C., Hagenaars, M. A., Batelaan, N. M., Bockting, C. L. H., van den Heuvel, R. M., Cuijpers, P., & Engelhard, I. M. (2020). Long-term outcomes of cognitive behavioral therapy for anxiety-related disorders: A systematic review and meta-analysis. *JAMA Psychiatry, 77* (3), 265–273. https://doi.org/10.1001/jamapsychiatry.2019.3986

van Kraaij, A. W. J., Schiavone, G., Lutin, E., Claes, S., & Van Hoof, C. (2020). Relationship between chronic stress and heart rate over time modulated by gender in a cohort of office workers: Cross-sectional study using wearable technologies. *Journal of Medical Internet Research, 22* (9). https://doi.org/10.2196/18253

van Nes, Y., Bloemers, J., van der Heijden, P. M., van Rooij, K., Gerritsen, J., Kessels, R., . . . Tuiten, A. (2017). The Sexual Event Diary (SED): Development and validation of a standardized questionnaire for assessing female sexual functioning during discrete sexual events. *Journal of Sexual Medicine, 14* (11), 1438–1450. https://doi.org/10.1016/j.jsxm.2017.09.008

Van Nieuwenhove, K., Truijens, F., Meganck, R., Cornelis, S., & Desmet, M. (2020). Working through childhood trauma-related interpersonal patterns in psychodynamic treatment: An evidence-based case study. *Psychological Trauma: Theory, Research, Practice, and Policy, 12* (1), 64–74. https://doi.org/10.1037/tra0000438

Van Wert, M., McVey, K., Donohue, T., Wasserstein, T., Curry, J., Goldstick Rosner, N., Kimchi, E., & McCann, U. (2021). Foam rubber pica and cautopyreiophagia in a highly educated woman: A clinical case study. *Clinical Case Studies, 20* (6), 468–481. https://doi.org/10.1177/15346501211014284

Vandeleur, C. L., Fassassi, S., Castelao, E., Glaus, J., Strippoli, M.-P. F., Lasserre, A. M., . . . Preisig, M. (2017). Prevalence and correlates of *DSM-5* major depressive and related disorders in the community. *Psychiatry Research, 250*, 50–58. https://doi.org/10.1016/j.psychres.2017.01.060

Vasileva, M., Graf, R. K., Reinelt, T., Petermann, U., & Petermann, F. (2020). Research review: A meta-analysis of the international prevalence and comorbidity of mental disorders in children between 1 and 7 years. *Journal of Child Psychology and Psychiatry*. https://doi.org/10.1111/jcpp.13261

Veale, D. & Roberts, A. (2014). Obsessive-compulsive disorder. *British Medical Journal*, 348:g2183. https://doi.org/10.1136/bmj.g218

Veale, D., Gledhill, L. J., Christodoulou, P., & Hodsoll, J. (2016). Body dysmorphic disorder in different settings: A systematic review and estimated weighted prevalence. *Body Image, 18*, 168–186. https://doi.org/10.1016/j.bodyim.2016.07.003

Vecera, C. M., Fries, G. R., Shahani, L. R., Soares, J. C., & Machado-Vieira, R. (2021). Pharmacogenomics of lithium response in bipolar disorder. *Pharmaceuticals (Basel), 14* (4). https://doi.org/10.3390/ph14040287

Vera-Gray, F., McGlynn, C., Kureshi, I., & Butterby, K. (2021). Sexual violence as a sexual script in mainstream online pornography. *British Journal of Criminology, 61* (5), 1243–1260. https://doi.org/10.1093/bjc/azab035

Verginer, L., & Juen, B. H. (2019). Spiritual explanatory models of mental illness in West Nile, Uganda. *Journal of Cross-Cultural Psychology, 50* (2), 233–253. https://doi.org/10.1177/0022022118813652

Vermeulen, J., van Rooijen, G., Doedens, P., Numminen, E., van Tricht, M., & de Haan, L. (2017). Antipsychotic medication and long-term mortality risk in patients with schizophrenia: A systematic review and meta-analysis. *Psychological Medicine, 47* (13), 2217–2228. https://doi.org/10.1017/S0033291717000873

Vestito, L., Mori, L., Trompetto, C., Tomatis, M., Alessandria, G., De Carli, F., Cocito, L., & Bandini, F. (2023). The 15-item version of the Boston Naming Test in Italian: Normative data for adults. *Aphasiology, 37* (1), 83–98. https://doi.org/10.1080/02687038.2021.1988506

Veterans Administration Office of Research and Development. (2021). VA research on traumatic brain injury. https://www.research.va.gov/topics/tbi.cfm#:~:text=The%20Defense%20and%20Veterans%20Brain,TBIs%20were%20classified%20as%20mild. Accessed 3/16/21.

Vigil, K. E., de Jong, D. C., & Poovey, K. N. (2021). Roles of genital self-image, distraction, and anxiety in women's sexual pleasure: A preregistered study. *Journal of Sex & Marital Therapy, 47* (4), 325–340. https://doi.org/10.1080/0092623X.2021.1874581

Vigo, L., Ilzarbe, D., Baeza, I., Banerjea, P., & Kyriakopoulos, M. (2019). Shared psychotic disorder in children and young people: A systematic review. *European Child & Adolescent Psychiatry, 28* (12), 1555–1566. https://doi.org/10.1007/s00787-018-1236-7

Villain, N., Planche, V., & Levy, R. (2022). High-clearance anti-amyloid immunotherapies in Alzheimer's disease. Part 1: Meta-analysis and review of efficacy and safety data, and medico-economical aspects. *Revue Neurologique, 178* (10), 1011–1030. https://doi.org/10.1016/j.neurol.2022.06.012

Voigt, R. G., Katusic, S. K., Colligan, R. C., Killian, J. M., Weaver, A. L., & Barbaresi, W. J. (2017). Academic achievement in adults with a history of childhood Attention-Deficit/Hyperactivity Disorder: A population-based prospective study. *Journal of Developmental and Behavioral Pediatrics, 38* (1), 1–11. https://doi.org/10.1097/dbp.0000000000000358

Völlm, B. A., Clarke, M., Herrando, V. T., Seppänen, A. O., Gosek, P., Heitzman, J., & Bulten, E. (2018). European Psychiatric Association (EPA) guidance on forensic psychiatry: Evidence based assessment and treatment of mentally disordered offenders. *European Psychiatry, 51*, 58–73. https://doi.org/10.1016/j.eurpsy.2017.12.007

von Gontard, A., Baeyens, D., Van Hoecke, E., Warzak, W. J., & Bachmann, C. (2011). Psychological and psychiatric issues in urinary and fecal incontinence. *Journal of Urology, 185* (4), 1432–1436. https://doi.org/10.1016/j.juro.2010.11.051

Vukasović, T., & Bratko, D. (2015). Heritability of personality: A meta-analysis of behavior genetic studies. *Psychological Bulletin, 141* (4), 769–785. https://doi.org/10.1037/bul0000017 10.1037/bul0000017.supp (Supplemental)

Vyas, N. S., Buchsbaum, M. S., Lehrer, D. S., Merrill, B. M., DeCastro, A., Doninger, N. A.,... Mukherjee, J. (2017). D2/D3 dopamine receptor binding with [F-18] fallypride correlates of executive function in medication-naïve patients with schizophrenia. *Schizophrenia Research, 192*, 442–456. https://doi.org/10.1016/j.schres.2017.05.017

Wagenmakers, M. J., Vansteelandt, K., van Exel, E., Postma, R., Schouws, S. N. T. M., Obbels, J., . . . Oudega, M. L. (2021). Transient cognitive impairment and white matter hyperintensities in severely depressed older patients treated with electroconvulsive therapy. *The American Journal of Geriatric Psychiatry*. https://doi.org/10.1016/j.jagp.2020.12.028

W

Walker, J. R., Korte, J. E., McRae-Clark, A. L., & Hartwell, K. J. (2019). Adherence across FDA-approved medications for alcohol use disorder in a Veterans Administration population. *Journal of Studies on Alcohol and Drugs, 80* (5), 572–577. https://doi.org/10.15288/jsad.2019.80.572

Walsh, B. M., Grobbel, H., Christ, S. L., Tichenor, S. E., & Gerwin, K. L. (2023). Exploring the relationship between resilience and the adverse impact of stuttering in children [Article]. *Journal of Speech, Language & Hearing Research, 66* (7), 2278–2295. https://doi.org/10.1044/2023_JSLHR-23-00012

Walter, H., Ciaramidaro, A., Adenzato, M., Vasic, N., Ardito, R. B., Erk, S., & Bara, B. G. (2009). Dysfunction of the social brain in schizophrenia is modulated by intention type: An fMRI study. *Social Cognitive and Affective Neuroscience, 4,* 166–176. https://doi.org/10.1093/scan/nsn047

Walton, C., & Kerr, M. (2015). Down syndrome: Systematic review of the prevalence and nature of presentation of unipolar depression. *Advances in Mental Health and Intellectual Disabilities, 9* (4), 151–162. https://doi.org/10.1108/AMHID-11-2014-0037

Wang, H.-I., Wright, B., Tindall, L., Cooper, C., Biggs, K., Lee, E., . . . Parrott, S. (2022). Cost and effectiveness of one session treatment (OST) for children and young people with specific phobias compared to multi-session cognitive behavioural therapy (CBT): Results from a randomised controlled trial. *BMC Psychiatry, 22.* https://doi.org/10.1186/s12888-022-04192-8

Wang, L., Yin, Y., Bian, Q., Zhou, Y., Huang, J., Zhang, P., . . . Tan, Y. (2021). Immature defense mechanisms mediate the relationship between childhood trauma and onset of bipolar disorder. *Journal of Affective Disorders, 278,* 672–677. https://doi.org/10.1016/j.jad.2020.10.029

Wang, M., & Kenny, S. (2014). Longitudinal links between fathers' and mothers' harsh verbal discipline and adolescents' conduct problems and depressive symptoms. *Child Development, 85,* 908–923. https://doi.org/10.1111/cdev.12143

Wang, X., Wang, C., Zhang, Y., & An, Z. (2023). Effect of pharmacogenomics testing guiding on clinical outcomes in major depressive disorder: A systematic review and meta-analysis of RCT. *BMC Psychiatry, 23* (1). https://doi.org/10.1186/s12888-023-04756-2

Wani, W. Y., Chatham, J. C., Darley-Usmar, V., McMahon, L. L., & Zhang, J. (2017). O-GlcNAcylation and neurodegeneration. *Brain Research Bulletin, 133,* 80–87. https://doi.org/10.1016/j.brainresbull.2016.08.002

Wardenaar, K. J., Lim, C. W., Al-Hamzawi, A. O., Alonso, J., Andrade, L. H., Benjet, C., . . . de Jonge, P. (2017). The cross-national epidemiology of specific phobia in the World Mental Health Surveys. *Psychological Medicine, 47* (10), 1744–1760. https://doi.org/10.1017/S0033291717000174

Warner, E. N., Ammerman, R. T., Glauser, T. A., Pestian, J. P., Agasthya, G., & Strawn, J. R. (2023). Developmental epidemiology of pediatric anxiety disorders. *Child and Adolescent Psychiatric Clinics of North America, 32* (3), 511–530. https://doi.org/10.1016/j.chc.2023.02.001

Watanabe, Y., Urakami, T., Hongo, S., & Ohtsubo, T. (2015). Frontal lobe function and social adjustment in patients with schizophrenia: Near-infrared spectroscopy. *Human Psychopharmacology: Clinical and Experimental, 30,* 28–41. https://doi.org/10.1002/hup.2448

Wechsler, D. (2008). *Wechsler adult intelligence scale* (4th ed.). American Psychological Corporation.

Wechsler, D. (2009). *Wechsler Memory Scale–Fourth Edition*. Pearson.

Wechsler, D. (2012). *Wechsler preschool and primary scale of intelligence, fourth edition (WPPSI-IV)*. Pearson.

Wechsler, D. (2014). *Wechsler intelligence scale for children, fifth edition (WISC-V)*. Pearson.

Wechsler, D. (2024). *Wechsler Adult Intelligence Scales*- 5. Pearson. https://www.pearsonassessments.com/store/usassessments/en/Store/Professional-Assessments/Cognition-%26-Neuro/Wechsler-Adult-Intelligence-Scale-%7C-Fifth-Edition/p/P100071002.html

Weinstock, R., Darby, W. C., Bonnici, D. M., Seroussi, A., & Leong, G. B. (2015). The ever-evolving duty to protect in California. *Journal of the American Academy of Psychiatry and the Law, 43* (2), 262–262.

Weiss, K. J., & Van Dell, L. (2017). Liability for diagnosing malingering. *Journal of the American Academy of Psychiatry and the Law, 45* (3), 339–347.

Weissman, M. M. (2007). Recent non-medication trials of interpersonal psychotherapy for depression. *International Journal of Neuropsychopharmacology, 10,* 117–122.

Wertag, A., Ribar, M., & Sučić, I. (2023). A look through dark-colored glasses: The dark tetrad and affective processing. *Scandinavian Journal of Psychology*. https://doi.org/10.1111/sjop.12951

West, A. L. (2015). Associations among attachment style, burnout, and compassion fatigue in health and human service workers: A systematic review. *Journal of Human Behavior in the Social Environment, 25,* 571–590. https://doi.org/10.1080/10911359.2014.988321

Wetzel, E., Brown, A., Hill, P. L., Chung, J. M., Robins, R. W., & Roberts, B. W. (2017). The narcissism epidemic is dead; long live the narcissism epidemic. *Psychological Science, 28* (12), 1833–1847. https://doi.org/10.1177/0956797617724208

Wetzel, E., Grijalva, E., Robins, R. W., & Roberts, B. W. (2020). You're still so vain: Changes in narcissism from young adulthood to middle age. *Journal of Personality and Social Psychology, 119* (2), 479–496. https://doi.org/10.1037/pspp0000266.supp (Supplemental)

Whitbourne, S. K., & Martins, B. (2020). Psychotherapy with the underserved older adult population. In J. Zimmerman, J. E. Barnett, & L. F. Campbell (Eds.), *Bringing psychotherapy to the underserved: Challenges and strategies.* (pp. 263–280). New York, NY: Oxford University Press.

Whitbourne, S. K., & Meeks, S. (2011). Psychopathology, bereavement, and aging. In K. W. Schaie & S. L. Willis (Eds.), *Handbook of the psychology of aging* (7th ed, pp. 311–324). Elsevier.

White, K. S., Brown, T. A., Somers, T. J., & Barlow, D. H. (2006). Avoidance behavior in panic disorder: The moderating influence of perceived control. *Behaviour Research and Therapy, 44,* 147–157.

Wilcox, S. L., Redmond, S., & Davis, T. L. (2015). Genital image, sexual anxiety, and erectile dysfunction among young male military personnel. *Journal of Sexual Medicine, 12,* 1389–1397. https://doi.org/10.1111/jsm.12880

Williams, R. J., Shaw, C. A., Belanger, Y. D., Christensen, D. R., el-Guebaly, N., Hodgins, D. C., McGrath, D. S., & Stevens, R. M. G. (2023). Etiology of problem gambling in Canada. *Psychology of Addictive Behaviors, 37* (3), 483–498. https://doi.org/10.1037/adb0000843

Willroth, E. C., Luo, J., Atherton, O. E., Weston, S. J., Drewelies, J., Batterham, . . . Graham, E. K. (2023). Personality traits and health care use: A coordinated analysis of 15 international samples. *Journal of Personality and Social Psychology, 125* (3), 629–648. https://doi.org/10.1037/pspp0000465 10.1037/pspp0000465.supp (Supplemental)

Wilson, D. K. (2015). Behavior matters: The relevance, impact, and reach of behavioral medicine. *Annals of Behavioral Medicine, 49,* 40–48. https://doi.org/10.1007/s12160-014-9672-1

Wilson, H. A. (2014). Can antisocial personality disorder be treated? A meta-analysis examining the effectiveness of treatment in reducing recidivism for individuals diagnosed with ASPD. *The International Journal of Forensic Mental Health, 13,* 36–46. https://doi.org/10.1080/14999013.2014.890682

Wilson, L. C., & Liss, M. (2020). Safety and belonging as explanations for mental health disparities among sexual minority college students. *Psychology of Sexual Orientation and Gender Diversity*. https://doi.org/10.1037/sgd0000421

Winsper, C., Bilgin, A., Thompson, A., Marwaha, S., Chanen, A. M., Singh, S. P., . . . Furtado, V. (2020). The prevalence of personality disorders in the community: A global systematic review and meta-analysis. *The British Journal of Psychiatry, 216* (2), 69–78. https://doi.org/10.1192/bjp.2019.166

Winsper, C., Marwaha, S., Lereya, S. T., Thompson, A., Eyden, J., & Singh, S. P. (2015). Clinical and psychosocial outcomes of borderline personality disorder in childhood and adolescence: A systematic review. *Psychological Medicine, 45,* 2237–2251. https://doi.org/10.1017/S0033291715000318

Witlox, M., Kraaij, V., Garnefski, N., Bohlmeijer, E., Smit, F., & Spinhoven, P. (2022). Cost-effectiveness and cost-utility of an Acceptance and Commitment Therapy intervention vs a Cognitive Behavioral Therapy intervention for older adults with anxiety symptoms: A randomized controlled trial. *PLoS ONE, 17* (1). https://doi.org/10.1371/journal.pone.0262220

Wittchen, H. U., Gloster, A. T., Beesdo-Baum, K., Fava, G. A., & Craske, M. G. (2010).

Agoraphobia: A review of the diagnostic classificatory position and criteria. *Depression and Anxiety, 27,* 113–133.

Wium-Andersen, M. K., Dalgaard Villumsen, M., Wium-Andersen, I. K., Jørgensen, M. B., Hjelmborg, J. B., Christensen, K., & Osler, M. (2020). Familial risk and heritability of depression by age at first diagnosis in Danish twins. *Acta Psychiatrica Scandinavica.* https://doi.org/10.1111/acps.13238

Wonderlich, S. A., Gordon, K. H., Mitchell, J. E., Crosby, R. D., & Engel, S. G. (2009). The validity and clinical utility of binge eating disorder. *International Journal of Eating Disorders, 42,* 687–705.

World Health Organization. (2019a). *International statistical classification of diseases and related health problems (ICD).* https://www.who.int/standards/classifications/classification-of-diseases

World Health Organization. (2019b). The WHO special initiative for mental health (2019–2023): Universal health coverage for mental health. License: CC BY-NC-SA 3.0 IGO. https://apps.who.int/iris/handle/10665/310981

World Health Organization. (2021). The global health observatory. https://www.who.int/data/gho/data/themes/mental-health#:~:text=Age%2Dstandardized%20suicide%20rates%3A%20There,10.5%20per%20100%20000%20population.

Wu, Y., Wang, Y., Zhang, Y., Yuan, X., & Gao, X. (2023). A preliminary study of the Saint Louis University Mental Status examination (SLUMS) for the assessment of cognition in moderate to severe traumatic brain injury patients. *Applied Neuropsychology: Adult, 30* (4), 409–413. https://doi.org/10.1080/23279095.2021.1952414

Wyatt v. Stickney. (1971). 325 F. Supp. 781 (M.D. Ala.); (1972) 344 F. Supp. (M.D. Ala.)

Wylie, K., Knudson, G., Khan, S. I., Bonierbale, M., Watanyusakul, S., & Baral, S. (2016). Serving transgender people: Clinical care considerations and service delivery models in transgender health. *The Lancet, 388* (10042), 401–411. https://doi.org/10.1016/S0140-6736(16)00682-6

X

Xie, R., Sun, X., Yang, L., & Guo, Y. (2020). Characteristic executive dysfunction for high-functioning autism sustained to adulthood. *Autism Research, 13* (12), 2102–2121. https://doi.org/10.1002/aur.2304

Y

Yakushko, O. (2018). Witches, charlatans, and old wives: Critical perspectives on history of women's indigenous knowledge. *Women & Therapy, 41* (1–2), 18–29. https://doi.org/10.1080/02703149.2017.1323474

Yalch, M. M., Hebenstreit, C. L., & Maguen, S. (2018). Influence of military sexual assault and other military stressors on substance use disorder and PTS symptomology in female military veterans. *Addictive Behaviors, 80,* 28–33. https://doi.org/10.1016/j.addbeh.2017.12.026

Yan, H., Ding, Y., & Guo, W. (2021). Suicidality in patients with premenstrual dysphoric disorder—A systematic review and meta-analysis. *Journal of Affective Disorders, 295,* 339–346. https://doi.org/10.1016/j.jad.2021.08.082

Yap, K. H., Abdul Manan, H., & Sharip, S. (2021). Heterogeneity in brain functional changes of cognitive processing in ADHD across age: A systematic review of task-based fMRI studies. *Behavioural Brain Research, 397.* https://doi.org/10.1016/j.bbr.2020.112888

Yazici, H., Ozdemir, M., & Koca, F. (2020). Impact of posttraumatic stress disorder symptoms on posttraumatic growth. *Journal of Loss and Trauma.* https://doi.org/10.1080/15325024.2020.1801240

Yeo, G. C., Hong, R. Y., & Riskind, J. H. (2020). Looming cognitive style and its associations with anxiety and depression: A meta-analysis. *Cognitive Therapy and Research, 44* (3), 445–467. https://doi.org/10.1007/s10608-020-10089-1

Yi-Feng Chen, N., Crant, J. M., Wang, N., Kou, Y., Qin, Y., Yu, J., & Sun, R. (2021). When there is a will there is a way: The role of proactive personality in combating COVID-19. *Journal of Applied Psychology.* https://doi.org/10.1037/apl0000865

Young, S. (2017). NFL star Brandon Marshall on his borderline personality disorder diagnosis and removing the stigma of mental illness. *People.* https://people.com/human-interest/nfl-star-brandon-marshall-on-his-borderline-personality-disorder-diagnosis-and-removing-the-stigma-of-mental-illness. Accessed 3/18/21.

Young, S. (2017). NFL star Brandon Marshall on his borderline personality disorder diagnosis and removing the stigma of mental illness. *People.* https://people.com/human-interest/nfl-star-brandon-marshall-on-his-borderline-personality-disorder-diagnosis-and-removing-the-stigma-of-mental-illness. Accessed 3/18/21.

Young, S., Adamo, N., Ásgeirsdóttir, B. B., Branney, P., Beckett, M., Colley, W., . . . Woodhouse, E. (2020). Females with ADHD: An expert consensus statement taking a lifespan approach providing guidance for the identification and treatment of attention-deficit/ hyperactivity disorder in girls and women. *BMC Psychiatry, 20.* https://doi.org/10.1186/s12888-020-02707-9

Youngberg v. Romeo. (1982). 457 U.S. 307.

Yovita, M., & Asih, S. R. (2018). The effects of academic stress and optimism on subjective well-being among first-year undergraduates. In A. A. Ariyanto, H. Muluk, P. Newcombe, F. P. Piercy, E. K. Poerwandari & S. R. Suradijono (Eds.), *Diversity in unity: Perspectives from psychology and behavioral sciences* (pp. 559–563). Routledge/Taylor & Francis Group.

Yrondi, A., Péran, P., Sauvaget, A., Schmitt, L., & Arbus, C. (2018). Structural-functional brain changes in depressed patients during and after electroconvulsive therapy. *Acta Neuropsychiatrica, 30* (1), 17–28. https://doi.org/10.1017/neu.2016.62

Z

Zablotsky, B., & Black, L. I. (2020). Prevalence of children aged 3–17 years with developmental disabilities, by urbanicity: United States, 2015–2018. National Health Statistics Reports, No. 139. https://www.cdc.gov/nchs/data/nhsr/nhsr139-508.pdf

Zablotsky, B., Ng, A. E., Black, L. I., & Blumberg, S. J. (2023). Diagnosed developmental disabilities in children aged 3-17 years: United States 2019-2021.NCHS Data Brief. No. 273. National Center for Health Statistics. https://doi.org/https://dx.doi.org/10.15620/cdc:129520

Zhao, T., Wei, B., Long, J., Tang, X., Zhou, M., & Dang, C. (2015). Cognitive disorders in HIV-infected and AIDS patients in Guangxi, China. *Journal of Neurovirology, 21,* 32–42. https://doi.org/10.1007/s13365-014-0295-x

Zheng, J., Islam, R. M., Bell, R. J., Skiba, M. A., & Davis, S. R. (2020). Prevalence of low sexual desire with associated distress across the adult life span: An Australian cross-sectional study. *Journal of Sexual Medicine, 17* (10), 1885–1895. https://doi.org/10.1016/j.jsxm.2020.07.007

Zhou, X., Feliciano, P., Shu, C., Wang, T., Astrovskaya, I., Hall, J. B., . . . The, S. C. (2022). Integrating de novo and inherited variants in 42,607 autism cases identifies mutations in new moderate-risk genes. *Nature Genetics, 54* (9), 1305–1319. https://doi.org/10.1038/s41588-022-01148-2

Zivanovic, O. (2017). Lithium: A classic drug—frequently discussed, but, sadly, seldom prescribed! *Australian and New Zealand Journal of Psychiatry, 51* (9), 886–896. https://doi.org/10.1177/0004867417695889

Zuchner, S., Wendland, J. R., Ashley-Koch, A. E., Collins, A. L., Tran-Viet, K. N., Quinn, K., . . . Murphy, D. L. (2009). Multiple rare SAPAP3 missense variants in trichotillomania and OCD. *Molecular Psychiatry, 14,* 6–9.

Zugliani, M. M., Martin-Santos, R., Nardi, A. E., & Freire, R. C. (2017). Personality traits in panic disorder patients with and without comorbidities. *Journal of Nervous and Mental Disease, 205* (11), 855–858. https://doi.org/10.1097/NMD.0000000000000745

Zwicker, J. G., Missiuna, C., Harris, S. R., & Boyd, L. A. (2012). Developmental coordination disorder: A review and update. *European Journal of Pediatric Neurology, 16* (6), 573–581. https://doi.org/10.1016/j.ejpn.2012.05.005

Zwickl, S., Burchill, L., Wong, A. F. Q., Leemaqz, S. Y., Cook, T., Angus, L. M., . . . Cheung, A. S. (2023). Pelvic pain in transgender people using testosterone therapy. *LGBT Health, 10* (3), 179–190. https://doi.org/10.1089/lgbt.2022.0187

NAME INDEX

T

U

V

W

SUBJECT INDEX

Bold locators indicate definitions of terms.

A

B

C

G

H

N

T

U

V

W

Y

Z